Pharmaceutics: The Science of Dosage Form Design

Pharmaceutics: The Science of Dosage Form Design

EDITED BY

Michael E. Aulton BPharm PhD MPS
Reader in Pharmacy, Leicester Polytechnic, Leicester, UK

CHURCHILL LIVINGSTONE
EDINBURGH LONDON MELBOURNE AND NEW YORK 1988

CHURCHILL LIVINGSTONE
Medical Division of Longman Group UK Limited
Distributed in the United States of America by
Churchill Livingstone Inc., 1560 Broadway, New
York, N.Y. 10036, and by associated companies,
branches and representatives throughout the world.

First published 1988
  Reprinted 1989
  Reprinted 1990

ISBN 0-443-03643-8

British Library Cataloguing in Publication Data
Pharmaceutics: the science of dosage form
   design.
   1. Pharmaceutics
   I. Aulton, Michael E.
   615'.19   RS403

Library of Congress Cataloging in Publication Data
Pharmaceutics: the science of dosage form design.
   Replaces: Cooper and Gunn's tutorial pharmacy.
6th ed. 1972.
   Includes bibliographies and index.
   1. Drugs — Design of delivery systems. 2. Drugs
— Dosage forms. 3. Biopharmaceutics.
4. Pharmaceutical technology. 5. Chemistry,
Pharmaceutical. 6. Microbiology, Pharmaceutical.
I. Aulton, Michael E.
[DNLM: 1. Biopharmaceutics. 2. Chemistry,
Pharmaceutical. 3. Dosage Forms. 4. Technology,
Pharmaceutical. 5. Microbiology, Pharmaceutical.
QV 785 P5366]
RS420.P48   1987   615.5'8   86–25888

Produced by Longman Group (FE) Ltd
Printed in Hong Kong

Contents

Preface

The first edition of *Pharmaceutics* has replaced the 6th edition of *Cooper and Gunn's Tutorial Pharmacy* published by Pitman in 1972. Since then, there has been a change in editorship, a change in the title of the book, a change in some of the authors and a completely redesigned content. But all is not new and disjointed, the editorial link with Leicester School of Pharmacy continues. Sidney Carter recently retired as Deputy Head of Leicester School of Pharmacy and passed on the book to me. He in turn had inherited the book from one of its founders, the late Colin Gunn who was formerly Head of Leicester School of Pharmacy but sadly died on 25 February 1983.

There are a greater number and a wider range of authors in this edition, each an accepted expert in the field on which they have written and, just as important, each has experience and ability in imparting that information to undergraduate pharmacy students.

The philosophy of the subject matter which the book covers has changed because pharmaceutics has changed. Since the last edition of *Tutorial Pharmacy* there have been very marked changes in the concept and content of pharmaceutics. Those changes are reflected in this edition. The era of biopharmaceutics was in its infancy at the time of the previous edition. Since then we have become increasingly concerned with not merely producing elegant and accurate dosage forms but also ensuring that the optimum amount of drug reaches the required place in the body and stays there for the optimum amount of time. Now we are concerned much more with designing dosage forms and with all aspects of drug delivery. This book reflects that concern.

Dr M E Aulton
School of Pharmacy
Leicester Polytechnic

Contributors

Dr N A Armstrong
Senior Lecturer in Pharmaceutics, Welsh School of Pharmacy, University of Wales Institute of Science and Technology, Cardiff, Wales.

Dr M E Aulton
Reader in Pharmacy, School of Pharmacy, Leicester Polytechnic, Leicester, England.

Professor B W Barry
Professor of Pharmaceutical Technology, Postgraduate School of Studies in Pharmacy, University of Bradford, Bradford, England.

M R Billany
Senior Lecturer in Pharmaceutics, School of Pharmacy, Leicester Polytechnic, Leicester, England.

D A Dean
Science and Technology Laboratories, Pharmaceutical Division, Fisons plc, Loughborough, England.

Dr C J de Blaey
Secretary for Scientific Affairs, Royal Dutch Association for Advancement in Pharmacy (K.N.M.P.), 's-Gravenhage (The Hague), Netherlands. Formerly Professor of Subfaculty of Pharmacy, University of Utrecht, Utrecht, Netherlands.

Dr J T Fell
Lecturer in Pharmacy, Department of Pharmacy, University of Manchester, Manchester, England.

Dr J L Ford
Lecturer in Dosage Form Design and Microbiology, School of Pharmacy, Liverpool Polytechnic, Liverpool, England.

Dr I Gonda
Lecturer in Industrial Pharmacy, Department of Pharmacy, University of Sidney, Sidney, Australia and Honorary Member of Staff, Department of Pharmacy, University of Aston in Birmingham, Birmingham, England.

Dr G W Hanlon
Senior Lecturer in Microbiology, Department of Pharmacy, Brighton Polytechnic, Brighton, England.

Dr N A Hodges
Senior Lecturer in Microbiology, Department of Pharmacy, Brighton Polytechnic, Brighton, England.

Dr J E Hogan
Director of Scientific Affairs, Colorcon Ltd, Orpington, England.

B E Jones
Technical Services, Elanco Division, Eli Lilly and Company Ltd, Basingstoke, England.

Dr J B Kayes
At time of writing, visiting Professor, School of Pharmaceutical Sciences, Universiti Sains Malaysia, Pulau Pinang, Malaysia. Formerly Senior Lecturer in Physical Pharmacy, Department of Pharmacy, University of Aston in Birmingham, Birmingham, England.

Professor C Marriott
Reader in Pharmacy, Department of Pharmacy, Brighton Polytechnic, Brighton, England.

Dr F S S Morton
Pharmaceutical Services Manager, R P Scherer Ltd, Swindon, England.

Professor M S Parker
Head of Department, Department of Pharmacy, Brighton Polytechnic, Brighton, England.

Dr S G Proudfoot
Senior Lecturer in Pharmaceutics, School of Pharmacy, Leicester Polytechnic, Leicester, England.

Dr J H Richards
Principal Lecturer in Pharmaceutics, School of Pharmacy, Leicester Polytechnic, Leicester, England.

Dr M H Rubinstein
Reader, School of Pharmacy, Liverpool Polytechnic, Liverpool, England.

Dr H Seager
Research and Development Director (Europe), R P Scherer Ltd, Swindon, England.

Dr C J Soper
Lecturer in Pharmaceutics, School of Pharmacy and Pharmacology, University of Bath, Bath, England.

Dr J N Staniforth
Lecturer in Pharmaceutics, School of Pharmacy and Pharmacology, University of Bath, Bath, England.

Dr M P Summers
Lecturer in Pharmaceutics, School of Pharmacy, University of London, London, England.

D N Travers
Principal Lecturer in Pharmaceutical Technology, School of Pharmacy, Leicester Polytechnic, Leicester, England.

Dr J J Tukker
Subfaculty of Pharmacy, University of Utrecht, Utrecht, Netherlands.

Dr J I Wells
Pharmaceutical Research and Development, Pfizer Central Research, Sandwich, Kent, England.

Dr P York
Senior Lecturer in Pharmaceutics, Postgraduate School of Studies in Pharmacy, University of Bradford, Bradford, England.

Acknowledgements

The Editor wishes to take this opportunity to thank the following who have assisted with the preparation of this text:

Mr Sidney Carter, who edited this book's predecessor, *Cooper and Gunn's Tutorial Pharmacy*, for passing on to me the opportunity to edit the first edition of this new textbook. His invaluable experience and guidance aided me throughout the preparation of this edition and are greatly appreciated.

The authors for the work and time that they put into their texts, often under pressure from numerous other commitments, and from me. The many unnamed typists and artists who assisted the authors.

My wife Christine, for typing and other secretarial assistance, and help in many other ways which enabled me to spend time on this book.

My BBC micro.

Katharine Watts and Alison Walsh of Churchill Livingstone, and Howard Bailey of Pitman, for their special expertise and assistance in introducing me to the world of publishing.

The many academic and industrial pharmacists who helped during the design of the contents of this edition to ensure that it corresponds as closely as possible with modern practice and with the syllabuses of most schools of pharmacy.

Those publishing companies who have given their permission to reproduce material here.

About this book

One of the earliest impressions that many new pharmacy students have of their chosen subject is the large number of long and sometimes unusual sounding names that are used to describe the various subject areas within pharmacy. The aim of this section is to explain to the reader what is meant by the term 'pharmaceutics', how the term has been interpreted for the purpose of this book and how pharmaceutics fits into the overall scheme of pharmacy. It will also lead the reader through the organization of this book and explain the necessity of an understanding of the material contained in its chapters.

The word pharmaceutics is used in pharmacy to encompass many subject areas which are all associated with the steps to which a drug is subjected towards the end of its development — i.e. after its discovery or synthesis, isolation and purification, and testing for advantageous pharmacological effects and absence from serious toxicological properties. Pharmaceutics is arguably the most diverse of all the subject areas in pharmacy and traditionally encompasses the design and formulation of medicines (physical pharmaceutics, dosage form design), the manufacture of these medicines on both a small (compounding) and large (pharmaceutical technology) scale, the cultivation, avoidance and elimination of microorganisms (microbiology) and the distribution of medicines to patients (dispensing and pharmacy practice).

As the subtitle of this edition indicates, this book concentrates on that part of pharmaceutics which is concerned with the conversion of a drug chemical into a medicine — the design of dosage forms. Medicines are drug delivery systems; they are means of getting drugs into the body in a safe, efficient, reproducible and convenient manner. The first chapter in the book describes, in a general way, the considerations that must be made so that this conversion of drug to medicine can take place. It emphasizes the fact that medicines are rarely drugs alone but require additives to make them into dosage forms and this in turn introduces the concept of formulation. The chapter explains that there are three major considerations in the design of dosage forms:

1 the physicochemical properties of the drug itself,
2 biopharmaceutical considerations, such as how the route of administration of a dosage form affects the rate and extent of drug absorption into the body,
3 therapeutic considerations of the disease state to be treated, which in turn decide the most suitable type of dosage form, possible routes of administration and the most suitable duration of action and dose frequency for the drug in question.

As a consequence of the first of these points, Part 1 of this book describes some of the more important physicochemical properties that one needs to know about in order to study and understand the design and preparation of dosage forms. The chapters have been designed to give the reader an insight into those physicochemical principles which are important to the formulation scientist. They are not intended as a substitute for a thorough understanding of physical chemistry and specific more detailed texts are recommended throughout. For many reasons, which are discussed in the book, the vast majority of dosage forms are orally administered in the form of solid products such as tablets and capsules. This means that one of the most important stages in drug administration is the dissolution of solid particles to form a solution in the gastrointestinal tract. This necessitates that the formulation scientist has a knowledge of both liquid and solid materials and particularly the properties of drugs in solution and the factors influencing drug dissolution from solid particles. However, before these subjects can be examined, the reader must first understand the way in which fluids flow and know a little about some of the resulting problems (additionally, solutions and semisolids are dosage forms in their own right). The properties of solutions are discussed next. The reader will see later in the book how drug release and absorption are strongly dependent on solution properties such as solute dissociation and diffusion. The properties of interfaces are described in the following chapter. These are important to an understanding of adsorption onto solid surfaces and as a prelude to the dissolution of solid particles and the study of disperse systems such as colloids, suspensions and emulsions. Before finalizing on a possible dosage form there must be a clear understanding of the stability of the drug(s) and other additives in the formulation with respect to the reasons why and the rates at which they degrade and there must be an awareness of means of inhibiting decomposition and increasing the shelf life of a product.

Even with this fundamental knowledge it is not possible to begin to design a dosage form without having an understanding of how drugs are absorbed into the body, the various routes that can be used for this purpose and the fate of the drugs once they enter the body and reach their site of action. This book concentrates on the preparation, administration, release and absorption of drugs, but stops short at the cellular level and leaves to other texts the detail of how drugs enter individual cells, how they act, how they are metabolized and how they are eliminated. These cellular considerations are not within the remit of this book.

The terms bioavailability and biopharmaceutics are defined and explained in Part 2 of the book. The factors influencing the bioavailability of a drug and methods of assessing it are described. Finally in that section consideration is given to the manner in which the frequency of administration of a drug affects its level in the blood at any given time.

In Part 3, the book then goes on to discuss the actual drug delivery systems which are available. It covers their formulation, the release of drugs from them, and their advantages and disadvantages as a dosage form. This part starts with a consideration of the pack into which the medicine is put. This may seem odd since packaging is often the last stage in a manufacturing process but the pack and any possible interactions between it and the drug or medicine it contains are so vitally linked that it must not be considered as an afterthought; these should be uppermost in the minds of the formulators as soon as they receive the drug powder on which to work. The steps that need to be considered before formulation itself can begin — preformulation — are discussed next. Results of tests carried out at this stage can give a much clearer indication of the possible dosage forms for a new drug candidate. Part 3 then considers existing dosage forms suitable for the administration of drugs through almost every possible body orifice and external surface, as well as an intimation to novel or future drug delivery systems.

Microbiology is a very wide ranging subject that is traditionally associated with pharmaceutics in schools of pharmacy. This book, in Part 4, has concentrated only on those aspects of microbiology that are directly relevant to the design, production and distribution of dosage forms. This mainly involves avoiding (asepsis) and eliminating (sterilization) their presence in medicines (contamination), and preventing the growth of any microorganism which might enter the product during storage and use (preservation). Techniques for testing that these intentions have been achieved are also described.

The actual production of medicines on a large scale is dealt with in the final part of the book, pharmaceutical technology. This begins with a consideration of the reaction vessels that are used during the manufacture of the drug chemical, other additives and the dosage form itself.

There then follows an examination of those aspects of production mainly associated with liquids, i.e. heat transfer and filtration. The technological problems associated with the manufacture of solid dosage forms are then described. The reader will quickly realize that a major problem in preparing solid dosage forms is the handling of powders and thus the book explains the concept of particle size of powders and its measurement, size reduction and size separation of powders from those of other sizes and the many problems associated with the flow of powders. In tablet and capsule production, for example, it is not simply enough to achieve fast flow, but that flow must also be uniform. We then see how powders are effectively enlarged in size (granulation). This is necessary partly to overcome some powder flow and tableting problems and also because granules are themselves a dosage form. Granulation most commonly involves the wetting of dry powders and so the drying of this wet material is described next. The book then moves on to tableting, tablet coating and encapsulation.

Following this, techniques associated with the microbiological aspects of production are discussed. These are necessary in industry to eliminate microorganisms from the product both before or during manufacture. The technology of packaging and filling of products completes the book since this is the final production stage before warehousing, distribution and finally dispensing to the public.

At this point the pharmaceutical technologist passes the product on to that other aspect of pharmaceutics — the interface with the patient, i.e. dispensing and pharmacy practice. These aspects are dealt with in the companion volume Cooper and Gunn's *Dispensing for Pharmaceutical Students* later to become *Pharmaceutical Practice*.

The design of dosage forms

PRINCIPLES OF DOSAGE FORM DESIGN

Drugs are rarely administered solely as pure chemical substances but are almost always given in formulated preparations. These can vary from relatively simple solutions to complex drug delivery systems, through the use of appropriate additives or excipients in the formulations to provide varied and specialized pharmaceutical functions. It is the formulation additives that, amongst other things, solubilize, suspend, thicken, preserve, emulsify, improve the compressibility and flavour drug substances to form various preparations or dosage forms.

The principal objective of dosage form design is to achieve a predictable therapeutic response to a drug included in a formulation which is capable of large scale manufacture with reproducible product quality. To ensure product quality, numerous features are required — chemical and physical stability, with suitable preservation against microbial contamination if appropriate, uniformity of dose of drug, acceptability to users including both prescriber and patient, as well as suitable packaging and labelling. Ideally, dosage forms should also be independent of patient to patient variation although in practice this feature remains difficult to achieve. Future developments in dosage form design may well attempt to accommodate to some extent this requirement.

Reference is made in Part 2 of this book to differences in bioavailability between apparently similar formulations and possible causative reasons. In recent years increasing attention has therefore been directed towards eliminating variation in bioavailability characteristics, particularly for chemically equivalent products since it is recognized that formulation factors can influence their therapeutic performance. To optimize the bioavailability of drug substances it is often necessary to carefully select the most appropriate chemical derivative of the drug, for example to obtain a specific solubility requirement, as well as its particle size and physical form, to combine it with appropriate additives and manufacturing aids that will not significantly alter the properties of the drug, to select the most appropriate administration route(s) and dosage form(s) and to consider aspects of manufacturing processes and suitable packaging.

There are numerous dosage forms into which a drug substance can be incorporated for the convenient and efficacious treatment of a disease. Dosage forms can be designed for administration by all possible delivery routes to maximize therapeutic response. Preparations can be taken orally or injected, as well as being applied to the skin or inhaled, and Table 1.1 lists the range of dosage forms which can be used to deliver drugs by the various administration routes. However, it is necessary to relate the drug substance and the disease state before the correct combination of drug and dosage form can be made since each disease or illness will require a specific type of drug therapy. In addition factors governing choice of administration route and the specific require-

Table 1.1 Range of dosage forms available for different administration routes

Administration route	Dosage forms
Oral	Solutions, syrups, elixirs, suspensions, emulsions, gels, powders, granules, capsules, tablets
Rectal	Suppositories, ointments, creams, powders, solutions
Topical	Ointments, creams, pastes, lotions, gels, solutions, topical aerosols
Parenteral	Injections (solution, suspension, emulsion forms), implants, irrigation and dialysis solutions
Lungs	Aerosols (solution, suspension, emulsion, powder forms), inhalations, sprays, gases
Nasal	Solutions, inhalations
Eye	Solutions, ointments
Ear	Solutions, suspensions, ointments

ments of that route which affect drug absorption need to be taken into account when designing dosage forms.

Versatile drugs are often formulated into several dosage forms of varying strengths, each having particular pharmaceutical characteristics which are suitable for a specific application. One such drug is the glucocorticoid prednisolone. Through the use of different chemical forms and formulation additives a range of effective anti-inflammatory preparations are available including tablet, enteric coated tablet, injections, eye drops and enema. The extremely low aqueous solubility of the base prednisolone and acetate salt makes these forms useful in tablet and slowly absorbed intramuscular suspension injection forms, whilst the soluble sodium phosphate salt enables a soluble tablet form, and solutions for eye drops, enema and intravenous injection to be prepared. The antibacterial drug combination co-trimoxazole, consisting of a mixture of five parts of sulphamethoxazole and one part trimethoprim, is also available in a range of dosage forms and strengths to meet specific needs of the user, including tablets, dispersible tablets, double strength tablets, double strength dispersible tablets, paediatric mixture, intramuscular injection, and a strong sterile solution for the preparation of an intravenous infusion. Because of the low aqueous solubility of both drug substances, specialized solvents are used for the intramuscular injection: 52% glycofurol, and strong sterile solution, 40% propylene glycol.

It is therefore apparent that before a drug substance can be successfully formulated into a dosage form many factors must be considered. These can be broadly grouped into three categories:

1 biopharmaceutical considerations, including factors affecting the absorption of the drug substance from different administration routes,
2 drug factors, such as the physical and chemical properties of the drug substance, and
3 therapeutic considerations including consideration of the disease to be treated and patient factors.

Appropriate and efficacious dosage forms will be prepared only when all these factors are considered and related to each other. This is the underlying principle of dosage form design.

BIOPHARMACEUTICAL CONSIDERATIONS IN DOSAGE FORM DESIGN

Biopharmaceutics can be regarded as the study of the relationship between the physical, chemical and biological sciences applied to drugs, dosage forms and drug action. Clearly, understanding of the principles of this subject is important in dosage form design particularly with regard to drug absorption, as well as drug distribution, metabolism and excretion. In general, a drug substance must be in solution form before it can be absorbed via absorbing membranes of the skin, gastrointestinal tract and lungs into body fluids. Drugs penetrate these membranes in two general ways — by passive diffusion and by specialized transport mechanisms. In passive diffusion, which is thought to control the absorption of most drugs, the process is driven by the concentration gradient existing across the membrane with drug molecules passing from regions of high to low concentration. The lipid solubility and degree of ionization of the drug at the absorbing site influence the rate of diffusion. Several specialized transport mechanisms are postulated including active and facilitated transport. Once absorbed, the drug can exert a therapeutic effect yet the site of action is often remote from the site of administration and has to be transported in body fluids (see Fig. 1.1).

When the drug is administered from dosage

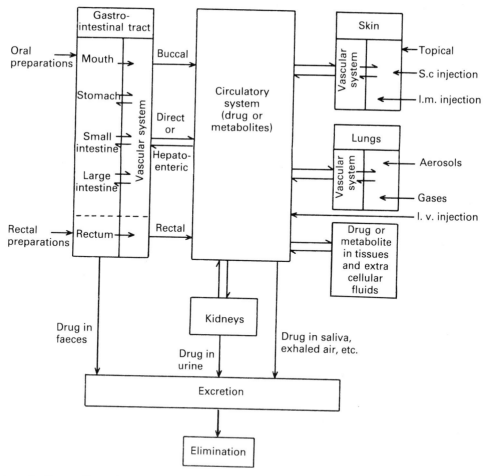

Fig. 1.1 Schematic diagram illustrating pathways a drug may take following administration of a dosage form by different routes

forms designed to deliver drugs via the buccal, rectal, intramuscular or subcutaneous routes, the drug passes directly into the circulation blood from absorbing tissues, whilst the intravenous route provides the most direct route of all. When delivered by the oral route onset of drug action will be delayed because of required transit time in the gastrointestinal tract, the absorption process and hepatoenteric blood circulation features. The physical form of the oral dosage form will also influence onset of action with solutions acting faster than suspensions which in turn generally act faster than capsules and tablets. Dosage forms can thus be listed in order of speed of onset of therapeutic effect (see Table 1.2). However, all drugs irrespective of their delivery route remain foreign substances to the human body and distribution, metabolic and elimination processes commence immediately following drug absorption until the drug has been eliminated from the body via the urine, faeces, saliva, skin or lungs in unchanged or metabolized form.

Table 1.2 Variation in time of onset of action for different dosage forms

Time of onset of action	Dosage form
Seconds	I.v. injections
Minutes	I.m. and s.c. injections, buccal tablets, aerosols, gases
Minutes to hours	Short term depot injections, solutions, suspensions, powders, granules, capsules, tablets, sustained release tablets
Several hours	Enteric coated formulations
Days	Depot injections, implants
Varies	Topical preparations

Routes of drug administration

The absorption pattern of drugs varies considerably between one another as well as between each potential administration route. Dosage forms are designed to provide the drug in a suitable form for absorption from each selected route of administration. The following discussion considers briefly the routes of drug administration and whilst dosage forms are mentioned, this is intended only as an introduction since they will be dealt with in greater detail in the chapters of Part 3.

Oral route

The oral route is the most frequently used route for drug administration. Oral dosage forms are usually intended for systemic effects resulting from drug absorption through the various mucosa of the gastrointestinal tract. A few drugs, however, are intended to dissolve in the mouth for rapid absorption, or for local effect in the tract due to poor absorption by this route or low aqueous solubility. Compared with other routes, the oral route is the simplest, most convenient and safest means of drug administration. Disadvantages, however, include relatively slow onset of action, possibilities of irregular absorption and destruction of certain drugs by the enzymes and secretions of the gastrointestinal tract. For example, insulin-containing preparations are inactivated by the action of stomach fluids.

Whilst drug absorption from the gastrointestinal tract follows the general principles outlined in Chapter 9, several specific features should be emphasized. Changes in drug solubility can result from reactions with other materials present in the gastrointestinal tract, as for example the interference of absorption of tetracyclines through the formation of insoluble complexes with calcium which can be available from foodstuffs or formulation additives. Gastric emptying time is an important factor for effective drug absorption from the intestine. Slow gastric emptying can be detrimental to drugs inactivated by the gastric juices, or slow down absorption of drugs more effectively absorbed from the intestine. In addition, since environmental pH can influence the ionization and lipid solubility of drugs, the pH change occurring along the gastrointestinal tract, from a pH of about 1 in the stomach to approximately 7 or 8 in the large intestine, is important to both degree and site of drug absorption. Since membranes are more permeable to unionized rather than ionized forms and since most drugs are weak acids or bases, it can be shown that weak acids being largely unionized are well absorbed from the stomach. In the small intestine (pH about 6.5) with its extremely large absorbing surface both weak acids and weak bases are well absorbed.

The most popular oral dosage forms are tablets,

capsules, suspensions, solutions and emulsions. Tablets are prepared by compression and contain drugs and formulation additives which are included for specific functions, such as disintegrants which promote tablet break-up into granules and powder particles in the gastrointestinal tract facilitating drug dissolution and absorption. Tablets are often coated, either to provide a protective coat from environmental factors for drug stability purposes or to mask unpleasant drug taste, as well as to protect drugs from the acid conditions of the stomach (enteric coating). Specialized tablet formulations are also available to provide controlled drug release systems through, for example, the use of tablet core matrices or polymeric coating membranes.

Capsules are solid dosage forms containing drug and usually appropriate filler(s), enclosed in a hard or soft shell composed of gelatin. As with tablets, uniformity of dose can be readily achieved and various sizes, shapes, and colours of shell are commercially available. The gelatin shell readily ruptures and dissolves following oral administration and in most cases drugs are released from capsules faster than from tablets. Recently, renewed interest has been shown in filling semi-solid formulations into hard gelatin capsules to provide rapidly dispersing dosage forms for poorly soluble drugs.

Suspensions, which contain finely divided drugs suspended in a suitable vehicle, are a useful means of administering large amounts of drugs which would be inconvenient if taken in tablet or capsule form. They are also useful for patients who experience difficulty in swallowing tablets and capsules and for paediatric use. Whilst dissolution of drug is required prior to absorption following administration of a dose of drug, fine particles with a large surface area are presented to dissolving fluids which facilitates drug dissolution and thereby the onset of drug action. Not all oral suspensions, however, are formulated for systemic effects and several, for example Kaolin and Morphine Mixture B.P.C., are designed for local effects in the gastrointestinal tract. Solutions, including formulations such as elixirs, syrups and linctuses, on the other hand are absorbed more rapidly than solid dosage forms or suspensions since drug dissolution is not required.

Rectal route

Drugs given rectally in solution, suppository or emulsion form, are generally administered for local rather than systemic effects. Suppositories are solid forms intended for introduction into body cavities (usually rectal, but also vaginal and urethral) where they melt, releasing the drug, and the choice of suppository base or drug carrier can greatly influence the degree and rate of drug release. This route of drug administration is indicated for drugs inactivated when given orally by the gastrointestinal fluids, when the oral route is precluded, as for example when a patient is vomiting or unconscious. Drugs administered rectally also enter the systemic circulation without passing through the liver, an advantage for drugs significantly inactivated by the liver following oral route absorption. Disadvantageously the rectal route is inconvenient and drug absorption is often irregular and difficult to predict.

Parenteral route

A drug administered parenterally is one injected via a hollow needle into the body at various sites and to varying depths. The three main parenteral routes are subcutaneous (s.c.), intramuscular (i.m.) and intravenous (i.v.), although other routes are less frequently used such as intracardiac and intrathecal. The parenteral route is preferred when rapid absorption is essential, as in emergency situations or when patients are unconscious or unable to accept oral medication, and in cases when drugs are destroyed or inactivated or poorly absorbed following oral administration. Absorption after parenteral drug delivery is rapid and, in general, blood levels attained are more predictable than those achieved by oral dosage forms.

Injectable preparations are usually sterile solutions or suspensions of drugs in water or other suitable physiologically acceptable vehicles. As referred to previously, drugs must be in solution to be absorbed and thus injection suspensions are slower acting than solution injections. In addition, since body fluids are aqueous, by using suspended drugs in oily vehicles a preparation exhibiting slower absorption characteristics can be formulated to provide a depot preparation providing a reservoir of drug which is slowly released into the systemic circulation. Such preparations are administered by intramuscular injection deep into skeletal muscles (e.g. several penicillin-containing injections). Alternatively, depot preparations can be achieved by subcutaneous implants or pellets, which are compressed or moulded discs of drug placed in loose subcutaneous tissue under the outer layers of the skin. More generally, subcutaneous injections are aqueous solutions or suspensions which allow the drug to be placed in the immediate vicinity of blood capillaries. The drug then diffuses into the capillary. Inclusion of vasoconstrictors or vasodilators in subcutaneous injections will clearly influence blood flow through the capillaries, thereby modifying the capacity for absorption. This principle is often used in the administration of local anaesthetics with the vasoconstrictor adrenaline which delays drug absorption. Conversely improved drug absorption can result when vasodilators are included. Intravenous administration involves injection of sterile aqueous solutions directly into a vein at an appropriate rate. Volumes delivered can range from a few millilitres, as in emergency treatment or for hypnotics, up to litre quantities as in replacement fluid treatment or nutrient feeding.

Topical route

Drugs are applied topically, that is to the skin, mainly for local action. Whilst this route can also be used for systemic drug delivery, percutaneous absorption is generally poor and erratic. Drug absorption is via the sweat glands, hair follicles, sebaceous glands and through the stratum corneum and drugs applied to the skin for local effect include antiseptics, antifungals, antiinflammatory agents, as well as skin emollients for protective effects.

Pharmaceutical topical formulations — ointments, creams and pastes — are composed of drug in a suitable semisolid base which is either hydrophobic or hydrophilic in character. The bases play an important role in determining the drug release character from the formulation. Ointments are hydrophobic, oleaginous-based dosage forms whereas creams are semisolid emulsions. Pastes contain more solids than ointments and thus are stiffer in consistency. For topical application in liquid form other than solution, lotions, suspensions of solids in aqueous solution or emulsions, are used.

Application of drugs to other topical surfaces such as the eye, ear and nose is common and ointments, suspensions and solutions are utilized. Ophthalmic preparations are required amongst other features to be sterile. Nasal dosage forms include solutions or suspensions delivered by drops or fine aerosol from a spray. Ear formulations in general are viscous to prolong contact with affected areas.

Respiratory route

The lungs provide an excellent surface for absorption when the drug is delivered in gaseous or aerosol mist form. For drug particles presented as an aerosol, droplet particle size largely determines the extent to which they penetrate the alveolar region, the zone of rapid absorption. Soluble drug particles that are in the range $0.5-1$ μm diameter reach the alveolar sacs. Particles outside this range are either expired or deposited upon larger bronchial airways. This delivery route has been found particularly useful for the treatment of asthmatic problems, using both powder aerosols (e.g. sodium cromoglycate) and metered aerosols containing the drug in liquefied inert propellant (e.g. isoprenaline sulphate aerosol and salbutamol aerosol).

DRUG FACTORS IN DOSAGE FORM DESIGN

Each type of dosage form requires careful study of the physical and chemical properties of drug substances to achieve a stable, efficacious product. These properties, such as dissolution, crystal size and polymorphic form, solid state stability and drug-additive interaction, can have profound effects on the physiological availability and physical and chemical stability of the drug. By combining such data with those from pharmacological and biochemical studies, the most suitable drug form and additives can be selected for the formulation of chosen dosage forms. Whilst comprehensive property evaluation will not be required for all types of formulations those properties which are recognized as important in dosage form design and processing are listed in Table 1.3. Also listed in Table 1.3 are the stresses to which the formulation might be exposed during processing or manipulation into dosage forms, as well as the procedures involved. Variations in physicochemical properties, occurring for example between batches of the same material or resulting from alternative treatment procedures can modify formulation requirements as well as processing and dosage form performance. For instance the fine milling of poorly soluble drug substances can modify their wetting and dissolution characteristics, important properties during granulation and product performance respectively. Careful evaluation of these properties and understanding of the effects of these stresses upon these parameters is therefore important in dosage form design and processing as well as product performance.

Table 1.3 Physical and chemical properties of drug substances important in dosage form design and potential stresses with range of manufacturing procedures used in processing

Properties	Processing stresses	Manufacturing procedures
Organoleptic	Temperature	Crystallization
Particle size, surface area	Pressure	Precipitation
	Mechanical	Filtration
Solubility	Radiation	Emulsification
Dissolution	Exposure to liquids	Milling
Partition coefficient	Exposure to gases and liquid vapours	Mixing
Ionization constant		Drying
Crystal properties, polymorphism		Granulation
		Compression
Stability		Autoclaving
(Other properties)		Handling
		Storage
		Transport

Organoleptic properties

Modern medicines require that pharmaceutical dosage forms are acceptable to the patient. Unfortunately many drug substances in use today are unpalatable and unattractive in their natural state

and dosage forms, particularly oral preparations, containing such drugs may require the addition of approved flavours, perfumes and/or colours.

The use of flavours and perfumes applies primarily to liquid dosage forms intended for oral administration. Available as concentrated extracts, solutions, adsorbed onto powders or microencapsulated, flavours and perfumes are usually composed of mixtures of natural and synthetic materials. The taste buds of the tongue respond quickly to bitter, sweet, salt or acid elements of a flavour. All other elements are recognized by smell, which can be altered more readily than taste using perfumes. Unpleasant taste can be overcome by using water-insoluble derivatives of drugs which have little or no taste. Examples are the use of chloramphenicol palmitate and amitriptyline pamoate, although other factors, such as bioavailability, must remain unchanged. If an insoluble derivative is unavailable or cannot be used, a flavour or perfume can be used. However, unpleasant drugs in capsules or prepared as coated tablets may be easily swallowed avoiding the taste buds.

Selection of flavour depends upon several factors but particularly on the taste of the drug substance. Certain flavours are more effective at masking various taste elements — for example citrus flavours are frequently used to combat sour or acid tasting drugs. Solubility and stability of the flavour in the vehicle are also important. In addition the age of the intended patient should also be considered, since children for example prefer sweet tastes, as well as the psychological links between colours and flavours (e.g. yellow colour is associated with lemon flavour). Sweetening agents may also be required to mask bitter tastes. Sucrose remains widely used but alternatives, such as sodium saccharin which is 200–700 times sweeter depending on concentration, are available. Sorbitol is recommended for diabetic preparations.

Colours are employed to standardize or improve an existing drug colour, to mask a colour change, or complement a flavour or perfume. Whilst colours are obtained both from natural sources (e.g. carotenoids) or synthesized (e.g. amaranth), the majority used are synthetically produced. Dyes may be aqueous (e.g. amaranth) or oil soluble (e.g. Sudan III) or insoluble in both (e.g. aluminium lakes). Lakes which are generally calcium or aluminium complexes of water-soluble dyes are particularly useful in tablets and tablet coatings because of greater stability to light than corresponding dyes, which also vary in their stability to pH and reducing agents. However, in recent years, the inclusion of colours in formulations has become extremely complex because of the banning of many traditionally used colours in some countries and not others. (A useful summary on colours is given in Martindale, *The Extra Pharmacopoeia*).

Particle size and surface area

Particle size reduction results in an increase in the specific surface (i.e. surface area per unit weight) of powders. Drug dissolution rate, absorption rate, dosage form content uniformity and stability are all dependent to varying degrees on particle size, size distribution and interactions of solid surfaces. In many cases for both drugs and additives particle size reduction is required to achieve the desired physicochemical characteristics.

It is now generally recognized that poorly soluble drugs showing a dissolution rate-limiting step in the absorption process will be more readily bioavailable when administered in a finely subdivided form with larger surface than as a coarse material. Examples include griseofulvin, phenothiazine, diphenylhydantoin, chloramphenicol, tolbutamide, indomethacin and spironolactone. The fine material often in micronized form with larger specific surface dissolves at faster rates which can lead to improved drug absorption by passive diffusion. On the other hand, with formulated nitrofurantoin preparations an optimal particle size of 150 μm reduced gastrointestinal distress whilst still permitting sufficient urinary excretion of this urinary antibacterial agent.

Rates of drug dissolution can be adversely affected, however, by unsuitable choice of formulation additives even though solids of appropriate particle size are used. Tableting lubricant powders, for example, can impart hydrophobicity to a formulation which inhibits drug dissolution. Fine powders can also increase air adsorption or static charge leading to wetting or agglomeration problems. Micronizing drug powders can lead to polymorphic and surface energy changes which cause reduced chemical stability. Drug particle size also influences content uniformity in solid dosage forms, particularly for low dose formulations. It is important in such cases to have as many particles as possible per dose to minimize potency variation between dosage units. Other dosage forms are also affected by particle size including suspensions (for controlling flow properties and particle interactions), inhalation aerosols (for optimal penetration of drug particles to absorbing mucosa) and topical formulations (for freedom from grittiness).

Solubility

All drugs, whatever route they are administered by, must exhibit at least limited aqueous solubility for therapeutic efficiency. Thus relatively insoluble compounds can exhibit erratic or incomplete absorption, and it might be appropriate to use more soluble salt or ester derivatives. Alternatively, micronizing, complexation or solid dispersion techniques might be employed. Solubility can also be important in the absorption of drugs already in solution in liquid dosage forms since precipitation in the gastrointestinal tract can occur and bioavailability modified.

Solubilities of acidic or basic compounds are pH dependent and can be altered by forming salts, with different salts exhibiting different equilibrium solubilities. However, the solubility of a salt of a strong acid is less affected by changes in pH than the solubility of a salt of a weak acid. In the latter case, when pH is low, the salt hydrolyses to an extent dependent of pH and pK_a resulting in decreased solubility. Reduced solubility can also occur for slightly soluble salts of drugs through the common ion effect. If one of the ions involved is added as a different more soluble salt, the solubility product can be exceeded and a portion of the drug precipitates.

Dissolution

As mentioned above, for a drug to be absorbed it must first be dissolved in the fluid at the site of absorption. For example, an orally administered drug in tablet form is not absorbed until drug particles are dissolved or solubilized by the fluids at some point along the gastrointestinal tract, depending on the pH–solubility profile of the drug substance. Dissolution describes the process by which the drug particles dissolve.

During dissolution, the drug molecules in the surface layer dissolve to form a saturated solution around the particles to form the diffusion layer. Dissolved drug molecules then pass throughout the dissolving fluid to contact absorbing mucosa and are absorbed. Replenishment of diffusing drug molecules in the diffusion layer is achieved by further drug dissolution and the absorption process continues. If dissolution is fast or the drug is delivered and remains in solution form, the rate of absorption is primarily dependent upon its ability to transverse the absorbing membrane. If, however, drug dissolution is slow due to its physicochemical properties or formulation factors, then dissolution may be the rate-limiting step in absorption and influence drug bioavailability. The dissolution of a drug is described by the general Noyes–Whitney equation:

$$\frac{dm}{dt} = kA \, (C_s - C)$$

where $\frac{dm}{dt}$ is the dissolution rate, k is the dissolution rate constant, A is the surface area of dissolving solid, C_s is the concentration of drug in the saturated diffusing layer and C is the concentration of drug in the dissolution medium at time t. The equation reveals that dissolution rate can be raised by increasing the surface area (reducing particle size) of the drug, by increasing the solubility of the drug in the diffusing layer and by increasing k which incorporates the drug diffusion coefficient and diffusion layer thickness. During the early phases of dissolution, $C_s \geqslant C$ and if the surface area, A, and experimental conditions are kept constant then k can be determined for compacts containing drug alone. The constant k is now termed the intrinsic dissolution rate constant and is a characteristic of each solid drug compound in a given solvent under fixed hydrodynamic condition. (See Chapter 5 for description of a suitable apparatus and technique.)

Drugs with values of k below $0.1 \, \text{mg}^{-1} \, \text{cm}^{-2}$ usually exhibit dissolution rate-limiting absorption. Particulate dissolution can also be examined where an effort is made to control A, and formulation effects can be studied.

Dissolution rate data when combined with solubility, partition coefficient and pK_a results provide an insight to the formulator into the potential *in vivo* absorption characteristics of a drug. However, *in vitro* tests only have significance if they can be related to *in vivo* results. Once such a relationship has been established, *in vitro* dissolution tests can be used as a quality control test. Nevertheless the importance of dissolution testing has been recognized recently by official compendia with the inclusion in recent editions of dissolution specification using standardized testing procedures for a range of official preparations.

Partition coefficient and pK_a

As pointed out earlier, for relatively insoluble compounds the dissolution rate is often the rate-determining step in the overall absorption process. Alternatively, for soluble compounds the rate of permeation across biological membranes is the rate-determining step. Whilst dissolution rate can be changed by modifying the physicochemical properties of the drug and/or by altering the formulation composition, the permeation rate is dependent upon the size, relative aqueous and lipid solubility and ionic charge of drug molecules, factors which can be altered through molecular modifications. The absorbing membrane acts as a lipophilic barrier to the passage of drugs which is related to the lipophilic nature of the drug molecule. The partition coefficient, for example between oil and water, is a measure of lipophilic character.

The majority of drugs are weak acids or bases and depending on the pH exist in an ionized or unionized form. Membranes of absorbing mucosa are more permeable to unionized forms of drugs than to ionized species because of the greater lipid solubility of the unionized forms and to the highly charged nature of the cell membrane which results in the binding or repelling of the ionized drug, thereby decreasing penetration.

The factors therefore that influence the absorption of weak acids and bases are the pH at the site of absorption and the lipid solubility of the unionized species. These factors, together with the Henderson–Hasselbalch equations for calculating the proportions of ionized and unionized species at a particular pH, constitute the widely accepted pH–partition theory for drug absorption (see Chapter 9). However, these factors do not describe completely the process of absorption since certain compounds with low partition coefficients and/or which are highly ionized over the entire physiological pH range show good bioavailability and therefore other factors are involved.

Crystal properties; polymorphism

Practically all drug substances are handled in powder form at some stage during manufacture into dosage forms. However, for those substances composed of, or containing, powders or compressed powders in the finished product the crystal properties and solid state form of the drug must be carefully considered. It is well recognized that drug substances can be amorphous (i.e. without regular molecular lattice arrangements), crystalline, anhydrous, at various degrees of hydration or solvated with other entrapped solvent molecules, as well as varying in crystal hardness, shape and size. In addition many drug substances can exist in more than one crystalline form with different lattice arrangements. This property is termed polymorphism and different polymorphs may be prepared by manipulation of conditions of crystallization such as solvent, temperature and rate of cooling. It is known that only one form of a pure drug substance is stable at a given temperature and pressure with the other forms, termed metastable, converting at different rates to the stable crystalline form. The different polymorphs vary in physical properties such as solubility, dissolution, solid state stability as well as processing behaviour in terms of powder flow and compaction during tableting.

These different crystalline forms can be of considerable importance in relation to ease or difficulty of formulation and as regards stability and biological activity. As might be expected, higher dissolution rates and solubilities are obtained for metastable polymorphic forms; for

example the metastable forms of chloramphenicol palmitate and chlortetracycline hydrochloride exhibit improved rate and extent of bioavailability. In some cases such as novobiocin, amorphous forms are more active than crystalline forms.

The widely used hormonal substance insulin also demonstrates how differing degrees of activity can result from the use of different crystalline forms of the same agent. In the presence of acetate buffer, zinc combines with insulin to form an extremely insoluble complex of the proteinaceous hormone. This complex is an amorphous precipitate (termed semi-lente) or crystalline product depending on environmental pH. The semi-lente form is rapidly absorbed following i.m. or s.c. injection and has a short duration of action, whilst the large crystalline product called ultra-lente, is more slowly absorbed and is of longer duration of action. A physical mixture of 7 parts ultra-lente and 3 parts semi-lente provides lente insulin which is intermediate in duration of action.

Polymorphic transitions can also occur during milling, granulating, drying and compressing operations (e.g. transitions during milling for digoxin, spironolactone; transitions during compression for phenylbutazone and some sulphonamides). Granulation can result in solvate formation or, during drying a solvated or hydrated molecule may be lost to form an anhydrous material. Consequently, the formulator must be aware of these potential transformations which can result in undesirable modified product performance, even though routine chemical analyses may not reveal any changes. Reversion from metastable forms, if used, to the stable form may also occur during the lifetime of the product. In suspensions, this may be accompanied by changes in the consistency of the preparation which affects its shelf life and stability. Such changes can often be prevented by additives, such as hydrocolloids and surface-active agents which appear to poison the crystal lattice.

Stability

The chemical aspects of formulation generally centre around the chemical stability of the drug and its compatability with the other formulation ingredients. In addition it should be stressed that the packaging of the dosage form is an important contributing factor to product stability and must be an integral part of stability testing programmes. Chapter 7 examines these aspects and only a brief summary is given at this point. It has been mentioned previously that one of the principles of dosage form design is to ensure that the chemical integrity of drug substances is maintained during the usable life of the product. At the same time chemical changes involving additive and any physical modifications to the product must be carefully monitored to optimize formulation stability.

In general drug substances decompose as a result of the effects of heat, oxygen, light and moisture. For example, esters such as aspirin and procaine are susceptible to solvolytic breakdown, whilst oxidative decomposition occurs for substances such as ascorbic acid. Drugs can be classified according to their sensitivity to breakdown:

1 stable at all conditions (e.g. kaolin),
2 stable if handled correctly (e.g. aspirin),
3 moderately unstable even with special handling (e.g. vitamins),
4 very unstable (e.g. certain antibiotics in solution form).

Whilst the mechanisms of solid-state degradation are complex and difficult to analyse, a full understanding is not a prerequisite in the design of a suitable formulation containing solids. For example, in cases where drug substances are sensitive to hydrolysis, steps such as minimum exposure to moisture during preparation, low moisture content specifications in the final product and moisture resistant packaging can be used. For oxygen-sensitive drugs antioxidants can be included in the formulation and, as with light-sensitive materials, suitable packaging can reduce or eliminate the problem. For drugs administered in liquid form, the stability in solution as well as the effects of pH over the physiological range of 1–8 should be understood. Buffers may be required to control the pH of the preparation to improve stability, or where liquid dosage forms are sensitive to microbial attack preservatives are required. In these formulations, and indeed in all dosage forms incorporating additives, it is also important to ensure that the components, which may include additional drug substances as in multivitamin preparations, do not produce chemical interactions themselves. Interactions between drug(s) and added excipients such as antioxidants, preservatives, suspending agents, colourants, tablet lubricants, packaging materials, do occur and must be checked for during formulation. Over recent years thermal analysis techniques, particularly differential scanning calorimetry (DSC), have been found to be particularly useful in screening for possible drug–additive and drug–drug interactions. For example, using DSC it has been demonstrated that the widely used tableting lubricant magnesium stearate interacts with aspirin and sodium dicloxacillin and should be avoided in formulations containing these drug substances.

Other drug properties

At the same time as ensuring that dosage forms are chemically and physically stable and are therapeutically efficacious, it is also relevant to establish that the selected formulation is capable of efficient and, in most cases, large scale manufacture. In addition to those properties previously discussed such as particle size and crystal form, other characteristics such as hygroscopicity, flowability and compressibility are particularly valuable when preparing solid dosage forms where the drugs constitute a large percentage of the formulation. Hygroscopic drugs can require low moisture manufacturing environments and need to avoid water during preparation. Poorly flowing formulations may require the addition of flow agents (e.g. fumed silica). Studies of the compressibility of drug substances are frequently undertaken using instrumented tablet machines in formulation laboratories to examine the tableting potential of the material in order to foresee any potential problems during compaction such as lamination or sticking which may require modification to the formulation or processing conditions.

THERAPEUTIC CONSIDERATIONS IN DOSAGE FORM DESIGN

The nature of the disease or illness against which the drug is intended is an important factor when selecting the range of dosage forms to be prepared. Factors such as the need for systemic or local therapy, duration of action required, and whether the drug will be used in emergency situations, need to be considered. In the vast majority of cases a single drug substance is prepared into a number of dosage forms to satisfy both the particular preferences of the patient or physician and the specific needs of a certain situation. For example many asthmatic patients use inhalation aerosols from which the drug is rapidly absorbed into the systematic circulation following deep inhalation.

Patients requiring relief from angina pectoris, a coronary circulatory problem, place tablets of nitroglycerin sublingually for rapid drug absorption from the buccal cavity. Thus, whilst systemic effects are generally obtained following oral and parenteral drug administration, other routes can be employed as the drug and situation demands. Local effects are generally restricted to those dosage forms applied directly such as those applied to the skin, ear, eye and throat. Some drugs may be well absorbed by one route and not another and must therefore be considered individually.

Recently interest has been growing in the design of drug-containing formulations which deliver drugs to specific 'targets' in the body, for example the use of liposomes and nanoparticles, as well as providing drugs over longer periods of time at controlled rates and several products such as the topical adhesive patches containing nitroglycerin have been marketed. Undoubtedly more of these sophisticated formulations will be developed and interest is likely to be directed to individual patient requirements such as age, weight, and physiological and metabolic factors, features which can influence drug absorption and bioavailability.

The age of the patient does play an important role in the types of dosage form prepared. Infants generally prefer liquid dosage forms, usually solutions and mixtures, given orally. Also, by having liquid preparations the amount of drug administered can be readily adjusted by dilution to give the required dose for the particular patient, taking weight, age and patient's condition into account. Children can have difficulty in swallowing solid dosage forms and for this reason many oral preparations are prepared as pleasantly flavoured syrups or mixtures. Adults generally prefer solid dosage forms, primarily because of their convenience. However alternative liquid preparations are usually available for those unable to take tablets and capsules.

SUMMARY

This chapter has demonstrated that the formulation of drugs into dosage forms requires the interpretation and application of a wide range of information from several study areas. Whilst the physical and chemical properties of drugs and additives need to be understood, the factors influencing drug absorption and the requirements of the disease to be treated also have to be taken into account when identifying potential delivery routes. The formulation and associated preparation of dosage forms demands careful examination, analysis and evaluation of wide ranging information by pharmaceutical scientists to achieve the objective of creating high quality and efficacious dosage forms.

BIBLIOGRAPHY

Ansel, H. C. (1976) General considerations in dosage form design. In: *Introduction to Pharmaceutical Dosage Forms*, 2nd edn, Chap. 3, pp. 61–106, Lea and Febiger, . Philadelphia.

Carstensen, J. T. (1974) Stability of solids and solid dosage forms. *J. pharm. Sci.*, **63**, 1–14.

Florence, A. T. and Attwood, D. (1981) Principles of drug absorption and routes of administration. In *Physicochemical Principles of Pharmacy*, Chap. 9, pp. 325–400, The Macmillan Press, London.

Habelain, J. (1975) Characterisation of habits and crystalline modifications of solids and their pharmaceutical applications. *J. pharm. Sci.*, **64**, 1269–1288.

Lowenthal, W. (1976) Bioavailability. In: *Dispensing of Medication* (Ed. J. E. Hoover), Chap. 2, pp. 39–83.

Martindale, *The Extra Pharmacopoeia* (1982) (Ed. J. E. F. Reynolds), Pharmaceutical Press, London, pp. 423–433.

Macek, T. J. (1975) Formulation. In: *Remington's Pharmaceutical Sciences*, 15th edn (Eds A. Osol, et al.), Chap. 75, pp. 1355–1367, Mack Publishing Co.,

Easton, Pennsylvania.

Polderman, J. (Ed.) (1977) *Formulation and Preparation of Dosage Forms*, Elsevier, Netherlands.

Shami, E.G., Dubzinski, J. R. and Lantz, R. J. (1976) Preformulation. In: *Theory and Practice of Industrial Pharmacy*, 2nd edn (Eds L. Lachman, H. A. Lieberman and J. L. Kanig), Chap. 1, pp. 1–31, Lea and Febiger, Philadelphia.

Talman, F. A. J. (1977) Formulation. In: *Bentley's Textbook of Pharmaceutics*, 8th edn (Ed. E. A. Rawlins), Chap. 37, pp. 641–668.

Wadke, D. A. and Jacobson, H. (1981) Preformulation. In: *Pharmaceutical Dosage Forms — Tablets* (Eds H. A. Lieberman and L. Lachman), Vol. 1, Chap. 1, pp. 1–59, Marcel Dekker, New York, 1–59.

York, P. (1983) Solid state properties of powders in the formulation and processing of solid dosage forms. *Int. J. Pharm.*, **14**, 1–28.

PART ONE

Physicochemical principles of pharmaceutics

Rheology and the flow of fluids

VISCOSITY, RHEOLOGY AND THE FLOW OF FLUIDS

The viscosity of a fluid may be described simply as its resistance to flow or movement. Thus, water which is easier to stir than syrup is said to have the lower viscosity.

Historically the importance of rheology, which may be defined as the study of the flow properties of materials, in pharmacy was merely as a means of characterizing and classifying fluids and semi-solids. For example, in the British Pharmacopoeia substances such as liquid paraffin have been controlled by a viscosity standard for many years whereas a yield value test for carbomer gels has only been introduced more recently. However, the development and adoption of dissolution testing has given added importance to a knowledge of solution viscosity since it may enable mechanisms of dissolution and absorption to be determined. Furthermore, advances in the methods of evaluation of the viscoelastic properties of semi-solids and biological materials have produced useful correlations with bioavailability and function.

The need for a proper understanding of the rheological properties of pharmaceutical materials is an essential fundamental to the preparation, development and evaluation of pharmaceutical dosage forms. This chapter will describe rheological behaviour and techniques of measurement and will form a basis for the applied studies described in later chapters.

NEWTONIAN FLUIDS

Viscosity values for Newtonian fluids

Dynamic viscosity

The definition of viscosity was put on a quantitative basis by Newton who was the first to realize that the rate of flow (D) was directly related to the applied stress (τ); the constant of proportionality is the coefficient of dynamic viscosity, η, more usually referred to simply as the viscosity. Simple fluids which obey the relationship are referred to as Newtonian fluids and fluids which deviate are known as non-Newtonian fluids.

The phenomenon of viscosity is best understood by a consideration of a hypothetical cube of fluid made up of infinitely thin layers (laminae) which are able to slide over one another like a pack of playing cards (Fig. 2.1(a)).

When a tangential force is applied to the uppermost layer it is assumed that each subsequent layer will move at progressively decreasing velocity and that the bottom layer will be stationary (Fig. 2.1(b)). A velocity gradient will therefore exist and this will be equal to the velocity of the upper layer in m s^{-1} divided by the height of the cube in m.·.The resultant gradient, which is effectively the rate of flow but is usually referred to as the rate of shear, D, will have units of reciprocal seconds (s^{-1}). The applied stress, known as the shear stress, is derived by dividing the applied force by the area of the upper layer and will have units of N m^{-2}.

Since Newton's law can be expressed as

$$\tau = \eta D \tag{2.1}$$

then
$$\eta = \tau/D \tag{2.2}$$

and η will have units of N m^{-2} s. Thus by reference to Eqn 2.1, it can be seen that a Newtonian fluid of viscosity 1 N m^{-2} s would produce a velocity of 1 m s^{-1} for a cube of 1 m dimension with an applied force of 1 N. Since the special name for the derived unit of force per unit area in the SI system is the pascal (Pa) then viscosity should be referred to in Pa.s. If this definition is modified by replacement of SI units by the c.g.s. equivalents then the viscosity would be in dyn cm^{-2} s which may also be referred to as poise (P). This latter unit is still used and 1 poise = 0.1 Pa.s. Even the poise is a relatively large unit and it is more normal to use the centipoise (cP) (= 1 mPa.s). A factor which may influence the continued use of this unit is that at 20 °C the viscosity of pure water is about 1 cP.

A summary of units is given in Table 2.1 and the values of the viscosity of water and some examples of other fluids of pharmaceutical interest are given in Table 2.2.

Kinematic viscosity

The dynamic viscosity is not the only coefficient which can be used to characterize a fluid. The

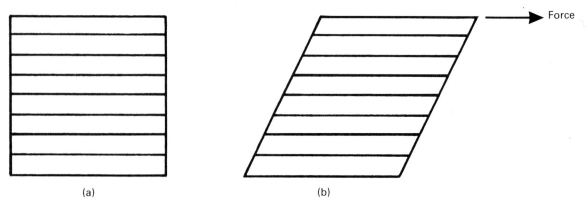

(a)   (b)

Fig. 2.1 Representation of the effect of shearing a 'block' of fluid

Table 2.1 Summary of units of viscosity coefficients

Viscosity coefficient	Units		
	SI	c.g.s.	Alternative
Dynamic viscosity	Pa.s	dyn cm^{-2} s	Poise (P) = 0.1 Pa.s
Kinematic viscosity	m^2 s^{-1}	cm^2 s^{-1}	Stoke (St) = 10^{-4} m^2 s^{-1}

Table 2.2 Viscosities of some fluids of pharmaceutical interest

Fluid	Dynamic viscosity at 20 °C (mPa.s)
Chloroform	0.58
Water	1.002
Ethanol	1.20
Glyceryl trinitrate	36.0
Olive oil	84.0
Castor oil	986.0
Glycerol	1490

kinematic viscosity (v) is also used and may be defined as the dynamic viscosity divided by the density of the fluid (ρ):

$$v = \frac{\eta}{\rho} \qquad (2.3)$$

and the SI units will be m^2 s^{-1} (or cm^2 s^{-1} in the c.g.s system). This latter unit may be referred to as the stoke (St) (= 10^{-4} m^2 s^{-1}) or more usefully the centistoke (cSt) (= 10^{-6} m^2 s^{-1}). The kinematic viscosity of water at 20 °C will be about 1 cSt.

Relative and specific viscosities

The viscosity ratio or relative viscosity (η_r) of a solution is the ratio of the solution viscosity to the viscosity of the solvent (η_o)

$$\eta_r = \frac{\eta}{\eta_o} \qquad (2.4)$$

and the specific viscosity (η_{sp}) is given by

$$\eta_{sp} = \eta_r - 1 \qquad (2.5)$$

In these calculations the solvent can be of any nature although in pharmaceutical products it is often water.

For a colloidal dispersion the equation derived by Einstein may be used:

$$\eta = \eta_o (1 + 2.5 \, \phi) \qquad (2.6)$$

where ϕ is the volume fraction of the colloidal phase (the volume of the dispersed phase divided by the total volume of the dispersion). The Einstein equation may be rewritten as

$$\frac{\eta}{\eta_o} = 1 + 2.5 \, \phi \qquad (2.7)$$

when, from Eqn 2.4, it can be seen that the left hand side of Eqn 2.7 is equal to the relative viscosity. It can also be rewritten as

$$\frac{\eta}{\eta_o} - 1 = \frac{\eta - \eta_o}{\eta_o} = 2.5 \, \phi \qquad (2.8)$$

when the left hand side equals the specific viscosity. Eqn 2.8 can be rearranged to produce

$$\frac{\eta_{sp}}{\phi} = 2.5 \qquad (2.9)$$

and since the volume fraction will be directly related to concentration then Eqn 2.9 can be rewritten as

$$\frac{\eta_{sp}}{C} = k \qquad (2.10)$$

When the dispersed phase is a high molecular mass polymer then a colloidal solution will result and provided moderate concentrations are used then Eqn 2.10 can be expressed as a power series.

$$\frac{\eta_{sp}}{C} = k_1 + k_2 C + k_3 C^2 \qquad (2.11)$$

Intrinsic viscosity

If $\frac{\eta_{sp}}{C}$, the viscosity number or reduced viscosity is determined at a range of polymer concentrations and plotted as a function of concentration (Fig. 2.2), then a linear relationship should be obtained and the intercept produced on extrapolation of the line to the ordinate will yield the constant k_1 which is referred to as the limiting viscosity number or the intrinsic viscosity, $[\eta]$, when the units of concentration are in g dl^{-1}.

The limiting viscosity number may be used to determine the approximate molecular mass (M) of polymers using the Mark–Houwink equation:

$$[\eta] = K \, M^\alpha \qquad (2.12)$$

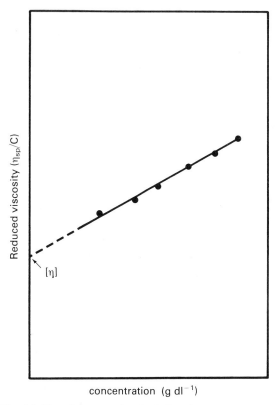

Reduced viscosity (η_{sp}/C)

[η]

concentration (g dl^{-1})

Fig. 2.2 Plot of concentration (g dl^{-1}) against reduced viscosity (η_{sp}/C) which by extrapolation gives the limiting viscosity number or intrinsic viscosity ([η])

where K and α are constants that must be obtained at a given temperature for the specific polymer–solvent system. However, once these constants are known then viscosity determinations provide a quick and precise method of molecular mass determination of pharmaceutical polymers such as dextran which is used as a plasma extender. Also the values of the two constants provide an indication of the shape of the molecule in solution; spherical molecules yield values of $\alpha = 0$ whilst extended rods have values of greater than 1.0. A randomly coiled molecule will yield an intermediate value (≈ 0.5).

The specific viscosity may be used in the following equation to determine the volume of a molecule in solution

$$\eta_{sp} = 2.5 \, C \, \frac{NV}{M} \qquad (2.13)$$

where C is concentration, N is Avogadro's number, V is the volume of each molecule and M is the molecular mass. However, it does suffer from the obvious disadvantage that the assumption is made that all polymeric molecules form spheres in solution.

Huggins' constant

Finally, the constant k_2 in Eqn 2.11 is referred to as the Huggins' constant and is equal to the slope of the plot shown in Fig. 2.2. Its value gives an indication of the interaction between the polymer and the solvent such that a positive slope is produced for a polymer which interacts weakly with the solvent and the slope becomes less positive as the interaction increases. A change in the value of the Huggins' constant can be used to evaluate the interaction of drug molecules with polymers.

Boundary layers

From Fig. 2.1 it can be seen that the rate of flow of a fluid over an even surface will be dependent upon the distance from the surface. The velocity, which will be almost zero at the surface, increases with increasing distance from the surface until the bulk of the fluid is reached and the velocity becomes constant. The region over which differences in velocity are observed is referred to as the boundary layer. Its depth is dependent upon the viscosity of the fluid and the rate of flow in the bulk fluid: high viscosity and a low flow rate would result in a thick boundary layer which will become thinner as either the viscosity falls or the flow rate is increased. The boundary layer, which arises because of the intermolecular forces between the liquid molecules and those of the surface resulting in reduction of movement of the layer adjacent to the wall to zero, represents an important barrier to heat and mass transfer. In the case of a capillary tube then the two boundary layers meet at the centre of the tube such that the velocity distribution is parabolic (Fig. 2.3). With increase either in diameter of the tube or the fluid velocity then the proximity of the two boundary layers is reduced and the velocity profile becomes flattened at the centre (Fig. 2.3).

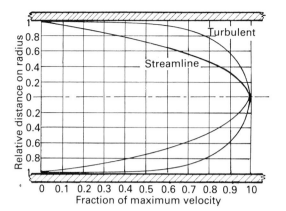

Fig. 2.3 Velocity distributions across a pipe

Laminar, transitional and turbulent flow

The conditions under which a fluid flows through, for example, a pipe can markedly affect the character of the flow. The type of flow which occurs can be best understood by reference to experiments which were conducted by Reynolds in 1883. The apparatus used (Fig. 2.4) consisted of a straight glass tube through which the fluid flowed under the influence of a force provided by a constant head of water. In the inlet of the tube a fine stream of dye was introduced at the centre of the tube.

At low flow rates the dye formed a coherent thread which remained undisturbed in the centre of the tube and grew very little in thickness along the length of the tube. This type of flow is described as *streamlined* or *laminar flow* and the liquid is considered to flow as a series of concentric cylinders in an analogous manner to an extending telescope.

If the speed of the fluid is increased a critical velocity is reached at which the thread begins to waver and then to break up, although no mixing occurs. This is known as *transitional flow*. When the velocity is increased to high values the dye instantaneously mixes with the fluid in the tube since all order is lost and irregular motions are imposed on the overall movement of the fluid. Such flow is described as *turbulent*. In this type of flow the movement of molecules is totally haphazard although the average movement will be in the direction of flow.

Reynolds' experiments indicated that the flow conditions were affected by four factors namely the diameter of the pipe and the viscosity, density and velocity of the fluid. Furthermore, it was shown that these factors could be combined to give the following equation.

$$Re = \frac{\rho \, u \, d}{\eta} \qquad (2.14)$$

where ρ is the density, u is the velocity and η is the dynamic viscosity of the fluid; d is the diameter of the pipe. Re is known as Reynolds' number and provided compatible units are used it will be dimensionless.

Values of Reynolds' number have been determined which can be associated with a particular type of flow. If it is below 2000 then streamline flow will occur whilst if it is above 4000 then flow will be turbulent. In between these two values the nature of the flow will depend upon the surface over which the fluid is flowing. For example, if the surface is smooth then streamline flow may not be disturbed and may exist at values of Reynolds'

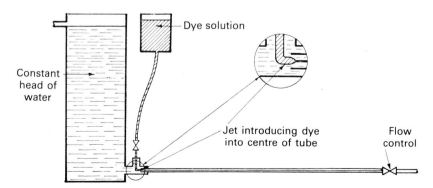

Fig. 2.4 Reynolds' apparatus

number above 2000. However, if the surface is rough or the channel tortuous then flow may well be turbulent at values below 4000 and even as low as 2000. Consequently, although it is tempting to state that values of Reynolds' number between 2000 and 4000 are indicative of transitional flow such a statement would only be correct for a specific set of conditions. This fact also explains why it is difficult to demonstrate transitional flow practically. However, Reynolds' number is still an important parameter and can be used to predict the type of flow which will occur in a particular situation. The importance of knowing the type of flow lies in the fact that with streamline flow there is no component at right angles to the direction of flow so that fluid cannot move across the tube. This component is strong for turbulent flow and interchange across the tube is rapid. Thus, for example, mass will be rapidly transported in the latter case whereas the fluid layers in streamline flow will act as a barrier to such transfer which can only occur by molecular diffusion.

Determination of the flow properties of simple fluids

A wide range of instruments exist which may be used to determine the flow properties of Newtonian fluids. However, only some of these are capable of providing data which can be used to calculate viscosities in fundamental units: the design of many instruments precludes the calculation of absolute viscosities since they are capable of providing data only in terms of empirical units.

It would be impossible to review all the instruments which could be used to measure viscosity and consequently this section will be limited to those instruments which are mentioned in the *British Pharmacopoeia* (BP) 1980 together with others which are commonly used for simple fluids and dilute colloidal solutions.

Capillary viscometers

A capillary viscometer can be used to determine viscosity provided that the fluid is Newtonian and the flow is streamlined. The rate of flow of the fluid through the capillary is measured under the influence of gravity or an externally applied pressure.

Ostwald U-tube viscometer   Such instruments are described in the BP 1980 and are the subject of a specification of the British Standards Institute. A range of capillary bores is available and an appropriate one should be selected such that a flow time of approximately 200 s is obtained: thus, the wider bore viscometers are for use with fluids of higher viscosity. For fluids where there is a viscosity specification in the BP, it states the size of instrument which must be used in the determination of their viscosity. These include liquid paraffin, dextran injection, the macrogols and iron sorbitol injection.

The instrument is shown in Fig. 2.5 and flow through the capillary occurs under the influence of gravity. The liquid is introduced into the viscometer up to mark G through arm V using a pipette long enough to prevent wetting the sides of the tube.

The viscometer is then clamped vertically in a constant temperature water bath and allowed to attain the required temperature. The level of the liquid is adjusted and is then blown or sucked into tube W until the meniscus is just above mark E. The time for the meniscus to fall between marks E and F is recorded. Determinations should be repeated until three readings all within 0.5 s are obtained. Care should be taken not to introduce air bubbles and that the capillary does not become partially occluded with small particles.

Suspended level viscometer   This instrument is a modification of the U-tube viscometer which avoids the necessity of filling the instrument with a precise volume of fluid. Also, the fact that the pressure head in the U-tube is continually changing as the two menisci approach one another is avoided. Once more, it is described in the BP 1980 where it is used to determine the viscosity of an aqueous solution of methyl cellulose 450. It is shown in Fig. 2.6.

A volume of liquid which will at least fill bulb C is introduced via tube V. The only upper limit on the volume used is that it should not block the ventilating tube Z. The viscometer is clamped vertically in a constant temperature water bath and allowed to attain the required temperature. Tube Z is closed and fluid is drawn into bulb C by the application of suction through tube W until the meniscus is just above the mark E. Tube W is

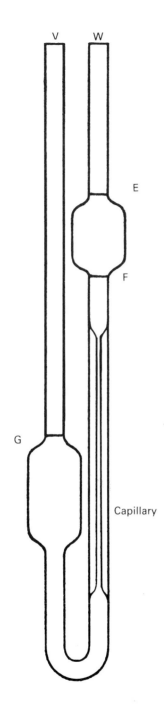

Fig. 2.5 A U-tube viscometer

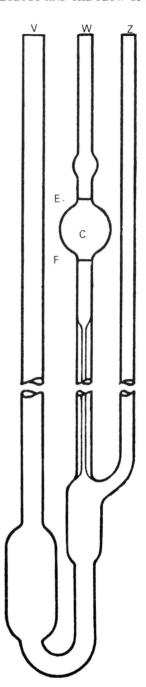

Fig. 2.6 A suspended level viscometer

then closed and tube Z opened so that liquid can be drawn away from the bottom of the capillary. The tube W is then opened and the time recorded for the fluid to fall between the marks E and F. If at any time during the determination the end

of the ventilating tube Z becomes blocked by the liquid then the experiment must be repeated. The same criteria for reproducibility of timings described with the U-tube viscometer must be applied.

Since the volume of fluid introduced into the instrument can vary between the limits described above then it means that measurements can be made at a range of temperatures without the need for adjustment of volume.

Calculation of viscosity from capillary viscometers

Poiseuille's law states that for a liquid flowing through a capillary tube

$$\eta = \frac{\pi r^4 t P}{8 L V} \tag{2.15}$$

where r is the radius of the capillary, t is the time of flow, P is the pressure difference across the ends of the tube, L is the length of the capillary and V is the volume of liquid. Since the radius and length of the capillary as well as the volume flowing are constants for a given viscometer then

$$\eta = K t P \tag{2.16}$$

where K is equal to $\dfrac{\pi r^4}{8LV}$

The pressure difference, P, depends upon the density, ρ, of the liquid, the acceleration due to gravity, g, and the difference in heights of the two menisci in the two arms of the viscometer. Since the value of g and the level of the liquids are constant these can be included in a constant and it can be written for the viscosities of an unknown and a standard liquid

$$\eta_1 = K' t_1 \rho_1 \tag{2.17}$$
$$\eta_2 = K' t_2 \rho_2 \tag{2.18}$$

Thus, when the flow times for two liquids are compared using the same viscometer, division of Eqn 2.17 by Eqn 2.18 gives

$$\frac{\eta_1}{\eta_2} = \frac{t_1 \rho_1}{t_2 \rho_2} \tag{2.19}$$

and reference to Eqn 2.4 will show that Eqn 2.19 will yield the viscosity ratio.

However, since Eqn 2.3 indicates that the kinematic viscosity is equal to the dynamic viscosity divided by the density then Eqn 2.19 may be rewritten as

$$\frac{v_1}{v_2} = \frac{t_1}{t_2} \tag{2.20}$$

For a given viscometer a standard fluid such as water can be used for the purposes of calibration. Then Eqn 2.20 may be rewritten as

$$v = c t \tag{2.21}$$

This is the equation which appears in the BP and explains the continued use of the kinematic viscosity since it means that liquids of known viscosity but of differing density from the test fluid can be used as the standard. A series of oils of given viscosity are available commercially and are recommended for calibration of viscometers for which water cannot be used.

Falling sphere viscometer

This viscometer is based upon Stokes' law (Chapter 6). When a body falls through a viscous medium it experiences a resistance or viscous drag which opposes the downward motion. Consequently if a body falls through a liquid under the influence of gravity, an initial acceleration period is followed by motion at a uniform terminal velocity when the gravitational force is balanced by the viscous drag. Eqn 2.22 will then apply to this terminal velocity when a sphere of density ρ_s and diameter d falls through a liquid of viscosity η and density ρ_1. The terminal velocity is u and g is the acceleration due to gravity:

$$3\pi\eta du = \frac{\pi}{6} d^3 g (\rho_s - \rho_1) \tag{2.22}$$

The viscous drag is given by the left hand side of equation whereas the right hand side represents the force responsible for the downward motion of the sphere under the influence of gravity. Eqn 2.22 may be used to calculate viscosity by rearranging to give:

$$\eta = \frac{d^2 g (\rho_s - \rho_1)}{18u} \tag{2.23}$$

Eqn 2.3 gives the relationship between η and the kinematic viscosity such that Eqn 2.23 may be rewritten as:

$$v = \frac{d^2 g (\rho_s - \rho_1)}{18u\rho_1} \tag{2.24}$$

In the derivation of these equations it is assumed

that the sphere is falling through a fluid of infinite dimensions. For practical purposes the fluid must be contained in a vessel of finite dimensions and therefore it is necessary to include a correction factor to allow for the end and wall effects. This correction used is due to Faxen and may be given as:

$$F = 1 - 2.104 \frac{d}{D} + 2.09 \frac{d^3}{D^3} - 0.95 \frac{d^5}{D^5} \quad (2.25)$$

when D is the diameter of the measuring tube. The last term in Eqn 2.25 accounts for the end effect and may be ignored if the middle third of the depth is used for measuring the velocity of the sphere. In fact the middle half of the tube can be used if D is at least ten times d and the second and third terms, which account for the wall effects, can be replaced by $2.1 \frac{d}{D}$.

The apparatus used to determine u is shown in Fig. 2.7. The liquid is placed in the fall tube which is clamped vertically in a constant temperature bath. A sufficient period of time must be allowed for temperature equilibration to occur and for air bubbles to rise to the surface. A steel sphere which has been cleaned and brought to the temperature of the experiment is introduced into the fall tube through a narrow guide tube. The passage of the sphere is monitored by means of a telescope and the time taken to fall between the etched marks A and B is recorded. It is usual to take the average of three readings, of which all are within 0.5%, as the fall time, t, to calculate the viscosity. If the same sphere and fall tube are used then Eqn 2.24 reduces to:

$$v = Kt \, (\rho_s/\rho_1 - 1) \quad (2.26)$$

where K is a constant that may be determined by use of a liquid of known kinematic viscosity.

The BP gives a detailed description of the falling sphere viscometer and specifies its use in the determination of the viscosity of a solution of pyroxylin in acetone. This type of viscometer is really only of use with Newtonian fluids and a variation has involved measurement of the time for a sphere to roll through the fluid contained in an inclined tube. This instrument can only be used after calibration with standard fluids since fundamental derivation of viscosity is impossible.

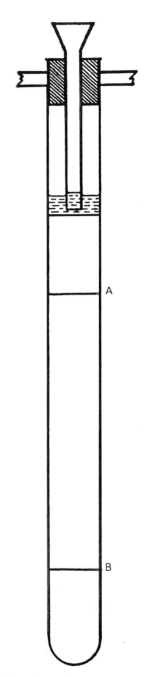

Fig. 2.7 A falling sphere viscometer

NON-NEWTONIAN FLUIDS

The characteristics described in the previous sections only apply to fluids which obey Newton's law and are consequently referred to as Newtonian.

However, most pharmaceutical fluids do not follow this law because the viscosity of the fluid varies with the rate of shear. The reason for these deviations is that the fluids concerned are not simple fluids like water and syrup but are disperse or colloidal systems including emulsions, suspensions and gels. These materials are known as non-Newtonian and with the increasing use of sophisticated polymer-based delivery systems more examples of such behaviour are found in pharmacy.

Types of non-Newtonian behaviour

More than one type of deviation from Newton's law can be recognized and it is the type of deviation which occurs that can be used to classify the particular material.

If a Newtonian fluid is subjected to an increasing rate of shear, D, and the corresponding shear stress, τ, recorded then a plot of τ against D will produce the linear relationship shown in Fig. 2.8(a). Such a plot is usually referred to as a flow curve or rheogram. The slope of this plot will give the 'fluidity' of the fluid and its viscosity may be determined from the reciprocal of the slope of the line. Eqn 2.1 implies that this line will pass through the origin.

Plastic (or Bingham) flow

Fig. 2.8(b) indicates an example of plastic or Bingham flow when the rheogram does not pass through the origin but intersects with the shear stress axis at a point usually referred to as the yield value, f_B. This infers that a plastic material does not flow until such a value of shear stress has been exceeded and at lower stresses the substance behaves as a solid (elastic) material. Plastic materials are often referred to as Bingham bodies in honour of the worker who carried out many of the original studies with such materials. The equation which he derived may be given as

$$U = \frac{(\tau - f_B)}{D} \qquad (2.27)$$

where U is the plastic viscosity and f_B the Bingham yield value (Fig. 2.8(b)). The equation implies that the rheogram is a straight line inter-

secting the shear stress axis at the yield value f_B. In practice flow occurs at a lower shear stress than f_B and the flow curve gradually approaches the extrapolation of the linear portion of the line shown in Fig. 2.8(b). This extrapolation will also give the Bingham yield value; the slope is 'the mobility' which can be considered to be analogous to the fluidity of a Newtonian fluid. The plastic viscosity will be given by the reciprocal of the mobility.

Plastic flow is exhibited by concentrated suspensions particularly if the continuous phase is of high viscosity or if the particles are flocculated.

Pseudoplastic flow

The rheogram shown in Fig. 2.8(c) arises at the origin and since no yield value exists then the material will flow as soon as a shear stress is applied and the slope of the curve gradually increases with increasing rate of shear. The viscosity is derived from the reciprocal of the slope and therefore decreases as the shear rate is increased. Materials exhibiting this behaviour are said to be pseudoplastic and no single value of viscosity can be considered as characteristic. The viscosity can only be calculated from the reciprocal of the slope of a tangent drawn to the curve at a specific point. Such viscosities are known as apparent viscosities (η_{app}) and are only of any use if quoted in conjunction with the shear rate at which the determination was made. Since it would need several apparent viscosities to characterize a pseudoplastic material then the most satisfactory representation of the material is by means of the entire flow curve. However, it is frequently noted that at higher shear stresses the flow curve tends towards linearity indicating that a minimum viscosity has been attained. When this is the case then such a viscosity can be a useful means of classification.

Not surprisingly, there is no satisfactory quantitative explanation of pseudoplastic flow. The relationship which is claimed to be the most frequently used is empirical and is given as

$$\tau^n = \eta'D \qquad (2.28)$$

where η' is a viscosity coefficient and the exponent n an index of pseudoplasticity in that as

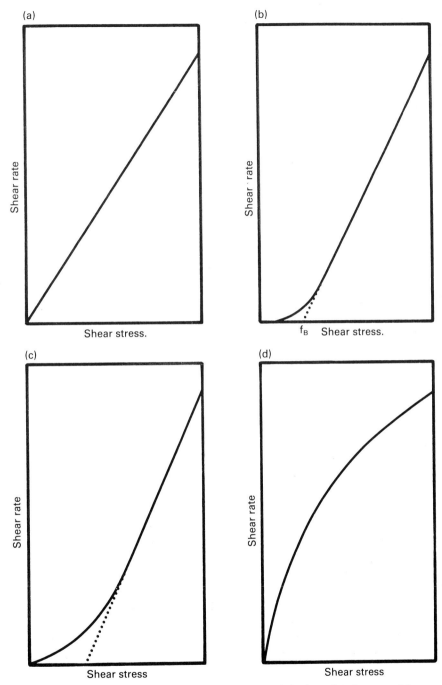

Fig. 2.8 Flow curves or rheograms representing the behaviour of various materials

its value falls from one, the flow becomes increasingly non-Newtonian since when the value of n is 1 then Eqn 2.28 is the same as Eqn 2.1. In order to obtain the values of the constants then log D must be plotted against log τ from which the slope will produce n and the intercept log η'. This equation can only be used over limited ranges of shear stress and does not find application for all pharmaceutical materials which exhibit pseudo-plastic flow. Such materials are most usually typified by aqueous dispersions of hydrocolloids such as tragacanth, alginates, methyl cellulose and synthetic materials such as polyvinylpyrrolidone. The presence of long high molecular weight molecules in solution results in entanglement together with the association of immobilized solvent. Under the influence of shear the molecules tend to become disentangled and align themselves in the direction of flow. The molecules thus offer less resistance to flow and this together with the release of some of the entrapped water accounts for the lower viscosity. At any particular shear rate an equilibrium will be established between the shearing force and the re-entanglement brought about by Brownian motion.

Dilatant flow

The opposite type of flow to pseudoplasticity is depicted by curve (d) in Fig. 2.8 in that the viscosity increases with increase in shear rate. Since such materials increase in volume during shearing then they are referred to as dilatant and exhibit shear thickening. An equation similar to that for pseudoplastic flow (Eqn 2.28) may be used to describe dilatant behaviour but the value of the exponent n will be greater than 1 and will increase as dilatancy increases.

This type of behaviour is less common than plastic or pseudoplastic flow but may be exhibited by dispersions containing a high concentration ($\simeq 50\%$) of small, deflocculated particles. Under conditions of zero shear, the particles are closely packed and the interparticulate voids are at a minimum (Fig. 2.9) which the vehicle is sufficient to fill. Consequently at low shear rates such as those created during pouring this fluid can adequately lubricate the relative movement of the particles. As the shear rate is increased the particles become displaced from their even distribution and the clumps which are produced result in the creation of larger voids into which the vehicle drains so that the resistance to flow is increased and viscosity rises. The effect is progressive with increase in shear rate until eventually the material may appear paste-like as flow ceases. Fortunately, the effect is reversible and removal of the shear stress results in the re-establishment of the fluid nature.

Dilatancy can be a problem during the processing of dispersions and granulation of tablet masses when high speed blenders and mills are employed. If the material being processed becomes dilatant in nature then the resultant solidification could overload and damage the motor. Changing of the batch or supplier of the material used could lead to processing problems which can only be avoided by rheological evaluation of the dispersions prior to introduction to the production process.

Time-dependent behaviour

In the description of the different types of non-Newtonian behaviour it was implied that although the viscosity of a fluid might vary with shear rate it was independent of the length of time that the shear rate was applied and also that replicate

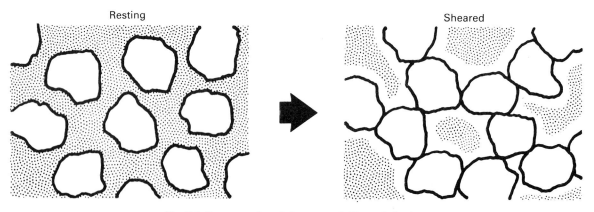

Fig. 2.9 Representation of the cause of dilatant behaviour

determinations at the same shear rate would always produce the same viscosity. This must be considered as the ideal situation since most non-Newtonian materials are colloidal in nature and as such the flowing elements, whether particles or macromolecules, may not adapt immediately to the new shearing conditions. Therefore, when such a material is subjected to a particular shear rate the shear stress and consequently the viscosity will decrease with time. Furthermore, once the shear stress has been removed even if the structure which has been broken down is reversible, it may not return to its original structure (rheological ground state) instantly. The common feature of all these materials is that if they are subjected to a gradually increasing shear rate followed immediately by a shear rate decreasing to zero then the downcurve will be displaced with regard to the upcurve and the rheogram will exhibit a hysteresis loop (Fig. 2.10). In the case of plastic and pseudoplastic materials the downcurve will be displaced to the left of the upcurve (Fig. 2.10) whereas for dilatant substances the reverse will be true (Fig. 2.11). The presence of the hysteresis loop indicates that a breakdown in structure has occurred and the area within the loop may be used as an index of the degree of breakdown.

The term which is used to describe such behaviour is thixotropy which means 'to change by touch' although strictly this term should only be applied to an isothermal sol–gel transformation. However, it has become common to describe as thixotropic any material which exhibits a reversible time-dependent decrease in apparent viscosity. Thixotropic systems are usually composed of asymmetric particles or macromolecules which are capable of interacting by numerous secondary bonds to produce a loose three-dimensional structure so that the material is gel-like when unsheared. The energy which is imparted during

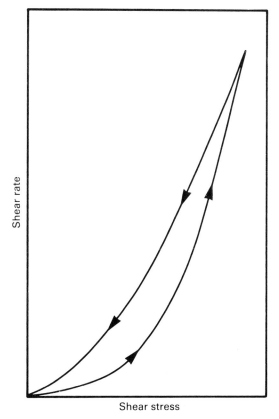

Fig. 2.10 A rheogram produced by a thixotropic pseudoplastic substance

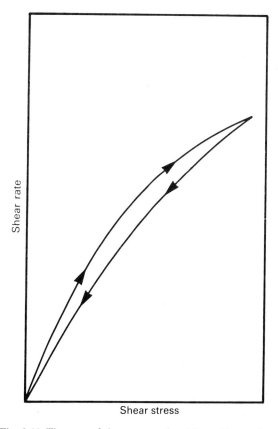

Fig. 2.11 The type of rheogram produced by a thixotropic dilatant material

shearing disrupts these bonds so that the flowing elements become aligned and the viscosity falls since a gel–sol transformation has occurred. When the shear stress is eventually removed the structure will tend to reform although the process is not immediate and will increase with time as the molecules return to the original state under the influence of Brownian motion. Furthermore, the time taken for recovery, which can vary from minutes to days depending upon the system, will be directly related to the length of time that the material was subjected to the shear stress since this will affect the degree of breakdown.

In some cases the structure which has been destroyed is never recovered no matter how long the system is left unsheared. Repeat determinations of the flow curve will then only produce the downcurve which was obtained in the experiment that resulted in the destruction. It is suggested that such behaviour be referred to as 'shear destruction' rather than thixotropy which as will be appreciated from above is a misnomer in this case.

An example of such behaviour are the gels produced by high molecular weight polysaccharides which are stabilized by large numbers of secondary bonds. Such systems undergo extensive reorganization during shearing such that the three-dimensional structure is reduced to a two-dimensional one: the gel-like nature of the original is then never recovered.

The occurrence of such complex behaviour creates problems in the quantitative classification because not only will the apparent viscosity change with shear rate but there will also be two viscosities which can be calculated for any given shear rate (i.e. from the upcurve and the downcurve). It is usual to attempt to calculate one viscosity for the upcurve and another for the downcurve. This must assume of course that each of the curves achieves linearity over some of its length otherwise a defined shear rate must be used: only the former situation is truly satisfactory. Each of the lines used to derive the viscosity may be extrapolated to the shear stress axis to give an associated yield value. However, only the one derived from the upcurve has any significance since that derived from the downcurve will relate to the broken down system. Consequently the

most useful index of thixotropy can be obtained by integration of the area contained within the loop. This will not of course take into account the shape of the up- and downcurves and consequently two materials may produce loops of similar area but which have completely different shapes representing totally different flow behaviour. In order to prevent confusion it is best to adopt a method whereby an estimate of area is accompanied by yield value(s). This is of particular importance with flow curves which exhibit complex upcurves such as that shown in Fig. 2.12. It is typical of the type of loop obtained with, for example, some samples of white soft paraffin where the upcurve exhibits a number of bulges. Those at lower shear rate are thought to be associated with the initial loss of three-dimensional structure whilst the smoother deviations occurring at the higher shear rates are associated with molecular reorientation. Such be-

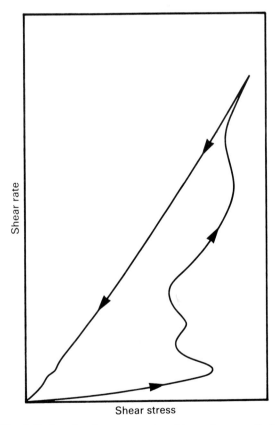

Fig. 2.12 Complex rheogram produced by a pharmaceutical gel

haviour is common in pharmaceutical systems and is one of the major causes of difficulties in their evaluation.

Determination of the flow properties of non-Newtonian fluids

With such a wide range of rheological behaviour it is extremely important to carry out measurements which will produce meaningful results. It is crucial therefore not to use a determination of viscosity at one shear rate (such as would be acceptable for a Newtonian fluid) since it could lead to completely erroneous comparative results. Figure 2.13 shows rheograms which are an example of the four different types of flow behaviour all of which intersect at point A which is equivalent to a shear rate of 100 s^{-1}. Therefore if a measurement were made at this one shear rate then all four materials would be shown to have the same viscosity although they all possess different properties and behaviour. Single point determinations are probably an extreme example but are used to emphasize the importance of properly designed experiments.

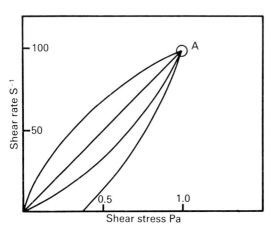

Fig. 2.13 Explanation of the effect of single point viscosity determination and the resultant errors

Rotational viscometers

These instruments rely on the viscous drag exerted on a body when it is rotated in the fluid to determine the viscosity. The major advantage of such instruments is that wide ranges of shear

rate can be achieved and often a programme of shear rates can be produced automatically. Thus, the flow curve of a material may be obtained directly. A number of commercial instruments are available but each shares a common feature in that two different measuring geometries are utilized: these are concentric cylinder (or couette) and cone–plate.

Concentric cylinder In this geometry there are two coaxial cylinders of different diameters, the outer forming the cup containing the fluid in which the inner cylinder or bob is positioned centrally (Fig. 2.14). In older types of instrument the outer cylinder is rotated and the viscous drag exerted by the fluid is transmitted to the inner cylinder as a torque so that it rotates against its torsion wire suspension. The stress on this inner cylinder is indicated by the angular deflection, θ, once equilibrium (i.e. steady flow) has been attained. The torque, T, can then be calculated from

$$C \theta = T \qquad (2.29)$$

where C is the torsional constant of the wire. The viscosity is then given by equation

$$\eta = \frac{\left(\dfrac{1}{r_1{}^2} - \dfrac{1}{r_2{}^2}\right)T}{4 \pi h \omega} \qquad (2.30)$$

where r_1 and r_2 are the radii of the inner and outer cylinders respectively, h is the height of the inner cylinder and ω is the angular velocity of the outer cylinder.

Cone-plate This geometry is composed of a flat circular plate with a wide angle cone placed centrally above (Fig. 2.15). The tip of the cone just touches the plate and the sample is loaded into the included gap. If the plate is rotated then the cone will be caused to rotate against a torsion wire in the same way as the inner cylinder as described above. Provided the angle is small (of the order of 1°) then the viscosity will be given by

$$\eta = \frac{3 \omega T}{2\pi r^3 \alpha} \qquad (2.31)$$

where ω is the angular velocity of the plate, T is the torque, r is the radius of the cone and α is the angle between the cone and plate.

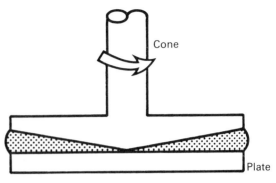

Fig. 2.15 Cone–plate geometry

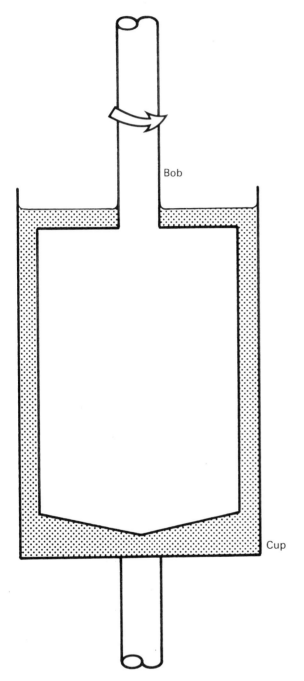

Fig. 2.14 Concentric cylinder geometry

part of the geometry, usually the plate or the outer cylinder, stationary and to rotate the other member at a constant speed. The developed shear stress can then be measured. An alternative is to rotate the upper member under a constant stress when the developed shear rate is measured. Either method has been the subject of considerable sophistication and having one part of the geometry stationary means that it can be circulated with water or other fluid at a temperature appropriate to the measurement.

Concentric cylinder viscometers are very useful for Newtonian and non-Newtonian fluids provided the latter are not too solid-like in nature. Wide ranges of shear rate can be achieved by varying the diameters of the cylinders. However, this geometry does suffer from disadvantages, the major one being that the shear rate across the gap is not constant and this is especially the case when the gap is large. Also, the end effects can be significant since Eqn 2.30 only takes into account the surfaces of the walls of the cylinders and not the ends. These end effects are usually accounted for by calibration of the instrument with a fluid of known viscosity. Frictional heating can be a problem at high shear rates and thus temperature control is essential with such instruments. Filling and cleaning are often difficult when the gap is small but if it is large then the volume of sample required may be prohibitive.

Whether cone–plate or concentric cylinder geometry is used, instruments, particularly the more modern examples, have been modified to make measurements both easier and more accurate. The common modification is to make one

Viscoelasticity

In the experiments described under rotational viscometers two observations are often made with pharmaceutical materials:

1 With cone–plate geometry the sample appears to 'roll-up' and at high shear rates becomes ejected from the gap.

2 With concentric cylinder geometry the sample will climb up the spindle of the rotating inner cylinder (Weissenberg effect).

The reason for both these phenomena is the same in that the liquids are not exhibiting purely viscous behaviour but are viscoelastic. Such materials display solid and liquid properties simultaneously and the factor which governs the actual behaviour is time. A whole spectrum of viscoelastic behaviour exists from materials which are predominantly liquid to those which are predominantly solid. Under a constant stress all of these materials will dissipate some of the energy in viscous flow and store the remainder which will be recovered when the stress is removed. The type of response can be seen in Fig. 2.16(a) where a small, constant stress has been applied to a 2% gelatin gel and the resultant change in shape (strain) is measured. In the region A–B an initial elastic jump is observed followed by a curved region B–C when the material is attempting to flow as a viscous fluid but is being retarded by its solid characteristics. At longer times an equilibrium is established such that for a system like this which is ostensibly liquid, viscous flow will eventually predominate and the curve will become linear (C–D). If the concentration of gelatin in the gel had been increased to 30% then the resultant material would be more solid-like and no flow

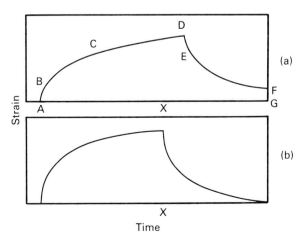

Fig. 2.16 Creep (or compliance) curves for (a) an uncrosslinked system and (b) a crosslinked system

would be observed at longer times and the curve would level out as shown in Fig. 2.16(b). In the case of the liquid system, when the stress is removed then only the stored energy will be recovered and this is exhibited by an initial elastic recoil (D–E, Fig. 2.16(a)) equivalent to the region A–B and a retarded response E–F equivalent to B–C. There will be a displacement from the starting position (F–G) and this will be related to the amount of energy lost in viscous flow. For the higher concentration gel, all the energy will be recovered so that only the regions D–E and E–F are observed.

This significance of time can be observed from the point X on the time axis. Although both systems are viscoelastic and indeed are produced by different concentrations of the same biopolymer in Fig. 2.16(a) the sample is flowing like a high viscosity fluid whereas in Fig. 2.16(b) it is behaving like a solid.

Creep testing

Both the experimental curves shown in Fig. 2.16 are examples of a phenomenon known as creep. If the measured strain is divided by the stress, which it should be remembered is constant, then a compliance will be produced. The resultant curve which will have the same shape as the original strain curve then becomes known as a creep compliance curve and since compliance is the reciprocal of elasticity it will have the units m^2 N^{-1} or Pa^{-1}. If the applied stress is below a certain limit (known as the linear viscoelastic limit) then it will be directly related to the strain and the creep compliance curve will have the same shape and magnitude regardless of the stress used to obtain it. This curve therefore represents a fundamental property of the system and derived parameters are characteristic and independent of the experimental method. For example, although it is common to use either cone–plate or concentric cylinders with viscoelastic pharmaceuticals, almost any measuring geometry can be used provided the shape of the sample can be defined.

It is common to analyse the creep compliance curve in terms of a mechanical model. An example of such a model is shown in Fig. 2.17. This figure also indicates the regions on the curve shown in

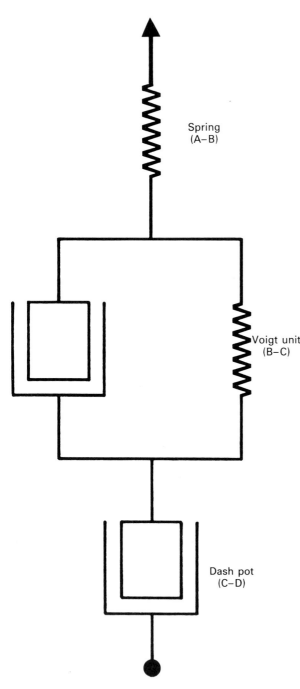

Fig. 2.17 Mechanical model representation of a creep compliance curve

Fig. 2.16(a) to which the components of the model relate. Thus, the instantaneous jump can be described by a perfectly elastic spring and the region of viscous flow by a piston fitted into a

cylinder containing an ideal Newtonian fluid (this arrangement is referred to as a dashpot). In order to describe the behaviour in the intermediate region it is necessary to combine both these elements in parallel such that the movement of the spring is retarded by the piston: this combination is known as a Voigt unit. It is implied that the elements of the model do not move until the preceding one has become fully extended and although it is not feasible to associate the elements of the model with the molecular arrangement of the material it is possible to ascribe viscosities to the fluids in the cylinders and elasticities (or compliances) to the springs. Thus, a viscosity can be calculated for the single dashpot (Fig. 2.17) from the reciprocal of the slope of the linear part of the creep compliance curve. This viscosity will be several orders of magnitude greater than that obtained by the conventional rotational techniques and may be considered to be that of the rheological ground state (η_o) since the creep test is non-destructive and should produce the same viscosity however many times it is repeated on the same sample. This is in direct contrast to continuous shear measurements which destroy the structure being measured and with which it is seldom possible to obtain the same result on subsequent experiments on the same sample. The compliance $(\mathcal{J}_o)$ of the spring can be measured directly from the height of region A–B (Fig. 2.16(a)) and the reciprocal of this value will yield the elasticity, E_o. It is often the case that this value together with η_o provides an adequate characterization of the material. However, the remaining portion of the curve can be used to derive the viscosity and elasticity of the elements of the Voigt unit. The ratio of the viscosity to the elasticity is known as the retardation time, τ, and is a measure of the time for the unit to deform to $1/e$ of its total deformation. Consequently more rigid materials will have longer retardation times and the more complex the material then the greater number of Voigt units that are necessary to describe the creep curve.

It is also possible to use a mathematical expression to describe the creep compliance curve:

$$\mathcal{J}(t) = \mathcal{J}_o - \sum_{i=1}^{n} \mathcal{J}_i \left(1 - e^{t/\tau_i}\right) + t/\eta_o \qquad (2.32)$$

where $\mathcal{J}(t)$ is the compliance at time t, $\mathcal{J}_i$ and τ_i are the compliance and retardation time of the 'ith' Voigt unit. Both the model and the mathematical approach interpret the curve in terms of a line spectrum. It is also possible to produce a continuous spectrum in terms of the distribution of retardation times (see Barry, 1974).

What is essentially the reverse of the creep compliance test is the stress relaxation test where the sample is subjected to a predetermined strain and the stress required to maintain this strain is measured as a function of time. In this instance a spring and dashpot in series (Maxwell unit) can be used to describe the behaviour. Initially the spring will extend and will then contract as the piston flows in the dashpot. Eventually the spring will be completely relaxed but the dashpot will be displaced and in this case the ratio of viscosity to elasticity is referred to as the relaxation time.

Dynamic testing

Both creep and relaxation experiments are considered to be static tests. Viscoelastic materials can also be evaluated by means of dynamic experiments whereby the sample is exposed to a forced sinusoidal oscillation and the transmitted stress measured. Once again, if the linear viscoelastic limit is not exceeded then the stress will also vary sinusoidally (Fig. 2.18). However, because of the nature of the material, energy will be lost so that the amplitude of the stress wave will be less than that of the strain wave: it will also lag behind the strain wave. If the amplitude ratio and the phase

lag can be measured then the elasticity, referred to as the storage modulus, G', is given by

$$G' = \left(\frac{\sigma}{\gamma}\right) \cos \delta \qquad (2.33)$$

where σ is the stress, γ is the strain and δ the phase lag. A further modulus G'', known as the loss modulus is given by

$$G'' = \left(\frac{\sigma}{\gamma}\right) \sin \delta \qquad (2.34)$$

This can be related to viscosity η' by

$$\eta' = \frac{G''}{\omega} \qquad (2.35)$$

where ω is the frequency of oscillation in rad (s^{-1}). From Eqns 2.33 and 2.34 it can be seen that

$$\frac{G''}{G'} = \tan \delta \qquad (2.36)$$

and $\tan \delta$ is known as the loss tangent.

Thus, a phase lag of $0°$ would be produced by a perfectly elastic material whereas a perfect fluid would give a phase lag of $90°$.

Suspensions

The rheological properties of suspensions are markedly affected by the degree of flocculation (see Chapter 6). The reason for this is that the amount of free continuous phase is reduced since it becomes entrapped in the diffuse floccules. Consequently the apparent viscosity of a floccu-

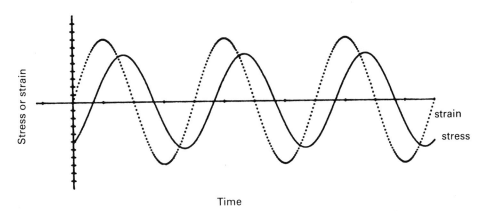

Fig. 2.18 Sine waves showing the stress wave lagging behind the strain wave by $60°$ during dynamic viscosity testing

lated suspension is normally higher than that of a suspension which is in all ways similar with the exception that it is deflocculated. In addition, when a disperse system is highly flocculated then the possibility of interaction between floccules occurs and structured systems result. If the forces bonding floccules together are capable of withstanding weak stresses then a yield value will result and below this value the suspension will behave like a solid. Once the yield value has been exceeded the amount of structural breakdown increases with increased shear stress. Therefore, flocculated suspensions will exhibit plastic or, more usually, pseudoplastic behaviour. Obviously, if the breakdown and reformation of the bonds between floccules is time dependent then thixotropic behaviour will also be observed.

The formation of structures does not occur in deflocculated suspensions so that their rheological behaviour is determined by that of the continuous phase together with the effect of distortion of the flow lines around the particles: in this situation the Einstein equation (Eqn 2.6) may apply. As the suspension becomes more concentrated and the particles come into contact then dilatancy will occur.

Many pharmaceutical products, particularly those for children, are presented as suspensions and their rheological properties are important. In general these properties must be adjusted so that:

1 The product is easily administered (e.g. easily poured from a bottle or forced through a syringe needle).
2 Sedimentation is either prevented or retarded; if it does occur, redispersion is easy.
3 The product has an elegant appearance.

Deflocculated particles in Newtonian vehicles

When such systems sediment then a compact sediment or cake is produced which is difficult to redisperse. The rate of sedimentation can be reduced by increasing the viscosity of the continuous medium which will remain Newtonian. However, there is a limit to which this viscosity can be increased because difficulty will be experienced, for example, in pouring the supension from a bottle. Furthermore, if sedimentation does occur then subsequent redispersion may be even more difficult.

Deflocculated particles in non-Newtonian vehicles

Only pseudoplastic or plastic dispersion media can be used in the formulation of suspensions and both will retard the sedimentation of small particles since their apparent viscosities will be high under the small stresses associated with sedimentation. Also, as the medium will undergo structural breakdown under the higher stresses involved in shaking and pouring both these processes are facilitated.

The hydrocolloids used as suspending agents such as acacia, tragacanth, methyl cellulose, gelatin and sodium carboxymethylcellulose all impart non-Newtonian properties, normally pseudoplasticity, to the suspensions. Thixotropy can occur and this is particularly the case with the mineral clays such as bentonite (which must only be used in suspensions for external use). The three-dimensional gel network traps the deflocculated particles at rest and their sedimentation is retarded and may be completely prevented. The gel network is destroyed during shaking so that administration is facilitated. It is desirable that the gel network is reformed quickly so that dispersion of the particles is maintained.

Flocculated particles in Newtonian vehicles

Such particles will still sediment but since the aggregates are diffuse, a large volume sediment is produced and as such is easier to disperse. These systems are seldom improved by an increase in the viscosity of the continuous phase since this will only influence the rate of sedimentation. The major problem is one of pharmaceutical inelegance in that the sediment does not fill the whole of the fluid volume. Methods of improving such products are given in Chapters 6 and 15.

Flocculated particles in non-Newtonian vehicles

These systems combine the advantages of both methods. Furthermore, variations in the properties of the raw materials to be suspended are unlikely to influence the performance of a product made on production scale. Consequently, less difference will be observed between batches made by the same method and plant.

Emulsions

Because nearly all but the most dilute of medicinal emulsions exhibit non-Newtonian behaviour, their rheological characteristics have a marked effect on their usefulness. The fluid emulsions are usually pseudoplastic and those approaching semisolid nature behave plastically and exhibit marked yield values. The semisolid creams are usually visco-elastic. A considerable variety of pharmaceutical products can be formulated by altering the concentration of the disperse phase and the nature and concentration of the emulsifying agent. The latter can be used to confer viscoelastic properties on a topical cream merely by variation of the ratio of surface-active agent to long chain alcohol. These aspects will be further discussed in Chapters 16 and 22.

THE EFFECT OF RHEOLOGICAL PROPERTIES ON BIOAVAILABILITY

The presence of the diffusion coefficient which is inversely related to viscosity in the constant k of the Noyes–Whitney equation (Chapter 5) means that the rate of dissolution of a drug particle will be decreased as the viscosity of the dissolution medium is increased. This will apply to both *in vitro* and *in vivo* situations and usually the medium into which the drug is dissolving will exhibit Newtonian behaviour. However, in the stomach the presence of the high molecular weight glyco-proteins from mucus in acid solution will only be Newtonian up to a concentration of about 2% beyond which it will exhibit non-Newtonian behaviour. In addition, the use of hydrocolloids will contribute to this effect and it has been shown the administration of a drug like griseofulvin in concentrations of methyl cellulose which will exhibit pseudoplastic behaviour does significantly delay absorption.

Attempts to predict this decrease in absorption have been made by the inclusion of natural or synthetic polymers in the dissolution medium used for *in vitro* studies. Some studies have shown that it is not the bulk viscosity of the dissolution medium which is of importance but the 'effective viscosity'. Also, it is by no means certain that these polymers will behave in the same manner as the macromolecules which will be encountered in the gastrointestinal tract. Furthermore, it is impossible to carry out a dissolution test in an environment which relates to conditions in the region of the gut wall.

This viscosity effect will also operate at other drug delivery sites. For example the absorption of drugs by the skin and from injection sites will be decreased by increase in the viscosity of the vehicle. Indeed, in the case of injections the creation of a depot with a highly viscoelastic nature should result in prolonged delivery of the drug.

A proper understanding of the rheological behaviour which exists both in the formulation and, if possible, at the absorption site is essential in any evaluation of bioavailability.

BIBLIOGRAPHY

Barry, B. W. (1974) *Advances in Pharmaceutical Sciences*, (eds H. S. Bean, A. H. Beckett and J. E. Carless), Vol. 4, Chapter 1, Academic Press, London.

Ferry, J. D. (1980) *Viscoelastic Properties of Polymers*, John Wiley & Sons, New York.

Martin, A. N., Swarbrick, J. and Camarata, A. (1970) *Physical Pharmacy*, 2nd edn, Chapter 18, Lea and Febiger, Philadelphia.

Schott, H. (1985) In: *Remington's Pharmaceutical Sciences*, 17th edn (ed. R. Gennaro), Chapter 22, Mack Publishing Co., Easton, Pennsylvania.

Scott-Blair, G. W. (1969) *Elementary Rheology*, Academic Press, London.

Sherman, P. (1970) *Industrial Rheology*, Academic Press, London.

van Wazer, J. R., Lyons, J. W., Kim, K. Y. and Colwell, R. E. (1963) *Viscosity and Flow Measurement*, Interscience, New York.

Solutions and their properties

The main aim of this chapter and Chapter 5 is to provide information on certain physicochemical principles that relate to the applications and implications of solutions in pharmacy. For the purposes of the present discussion these principles have been classified in a somewhat arbitrary manner. Thus, this chapter deals mainly with the physicochemical properties of solutions that are important with respect to systems and processes described in other parts of this book or in the companion volume, *Dispensing for Pharmaceutical Students* by Carter (1975) (new edition in preparation). Chapter 5 on the other hand is concerned with the principles underlying the formation of solutions and the factors that affect the rate and extent of this dissolution process. Because of limitations of space and the number of principles and properties that need to be considered the contents of each of these chapters should only be regarded as introductions to the various topics. The student is encouraged, therefore, to refer to the bibliography cited at the end of each chapter in order to augment the present contents. The textbook written by Florence and Attwood (1981) is recommended particularly, because of the large number of pharmaceutical examples that are used to aid understanding of physicochemical principles.

DEFINITION OF TERMS

A solution may be defined as a mixture of two or more components that form a single phase, which is homogeneous down to the molecular level. The component that determines the phase of the solution is termed the solvent and usually constitutes the largest proportion of the system. The other components are termed solutes and these are dispersed as molecules or ions throughout the solvent; i.e. they are said to be dissolved in the solvent. The extent to which the dissolution proceeds under a given set of experimental conditions is referred to as the solubility of the solute in the solvent. Thus, the solubility of a substance is the amount of it that passes into solution when an equilibrium is established between the solution and excess, i.e. undissolved, substance. The solution that is obtained under these conditions is said to be saturated. Since the above definitions are general ones they may be applied to all types of solution. However, when the two components forming a solution are either both gases or both liquids then it is more usual to talk in terms of miscibility rather than solubility.

Methods of expressing concentration

Quantity per quantity

Concentrations are often expressed simply as the weight or volume of solute that is contained in a given weight or volume of the solution. The majority of solutions encountered in pharmaceutical practice consist of solids dissolved in liquids. Consequently, concentration is expressed most commonly by the weight of solute contained in a given volume of solution. Although the SI unit is kg m^{-3} the terms that are used in practice are based on more convenient or appropriate weights and volumes. For example, in the case of a solution with a concentration of 1 kg m^{-3} the strength may be denoted by any one of the following concentration terms depending on the circumstances:

$$1 \text{ g l}^{-1}, 0.1 \text{ g per } 100 \text{ ml}, 1 \text{ mg ml}^{-1}, 5 \text{ mg in } 5 \text{ ml}$$
$$\text{or } 1 \text{ } \mu\text{g } \mu\text{l}^{-1}.$$

Percentage

The British and European Pharmacopoeias use the same method as a basis for their percentage expressions of the strengths of solutions. For example, the concentration of a solution of a solid in a liquid would be given by

$$\text{concentration in } \% \text{ w/v} = \frac{\text{weight of solute}}{\text{volume of solution}} \times 100$$

Per cent v/w, % v/v and % w/w expressions are also referred to in the *General Notices* of the *British Pharmacopoeia* (1980) together with the statement that the latter two expressions are used for solutions of liquids in liquids and solutions of gases in liquids, respectively.

It should be realized that if concentration is expressed in terms of weight of solute in a given volume of solution then changes in volume caused by temperature fluctuations will alter the concentration.

Parts

The Pharmacopoeia also expresses some concentrations in terms of the number of 'parts' of solute dissolved in a stated number of 'parts' of solution. Use of this method to describe the strength of a solution of a solid in a liquid infers that a given number of parts by volume (ml) of solution contain a certain number of parts by weight (g) of solid. In the case of solutions of liquids in liquids parts by volume of solute in parts by volume of solution are intended whereas with solutions of gases in liquids parts by weight of gas in parts by weight of solution are inferred.

Molarity

This is the number of moles of solute contained in 1 dm^3 (or, more commonly in pharmacy, 1 litre) of solution. Thus, solutions of equal molarity contain the same number of solute molecules in a given volume of solution. The unit of molarity is mol l^{-1} (equivalent to 10^3 mol m^{-3} if converted to the SI unit). Although use of the term molar concentration and its symbol M to describe the molarity of a solution has been discouraged since the introduction of SI units the symbol M is still used in the current British and European Pharmacopoeias.

Molality

This is the number of moles of solute divided by the mass of the solvent, i.e. its SI unit is mol kg^{-1}. Although it is less likely to be encountered in pharmaceutical practice than the other terms it does offer a more precise description of concentration because it is unaffected by temperature.

Mole fraction

This is often used in theoretical considerations and is defined as the number of moles of solute divided by the total number of moles of solute and solvent, i.e.

$$\text{mole fraction of solute } (x_1) = \frac{n_1}{n_1 + n_2}$$

where n_1 and n_2 are the numbers of moles of solute and solvent, respectively.

Milliequivalents and normal solutions

The concentrations of solutes in body fluids and in solutions used as replacements for these fluids are usually expressed in terms of the number of millimoles (1 millimole = one thousandth of a mole) in a litre of solution. In the case of electrolytes, however, these concentrations may still be expressed in terms of milliequivalents per litre. A milliequivalent (mEq) of an ion is, in fact, one thousandth of the gram equivalent of the ion, which is, in turn, the ionic weight expressed in grams divided by the valency of the ion. Alternatively,

$$1 \text{ mEq} = \frac{\text{ionic weight in mg}}{\text{valency}}$$

A knowledge of the concept of chemical equivalents is also required in order to understand the use of 'normality' as a means of expressing concentration of solutions, because a normal solution, i.e. concentration = 1 N, is one that contains the equivalent weight of the solute, expressed in grams, in 1 litre of solution. It was thought that this term would disappear on the introduction of SI units but it is still encountered in some volumetric assay procedures, e.g. in *British Pharmacopoeias* preceding the 1980 edition and in the current *European Pharmacopoeia*. The student is referred to Beckett and Stenlake (1975) for an explanation of chemical equivalents.

TYPES OF SOLUTION

Solutions may be classified on the basis of the physical states, i.e. gas, solid or liquid, of the solute(s) and solvent. Although a variety of different types can exist, solutions of pharmaceutical interest virtually all possess liquid solvents. In addition, the solutes are predominantly solid substances. Consequently, most of the comments given in this chapter and in Chapter 5 are made with solutions of solids in liquids in mind. However, appropriate comments on other types, e.g. gases in liquids, liquids in liquids and solids in solids are included.

Vapour pressures of solids, liquids and solutions

An understanding of many of the properties of solutions requires an appreciation of the concept of an ideal solution and its use as a reference system, to which the behaviours of real (non-ideal) solutions can be compared. This concept is itself based on a consideration of vapour pressure. The present section is included, therefore, as an introduction to the later discussions on ideal and non-ideal solutions.

The kinetic theory of matter indicates that the thermal motions of molecules of a substance in its gaseous state are more than adequate to overcome the attractive forces that exist between the molecules, so that the molecules undergo a completely random movement within the confines of the container. The situation is reversed, however, when the temperature is lowered sufficiently so that a condensed phase is formed. Thus, the thermal motions of the molecules are now insufficient to overcome completely the intermolecular attractive forces and some degree of order in the relative arrangement of molecules occurs. If the intermolecular forces are so strong that a high degree of order, which is hardly influenced by thermal motions, is brought about then the substance is usually in the solid state.

In the liquid condensed state the relative influences of thermal motion and intermolecular attractive forces are intermediate between those in the gaseous and solid states. Thus, the effects of interactions between the permanent and induced dipoles, i.e. the so-called van der Waals forces of attraction, lead to some degree of coherence between the molecules of liquids. Consequently, liquids occupy a definite volume, unlike gases, and whilst there is evidence of structure within liquids such structure is much less apparent than in solids.

Although solids and liquids are condensed systems with cohering molecules some of the surface molecules in these systems will occasionally acquire sufficient energy to overcome the attractive forces exerted by adjacent molecules and so escape from the surface to form a vaporous phase. If temperature is maintained constant an equilibrium will be established eventually between the vaporous and condensed phases and the pressure exerted by the vapour at equilibrium is referred to as the vapour pressure of the substance.

All condensed systems have the inherent ability to give rise to a vapour pressure. However, the vapour pressures exerted by solids are usually much lower than those exerted by liquids, because the intermolecular forces in solids are stronger than those in liquids so that the escaping tendency for surface molecules is higher in liquids. Consequently, surface loss of vapour from liquids by the process of evaporation is more common than surface loss of vapour from solids via sublimation.

In the case of a liquid solvent containing a dissolved solute then molecules of both solvent and solute may show a tendency to escape from the surface and so contribute to the vapour pressure. The relative tendencies to escape will depend not only on the relative numbers of the different molecules in the surface of the solution but also on the relative strengths of the attractive forces between adjacent solvent molecules on the one hand and between solute and solvent molecules on the other hand. Thus, since the intermolecular forces between solid solutes and liquid solvents tend to be relatively strong such solute molecules do not generally escape from the surface of a solution and contribute to the vapour pressure. In other words the solute is non-volatile and the vapour pressure arises solely from the dynamic equilibrium that is set up between the rates of evaporation and condensation of solvent molecules contained in the solution. In a mixture of miscible liquids, i.e. a liquid in liquid solution, the molecules of both components are likely to evaporate and contribute to the overall vapour pressure exerted by the solution.

Ideal solutions; Raoult's Law

The concept of an ideal solution has been introduced in order to provide a model system that can be used as a standard, to which real or non-ideal solutions can be compared. In the model it is assumed that the strengths of all intermolecular forces are identical, i.e. solvent–solvent, solute–solvent and solute–solute interactions are the same and are equal, in fact, to the strength of the intermolecular interactions in either the pure solvent or pure solute. Because of this equality the relative tendencies of solute and solvent molecules to escape from the surface of the solution will be determined only by their relative numbers in the surface. Since a solution is homogeneous by definition then the relative numbers of these surface molecules will be reflected by the relative numbers in the whole of the solution. The latter can be expressed conveniently by the mole fractions of the components because, for a binary solution, i.e. one with two components, $x_1 + x_2 = 1$, where x_1 and x_2 are the mole fractions of the solute and solvent, respectively. Thus, the total vapour pressure (p) exerted by such a binary solution is given by Eqn 3.1:

$$p = p_1 + p_2 = p_1^o x_1 + p_2^o x_2 \qquad (3.1)$$

where p_1 and p_2 are the partial vapour pressures exerted above the solution by solute and solvent, respectively, and p_1^o and p_2^o are the vapour pressures exerted by pure solute and pure solvent, respectively.

If the total vapour pressure of the solution is described by Eqn 3.1 it follows that Raoult's law is obeyed by the system because this law states that the partial vapour pressure exerted by a volatile component in a solution at a given temperature is equal to the vapour pressure of the pure component at the same temperature, multiplied by its mole fraction in the solution, i.e.

$$p_1 = p_1^o x_1 \qquad (3.2)$$

One of the consequences of the preceding comments is that an ideal solution may be defined as one which obeys Raoult's law. In addition, ideal behaviour should only be expected to be exhibited by real systems comprised of chemically similar components, because it is only in such systems that the condition of equal intermolecular forces between components, that is assumed in the ideal model, is likely to be satisfied. Consequently, Raoult's law is obeyed over an appreciable concentration range by relatively few systems in reality. Mixtures of benzene + toluene, n-hexane + n-heptane and ethyl bromide + ethyl iodide are commonly mentioned systems that exhibit ideal behaviour, whilst a more pharmaceutically interesting example is provided by binary mixtures of fluorinated hydrocarbons. These latter mixtures are used as propellants in therapeutic aerosols and their approximation to ideal behaviour allows Eqn 3.1 to be used to calculate the total pressure exerted by a given mixture.

Real or non-ideal solutions

The majority of real solutions do not exhibit ideal behaviour because solute–solute, solute–solvent and solvent–solvent forces of interaction are unequal. These inequalities alter the effective concentration of each component so that it cannot be represented by a normal expression of concentration, such as the mole fraction term x that is used in Eqns 3.1 and 3.2. Consequently, deviations from Raoult's law are often exhibited by real solutions and the previous equations are not obeyed in such cases. The equations can be modified, however, by substituting each concentration term (x) by a measure of the effective concentration, which is provided by the so-called *activity* (or *thermodynamic activity*), a. Thus, Eqn 3.2 is converted into Eqn 3.3,

$$p_1 = p_1^0 a_1 \qquad (3.3)$$

which is applicable to all systems whether they be ideal or non-ideal. It should be noted that if a solution exhibits ideal behaviour then $a = x$, whereas $a \neq x$ if deviations from such behaviour are apparent. The ratio of activity/concentration is termed the *activity coefficient* (f) and it provides a measure of the deviation from ideality. (The

student is encouraged to study relevant parts of the bibliography for further information on thermodynamic terms such as activity, activity coefficient, free energy and chemical potential.)

If the attractive forces between solute and solvent molecules are weaker than those exerted between the solute molecules themselves or the solvent molecules themselves then the components will have little affinity for each other. The escaping tendency of the surface molecules in such a system is increased when compared with an ideal solution. In other words p_1, p_2 and p are greater than expected from Raoult's law and the thermodynamic activities of the components are greater than their mole fractions, i.e. $a_1 > x_1$ and $a_2 > x_2$. This type of system is said to show a positive deviation from Raoult's law and the extent of the deviation increases as the miscibility of the components decreases. For example, a mixture of alcohol and benzene shows a smaller deviation than the less miscible mixture of water + diethyl ether whilst the virtually immiscible mixture of benzene + water exhibits a very large positive deviation.

Conversely, if the solute and solvent have a strong mutual affinity that results in the formation of a complex or compound then a negative deviation from Raoult's law occurs. Thus, p_1, p_2 and p are lower than expected and $a_1 < x_1$ and $a_2 < x_2$. Examples of systems that show this type of behaviour include chloroform + acetone, pyridine + acetic acid and water + nitric acid.

Even though most systems are non-ideal and deviate either positively or negatively from Raoult's law, such deviations are small when a solution is dilute because the effects of a small amount of solute on interactions between solvent molelcules are minimal. Thus, dilute solutions tend to exhibit ideal behaviour and the activities of their components approximate to their mole fractions, i.e. $a_1 \approx x_1$ and $a_2 \approx x_2$. Conversely, large deviations may be observed when the concentration of a solution is high. Knowledge of the consequences of such marked deviations is particularly important in relation to the distillation of liquid mixtures. For example, the complete separation of the components of a mixture by fractional distillation may not be achievable if large positive or negative deviations from Raoult's law give rise to the formation of so-called azeotropic mixtures with minimum and maximum boiling points, respectively. Such knowledge is obviously important to the pharmaceutical chemist but is beyond the scope of the present chapter.

IONIZATION OF SOLUTES

Many solutes dissociate into ions if the dielectric constant of the solvent is high enough to cause sufficient separation of the attractive forces between the oppositely charged ions. Such solutes are termed electrolytes and their ionization (or dissociation) has several consequences that are often important in pharmaceutical practice. Some of these consequences are indicated below whilst others that relate to solubilities and dissolution rates are referred to in Chapter 5.

Hydrogen ion concentration and pH

The dissociation of water can be represented by Eqn 3.4:

$$H_2O \rightleftharpoons H^+ + OH^- \qquad (3.4)$$

although it should be realized that this is a simplified representation because the hydrogen and hydroxyl ions do not exist in a free state but combine with undissociated water molecules to yield more complex ions such as H_3O^+ and $H_7O_4^-$.

In pure water the concentrations of H^+ and OH^- ions are equal and at 25 °C both have the values of 1×10^{-7} mol l^{-1}. Since the Lowry–Brönsted theory of acids and bases defines an acid as a substance which donates a proton (or hydrogen ion) it follows that the addition of an acidic solute to water will result in a hydrogen ion concentration that exceeds this value. Conversely, the addition of a base, which is defined as a substance that accepts protons, will decrease the concentration of hydrogen ions.

The hydrogen ion concentration range that can be obtained decreases from 1 mol l^{-1} for a strong acid down to 1×10^{-14} mol l^{-1} for a strong base. In order to avoid the frequent use of low values that arise from this range the concept of pH has been introduced as a more convenient measure of hydrogen ion concentration. pH is defined as the negative logarithm of the hydrogen ion concentration $[H^+]$ as shown by Eqn 3.5:

$$pH = -\log_{10}[H^+] \qquad (3.5)$$

so that the pH of a neutral solution like pure water is 7, because the concentration of H^+ ions (and OH^-) ions $= 1 \times 10^{-7}$ mol l^{-1}, and the pHs of acidic and alkaline solutions will be less or greater than 7, respectively.

pH has several important implications in pharmaceutical practice. For example, in addition to its effects on the solubilities of drugs that are weak acids or bases, as indicated in Chapter 5, pH may have a considerable effect on the stabilities of many drugs, be injurious to body tissues and affect the ease of absorption of drugs from the gastrointestinal tract into the blood (see Chapter 9).

Dissociation (or ionization) constants and pK_a

Many drugs may be classified as weak acids or weak bases which means that in solutions of these drugs equilibria exist between undissociated molecules and their ions. Thus, in a solution of a weakly acidic drug HA the equilibrium may be represented by Eqn 3.6:

$$HA \rightleftharpoons H^+ + A^- \qquad (3.6)$$

although the proton H^+ would be better represented by H_3O^+ because it is always strongly solvated by a water molecule. Similarly, the protonation of a weakly basic drug B can be represented by Eqn 3.7:

$$B + H^+ \rightleftharpoons BH^+ \qquad (3.7)$$

Such equilibria are unlikely to occur in solutions of most salts of strong acids or bases in water because these compounds are completely ionized.

The ionization constant (or dissociation constant) K_a of a weak acid can be obtained by applying the Law of Mass Action to Eqn 3.6 to yield Eqn 3.8:

$$K_a = \frac{[H^+][A^-]}{[HA]} \qquad (3.8)$$

Taking logarithms of both sides of Eqn 3.8 yields

$$\log K_a = \log [H^+] + \log [A^-] - \log [HA]$$

and the signs in this equation may be reversed to give Eqn 3.9:

$$-\log K_a = -\log [H^+] - \log [A^-] + \log [HA]$$
$$(3.9)$$

The symbol pK_a is used to represent the negative logarithm of the acid dissociation constant K_a in the same way that pH is used to represent the negative logarithm of the hydrogen ion concentration $[H^+]$ and Eqn 3.9 may therefore be rewritten as Eqn 3.10:

$$pK_a = pH + \log [HA] - \log [A^-] \quad (3.10)$$

or

$$pK_a = pH + \log \frac{[HA]}{[A^-]} \quad (3.11)$$

Thus, a general equation, Eqn 3.12, that is applicable to any acidic drug with one ionizable group may be written, where c_u and c_i represent the concentrations of the unionized and ionized species, respectively. This equation is known as the *Henderson–Hasselbalch equation*.

$$pK_a = pH + \log \frac{c_u}{c_i} \quad (3.12)$$

From Eqn 3.7 it can be seen that the acid dissociation constant (K_a) of a protonated weak base is given by Eqn 3.13:

$$K_a = \frac{[H^+][B]}{[BH^+]} \quad (3.13)$$

Taking negative logarithms yields Eqn 3.14:

$$-\log K_a = -\log [H^+] - \log [B] + \log [BH^+]$$
$$(3.14)$$

or

$$pK_a = pH + \log \frac{[BH^+]}{[B]}$$

The Henderson–Hasselbalch equation for any weak base with one ionizable group may therefore be written as shown by Eqn 3.15:

$$pK_a = pH + \log \frac{c_i}{c_u} \quad (3.15)$$

where c_i and c_u refer to the concentrations of the protonated and unionized species, respectively.

Various analytical techniques, e.g. spectrophotometric and potentiometric methods, may be used to determine ionization constants but the temperature at which the determination is performed should be specified because the values of the constants vary with temperature.

Ionization constants are usually expressed in terms of pK_a values for both acidic and basic drugs and a list of pK_a values for a series of important drugs is given in the *Pharmaceutical Handbook* (1980).

The degree of ionization of a drug in a solution can be calculated from the Henderson–Hasselbalch equations for weak acids and bases (Eqns 3.12 and 3.15, respectively) if the pK_a value of the drug and the pH of the solution are known. Such calculations are particularly useful in determining the degree of ionization of drugs in various parts of the gastrointestinal tract and in the plasma (see Chapter 9). The following examples are therefore related to this type of situation.

1 The pK_a value of aspirin, which is a weak acid, is about 3.5, and if the pH of the gastric contents is 2.0 then from Eqn 3.12

$$\log \frac{c_u}{c_i} = pK_a - pH = 3.5 - 2.0 = 1.5$$

so that the ratio of the concentration of unionized acetylsalicyclic acid to acetylsalicylate anion is given by

$$c_u:c_i = \text{antilog } 1.5 = 31.62:1$$

2 The pH of plasma is 7.4 so that the ratio of unionized:ionized aspirin in this medium is given by

$$\log \frac{c_u}{c_i} = pK_a - pH = 3.5 - 7.4 = -3.9$$

and

$$c_u:c_i = \text{antilog } -3.9 = \text{antilog } \overline{4}.1$$
$$= 1.259 \times 10^{-4}:1$$

3 The pK_a of the weakly acidic drug sulphapyridine is about 8.0 and if the pH of the intestinal contents is 5.0 then the ratio of unionized:ionized drug is given by

$$\log \frac{c_u}{c_i} = pK_a - pH = 8.0 - 5.0 = 3.0$$

and

$$c_u:c_i = \text{antilog } 3.0 = 10^3:1$$

4 The pK_a of the basic drug amidopyrine is 5.0, and in the stomach the ratio of ionized:unionized drug is shown from Eqn 3.15 to be given by

$$\log\frac{c_i}{c_u} = pK_a - pH = 5.0 - 2.0 = 3.0$$

and

$$c_i:c_u = \text{antilog } 3.0 = 10^3:1$$

while in the intestine the ratio is given by

$$\log\frac{c_i}{c_u} = 5.0 - 5.0 = 0$$

and

$$c_i:c_u = \text{antilog } 0 = 1:1$$

Buffer solutions and buffer capacity

These solutions will maintain a constant pH even when small amounts of acid or alkali are added to the solution. They usually contain mixtures of a weak acid and its salt (i.e. its conjugate base) although mixtures of weak bases and their salts (i.e. their conjugate acids) may be used but suffer from the disadvantage that arises from the volatility of many of the bases.

The action of a buffer solution can be appreciated by considering a simple system such as a solution of acetic acid and sodium acetate in water. The acetic acid, being a weak acid, will be confined virtually to its undissociated form because its ionization will be suppressed by the presence of common acetate ions produced by complete dissociation of the sodium salt. The pH of this solution can be described by Eqn 3.16, which is a rearranged form of Eqn 3.12:

$$pH = pK_a + \log\frac{c_i}{c_u} \qquad (3.16)$$

It can be seen from Eqn 3.16 that the pH will remain constant as long as the logarithm of the ratio c_i/c_u does not change. When a small amount of acid is added to the solution it will convert some of the salt into acetic acid but if the concentrations of both acetate ion and acetic acid are reasonably large then the effect of the change will be negligible and the pH will remain constant. Similarly, the addition of a small amount of base will convert some of the acetic acid into its salt

form but the pH will be unaltered if the overall changes in concentrations of the two species are relatively small.

If large amounts of acid or base are added to a buffer then changes in the log c_i/c_u term become appreciable and the pH alters. The ability of a buffer to withstand the effects of acids and bases is an important property from a practical point of view. This ability is expressed in terms of a buffer capacity (β), which is equal to the amount of strong acid or strong base, expressed as moles of H^+ or OH^- ion, required to change the pH of 1 litre of the buffer by 1 pH unit. From the remarks in the previous paragraph it should be obvious that buffer capacity increases as the concentrations of the buffer components increase. In addition, the capacity is also affected by the ratio of the concentrations of weak acid and its salt, maximum capacity (β_{max}) being obtained when the ratio = 1. In such circumstances pH = pK_a of the acid and $\beta_{max} = 0.576$ (total buffer concentration).

The components of various buffer systems and the concentrations required to produce different pHs are listed in several reference books, such as the *British Pharmacopoeia* (1980), the *Pharmaceutical Handbook* (1980), the *Merck Index* (1983) and *Documenta Geigy* (1962). When selecting a suitable buffer the pK_a value of the acid should be close to the required pH and the compatibility of its components with other ingredients in the system should be considered. The toxicity of buffer components must be taken into account if the solution is to be used for medicinal purposes.

Various methods, e.g. pH meters and indicators, may be used to determine the pH of a given solution. These methods are discussed by Carter (1975) in relation to the adjustment of pH of pharmaceutical solutions for injection together with the reasons for such adjustment (see also Chapter 21).

COLLIGATIVE PROPERTIES

When a non-volatile solute is dissolved in a solvent certain properties of the resultant solution are largely independent of the nature of the solute and are determined by the concentration of solute particles. These properties are known as colligative properties. In the case of a non-electrolyte the solute particles will be molecules but if the solute is an electrolyte then its degree of dissociation will determine whether the particles will be ions only or a mixture of ions and undissociated molecules.

Osmotic pressure

The most important colligative property from a pharmaceutical point of view is referred to as osmotic pressure. However, since all colligative properties are related to each other by virtue of their common dependency on the solute concentration then the remaining colligative properties, which are lowering of vapour pressure of the solvent, elevation of its boiling point and depression of its freezing point, are of pharmaceutical interest because they offer alternative means to osmotic pressure determinations as methods of comparing the colligative properties of different solutions.

The osmotic pressure of a solution is the external pressure that must be applied to the solution in order to prevent it being diluted by the entry of solvent via a process that is known as osmosis. This process refers to the spontaneous diffusion of solvent from a solution of low concentration (or pure solvent) into a more concentrated one through a semipermeable membrane, which separates the two solutions and which is permeable only to solvent molecules.

Since the process occurs spontaneously at constant temperature and pressure the laws of thermodynamics indicate that it will be accompanied by a decrease in the so-called free energy (G) of the system. This free energy may be regarded as the energy available in the system for the performance of useful work and when an equilibrium position is attained then there is no difference between the states that are in equilibrium. The free energy of a solution will depend on the number of moles of solute and solvent and is termed an extensive property of the system as opposed to an intensive property such as temperature, which is independent of the amount of a substance. The rate of increase in free energy of a solution caused by an increase in the number of moles of one component is termed the partial molar free energy ($\bar{G}$) or chemical potential (μ) of

that component. For example, the chemical potential of the solvent in a binary solution is given by Eqn 3.17:

$$\left(\frac{\partial G}{\partial n_2}\right)_{T,P,n_1} = \bar{G}_2 = \mu_2 \qquad (3.17)$$

where the subscripts outside the bracket on the left hand side indicate that temperature, pressure and amount of component 1 (the solute in this case) remain constant.

Because only solvent can pass across the semipermeable membrane the driving force for osmosis arises from the inequality of the chemical potentials of the solvent on opposing sides of the membrane. Thus the direction of osmotic flow is from the dilute solution (or pure solvent), where the chemical potential of the solvent is highest because there are more moles of it, into the concentrated solution, where the number of moles and, consequently, the chemical potential of the solvent is reduced by the presence of more solute.

The chemical potential of the solvent in the more concentrated solution can be increased by forcing its molecules closer together under the influence of an externally applied pressure. Osmosis can be prevented, therefore, by such means, hence the definition of osmotic pressure.

The relationship between osmotic pressure (π) and concentration of a non-electrolyte is given for dilute solutions, which may be assumed to exhibit ideal behaviour, by the van't Hoff equation (Eqn 3.18):

$$\pi V = n_2 RT \qquad (3.18)$$

where V is the volume of solution, n_2 is the number of moles of solute, T is the thermodynamic temperature and R is the gas constant. This equation, which is similar to the ideal gas equation, was derived empirically but it does correspond to a theoretically derived equation if approximations based on low solute concentrations are taken into account.

If the solute is an electrolyte Eqn 3.18 must be modified in order to allow for the effect of ionic dissociation, because this will increase the number of particles in the solution. This modification is achieved by insertion of the van't Hoff correction factor (i) to give

$$\pi V = in_2 RT \qquad (3.19)$$

where $i = \dfrac{\text{observed colligative property}}{\text{colligative property expected if dissociation did not occur}}$

Osmolality and osmolarity

The amount of osmotically active particles in a solution is sometimes expressed in terms of osmoles or milliosmoles (1 osmol = 1×10^3 mosmol) and these particles may be either molecules or ions. The concentration of a solution may therefore be expressed in terms of its osmolality or its osmolarity, where osmolality is the number of osmoles per kilogram of water and osmolarity is the number of osmoles per litre of solution.

Iso-osmotic solutions

If two solutions are separated by a perfect semipermeable membrane, i.e. a membrane which is permeable only to solvent molecules, and no net movement of solvent occurs across the membrane then the solutions are said to be iso-osmotic and will have equal osmotic pressures.

Isotonic solutions

Biological membranes do not always function as perfect semipermeable membranes and some solute molecules as well as water are able to pass through them. However, if two iso-osmotic solutions remain in osmotic equilibrium when separated by a biological membrane they may be described as being isotonic with respect to that particular membrane.

The consequences of deviation from isotonicity (i.e. hypo- and hypertonicity) with serum in relation to the formulation of solutions for intravenous administration are described in Chapter 21. Reasons for adjusting the tonicity of formulations intended for other parenteral routes of administration are given in the same chapter.

DIFFUSION IN SOLUTION

By definition the components of a solution form a single phase, which is homogeneous. This homogeneity arises from the process of diffusion, which occurs spontaneously and is consequently accompanied by a decrease in the free energy (G) of the system. Diffusion may be defined as the spontaneous transference of a component from a region in the system where it has a high chemical potential into a region where its chemical potential is lower. Although such a gradient in chemical potential provides the driving force for diffusion the laws that describe this phenomenon are usually expressed in terms of concentration gradients. For example, Fick's first law, which indicates that the rate of diffusion is proportional to the concentration gradient, may be expressed by Eqn 3.20:

$$\mathscr{J} = \frac{\mathrm{d}m}{\mathrm{d}t} = -\mathrm{D}\frac{\mathrm{d}C}{\mathrm{d}x} \qquad (3.20)$$

where $\mathscr{J}$, the flux of a component, is given by the rate of diffusion of the component expressed in terms of amount ($\mathrm{d}m$) transported in time ($\mathrm{d}t$) across a plane of unit area and $\mathrm{d}C/\mathrm{d}x$ is the concentration gradient. The negative sign on the right hand side is necessary because diffusion occurs in the opposite direction to that of increasing concentration, i.e. $\mathrm{d}C/\mathrm{d}x$ is negative. D is known as the *diffusion coefficient* and is assumed to have a constant value for a particular system at a given temperature. This assumption is only strictly true at infinite dilution and D may therefore exhibit some concentration dependency. The dimensions of D are area per unit time, e.g. $cm^2\ s^{-1}$. In a given solvent the value of D decreases as the size of the diffusing solute molecule increases. In water, for example, D is of the order of $2 \times 10^{-5}\ cm^2\ s^{-1}$ for solutes with molecular weights of approximately 50 and it decreases to about $1 \times 10^{-6}\ cm^2\ s^{-1}$ when the molecular weight increases to a few thousand.

The most common explanation of the mechanism of diffusion in solution is based on the lattice theory of the structure of liquids. (It should be noted that other approaches to liquid structures have been considered, see, for example, Eyring *et al.* (1971) and Barker and Henderson (1972).) Various lattice theories have been proposed (Barker, 1963) the one receiving most attention being the significant structure theory of Eyring and his collaborators (e.g. Eyring and Jhon, 1969).

Lattice theories postulate that liquids have crystalline or quasicrystalline structures. The concept of a crystal type of lattice is only intended to provide a convenient starting point and should not be interpreted as a suggestion that liquids possess rigid structures. The theories also postulate that a reasonable proportion of the volume occupied by the liquid is, at any moment, empty, i.e. there are 'holes' in the liquid lattice network, which constitute the so-called free volume of the liquid. Such a hole is produced when the kinetic energy (the pressure), which tends to make a region expand, is balanced by the opposing potential energy density (the internal pressure), which tends to bring about collapse of the hole.

Diffusion can therefore be regarded as the process by which solute molecules move from hole to hole within a liquid lattice. In order to achieve such movement a solute molecule must acquire sufficient kinetic energy at the right time so that it can break away from any bonds that tend to anchor it in one hole and then jump into an adjacent hole. If the average distance of each jump is δ cm and the frequency with which the jumps occur is ϕ s^{-1} then the diffusion coefficient (D) is given by

$$D = \frac{\delta^2 \phi}{6} \ \text{cm}^2 \ \text{s}^{-1} \qquad (3.21)$$

The value of δ for a given solute is unlikely to alter very much from one liquid to another. Differences in the diffusion coefficient of a substance in solution in various solvents arise mainly from changes in jump frequency (ϕ), which is determined, in turn, by the free volume or looseness of packing in the solvent.

When the size of the solute molecules is not appreciably larger than that of the solvent molecules then Stein (1962) has shown that the diffusion coefficient of the former is related to its molecular weight (M) by the relationship

$$DM^{\frac{1}{2}} = \text{constant} \qquad (3.22)$$

When the solute is much greater in size than the solvent, diffusion arises largely from transport of solvent molecules in the opposite direction and the relationship becomes

$$DM^{\frac{1}{3}} = \text{constant} \qquad (3.23)$$

This latter equation agrees with the Stokes–Einstein equation (3.24) for the diffusion of spherical particles that are larger than surrounding liquid molecules, since the mass (m) of a spherical particle is proportional to the cube of its radius (r), i.e. $r \propto m^{\frac{1}{3}}$ and it follows from Eqn 3.23 that $Dm^{\frac{1}{3}}$ and consequently Dr are constants for such a system. The Stokes–Einstein equation is usually written in the form

$$D = \frac{kT}{6\pi r \eta} \qquad (3.24)$$

where k is the Boltzmann constant, T is the thermodynamic temperature and η is the viscosity of the liquid. The appearance of a viscosity term in this type of equation is not unexpected because the reciprocal of viscosity, which is known as the fluidity of a liquid, is proportional to the free volume in a liquid. Thus, jump frequency (ϕ) and diffusion coefficient (D) will increase as the viscosity of a liquid decreases or as the number of holes in its structure increases.

The experimental determination of diffusion coefficients of solutes in liquid solvents is not easy because the effects of other factors that may influence the movement of solute in the system, e.g. temperature and density gradients, mechanical agitation and vibration, must be eliminated. Students are recommended to consult the bibliography for descriptions of experimental techniques.

REFERENCES AND BIBLIOGRAPHY

Barker, J. A. (1963) Lattice Theories of the Liquid State, Pergamon Press, Oxford.
Barker, J. A. and Henderson, D. (1972) Ann. Rev. phys. Chem., 23, 439.
Beckett, A. H. and Stenlake, J. B. (1975) Practical Pharmaceutical Chemistry Part 1: General Pharmaceutical Chemistry, 3rd Edn, Athlone Press, London.

British Pharmacopoeia (1980) HMSO, London.
Carstensen, J. T. (1972) Theory of Pharmaceutical Systems, Vol. 1. General Principles, Academic Press, London.
Carter, S. J. (ed.) (1975) Dispensing for Pharmaceutical Students, 12th edn. Pitman, London.
Documenta Geigy (1962) 6th edn (Ed. K. Diem). Geigy Pharmaceutical Company, Manchester.

Eyring, H., Henderson, D. and Jost, W. (1971) *Physical Chemistry, An Advanced Treatise*, Volume VIIIA, *Liquid State*, Academic Press, London.

Eyring, H. and Jhon, M. S. (1969) *Significant Liquid Structure*, Wiley, New York.

Florence, A. T. and Attwood, D. (1981) *Physicochemical Principles of Pharmacy*, Macmillan Press Ltd, London.

Hildebrand, J. H., Prausnitz, J. M. and Scott, R. L. (1970) *Regular and Related Solutions: the Solubility of Gasses, Liquids and Solids*, Van Nostrand Reinhold, New York.

Merck Index (1983) 10th edn (Ed. M. Windholz), Merck.

Pharmaceutical Handbook (1980) 19th edn (Ed. A. Wade), The Pharmaceutical Press, London.

Price, N. C. and Dwek, R. A. (1979) *Principles and Problems in Physical Chemistry for Biochemists*, 2nd edn, Clarendon Press, Oxford.

Rowlinson, J. S. and Swinton, F. L. (1982) *Liquids and Liquid Mixtures*, 3rd edn, Butterworth Scientific, London.

Stein, W. D. (1962) In: *Comprehensive Biochemistry* (Ed. M. Florkin and E. Stotz), Vol. 2, Chapter III, Elsevier, Amsterdam.

Wallwork, S. C. and Grant, D. J. W. (1977) *Physical Chemistry for Students of Pharmacy and Biology*, 3rd edn, Longman, London.

Williams, V. R., Mattice, W. L. and Williams, H. B. (1978) *Basic Physical Chemistry for the Life Sciences*, 3rd edn, W.H. Freeman and Co., San Francisco.

Surface and interfacial phenomena

The boundary between two phases is generally described as an interface. When one of the phases is a gas or a vapour, the term surface is frequently applied. Matter at interfaces usually has different characteristics from that in the bulk of the media and as a consequence the study of interfaces has developed into a separate branch of chemistry — surface chemistry. In pharmacy, interfacial phenomena play an important role in the processing of a wide variety of formulations. The subsequent behaviour of these formulations *in vivo* is often governed by an interfacial process.

Interfaces are categorized according to the phases they separate as follows: liquid/liquid (L/L), liquid/vapour (L/V), solid/vapour (S/V) and solid/liquid (S/L). It is convenient to treat each interface separately.

SURFACE TENSION AND SURFACE FREE ENERGY

A drop of a single component liquid in equilibrium with its vapour takes the form of a sphere, so minimizing the surface to volume ratio. This implies that work must be carried out on the drop to increase the surface area and, since systems tend to a state of minimum free energy, the molecules at the surface must possess a higher free energy than those in the bulk. This can be explained by considering the attractive forces existing between molecules. In the bulk of a medium, each molecule will be surrounded by an equal number of nearest neighbours and hence will be subject to equal attraction in all directions. At an interface, however, the molecules have fewer nearest neighbours and hence are subjected

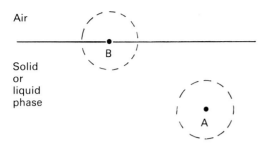

Air

Solid
or
liquid
phase

Fig. 4.1 Attractive forces at the surface and in the bulk of a material

to a net inward force of attraction normal to the surface (see Fig. 4.1).

Consequently, the formation of a liquid surface involves a free energy change, the surface free energy, which is defined as the work required to increase the surface area by 1 m². Typical units are mJ m⁻². The net inward attraction described above means that a surface is in a state of lateral tension, a concept known as surface tension. This is defined as the force acting parallel to the surface and at right angles to a line of 1 m length anywhere in the surface. Its units are typically mN m⁻¹. Surface free energy and surface tension are dimensionally equivalent, since $J = N \cdot m$ and are numerically equal. Interfacial phenomena in liquids are usually considered in terms of surface tension.

The above concepts were derived from a consideration of a liquid/vapour system. Identical arguments can be used for liquid/liquid systems, the terminology being changed to interfacial free energy and interfacial tension. In principle, the above argument also applies to solids, although it is easier to visualize the existence of the surface free energy of solids in terms of the unbalanced forces projecting from the interface, rather than the net inward attraction exerted on the molecules residing at the interface.

In this chapter, the symbol γ will be used to denote surface or interfacial tension. When it is necessary to distinguish between different surface or interfacial tensions, subscripts will be used. For example $\gamma_{L/L}$ is the interfacial tension between two liquids and $\gamma_{L/V}$ is the surface tension between a liquid and its vapour. For more specific cases, γ_A will represent the surface tension of a liquid A and $\gamma_{A/B}$ the interfacial tension between liquids A and B.

Liquid/vapour systems

Curved surfaces

A pressure drop exists across curved surfaces to balance the influence of surface tension. A knowledge of this is important in some methods of the measurement of surface tension.

Consider a bubble of vapour in a liquid. In the absence of any external forces the bubble will be spherical in shape and will remain the same size because the surface tension forces are balanced by an internal excess pressure. This excess pressure is given by

$$\Delta p = \frac{2\gamma}{r} \qquad (4.1)$$

where Δp is the excess pressure and r is the radius of the bubble. For non-spherical surfaces which can be described by two radii of curvature the equation becomes

$$\Delta p = \gamma \left(\frac{1}{r_1} + \frac{1}{r_2} \right) \qquad (4.2)$$

This is known as the Laplace equation. γ is always positive. For Δp to be positive, r must be positive which means that the pressure is always greater on the concave side.

These equations (4.1 and 4.2) apply to any curved liquid interface, e.g. the system described above, a liquid film around a bubble in air or the meniscus of a bulk liquid.

Influence of temperature

For the majority of liquids, an increase in temperature leads to a decrease in surface tension. The exceptions are some molten metals. The decrease in surface tension with temperature is approximately linear. As the temperature approaches the critical temperature for a liquid (i.e. the temperature when the liquid structure is lost), the intermolecular cohesion forces approach zero and the surface tension becomes very small.

Liquid/liquid systems

The interfacial tension between two immiscible liquids arises due to an imbalance of forces in an identical manner to the surface tension between

Table 4.1 The surface tensions of some common liquids and their interfacial tensions against water (mN m^{-1}), 20 °C

Liquid	Surface tension	Interfacial tension against water
Water	72	—
n-Octanol	27	8.5
Carbon tetrachloride	27	45
Chloroform	27	33
Olive oil	36	33
n-Hexane	18	51

a liquid and its vapour. Interfacial tensions generally lie between the surface tensions of the two liquids under consideration. Table 4.1 lists the surface tensions of several liquids and their interfacial tensions against water.

Spreading

If a small quantity of an immiscible liquid is placed on a clean surface of a second liquid, it may spread to cover the surface with a film or remain as a drop or lens (see Fig. 4.2). Which of the two applies depends on the achievement of a state of minimum free energy. The ability of one liquid to spread over another can be assessed in terms of the spreading coefficient (S):

$$S = \gamma_A - (\gamma_B + \gamma_{A/B}) \qquad (4.3)$$

A positive or zero value of S is required for spreading to occur.

An alternative approach is to examine spreading in terms of the work of cohesion and adhesion. The work of cohesion is for a single liquid and is the work required to pull apart a column of liquid of unit cross-sectional area and create two liquid/air interfaces.

$$W_{A/A} = 2\gamma_A \qquad (4.4)$$

The work of adhesion is the work required to separate unit cross-sectional area of a liquid/liquid interface to form two different liquid/air interfaces, and is given by the Dupré equation:

$$W_{A/B} = \gamma_A + \gamma_B - \gamma_{A/B} \qquad (4.5)$$

Hence, by substitution:

$$S = W_{A/B} - W_{A/A} \qquad (4.6)$$

Therefore, spreading occurs when the liquid placed on the water surface adheres to the water more strongly than it coheres to itself.

In practice, when two immiscible liquids are placed in contact, the bulk liquids eventually will become mutually saturated. This will change the values of the various surface and interfacial tensions. Hence, there is an initial spreading coefficient which is an immediate value, and a final spreading coefficient after mutual saturation has taken place. For benzene or hexanol on water, the initial spreading coefficients are positive. When mutual saturation has occurred, the values of the surface and interfacial tensions are reduced so that the final spreading coefficients are negative. Hence benzene or hexanol spread immediately on water, and then the spreading stops, leaving a monomolecular layer of benzene or hexanol with the remainder to the liquid in the form of flat lenses.

Measurement of surface and interfacial tension

There are several methods available for the measurement of surface and interfacial tension. Four will be described here. Further details and descriptions of other methods can be obtained by consulting the articles, etc. listed in the Bibliography.

Wilhelmy plate methods The apparatus consists of a thin mica, glass or platinum plate attached to a suitable balance (Fig. 4.3). When used as a detachment method, the plate is immersed in the liquid, and the liquid container is gradually lowered. The reading on the balance immediately prior to detachment is noted. The detachment force is equal to the surface tension multiplied by the perimeter of the surface detached.

$$W_L - W = 2 (L + T)\gamma \qquad (4.7)$$

Where W_L is the reading on the balance prior to

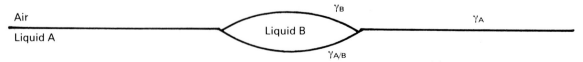

Fig. 4.2 Spreading of one liquid on another

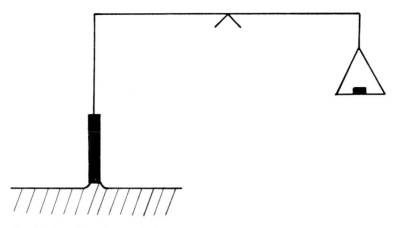

Fig. 4.3 Wilhelmy plate method

detachment, W is the weight of the plate in air, L and T are the length and the thickness of the plate, respectively. Immersion of the plate into the lower of two liquids in a container and subsequent detachment will give the interfacial tension.

Alternatively, the plate can be used in a static mode where the change in force required to keep the plate at a constant depth is measured. This is useful for measuring changes in surface tension with time.

The method requires the contact angle that the liquid makes with the plate to be zero. This can be achieved by scrupulous cleaning and by roughening the surface of the plate. In addition, it must be ensured that the edge of the plate lies in a horizontal plane.

Ring method (du Nuoy tensiometer) The method measures the force to detach a platinum ring from a surface or an interface. Figure 4.4 shows the set up for an interface. Again, the detachment force is equal to the surface tension multiplied by the perimeter of liquid detached, hence

$$F = 2\pi (R_1 + R_2)\gamma \qquad (4.8)$$

where F is the detachment force and R_1 and R_2 are the inner and outer radii of the ring.

Again a zero contact angle of the liquid on the ring must be assured or the equation will not hold. This can be achieved by careful cleaning and flaming of the platinum loop, or by the use of a silicone treated ring for oils. The ring must also lie horizontally in the surface.

As the shape of the liquid supported by the ring

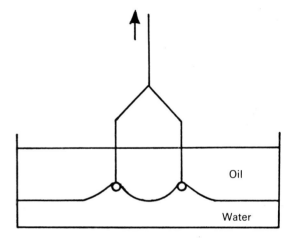

Fig. 4.4 du Nuoy tensiometer being used to measure interfacial tension

during detachment is complex and hence the surface tension forces do not act vertically, the above simple equation is in error and correction factors must be applied for accurate determinations.

Drop weight and drop volume methods If the volume or weight of a drop as it is detached from a tip of known radius is determined, the surface or interfacial tension can be calculated from

$$\gamma = \frac{\phi \, mg}{2\pi r} = \frac{\phi \, V\rho g}{2\pi r} \qquad (4.9)$$

where m is the mass of the drop, V is the volume of the drop, ρ is the density of the liquid, r is the radius of the tip, g is the acceleration due to gravity and ϕ is a correction factor. A typical apparatus is shown in Fig. 4.5. The method is

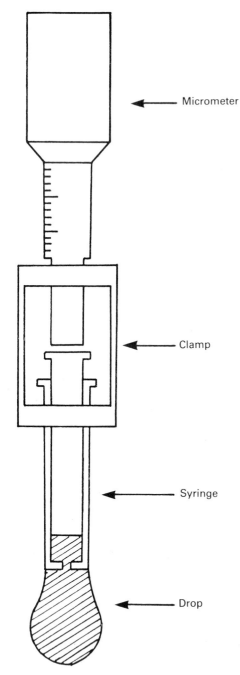

Fig. 4.5 Drop volume or weight method

easily adapted for both surface and interfacial tensions and is therefore popular. The correction factor is required as not all the drop leaves the tip on detachment. The correction factors are shown in Fig. 4.6 and depend on the radius of the tip

and the drop volume. It is important that the tip is completely wetted by the liquid, and that the drop does not 'climb' up the outside of the tube. The drop should also be formed slowly, especially in the stage immediately preceding detachment.

Capillary rise method   Although this method is used little in pharmaceutical research, it is considered to be the most accurate way of measuring surface tension and has been used to establish values for many liquids. As the surface of the liquid is undisturbed during the measurement, time effects can be followed.

If a capillary tube is placed in a liquid, providing the angle of contact that the liquid makes with the capillary tube is less than 90°, the liquid will rise in the tube to a certain height. Figure 4.7 shows a diagrammatic representation of this. If the tube is small in diameter, the meniscus can be considered to be hemispherical and the radius of curvature will be

$$r_t = r_m \cos \theta \qquad (4.10)$$

where r_t is the radius of the capillary tube, r_m is the radius of curvature of the meniscus and θ is the contact angle. Hence, from the Laplace equation (Eqn 4.2) for this system

$$\Delta p = \frac{2\gamma \cos \theta}{r_t} \qquad (4.11)$$

which is the pressure difference between atmospheric and that immediately below the meniscus. Referring to Fig. 4.7, the pressure at point B is atmospheric, whereas that at point A is less by an amount given in Eqn 4.11. At point C the pressure is atmospheric and as the liquid here is effectively flat, i.e. the radius of curvature of the meniscus is large, the pressure at point D is also atmospheric. The pressure difference between D and A causes the liquid to rise in the capillary tube until the pressure difference is balanced by the hydrostatic pressure of the column of liquid. At this equilibrium point:

$$\frac{2\gamma \cos \theta}{r_t} = h (\rho_L - \rho_V)g \qquad (4.12)$$

where θ is the contact angle of the liquid on the capillary tube, $\rho_L - \rho_V$ is the density difference between the liquid and its vapour, g is the accel-

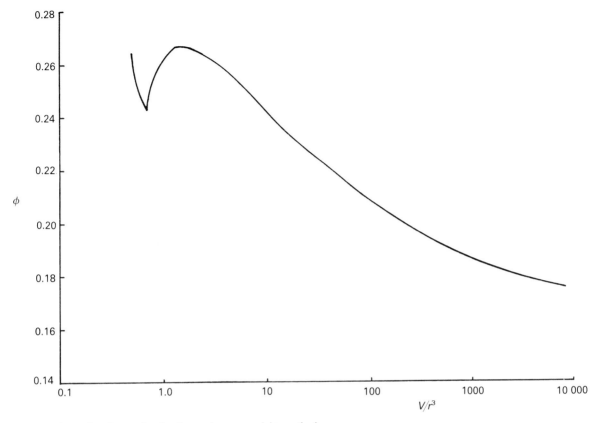

Fig. 4.6 Correction factors for the drop volume or weight method

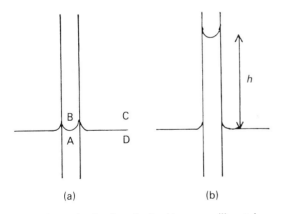

Fig. 4.7 Stages in the rise of a liquid up a capillary tube

eration due to gravity and h is the height of the liquid in the capillary tube.

As contact angles are difficult to reproduce, experiments are always run at $\theta = 0$, ($\cos \theta = 1$), achieved by careful cleaning. Hence the equation reduces to

$$\gamma = \frac{r_t\, h\, (\rho_L - \rho_V)g}{2} \qquad (4.13)$$

The capillaries used must be of circular cross-section and of uniform bore. As in all methods of measuring surface and interfacial tension, cleanliness at all stages of the experiment is vital and adequate temperature control must be ensured.

Solid/vapour and solid/liquid systems

Liquid surfaces and interfaces are open to direct, simple experimental procedures for determining surface and interfacial tensions. Methods for determining similar parameters for solids are indirect and difficult. The system of most interest pharmaceutically is the behaviour of a liquid in contact with a solid.

Contact angle

If a drop of liquid is placed on a flat, smooth horizontal surface it may spread completely, but

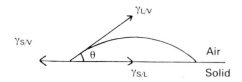

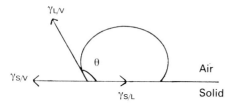

Fig. 4.8 The shapes of liquid drops in contact with solids

it is more likely to form a drop. This drop will exhibit a definite angle against the solid, known as the contact angle (Fig. 4.8). By equating the horizontal components of the various surface tensions, the following equation is derived (Young's equation):

$$\gamma_{S/V} = \gamma_{S/L} + \gamma_{L/V} \cos \theta \qquad (4.14)$$

The work of adhesion between the solid and the liquid is given by the appropriate form of the Dupré equation (Eqn 4.5):

$$W_{S/L} = \gamma_{S/V} + \gamma_{L/V} - \gamma_{S/L} \qquad (4.15)$$

Combining this with the equation above (Eqn 4.14) gives the following:

$$W_{S/L} = \gamma_{L/V} (1 + \cos \theta) \qquad (4.16)$$

which means that the work of adhesion between the solid and the liquid can be determined in terms of easily measurable quantities.

In a similar manner to two liquids, a spreading coefficient (S) for a liquid on a solid may be defined as

$$S = \gamma_{L/V} (\cos \theta - 1) \qquad (4.17)$$

which will give a measure of how well a liquid will spread on a solid. If a liquid is penetrating into a capillary in a solid, the value of interest is the adhesion tension (AT), given by

$$AT = \gamma_{L/V} \cos \theta \qquad (4.18)$$

As $\gamma_{L/V}$ is always positive, the spontaneity of the process will be controlled by $\cos \theta$. For example,

for penetration into capillaries under no extra applied pressure the adhesion tension must be positive, hence, $\cos \theta$ must be positive, i.e. θ must be below 90°.

The contact angle, θ, can be determined for materials of pharmaceutical interest. Examples illustrating the range of values obtained are shown in Table 4.2.

Table 4.2 The contact angles of some pharmaceutical solids against their saturated aqueous solutions

Material	Contact angle (degrees)
Acetylsalicylic acid	74
Amylobarbitone	102
Diazepam	83
Lactose	30
Magnesium stearate	121
Paracetamol	59
Phenacetin	78
Phenobarbitone	86
Phenylbutazone	109
Sulphanilamide	64

Values taken from Lerk *et al.*, 1976, 1977.

Pharmaceutical applications

Many pharmaceutical processes involve an interaction between a liquid and a solid. Granulation, prior to tableting, involves the mixing of a powder with a liquid binder and the success of the process will, in part, depend on the spreading of the liquid over the solid. Similarly, film coating requires the spread of liquid over a tablet surface. The successful dissolution of a tablet or capsule necessitates penetration of liquid into the pores of the dosage form. In all these examples, the contact angle and the surface tension of the liquid are of importance. Surface-active agents are commonly employed in formulation as they reduce the contact angle and hence aid in the wetting of a solid by reducing $\gamma_{L/V}$ and also adsorbing at the solid/liquid interface and reducing $\gamma_{S/L}$.

ADSORPTION

Liquid/vapour and liquid/liquid systems

Surface-active agents

Many compounds have structures that contain two separate regions, a hydrophilic region (water-liking) which confers on the compound a solubility in water, and a hydrophobic region (water-hating) which renders the material soluble in hydrocarbon solvents. Because of this dual structure, it is energetically favourable for these materials, when dissolved, to adsorb at interfaces, orientating themselves in such a manner that the regions are associated with the appropriate solvent (Fig. 4.9). Such materials are termed surface-active agents (or surfactants). Details of their structures and properties are given in Chapters 6 and 16. Because of the accumulation of surfactants at surfaces and interfaces, there will be an expansion which will reduce surface and interfacial tensions. The reduction will be by an amount equal to the surface pressure of an adsorbed layer of surfactant (see Chapter 6). Surfactants will lower surface tension to different degrees. An approximation, Traube's rule, states that for a particular homologous series of surfactants, in dilute solution, the concentration necessary to produce an equal lowering of surface tension decreases by a factor of three for each additional CH_2 group. The formation of the adsorbed surface layer will not be instantaneous, but will be governed by the diffusion of the surfactant to the interface. The time taken to reach equilibrium will depend on factors such as molecular size, shape and the presence of impurities. For immiscible liquids, the reduction in interfacial tension may be such that emulsification readily takes place. Detailed aspects of this are dealt with in Chapter 6.

In certain cases, a 'negative adsorption' may occur, i.e. the solute molecules migrate away from the surface. In these cases, examples of which are solutions of sugars and electrolytes, small increases in surface tension are observed.

Surface excess concentration

The extent of the distribution of a solute between an interface and the bulk phase is generally expressed in terms of a surface excess. This is the amount of a material present at the interface in excess of that which would have been there if the bulk phases extended to the interface without a change in composition, n.

The surface excess concentration Γ is $\dfrac{n}{A}$ where A is the area of the interface.

The adsorption of material at any interface is given by the Gibbs adsorption equation. Its general form is

$$d\gamma = -\Sigma\ \Gamma_i\ du_i \qquad (4.19)$$

where $d\gamma$ is the change in interfacial tension, Γ_i is the surface excess concentration of the ith component and u_i is the chemical potential of the ith component.

In the specific case of a solute partitioning between the surface and the bulk of a liquid, the equation becomes

$$\Gamma = -\ \frac{C}{RT} \cdot \frac{d\gamma_{L/V}}{dC} \qquad (4.20)$$

where C is the overall solute concentration, R is the gas constant, T is the absolute temperature and $\dfrac{d\gamma_{L/V}}{dC}$ is the change of surface tension with concentration. The above is applicable to dilute

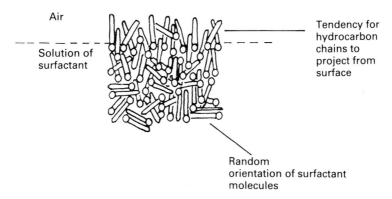

Air

Solution of surfactant

Tendency for hydrocarbon chains to project from surface

Random orientation of surfactant molecules

Fig. 4.9 The orientation of molecules at surfaces and interfaces

solutions. For concentrated solutions, activities must be substituted for concentrations. The above equation (Eqn 4.20) has been verified experimentally by direct measurement of surface concentrations after removal of the surface layer with a microtome blade. The equation enables calculation of the surface excess from surface tension data.

As the concentration of a surface-active agent in aqueous solution is increased, the surface layer will eventually become saturated. Figure 4.10 shows a typical plot of surface tension against concentration. When the surface layer is saturated, further increases in concentration can no longer change the surface tension, and the surfactant molecules form micelles (small aggregates of molecules) as an alternative means of 'protecting' the hydrophobic regions. Details of these are given in Chapter 6. The discontinuity of the plot in Fig. 4.10 is called the critical micelle concentration. Immediately before this, the surfactant molecules are closely packed at the surface and this gives a method of determining the surface area occupied by each molecule, A, from

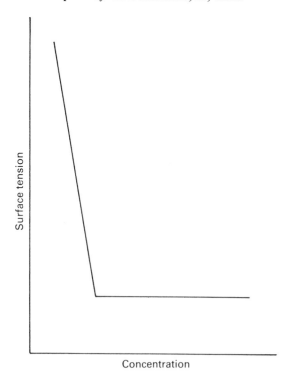

Fig. 4.10 The relationship between surface tension and concentration for a typical surfactant

$$A = \frac{1}{N_A \Gamma} \qquad (4.21)$$

where N_A is Avogadro's number and Γ is the surface excess concentration calculated from the slope of the plot $\mathrm{d}\gamma_{L/V}/\mathrm{d}\log C$ immediately before the critical micelle concentration (remember that Γ is a concentration expressed in terms of surface area).

Because of their structures, many drugs are surface active in nature and this activity may play a part in their pharmacological effects. Examples are some antihistamines, the phenothiazine tranquillizers and antidepressants.

Monomolecular films (monolayers)

Certain insoluble materials can, when dissolved in a suitable volatile solvent, be made to spread on the surface of water to form a film which is one molecule thick. This may be regarded as an extreme case of adsorption as all the molecules are at the surface. Surface excess concentrations can be calculated directly from a knowledge of the amount of material and the surface area. The monolayer will reduce the surface tension of the water by an amount equal to the surface pressure. The surface pressure, which is the expanding pressure due to the monolayer opposing the contracting tension of the water can be measured directly by enclosing the film between movable barriers.

$$\pi = \gamma_o - \gamma_m \qquad (4.22)$$

where π is the surface pressure, γ_o is the surface tension of the 'clean' liquid and γ_m, the surface tension of the liquid covered with a monolayer.

Monolayers exist in different physical states which in some way are analogous to the three states of matter: solids, liquids and gases. Pharmaceutically, monolayers have been used to study polymers which are used for film coating and packaging and as models for cell membranes (Zatz *et al.*, 1969; Cleary and Zatz, 1977).

Solid/vapour systems

Although adsorption in solid/liquid systems is of more interest pharmaceutically, the interpretation of results is often achieved using equations developed for solid/vapour systems. Hence this system will be described first.

If a gas or vapour is brought into contact with a solid, some of it will become attached to the surface. This reduces the imbalance of attractive forces and hence the surface free energy. (Adsorption here must be distinguished from absorption, where penetration into the solid may take place. In some cases it is impossible to distinguish between the two. Here the general term, sorption, is used.) Adsorption may be by relatively weak non-specific forces (van der Waals forces), this form of adsorption being termed physical adsorption. Alternatively, the adsorption may be by stronger specific valence forces, chemisorption. Physical adsorption is rapid, reversible and multilayer adsorption is possible. Chemisorption is specific, may require an activation energy and therefore be slow and not readily reversible and only monomolecular chemisorbed layers are possible.

Adsorption studies using gases or vapours generally involve the determination of the amount of gas or vapour adsorbed, x, by a given mass, m, of the adsorbent at constant temperature. Determinations are carried out at different equilibrium pressures p, (the pressure attained after adsorption has taken place) to yield an adsorption isotherm. When vapours are used, the results are generally expressed in terms of a relative vapour pressure p/p_0 where p_0 is the saturated vapour pressure. Prior to the studies, the solid adsorbent must have any adsorbed material removed by placing it under vacuum or heating.

The isotherms obtained can generally be classified into five types, shown in Fig. 4.11. Type I isotherms exhibit a rapid rise in adsorption up to a limiting value. They are referred to as Langmuir-type isotherms and are due to the adsorption being restricted to a monolayer. Hence adsorption of the chemisorption type will give this type of curve. Type II isotherms represent multilayer physical adsorption on non-porous materials. Types III and V occur when the adsorption in the first layer is weak and are rare. Type IV is

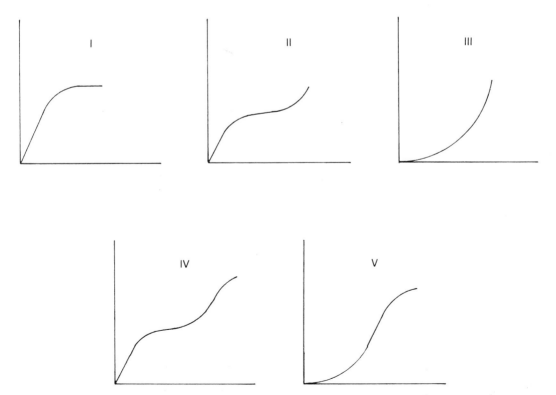

Fig. 4.11 Classification of isotherms for the adsorption of vapours by solids. Ordinates x/m, abscissae p/p_0

considered to be due to condensation of vapour in fine capillaries within a porous solid.

There have been many attempts to develop equations to fit the experimentally observed isotherms. Amongst the most widely used expressions are the following.

Langmuir adsorption isotherm

The equation was derived by assuming only monolayer coverage was possible, hence it is only applicable to type I isotherms. The equation is usefully written as

$$p\frac{m}{x} = \frac{1}{b}p + \frac{1}{ab} \qquad (4.23)$$

where p, m and x are as defined previously and b and a are constants, b being the amount of gas required to produce a monolayer over the whole surface of the absorbent. Hence plotting $\frac{pm}{x}$ against p should give a straight line with a slope $\frac{1}{b}$ and intercept $\frac{1}{ab}$.

Freundlich adsorption isotherm

This is given by

$$\frac{x}{m} = kp^{1/n} \qquad (4.24)$$

where n and k are constants for a particular system. Plots of $\log \frac{x}{m}$ against $\log p$ should therefore give straight lines. The equation does not predict a limiting value as does the Langmuir equation.

Brunauer, Emmett and Teller (BET) equation

This equation takes into account multilayer adsorption and hence describes type II isotherms. It is usually written in the form

$$\frac{p}{V(p_0 - p)} = \frac{1}{V_m \cdot c} + \frac{(c-1)}{V_m \cdot c} \cdot \frac{p}{p_0} \qquad (4.25)$$

where p_0 is the saturation vapour pressure, V is the equilibrium volume of gas adsorbed per unit

mass of adsorbent, V_m is the volume of gas required to cover unit mass of adsorbent with monolayer and c is a constant. The equation reduces to the Langmuir equation if adsorption is restricted to monolayer formation.

One direct practical application of the adsorption of gases of pharmaceutical interest is the determination of the surface area of powders. If the isotherm is determined and the point of monolayer formation identified, a knowledge of the surface area of the adsorbing species will give a value for the surface area of the powder.

Solid/liquid systems

The adsorption of most interest is that of a solute, in solution, on to a solid. The equations most widely used to interpret the data are those of Langmuir and Freundlich. The pressure terms are replaced by concentration terms; hence the Langmuir equation becomes

$$\frac{x}{m} = \frac{abC}{(1 + bC)} \qquad (4.26)$$

where x is the amount of solute adsorbed by a weight, m, of adsorbent, C is the concentration of the solution at equilibrium and b and a are constants.

Adsorption from solution

Several factors will affect the extent of adsorption from solution. These include the following.

Solute concentration An increase in the concentration of the solute will cause an increase in the amount of adsorption that occurs at equilibrium until a limiting value is reached. It should be noted that for most adsorptions from solution, the *relative* amount of solute removed from solution is greater in dilute solutions.

Temperature Adsorption is generally exothermic and hence an increase in temperature leads to a decrease in adsorption.

pH The influence of pH is usually through a change in the ionization of the solute and the influence will depend on which species is more strongly adsorbed.

Surface area of adsorbent An increased surface area, achieved by a reduction in particle size or the use of a porous material, will increase the extent of adsorption.

Pharmaceutical applications of adsorption from solution

The phenomenon of adsorption from solution finds practical application of pharmaceutical interest in chromatographic techniques and in the removal of unwanted materials. In addition adsorption may give rise to certain formulation problems.

The role of adsorption in chromatography is outside the scope of this book. Materials such as activated charcoal can be given in cases of orally taken poisons to adsorb the toxic materials. In addition, adsorbents may be used in haemodialysis to remove the products of dialysis from the dialysing solution and hence allowing the solution to be recycled. Adsorption may cause problems in formulation where drugs or other materials such as preservatives are adsorbed by containers, thus reducing the effective concentration. Glyceryl trinitrate is a volatile solid given in the form of tablets. The vapour may be sorbed by the container leading to further volatilization and loss of potency (Russell *et al.*, 1973). The adsorption of insulin on to intravenous administration sets has been reported (Hirsch *et al.*, 1977) as has the sorption of phenylmercuric acetate, used as a preservative in eyedrops, on to polyethylene containers (Aspinall *et al.*, 1980).

REFERENCES

Aspinall, J. D., Duffy, T. D., Saunders, M. B. and Taylor, C. G. (1980) The effect of low density polyethylene containers on some hospital manufactured eye-drop formulations: Sorption of phenyl mercuric acetate. *J. clin. hosp. Pharm.*, 5, 21–30

Cleary, G. W. and Zatz, J. L. (1977) Interaction of hydrocortisone with model membranes containing phospholipid and cholesterol. *J. pharm. Sci.*, 66 975–980.

Hirsch, J. I., Fratkin, M. J., Wood, J. H. and Thomas, R. B. (1977) Clinical significance of insulin adsorption by polyvinyl chloride infusion systems. *Am. J. hosp. Pharm.*, 34, 583–588.

Lerk, C. F., Lagas, M., Boelstra, J. P. and Broersma, P. (1977) Contact angles of pharmaceutical powders. *J. pharm. Sci.*, 66, 1480–1482.

Lerk, C. F., Schoonen, A. J. M., and Fell, J. T. (1976) Contact angles and wettability of pharmaceutical powders. *J. pharm. Sci.*, 65, 843–847.

Russell, V. A., Lund, W., and Lynch, M. (1973) Storage of glyceryl trinitrate tablets in dispensing containers. *Pharm. J.*, **211**, 466–468.

Zatz, J. L., Weiner, N. D. and Gibaldi, M. (1969) Monomolecular film properties of protective and enteric film formers. *J. pharm. Sci.*, 58, 1493–1496.

BIBLIOGRAPHY

Adamson, A. W. (1980) *Physical Chemistry of Surfaces*, 4th edn, John Wiley, New York.

Florence, A. T. and Attwood, D. (1981) *Physicochemical Principles of Pharmacy*, Macmillan Press, London.

Gregg, S. J. (1965) *The Surface Chemistry of Solids*, 2nd edn, Chapman and Hall, London.

Rosen, M. J. (1978) *Surfactants and Interfacial Phenomena*, John Wiley, New York.

Shaw, D. J. (1980) *Introduction to Colloid and Surface Chemistry*, 3rd edn, Butterworths, London.

Solubility and dissolution rate

THE PROCESS OF DISSOLUTION

The kinetic theory of matter indicates that in condensed phases the thermal motions of molecules are reduced sufficiently so that intermolecular forces of attraction result in the formation of coherent masses of molecules, unlike the situation in gaseous phases where the molecules move independently within the confines of the container. In solid condensed phases the thermal motions of molecules (or ions) are virtually restricted to vibrations about mean positions and the components tend to form three-dimensional arrangements or crystal lattices, in which the inter-component forces are best satisfied and the potential energy of the system is minimized. In liquid condensed systems the thermal motions of molecules are greater than those in solids but less than those in gases. The structure of liquids is intermediate, therefore, between those of solids and liquids. Thus, although the molecules can move within the confines of the liquid phase boundaries small groups of them tend to form regular arrangements in a transient manner. In addition, liquids are thought to contain a small amount of so-called 'free volume' in the form of 'holes' that, at a given instant, are not occupied by the solvent molecules themselves.

When a substance dissolves in a liquid the increase in volume of the latter is less than expected. The process of dissolution may be considered, therefore, to involve the relocation of a solute molecule from an environment where it is surrounded by other identical molecules, with which it forms intermolecular attractions, into a cavity in a liquid where it is surrounded by non-identical molecules, with which it may interact to a different degree.

In order for this process to occur spontaneously at a constant pressure the accompanying change in free energy or Gibbs free energy (ΔG) must be negative. This change is defined by the generally applicable thermodynamic equation

$$\Delta G = \Delta H - T\Delta S \qquad (5.1)$$

where ΔH, which is known as the change in the enthalpy of the system, is the amount of heat absorbed or evolved as the system changes its thermodynamic state, i.e. when dissolution occurs in this case, T is the thermodynamic temperature and ΔS is the change in the so-called entropy, which is a measure of the degree of disorder or randomness in the system.

The entropy change (ΔS) is usually positive for any process such as dissolution, that involves mixing of two or more components. In an ideal solution, there is, by definition, no net change in the intermolecular forces experienced by either solute or solvent when dissolution occurs. In such circumstances $\Delta H = 0$. Thus, the free energy change ΔG during the formation of an ideal solution is provided solely by the term $T\Delta S$.

In most real systems dissolution is accompanied by a change in the intermolecular forces experienced by the solute and solvent before and after the event. A change in enthalpy will therefore accompany dissolution in such systems. Equation 5.1 indicates that the likelihood of dissolution will depend on the sign of ΔH and, if this sign is positive, on the value of ΔH relative to that of $T\Delta S$. In other words it follows from Eqn 5.1 that since $T\Delta S$ is usually positive then

dissolution will occur if ΔH is either negative or if it is positive but less than $T\Delta S$.

The overall change in enthalpy of dissolution ΔH can be regarded as being made up of the change resulting from removal of a solute molecule from its original environment plus that resulting from its new location in the solvent. For example, in the case of a crystalline solid dissolving in a liquid these contributions can be described by Eqn 5.2

$$\Delta H = \Delta H_{cl} + \Delta H_{solv} \qquad (5.2)$$

where the change in crystal lattice enthalpy (ΔH_{cl}) is the heat absorbed when the molecules (or ions) of the crystalline solute are separated by an infinite distance against the effects of their intermolecular attractive forces. The enthalpy of solvation (ΔH_{solv}) is the heat absorbed when the solute molecules are immersed in the solvent.

ΔH_{cl} is always positive and ΔH_{solv} is negative. In most cases $\Delta H_{cl} > \Delta H_{solv}$ so that ΔH is also positive. In these cases heat is absorbed when dissolution occurs and the process is usually defined as an endothermic one. In some systems where marked affinity between solute and solvent occurs the negative ΔH_{solv} is so great that it exceeds the positive ΔH_{cl}. The overall enthalpy change then becomes negative so that heat is evolved and the process is an exothermic one.

SOLUBILITY

The free energy (G) is a measure of the energy available to the system to perform work. Its value decreases during a spontaneously occurring process until an equilibrium position is reached when no more energy can be made available, i.e. $\Delta G = 0$ at equilibrium.

The solution produced when equilibrium is established between undissolved and dissolved solute in a dissolution process is termed a saturated solution. The amount of substance that passes into solution in order to establish the equilibrium at constant temperature and pressure and so produce a saturated solution is known as the solubility of the substance. It is possible to obtain supersaturated solutions but these are unstable and precipitation of the excess solute tends to occur readily.

Methods of expressing solubility

Solubilities may be expressed by means of any of the concentration terms that are defined in Chapter 3. They are expressed most commonly, however, in terms of the maximum mass or volume of solute that will dissolve in a given mass or volume of solvent at a particular temperature. For example, the solubility of nitrofurantoin in water at 37 °C is 174 mg dm^{-3} (Cadwallader and Hung Won Jun, 1976).

The *British Pharmacopoeia* (1980) gives information on the approximate solubilities of official substances in terms of the number of parts by volume of solvent required to dissolve one part by weight of a solid or one part by volume of a liquid. Unless otherwise specified these solubilities apply at a temperature of 20 °C. Figures given under the side heading 'Solubility' in the pharmacopoeial monographs are only approximate and are not intended to be official requirements, whereas statements under side headings such as 'Solubility in Alcohol' are exact and form one of the official requirements for that substance. The *European Pharmacopoeia* (1982) also uses the expression 'parts' in defining the approximate solubilities that correspond to descriptive terms such as 'freely soluble' and 'sparingly soluble'.

Prediction of solubility

Similar types of intermolecular force may contribute to solute–solvent, solute–solute and solvent–solvent interactions. The attractive forces exerted between polar molecules are much stronger, however, than those that exist between polar and non-polar molecules or between non-polar molecules themselves. Consequently, a polar solute will dissolve to a greater extent in a polar solvent, where the strength of the solute–solvent interaction will be comparable to that between solute molecules, than in a non-polar solvent, where the solute–solvent interaction will be relatively weak. In addition, the forces of attraction between the molecules of a polar solvent will be too great to facilitate the separation of these molecules by the insertion of a non-polar solute between them, because the solute–solvent forces will again be relatively weak. Thus, solvents for non-polar solutes tend to be restricted to non-polar liquids.

The above considerations are often expressed in the very general manner that 'like dissolves like', i.e. a polar substance will dissolve in a polar solvent and a non-polar substance will dissolve in a non-polar solvent. Such a generalization should be treated with caution, because the intermolecular forces involved in the process of dissolution are influenced by factors that are not obvious from a consideration of the overall polarity of a molecule. For example, the possibility of intermolecular hydrogen-bond formation between solute and solvent may be more significant than polarity.

Solubility parameter Attempts have been made to define a parameter that indicates the ability of a liquid to act as a solvent. The most satisfactory approach, introduced by Hildebrand and Scott (1962), is based on the concept that the solvent power of a liquid is influenced by its intermolecular cohesive forces and that the strength of these forces can be expressed in terms of a solubility parameter. The initially introduced parameters, which are concerned with the behaviour of non-polar, non-interacting liquids, are referred to as Hildebrand solubility parameters. Whilst these provide good quantitative predictions of the behaviour of a small number of hydrocarbons they only provide a broad qualitative description of the behaviours of most liquids, because of the influence of factors such as hydrogen-bond formation and ionization. The concept has been extended, however, by the introduction of partial solubility parameters, e.g. Hansen parameters and interaction parameters, that have improved the quantitative treatment of systems in which polar effects and interactions occur.

Solubility parameters and other cohesive parameters are well reviewed by Barton (1983), who also indicates that the electrostatic properties of liquids, e.g. dielectric constant and dipole moment, have often been linked by empirical or semi-empirical relationships either to these parameters or to solvent properties. Studies on solubility parameters are sometimes reported in the pharmaceutical literature and those of Beerbower et al. (1984) and Martin et al. (1984) are recent examples. The use of dielectric constants as indicators of solvent power has also received attention in the pharmaceutical literature (e.g. Paruta *et al.*, 1964) but deviations from the behaviour predicted by such methods may occur (Ecanow and Takruri, 1970).

Mixtures of liquids are often used as solvents. If the two liquids have similar chemical structures, e.g. benzene and toluene, then neither tends to associate in the presence of the other and the solvent properties of a 50:50 mixture would be a mean of those of each pure liquid. If the liquids have dissimilar structures, e.g. water and propanol, then the molecules of one of them tend to associate with each other and so form regions of high concentration within the mixture. The solvent properties of this type of system are not so simply related to its composition as in the previous case. Williams and Amidon (1984) have presented a series of papers which describe the application of an approach, based on an excess free energy model, to the prediction of the solubilities of various compounds in ethanol–water mixtures and of phenobarbitone and hydrocortisone in ethanol–propylene glycol–water mixtures.

Solubility of gases in liquids

The amount of gas that will dissolve in a liquid is determined by the natures of the two components and by temperature and pressure.

Provided that no reaction occurs between the gas and liquid then the effect of pressure is indicated by Henry's law, which states that at constant temperature the solubility of a gas in a liquid is directly proportional to the pressure of the gas above the liquid. The law may be expressed by Eqn 5.3

$$w = kp \qquad (5.3)$$

where w is the mass of gas dissolved by unit volume of solvent at an equilibrium pressure p and k is a proportionality constant. Although Herny's law is most applicable at high temperatures and low pressures, when solubility is low, it provides a satisfactory description of the behaviour of most systems at normal temperatures and reasonable pressures, unless solubility is very high or reaction occurs. Equation 5.3 also applies to the solubility

of each gas in a solution of several gases in the same liquid provided that p represents the partial pressure of a particular gas.

The solubility of most gases in liquids decreases as the temperature rises. This provides a means of removing dissolved gases. For example, Water for Injections BP free from either carbon dioxide or air, as specified in some monographs of the *British Pharmacopoeia*, may be prepared by boiling Water for Injections with minimum exposure to air and prevention of access of air during cooling. The presence of electrolytes may also decrease the solubility of a gas in water by a 'salting out' process, which is caused by the marked attraction exerted between electrolyte and water.

Solubility of liquids in liquids

The components of an ideal solution are miscible in all proportions. Such complete miscibility is also observed in some real binary systems, e.g. ethanol and water, under normal conditions. However, if one of the components tends to self-associate because the attractions between its own molecules are greater than those between its molecules and those of the other component, i.e. if a positive deviation from Raoult's law occurs, the miscibility of the components may be reduced. The extent of the reduction depends on the strength of the self-association and, therefore, on the degree of deviation from Raoult's law. Thus, partial miscibility may be observed in some systems whereas virtual immiscibility may be exhibited when the self-association is very strong and the positive deviation from Raoult's law is large.

In those cases where partial miscibility occurs under normal conditions then the degree of miscibility is usually dependent on the temperature. This dependency is indicated by the Phase Rule, introduced by J. Willard Gibbs, which is expressed quantitatively by Eqn 5.4

$$F = C - P + 2 \qquad (5.4)$$

where P and C are the numbers of phases and components in the system, respectively, and F is the number of degrees of freedom, i.e. the number of variable conditions such as temperature, pressure and composition that must be stated in order to define completely the state of the system at equilibrium.

The overall effect of temperature variation on the degree of miscibility in these systems is usually described by means of phase diagrams, which are graphs of temperature versus composition at constant pressure. For convenience of discussion of their phase diagrams the partially miscible systems may be divided into the following types.

Systems showing an increase in miscibility with rise in temperature

A positive deviation from Raoult's law arises from a difference in the cohesive forces that exist between the molecules of each component in a liquid mixture. This difference becomes more marked as the temperature decreases and the positive deviation may then result in a decrease in miscibility sufficient to cause the separation of the mixture into two phases. Each phase consists of a saturated solution of one component in the other liquid. Such mutually saturated solutions are known as conjugate solutions.

The equilibria that occur in mixtures of partially miscible liquids may be followed either by shaking the two liquids together at constant temperature and analysing samples from each phase after equilibrium has been attained, or by observing the temperature at which known proportions of the two liquids, contained in sealed glass ampoules, become miscible, as shown by the disappearance of turbidity.

Phenol–water system The temperature–composition diagram of phenol and water at constant pressure (Fig. 5.1) is convenient to use in the explanation of the effects of partial miscibility in systems that show an increase in miscibility with rise in temperature.

The areas shown in Fig. 5.1 each correspond to the existence of various phases as shown in the diagram. The most important part of the diagram, for the purpose of the present discussion, is that indicated by the line *BCD*, which separates a single-phase system of one liquid from a two-phase system of two mutually saturated liquids. If gradually increasing amounts of phenol are added to water at 20 °C, the composition moves along the line *abcde*. Between *a* and *b* there is only one liquid phase, and application of the Phase Rule shows that there are three degrees of freedom:

$$F = 2 - 1 + 2 = 3$$

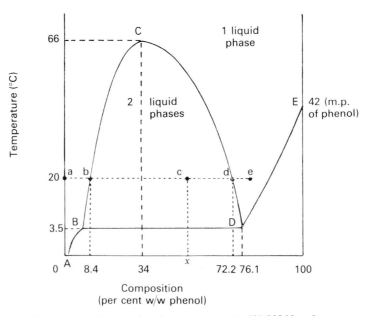

Fig. 5.1 Temperature–composition diagram for the phenol–water system (at 101 325 N m^{-2})

This means that temperature and composition must be specified in order to define the system completely at constant pressure. The aqueous solution is eventually saturated at a composition corresponding to *b* (containing 8.4% phenol). The line *BC* therefore represents the effect of temperature on the solubility of phenol in water. If more phenol is added, then a second layer separates. This is a saturated solution of water in liquid phenol. Thus, at a total composition corresponding to point *c* (i.e. containing *x*% phenol) two conjugate solutions will exist as separate phases. The compositions of these phases will correspond to points *b* and *d* respectively (i.e. one solution contains 8.4% phenol in water and the other contains 27.8% water in phenol). The relative amounts of these solutions at 20 °C are given by

Amount of saturated solution of phenol in water / Amount of saturated solution of water in phenol

$$= \frac{cd}{bc}$$

Application of the Phase Rule to the system at *c* shows that there are two degrees of freedom:

$$F = 2 - 2 + 2 = 2$$

Thus, the system is completely defined if the temperature is specified at constant pressure. For example, at 20 °C the system consists of one phase with a composition corresponding to *b* and another with a composition corresponding to *d*.

If more phenol is added, the point *d* is reached where the system consists of a saturated solution of phenol in water. Thus, the line *DC* represents the effect of temperature on the solubility of water in phenol. Further addition of phenol produces an unsaturated solution of water in phenol (i.e. at *e*).

It can be seen that *BC* and *DC* meet at *C*; i.e. above *C* only one liquid phase can exist. The two components are therefore miscible in all proportions above *C*, which is known as the upper critical temperature (upper CST). The composition at *C* corresponds to a mixture containing 34% phenol and such a mixture will remain separated into two layers up to a higher temperature than any other. Application of the Phase Rule to the system at *C* shows that this point is invariant; i.e.

the upper CST is fixed at 66 °C for the phenol–water system at atmospheric pressure (101 325 N m^{-2}).

The remaining part of the phenol–water phase diagram is of importance with regard to the formulation of a solution containing a large proportion of phenol. Such a solution is used in dispensing practice in preference to solid phenol, since the latter is deliquescent and therefore difficult to weigh accurately. In order to be satisfactory for dispensing purposes the liquid should remain homogeneous at normal room temperatures; i.e. it should not readily deposit crystalline phenol when the room temperature falls during cool periods. It can be seen from Fig. 5.1 that a solution containing 76.1% w/w phenol will meet this requirement most satisfactorily since this mixture will withstand the lowest possible temperature (3.5 °C) before solid phenol is deposited. On the basis of his investigation into this section of the phenol–water diagram Mulley (1959) has suggested that a solution containing 76.1% w/w phenol, which corresponds to an 80% w/v solution in water, should be used in dispensing. The percentage w/v concentration allows more rapid calculation of the weight of phenol in a given volume of solution than the official solution known as Liquefied Phenol BP 1980, which contains 77–81.5% w/w phenol in water. In addition, the official formulation deposits phenol at a higher temperature (about 10 °C).

Systems showing a decrease in miscibility with rise in temperature

A few mixtures, which probably involve compound formation, exhibit a lower critical solution temperature (lower CST), e.g. triethylamine plus water, paraldehyde plus water. The formation of a compound produces a negative deviation from Raoult's law, and miscibility therefore increases as the temperature falls, as shown in Fig. 5.2.

The effect of temperature on miscibility is of use in the preparation of paraldehyde enemas, which usually consist of a solution of paraldehyde in normal saline. Cooling the mixture during preparation allows more rapid solution, and storage of the enema in a cool place is recommended.

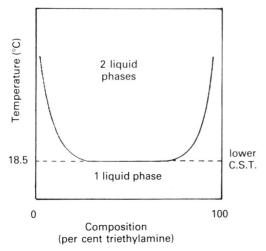

Fig. 5.2 Temperature–composition diagram for the triethylamine–water system (at 101 325 N m⁻²)

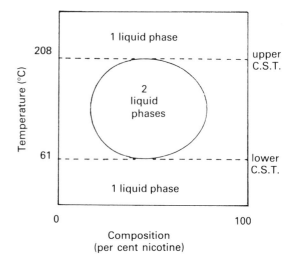

Fig. 5.3 Temperature–composition diagram for the nicotine–water system (at 101 325 N m⁻²)

Systems showing upper and lower critical solution temperatures

The decrease in miscibility with increase in temperature in systems having a lower CST is not indefinite. Above a certain temperature, positive deviations from Raoult's law become important and miscibility starts to increase again with further rise in temperature. This behaviour produces a closed-phase diagram as shown in Fig. 5.3, which represents the nicotine–water system.

In some mixtures where an upper and lower CST are expected, these points are not, in fact, observed since a phase change by one of the components occurs before the relevant CST is reached. For example, the ether–water system is expected to exhibit a lower CST, but water freezes before the temperature is reached.

The effects of added substances on critical solution temperatures

It has already been stated that a CST is an invariant point at constant pressure. These temperatures are very sensitive to impurities or added substances. In general, the effects of additives may be summarized by Table 5.1.

The increase in miscibility of two liquids caused by the addition of a third substance is referred to as blending.

The use of propylene glycol as a blending agent, which improves the miscibility of volatile

Table 5.1 The effects of additives on CST

Type of CST	Solubility of additive in each component	Effect on CST	Effect on miscibility
Upper	Approx. equally soluble in both components	Lowered	Increased
Upper	Readily soluble in one component but not in other	Raised	Decreased
Lower	Approx. equally soluble in both components	Raised	Increased
Lower	Readily soluble in one component but not in other	Lowered	Decreased

oils and water, is discussed by Wallwork and Grant (1977) in terms of a ternary phase diagram. This diagram is a triangular plot which indicates the effects of changes in the relative proportions of the three components at constant temperature and pressure and it presents a good example of the interpretation and use of such phase diagrams.

Solubility of solids in solids

If two solids are either melted together and then cooled or dissolved in a suitable solvent, which is then removed by evaporation, the solid that is redeposited from the melt or the solution will either be a one-phase solid solution or a two-phase eutectic mixture.

In a solid solution, as in other types of solution,

the molecules of one component (the solute) are dispersed molecularly throughout the other component (the solvent). Complete miscibility of two solid components is only achieved if

1 the molecular size of the solute is the same as that of the solvent so that a molecule of the former can be substituted for one of the latter in its crystal lattice structure, or
2 the solute molecules are much smaller than the solvent molecules so that the former can be accommodated in the spaces of the solvent lattice structure.

These two types of solvent mechanism are referred to as substitution and interstitial effects, respectively. Since these criteria are only satisfied in relatively few systems then partial miscibility of solids is observed more commonly. Thus, dilute solutions of solids in solids may be encountered in systems of pharmaceutical interest, for example, when the solvent is a polymeric material with large spaces between its intertwined molecules that can accommodate solute molecules.

Unlike a solution, a simple eutectic consists of an intimate mixture of the two microcrystalline components in a fixed composition. However, both solid solutions and eutectics provide a means of dispersing a relatively water-insoluble drug in a very fine form, i.e. as molecules or microcrystalline particles, respectively, throughout a water-soluble solid. When the latter carrier solid is dissolved away the molecules or small crystals of insoluble drug may dissolve more rapidly than a conventional powder because the contact area between drug and water is increased (see later in this Chapter). The rate of dissolution and, consequently, the bioavailabilities of poorly soluble drugs may be improved, therefore, by the use of solid solutions or eutectics. Students are recommended to refer to literature reports of studies on such systems (e.g. Sekiguchi and Obi, 1961; Sekiguchi *et al.*, 1964; Goldberg et al., 1965, 1966a, b, c) and to the bibliography for descriptions of their phase diagrams.

Solubility of solids in liquids

As indicated in Chapter 3 solutions of solids in liquids are the most important type of solution encountered in pharmaceutical practice. A pharmacist should therefore be aware of the general method of determining the solubility of a solid in a liquid and the various precautions that should be taken in the determination.

Determination of the solubility of a solid in a liquid

The following points should be observed in all solubility determinations.

1 The solvent and solute must be pure.
2 A saturated solution must be obtained before any solution is removed for analysis.
3 The method of separating a sample of saturated solution from undissolved solute must be satisfactory.
4 The method of analysing the solution must be reliable.
5 Temperature must be adequately controlled.

A saturated solution is obtained either by stirring excess powdered solute with solvent for several hours at the required temperature until equilibrium has been attained, or by warming the solvent with an excess of the solute and allowing the mixture to cool to the required temperature. It is essential that some undissolved solid should be present at the completion of this stage in order to ensure that the solution is saturated.

A sample of the saturated solution is obtained for analysis by separating the solution from the undissolved solid. Filtration is usually used, but precautions should be taken to ensure that:

1 it is carried out at the temperature of the solubility determination, in order to prevent any change in the equilibrium between dissolved and undissolved solute; and
2 loss of a volatile component does not occur.

The filtration process has been simplified by the introduction of membrane filters that can be used in conjunction with conventional syringes fitted with suitable adaptors.

The amount of solute contained in the sample of saturated solution may be determined by a variety of methods; e.g. gravimetric or volumetric analysis, electrical conductivity measurements, u.v. spectrophotometry and chromatographic methods. The selection of an appropriate method is affected by the natures of the solute and solvent and by the concentration of the solution.

Factors affecting the solubility of solids in liquids

Knowledge of these factors, which are discussed below together with their practical applications, is an important aspect of the pharmacist's expertise. Additional information, which shows how some of these factors may be used to improve the solubilities and bioavailabilities of drugs is given in Chapters 14 and 9, respectively.

Temperature   Earlier discussion centred on Eqn 5.1 shows that the free energy change (ΔG) that accompanies dissolution is dependent on the value and sign of the change in enthalpy (ΔH). The additional comments that referred to Eqn 5.2 indicate that the dissolution process is usually an endothermic one when ΔH is positive, i.e. heat is absorbed when dissolution occurs. If this type of system is heated it will tend to react in a way that will nullify the constraint imposed upon it, e.g. the rise in temperature. This tendency is an example of Le Chatelier's principle. Thus, a rise in temperature will lead to an increase in the solubility of a solid with a positive heat of solution.

Conversely, in the case of the less commonly occurring systems that exhibit exothermic dissolution then an increase in temperature will give rise to a decrease in solubility.

Plots of solubility versus temperature, which are referred to as *solubility curves*, are often used to describe the effect of temperature on a given system. Some examples are shown in Fig. 5.4. Most of the resultant curves are continuous ones. However, abrupt changes in slope may be observed with some systems if a change in the nature of the dissolving solid occurs at a specific transition temperature. For example, sodium sulphate exist as the decahydrate $Na_2SO_4.10H_2O$ up to 32.5 °C and its dissolution in water is an endothermic process. Its solubility therefore increases with rise in temperature until 32.5 °C is reached. Above this temperature the solid is converted into the anhydrous form Na_2SO_4 and the dissolution of this compound is an exothermic process. The solubility therefore exhibits a change from a positive to a negative slope as the temperature exceeds the transition value.

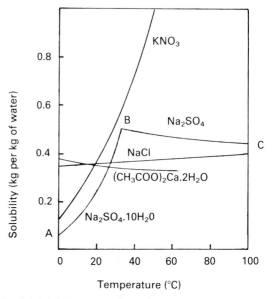

Fig. 5.4 Solubility curves for various substances in water

Molecular structure of solute   It should be appreciated from the previous comments in this chapter on the prediction of solubility that the natures of the solute and solvent will be of paramount importance in determining the solubility of a solid in a liquid. It should be realized, in addition, that even a small change in the molecular structure of a compound can have a marked effect on its solubility in a given liquid. For example, the introduction of a hydrophilic hydroxyl group can produce a large improvement in water solubility as evidenced by the more than 100-fold difference in the solubilities of phenol and benzene.

In addition, the conversion of a weak acid to its sodium salt leads to a much greater degree of ionic dissociation of the compound when it dissolves in water. The overall interaction between solute and solvent is increased markedly and the solubility consequently rises. A specific example of this effect is provided by a comparison of the aqueous solubilities of salicylic acid and its sodium salt, which are 1 in 550 and 1 in 1, respectively.

The reduction in aqueous solubility of a parent drug by its esterification may also be cited as an example of the effects of changes in the chemical structure of the solute. Such a reduction in solubility may provide a suitable method for:

1 masking the taste of a parent drug, e.g. chloramphenicol palmitate is used in paediatric suspensions rather than the more soluble and very bitter chloramphenicol base,
2 protecting the parent drug from excessive degradation in the gut, e.g. erythromycin propionate is less soluble and, consequently, less readily degraded than erythromycin, and
3 increasing the ease of absorption of drugs from the gastrointestinal tract, e.g. erythromycin propionate is also more readily absorbed than erythromycin.

Nature of solvent: cosolvents The importance of the nature of the solvent has already been discussed in terms of the statement 'like dissolves like' and in relation to solubility parameters. In addition, the point has been made that mixtures of solvents may be employed. Such mixtures are often used in pharmaceutical practice in order to obtain aqueous based systems that contain solutes in excess of their solubilities in pure water. This is achieved by using cosolvents such as ethanol or propylene glycol, which are miscible with water and which act as better solvents for the solute in question.

For example, the aqueous solubility of metronidazole is about 100 mg in 10 ml. Chien (1984) has shown, however, that the solubility of this drug can be increased exponentially by the incorporation of one or more water-miscible cosolvents so that a solution, containing 500 mg in 10 ml and suitable for parental administration in the treatment of anaerobic infection, can be obtained.

Crystal characteristics: polymorphism and solvation The value of the term ΔH_{cl} in Eqn 5.2 is determined by the strength of the interactions between adjacent molecules (or ions) in a crystal lattice. These interactions will depend on the relative positions and orientations of the molecules in the crystal. When the conditions under which crystallization is allowed to occur are varied then some substances produce crystals in which the constituent molecules are aligned in different ways with respect to one another in the lattice structure. These different crystalline forms of the same substance, which are known as *polymorphs*, consequently possess different lattice energies and this difference is reflected by changes in other properties. For example, the polymorphic form with the lowest free energy will be the most stable and possess the highest melting point. Other less stable (or metastable) forms will tend to transform into the most stable one at rates that depend on the energy differences between the metastable and stable forms.

The effect of polymorphism on solubility is particularly important from a pharmaceutical point of view, because it provides a means of increasing the solubility of a crystalline material and hence its rate of dissolution (see later in this chapter) by using a metastable polymorph.

Although the more soluble polymorphs are metastable and will convert to the stable form the rate of such conversion is often slow enough for the metastable form to be regarded as being sufficiently stable from a pharmaceutical point of view. The degree of conversion should obviously be monitored during storage of the drug product to ensure that its efficacy is not altered significantly. In addition, conversion to the less soluble and most stable polymorph may contribute to the growth of crystals in suspension formulations.

Many drugs exhibit polymorphism, e.g. steroids, barbiturates and sulphonamides. Examples of the importance of polymorphism with respect to the bioavailabilities of drugs and to the occurrence of crystal growth in suspensions are given in Chapters 9 and 15 respectively, whilst the general implications of polymorphism in pharmacy have been reviewed by Haleblian and McCrone (1969).

The absence of crystalline structure that is usually associated with a so-called amorphous powder may also lead to an increase in the solubility of a drug when compared with that of its crystalline form as Mullins and Macek (1960) demonstrated with the antibiotic novobiocin.

In addition to the effect of polymorphism the lattice structures of crystalline materials may be altered by the incorporation of molecules of the solvent from which crystallization occurred. The resultant solids are called *solvates* and the phenomenon is referred to as solvation although the term *pseudopolymorphism* is encountered sometimes. The alteration in crystal structure that accompanies solvation will affect ΔH_{cl} so that the solubilities of solvated and unsolvated crystals will differ.

If water is the solvating molecule, i.e. if a hydrate is formed, then the interaction between the substance and water that occurs in the crystal phase reduces the amount of energy liberated when the solid hydrate dissolves in water. Consequently, hydrated crystals tend to exhibit a lower aqueous solubility than their unhydrated forms. This decrease in solubility can lead to precipitation from solutions of drugs. For example, Suryanarayanan and Mitchell (1984) have shown that the precipitating tendency of solutions of calcium gluceptate, which is used in the treatment of calcium deficiency and which is very water soluble, is due in part to the formation of a sparingly soluble crystalline hydrate.

In contrast to the effect of hydrate formation, the aqueous solubilities of other, i.e. non-aqueous, solvates are often greater than those of the unsolvated forms. Examples of the effects of solvation and the attendant changes in solubilities of drugs on their bioavailabilities are given in Chapter 9.

Particle size of the solid The changes in interfacial free energy (see earlier in this chapter) that accompany the dissolution of particles of varying sizes cause the solubility of a substance to increase with decreasing particle size, as indicated by Eqn 5.5,

$$\log \frac{s}{s_0} = \frac{2\gamma M}{2.303 RT \rho r} \qquad (5.5)$$

where s is the solubility of small particles of radius r, s_0 is the normal solubility (i.e. of a solid consisting of fairly large particles), γ is the interfacial energy, M is the molecular weight of the solid, ρ is the density of the bulk solid, R is the gas constant, and T is the thermodynamic temperature.

This effect may be significant in the storage of pharmaceutical suspensions, since the smaller particles in such a suspension will be more soluble than the larger ones. As the small particles disappear, the overall solubility of the suspended drug will decrease, and growth of the larger particles will occur. The occurrence of crystal growth by this mechanism is of particular importance in the storage of suspensions intended for injection (Carter, 1975).

The increase in solubility with decrease in particle size ceases when the particles have a very small radius, and any further decrease in size causes a decrease in solubility. It has been postulated that this change arises from the presence of an electrical charge on the particles and that the effect of this charge becomes more important as the size of the particles decreases (Buckley, 1951).

pH If the pH of a solution of either a weakly acidic drug or a salt of such a drug is reduced then the proportion of unionized acid molecules in the solution increases. Precipitation may occur therefore, because the solubility of the unionized species is less than that of the ionized form. Conversely, in the case of solutions of weakly basic drugs or their salts precipitation is favoured by an increase in pH. Such precipitation is an example of one type of chemical incompatibility that may be encountered in the formulation of liquid medicines.

The relationship between pH and the solubility and pK_a' value of an acidic drug is given by Eqn 5.6, which is a modification of the Henderson–Hasselbalch equation Eqn 3.12,

$$pH = pK_a + \log \frac{S - S_0}{S_0} \qquad (5.6)$$

where S is the overall solubility of the drug and S_0 is the solubility of its unionized form, i.e. $S = S_0 +$ solubility of ionized form. If the pH of the solution is known then Eqn 5.6 may be used to calculate the solubility of an acidic drug at that pH. Alternatively, the equation allows determination of the minimum pH that must be maintained in order to prevent precipitation from a solution of known concentration.

In the case of basic drugs the corresponding relationship is given by Eqn 5.7:

$$pH = pK_a + \log \frac{S_0}{S - S_0} \qquad (5.7)$$

Details of the application of Eqn 5.6 to a solution of sodium phenobarbitone are given by Carter (1975) together with a table showing the relationship between the values of $pK_a - pH$ and S_0 for weakly acidic and weakly basic drugs.

Common ion effect The equilibrium in a saturated solution of a sparingly soluble salt in contact with undissolved solid may be represented by

$$AB \rightleftharpoons A^+ + B^-$$
$$\text{(solid)} \qquad \text{(ions)} \qquad\qquad (5.8)$$

From the Law of Mass Action the equilibrium constant K for this reversible reaction is given by Eqn 5.9,

$$K = \frac{[A^+]\,[B^-]}{[AB]} \qquad\qquad (5.9)$$

where the square brackets signify concentrations of the respective components. Since the concentration of a solid may be regarded as being constant then

$$K'_s = [A^+][B^-] \qquad\qquad (5.10)$$

where K'_s is a constant, which is known as the solubility product of compound AB.

If each molecule of the salt contains more than one ion of each type e.g. $A_x^+ B_y^-$, then in the definition of the solubility product the concentration of each ion is expressed to the appropriate power; i.e.

$$K'_s = [A^+]^x[B^-]^y$$

These equations for the solubility product are only applicable to solutions of sparingly soluble salts.

If K'_s is exceeded by the product of the concentration of the ions, i.e. $[A^+][B^-]$, then the equilibrium shown above, Eqn 5.8, moves towards the left in order to restore the equilibrium, and solid AB is precipitated. The product $[A^+][B^-]$ will be increased by the addition of more A^+ ions produced by the dissociation of another compound, e.g. $AX \rightarrow A^+ + X^-$, where A^+ is the common ion. Solid AB will be precipitated and the solubility of this compound is therefore decreased. This is known as the *common ion effect*. The addition of common B^- ions would have the same effect.

The precipitating effect of common ions is, in fact, less than that predicted from Eqn 5.10. The reason for this is explained in the following section.

Effect of indifferent electrolytes on the solubility product   The solubility of a sparingly sol-

uble electrolyte may be increased by the addition of a second electrolyte that does not possess ions common to the first; i.e. an different electrolyte.

The definition of the solubility product of a sparingly soluble electrolyte in terms of the concentration of ions produced at equilibrium, as indicated by Eqn 5.10 is only an approximation from the more exact thermodynamic relationship expressed by Eqn 5.11:

$$K_s = a_{A^+}.a_{B^-} \qquad\qquad (5.11)$$

where K_s is the solubility product of compound AB and a_{A^+} and a_{B^-} are known as the activities of the respective ions. The activity of a particular ion may be regarded as its 'effective concentration'. In general, this has a lower value than the actual concentration, because some ions produced by dissociation of the electrolyte are strongly associated with oppositely charged ions and do not contribute so effectively as completely unassociated ions to the properties of the system. At infinite dilution, the wide separation of ions prevents any interionic association, and the molar concentration (c_{A^+}) and activity (a_{A^+}) of a given ion (A^+) are then equal; i.e.

$$a_{A^+} = c_{A^+} \quad \text{or} \quad \frac{a_{A^+}}{c_{A^+}} = 1$$

As the concentration increases, the effects of interionic association are no longer negligible, and the ratio of activity to molar concentration becomes less than unity; i.e.

$$\frac{a_{A^+}}{c_{A^+}} = f_{A^+}$$

or

$$a_{A^+} = c_{A^+} . f_{A^+}$$

where f_{A^+} is known as the activity coefficient of A^+. If concentrations and activity coefficients are used instead of activities in Eqn 5.11 then

$$K_s = (c_{A^+}.c_{B^-})(f_{A^+}.f_{B^-})$$

The product of the concentrations, i.e. $(c_{A^+}.c_{B^-})$, will be a constant (K'_s) as shown by Eqn 5.10, and $(f_{A^+}.f_{B^-})$ may be equated to $f_{A^+B^-}$, where $f_{A^+B^-}$ is the mean activity coefficient of the salt AB, i.e.

$$K_s = K'_s f_{A^+B^-} \qquad\qquad (5.12)$$

Since $f_{A^+B^-}$ varies with the overall concentration of ions present in solution (the ionic strength), and since K_s is a constant, it follows that K'_s must also vary with the ionic strength of the solution in an inverse manner to the variation of $f_{A^+B^-}$. Thus, in a system containing a sparingly soluble electrolyte without a common ion, the ionic strength will have an appreciable value and the mean activity coefficient $f_{A^+B^-}$ will be less than one.

From Eqn 5.12 it will be seen that K'_s will, therefore, be greater than K'_s. In fact, the concentration solubility product K'_s will become larger and larger as the ionic strength of the solution increases. The solubility of AB will therefore increase as the concentration of added electrolyte increases.

This argument also accounts for the fact that if no allowance is made for the variation in activity with ionic strength of the medium, the precipitating effect of common ions is less than that predicted from the Law of Mass Action.

Effect of non-electrolytes on the solubility of electrolytes The solubility of electrolytes depends on the dissociation of dissolved molecules into ions. The ease of this dissociation is affected by the dielectric constant of the solvent, which is a measure of the polar nature of the solvent. Liquids with a high dielectric constant (e.g. water and formic acid) are able to reduce the attractive forces that operate between oppositely charged ions produced by dissociation of an electrolyte.

If a water-soluble non-electrolyte such as alcohol is added to an aqueous solution of a sparingly soluble electrolyte, the solubility of the latter is decreased because the alcohol lowers the dielectric constant of the solvent and ionic dissociation of the electrolyte becomes more difficult.

Effect of electrolytes on the solubility of non-electrolytes Non-electrolytes do not dissociate into ions in aqueous solution, and in dilute solution the dissolved species therefore consists of single molecules. Their solubility in water depends on the formation of weak intermolecular bonds (hydrogen bonds) between their molecules and those of water. The presence of a very soluble electrolyte (e.g. ammonium sulphate), the ions of which have a marked affinity for water, will reduce the solubility of a non-electrolyte by competing for the aqueous solvent and breaking the intermolecular bonds between the non-electrolyte and water. This effect is important in the precipitation of proteins.

Complex formation The apparent solubility of a solute in a particular liquid may be increased or decreased by the addition of a third substance which forms an intermolecular complex with the solute. The solubility of the complex will determine the apparent change in the solubility of the original solute. For example, the formation of the complexes between 3-aminobenzoic acid and various dicarboxylic acids has been shown to increase the apparent water solubility of the former compound (Wurster and Kilsig, 1965), and Kostenbauder and Higuchi (1956) have shown that soluble and insoluble complexes may be obtained by interactions between various amides and 4-hydroxybenzoic acid, salicylic acid, chloramphenicol, and phenol. Use is also made of complex formation as an aid to solubility in the preparation of solution of mercuric iodide (HgI_2). The latter is not very soluble in water but it is soluble in aqueous solutions of potassium iodide because of the formation of a water-soluble complex, $K_2(HgI_4)$.

Solubilizing agents These agents are capable of forming large aggregates or micelles in solution when their concentrations exceed certain values. In aqueous solution the centre of these aggregates resembles a separate organic phase and organic solutes may be taken up by the aggregates thus producing an apparent increase in their solubilities in water. This phenomenon is known as solubilization. A similar phenomenon occurs in organic solvents containing dissolved solubilizing agents because the centre of the aggregates in these systems constitutes a more polar region than the bulk of the organic solvent. If polar solutes are taken up into these regions their apparent solubilities in the organic solvents are increased.

DISTRIBUTION OF SOLUTES BETWEEN IMMISCIBLE LIQUIDS

Partition coefficients

If a substance, which is soluble in both components of a mixture of immiscible liquids, is dissolved in such a mixture, then, when equilibrium is attained at constant temperature, it is found that the solute is distributed between the two liquids in such a way that the ratio of the activities of the substance in each liquid is a constant. This is known as the Nernst distribution law, which can be expressed by Eqn 5.13:

$$\frac{a_A}{a_B} = \text{constant} \qquad (5.13)$$

where a_A and a_B are the activities of the solute in solvents A and B, respectively. When the solutions are dilute or when the solute behaves ideally, the activities may be replaced by concentrations (c_A and c_B),

$$\frac{c_A}{c_B} = K \qquad (5.14)$$

where the constant K is known as the distribution or partition coefficient. In the case of sparingly soluble substances, K is approximately equal to the ratio of the solubilities (s_A and s_B) of the solute in each liquid; i.e.

$$\frac{s_A}{s_B} = K \qquad (5.15)$$

In most other systems, however, deviation from ideal behaviour invalidates Eqn 5.15. For example, if the solute exists as monomers in solvent A and as dimers in solvent B, the distribution coefficient is given by Eqn 5.16, in which the square root of the concentration of the dimeric form is used:

$$K = \frac{c_A}{\sqrt{c_B}} \qquad (5.16)$$

If the dissociation into ions occurs in the aqueous layer, B, of a mixture of immiscible liquids, then the degree of dissociation (α) should be taken into account as indicated by Eqn 5.17:

$$K = \frac{c_A}{c_B(1 - \alpha)} \qquad (5.17)$$

The solvents, in which the concentrations of the solute — numerators and denominators of Eqns 5.14 to 5.17 — are expressed, should be indicated when partition coefficients are quoted. For example, a partition coefficient of 2 for a solute distributed between oil and water may also be expressed as a partition coefficient between water and oil of 0.5. This can be represented as $K_{water}^{oil} = 2$ and $K_{oil}^{water} = 0.5$. The abbreviation K_w^o is often used for the former.

DISSOLUTION RATES OF SOLIDS IN LIQUIDS

The dissolution of a solid in a liquid may be regarded as being composed of two consecutive stages. The first of these, which is an interfacial reaction that results in the liberation of solute molecules from the solid phase, is followed by transport of these molecules away from the interface into the bulk of the liquid phase under the influence of diffusion or convection. Like any reaction that involves consecutive stages the overall rate of mass transport, that occurs during dissolution, will be determined by the rate of the slowest stage. In the absence of a chemical reaction between solute and solvent then the slowest stage is usually the diffusion of dissolved solute across the static boundary layer of liquid that exists at a solid–liquid interface. Under these conditions the rate of dissolution of a solid in a liquid may be described quantitatively by the Noyes–Whitney equation (Eqn 5.18):

$$\frac{dm}{dt} = kA(C_s - C) \qquad (5.18)$$

where m is the mass of solute that has passed into solution in time t, i.e. dm/dt represents the rate of dissolution, A is the surface area of the undissolved solid in contact with the solvent, C_s is the concentration of solute required to saturate the solvent at the experimental temperature, C is the solute concentration at time t and k is the intrinsic dissolution rate constant or simply the dissolution rate constant. This constant has the dimensions of length^{-2} time^{-1} and it can be shown that

$$k = \frac{D}{Vh} \qquad (5.19)$$

where D is the diffusion coefficient of the solute in the dissolution medium (or solvent), V is the volume of the dissolution medium and h is the thickness of the boundary layer.

If the solute is removed from the dissolution

medium by some process at a faster rate than it passes into solution then the term $(C_s - C)$ in Eqn 5.18 may be approximated to C_s. Alternatively, if the volume of the dissolution medium is so large that C is not allowed to exceed 10% of the value of C_s then the same approximation may be made. In either of these circumstances dissolution is said to occur under 'sink' conditions and Eqn 5.18 may be simplified to

$$\frac{dm}{dt} = kAC_s \qquad (5.20)$$

It should be realized that such 'sink' conditions may arise *in vivo* when a drug is absorbed from its solution in the gastrointestinal fluids at a faster rate than it dissolves in those fluids from a solid dosage form such as a tablet.

If solute is allowed to accumulate in the dissolution medium to such an extent that the above approximation is no longer valid, i.e. when $C > C_s/10$, then 'non-sink' conditions are said to be in operation. When $C = C_s$ it is obvious from Eqn 5.18 that the overall dissolution rate will be zero because the dissolution medium is saturated with solute.

Factors affecting dissolution rates

These factors may be derived from a consideration of the terms that appear in the Noyes–Whitney equation (Eqn 5.18) and a knowledge of the factors that in turn affect these terms. Most of the effects of these latter factors have already been mentioned earlier in this chapter and are included in the summary given in Table 5.2. It should be borne in mind that pharmacists are often concerned with the rate of dissolution of a drug from a formulated product such as a tablet or a capsule, as well as with the dissolution rates of pure solids. The later chapters in this book should be consulted for information on the influence of formulation factors on the rates of release of drugs into solution from various dosage forms.

Measurement of dissolution rates

Many methods have been described in the literature, particularly in relation to the determination of the rate of release of drugs into solution from

tablet and capsule formulations, because such release may have an important effect on the therapeutic efficiency of these dosage forms (see Chapters 9, 18 and 19). Hersey (1969) and Swarbrick (1970) have reviewed the methods for determining dissolution rates and have attempted to classify them. These classifications are based mainly on whether or not the mixing processes that take place in the various methods occur by natural convection arising from density gradients produced in the dissolution medium, or by forced convection brought about by stirring or shaking the system. The following brief descriptions are given as examples of the more commonly used methods that are illustrated in Fig. 5.5. The student is referred to the above-mentioned reviews and to the book by Leeson and Carstensen (1974) for information on others.

Beaker method

The methodology described by Levy and Hayes (1960) forms the basis of this technique. In their initial work these authors used a 400 cm³ beaker containing 250 cm³ of dissolution medium, which was agitated by means of a three-bladed polyethylene stirrer with a diameter of 50 mm. The stirrer was immersed to a depth of 27 mm into the dissolution medium and rotated at 60 rpm. Tablets were dropped into the beaker and samples of the liquid were removed at known times, filtered and assayed.

Flask-stirrer method

This is similar to the previous method except that a round-bottomed flask is used instead of a beaker. The apparatus and methodology are described by Poole (1969). The use of a round-bottomed container helps to avoid the problems that may arise from the formation of 'mounds' of particles in different positions on the flat bottom of a beaker.

Rotating basket method

This was introduced by Searl and Pernarowski (1967) and forms the basis of the only method described in the *British Pharmacopoeia* (1980) and of one of those described in the *United States*

Table 5.2 Factors affecting *in vitro* dissolution rates of solids in liquids

Term in Noyes–Whitney equation	Affected by	Comments
A, surface area of undissolved solid	Size of solid particles	$A \propto 1/\text{particle size}$. Particle size will change during dissolution process, because large particles will become smaller and small particles will eventually disappear. Compacted masses of solid may also disintegrate into smaller particles
	Dispersibility of powdered solid in dissolution medium	If particles tend to form coherent masses in the dissolution medium then the surface area available for dissolution is reduced. This effect may be overcome by the addition of a wetting agent
	Porosity of solid particles	Pores must be large enough to allow access of dissolution medium and outward diffusion of dissolved solute molecules
C_s, solubility of solid in dissolution medium.	Temperature	Dissolution may be an exothermic or endothermic process
	Nature of dissolution medium	See previous comments on solubility parameters, cosolvents and pH
	Molecular structure of solute	See previous comments on sodium salts of weak acids and esterification
	Crystalline form of solid	See previous comments on polymorphism and solvation
	Presence of other compounds	See previous comments on common ion effect, complex formation and solubilizing agents
C, concentration of solute in solution at time t	Volume of dissolution medium	If volume is small C will approach C_s; if volume is large C may be negligible with respect to C_s, i.e. apparent 'sink' conditions will operate
	Any process that removes dissolved solute from the dissolution medium	For example, adsorption on to an insoluble adsorbent, partition into a second liquid that is immiscible with the dissolution medium, removal of solute by dialysis or by continuous replacement of solution by fresh dissolution medium
k, dissolution rate constant	Thickness of boundary layer	Affected by degree of agitation, which depends, in turn, on speed of stirring or shaking, shape, size and position of stirrer, volume of dissolution medium, shape and size of container, viscosity of dissolution medium
	Diffusion coefficient of solute in the dissolution medium	Affected by viscosity of dissolution medium and size of diffusing molecules.

Pharmacopoeia XX and National Formulary XV (1980) for the determination of the dissolution rates of drugs from tablets and capsules. Details of the apparatus and methods of operation are given in these official compendia. Basically these methods involve placing the tablet or capsule inside a stainless steel wire basket, which is rotated at a fixed speed whilst immersed in the dissolution medium that is contained in a wide-mouthed cylindrical vessel. The bottom of this vessel is flat in the BP apparatus and spherical in the USP and NF apparatus. Samples of the dissolution medium are removed at specified times, filtered and assayed. Various criticisms of this method that have appeared in the literature are referred to by Hersey and Marty (1975).

Paddle method

This is another official method of the *United States Pharmacopoeia XX and National Formulary XV* (1980). The dissolution vessel described in the rotating basket method, i.e. the cylindrical vessel with the spherical bottom, is also used in this method. Agitation is provided by a rotating paddle and the dosage form is allowed to sink to the bottom of the dissolution vessel before agitation is commenced.

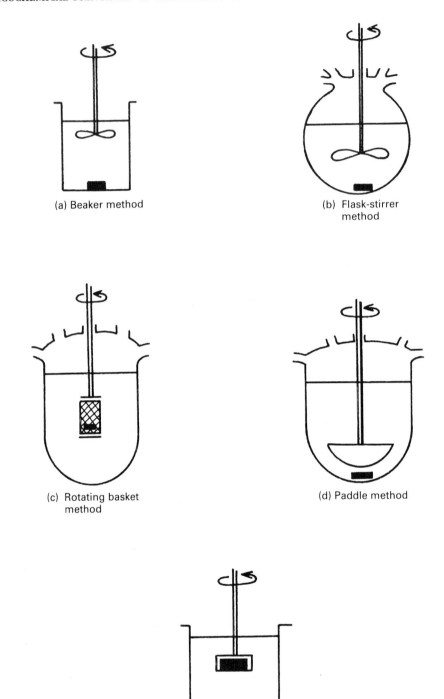

(a) Beaker method

(b) Flask-stirrer method

(c) Rotating basket method

(d) Paddle method

(e) Rotating disc method
Static disc method

Fig. 5.5 Methods of measuring dissolution rates

Rotating and static disc methods

In these methods the compound that is to be assessed for rate of dissolution is compressed into a non-disintegrating disc. This is mounted in a holder so that only one face of the disc is exposed. The holder and disc are immersed in the dissolution medium and either held in a fixed position in the static disc method or rotated at a given speed in the rotating disc method. Samples of dissolution medium are removed after known times, filtered and assayed.

In both methods it is assumed that the surface area, from which dissolution can occur, remains constant. Under these conditions the amount of substance dissolved per unit time and unit surface area can be determined. This is referred to as the intrinsic dissolution rate and should be distinguished from the measurement that is obtained from the previously described methods. In these latter methods the surface area of the drug that is available for dissolution changes considerably during the course of the determination because the dosage form usually disintegrates into many smaller particles and the size of these particles then decreases as dissolution proceeds. Since these changes are not usually monitored the dissolution rate is measured in terms of the total amount of drug dissolved per unit time.

It should be appreciated from a consideration of the comments made in Table 5.2 that not only will different dissolution rate methods yield different results but also changes in the experimental variables in a given method are likely to lead to changes in the results. This latter point is particularly important since dissolution rate tests are usually performed in a comparative manner to determine, for example, the difference between two polymorphic forms of the same compound or between the rate of release of a drug from two formulations. Thus, standardization of the experimental methodology is essential if such comparisons are to be meaningful.

Finally, it should also be realized that although the majority of dissolution testing is concerned with pure drugs or with conventional tablet or capsule formulations, knowledge of the rates of drug release from other types of dosage form is also important. Reference to the later chapters in Part 3 of this book for information on the dissolution methods applied to these other dosage forms should therefore be made.

REFERENCES

Barton, A. F. M. (1983) *Handbook of Solubility Parameters and Other Cohesion Parameters*, CRC Press, Inc., Boca Raton, Florida.
Beerbower, A., Wu, P. L. and Martin, A. (1984) *J. pharm. Sci.*, **73**, 179–188.
British Pharmacopoeia (1980) HMSO, London.
Buckley, H. E. (1951) *Crystal Growth*, pp. 29–31, Wiley, New York.
Cadwallader, D. E. and Hung Won Jun (1976) In *Analytical Profiles of Drug Substances*, K. Florey (ed.), 5, p. 346, Academic Press, London.
Carter, S. J. (1975) *Dispensing for Pharmaceutical Students*, 12th edn, Pitman Medical, London.
Chien, Y. W. (1984) *J. Parental Sci. Tech.*, **38**, 32–36.
Ecanow, B. and Takruri, H. (1970) *J. pharm. Sci.*, **59**, 1848.
European Pharmacopoeia (1982) 2nd edn, Maisonneuve S.A., France.
Goldberg, A. H., Gibaldi, M. and Kanig, J. L. (1965) *J. pharm. Sci.*, **54**, 1145–1148.
Goldberg, A. H., Gibaldi, M. and Kanig, J. L. (1966a) *J. pharm. Sci.*, **55**, 482–487.
Goldberg, A. H., Gilbaldi, M. and Kanig, J. L. (1966b) *J. pharm. Sci.*, **55**, 487–492.
Goldberg, A. H., Gibaldi, M., Kanig, J. L. and Mayersohn, M. (1966c) *J. pharm. Sci.*, **55**, 581–583.

Haleblian, J. and McCrone, W. (1969) *J. pharm. Sci.*, **58**, 911–929.
Hersey, J. A. (1969) *Mfg Chem Aerosol News*, **40**, 32–35.
Hersey, J. A. and Marty, J. J. (1975) *Mfg Chem Aerosol News*, **46**, 43–47.
Hildebrand, J. H. and Scott, R. L. (1962) *Regular Solutions*, Prentice-Hall, New Jersey.
Kostenbauder, H. B. and Higuchi, T. (1956) *J. pharm. Sci.*, **45**, 518–522, 810–813.
Leeson, L. and Carstensen, J. T. (1974) *Dissolution Technology*, I.P.T. Academy of Pharmaceutical Science, Washington DC.
Levy, G. and Hayes, B. A. (1960) *New Engl. J. Med.*, **21**, 1053–1058.
Martin, A., Wu, P. L. and Beerbower, A. (1984) *J. pharm. Sci.*, **73**, 188–194.
Mulley, B. A. (1959) *Drug Stand.*, **27**, 108–109.
Mullins, J. D. and Macek, T. J. (1960) *J. Am. Pharm. Ass. (Sci. Edn)*, **49**, 245–248.
Paruta, A. H., Sciarrone, B. J. and Lordi, N. G. (1964) *J. pharm. Sci.*, **53**, 1349–1353.
Poole, J. W. (1969) *Drug Inf. Bull.*, **3**, 8–16.
Searl, R. O. and Pernarowski. M. (1967) *Can. Med. Ass. J.*, **96**, 1513–1520.

Sekiguchi, K. and Obi, N. (1961) *Chem. pharm. Bull.*, **9**, 866–872.

Sekiguchi, K., Obi, N. and Ueda, Y. (1964) *Chem. pharm. Bull.* **12**, 134–144.

Suryanarayanan, R. and Mitchell, A. G. (1984) *J. pharm. Sci.*, **73**, 78–82.

Swarbrick, J. (1970) In *Current Concepts in the Pharmaceutical Sciences: Biopharmaceutics*, J. Swarbrick (ed.), pp. 265–296, Lea and Febiger, Philadelphia.

United States Pharmacopoeia XX and National Formulary XV (1980) The United States Pharmacopoeial Convention Inc., Rockville, Md.

Wallwork, S. C. and Grant, D. J. W. (1977) *Physical Chemistry for Students of Pharmacy and Biology*, 3rd edn. Longman, London.

Williams, N. A. and Amidon, G. L. (1984) *J. pharm. Sci.*, **73**, 9–13, 14–18, 18–23.

Wurster, D. E. and Kilsig, D. O. (1965) *J. pharm. Sci.*, **54**, 1491–1494.

BIBLIOGRAPHY

Barton, A. F. M. (1983) *Handbook of Solubility Parameters and other Cohesion Parameters*, CRC Press Inc., Boca Raton, Florida.

Carstensen, J. T. (1972) *Theory of Pharmaceutical Systems*, Vol. 1. *General Principles*, Academic Press, London.

Eyring, H., Henderson, D. and Jost, W. (1971) *Physical Chemistry, An Advanced Treatise*, Volume VIIIA *Liquid State*, Academic Press, London.

Florence, A. T. and Attwood, D. (1981) *Physicochemical Principles of Pharmacy*, Macmillan Press Ltd, London.

Hildebrand, J. H., Prausnitz, J. M. and Scott, R. L. (1970) *Regular and related solutions: the solubility of gases, liquids and solids*, Van Nostrand Reinhold, New York.

Leeson, L. and Cartsensen, J. T. (1974) *Dissolution Technology*, I.P.T. Academy of Pharmaceutical Science, Washington DC.

Pharmaceutical Handbook (1980) 19th edn (Ed. A. Wade), The Pharmaceutical Press, London.

Price, N. C. and Dwek, R. A. (1979) *Principles and Problems in Physical Chemistry for Biochemists*, 2nd edn, Clarendon Press, Oxford.

Rowlinson, J. S. and Swinton, F. L. (1982) *Liquids and Liquid Mixtures*, 3rd edn, Butterworth Scientific, London.

Swarbrick, J. (1970) in *Current Concepts in the Pharmaceutical Sciences: Biopharmaceutics*, (Ed. J. Swarbrick). Lea and Febiger, Philadelphia.

Wallwork, S. C. and Grant, D. J. W. (1977) *Physical Chemistry for Students of Pharmacy and Biology*, 3rd edn, Longman, London.

Williams, V. R., Mattice, W. L. and Williams, H. B. (1978) *Basic Physical Chemistry for the Life Sciences*, 3rd edn, W. H. Freeman and Co., San Francisco.

Disperse systems

Table 6.1 Types of disperse systems

Dispersed phase	Dispersion medium	Name	Examples
Liquid	Gas	Liquid aerosol	Fogs, mists, aerosols
Solid	Gas	Solid aerosol	Smoke, powder aerosols
Gas	Liquid	Foam	Foam on surfactant solutions
Liquid	Liquid	Emulsion	Milk, pharmaceutical emulsions
Solid	Liquid	Sol, suspension	Silver iodide sol, aluminium hydroxide suspension
Gas	Solid	Solid foam	Expanded polystyrene
Liquid	Solid	Solid emulsion	Liquids dispersed in soft paraffin, opals, pearls
Solid	Solid	Solid suspension	Pigmented plastics, colloidal gold in glass (ruby glass)

DISPERSE SYSTEMS

A disperse system may be defined as a system in which one substance, the disperse phase, is dispersed as particles throughout another, the dispersion medium.

Although systems in which the size of the dispersed particles are within the range of about 10^{-9} m (1 nm) to 10^{-6} m (1 μm) are termed colloidal, and have specific properties, there is no sharp distinction between colloidal and non-colloidal systems, particularly at the upper size limit. For example the droplet size in emulsions, the particle size in suspensions and the natural systems of micro-organisms and blood are normally in excess of 1 μm and yet such dispersions show many of the properties of colloidal systems. Some examples of the different disperse systems are given in Table 6.1.

The essential character common to all disperse systems is the large area to volume ratio for the particles involved, for example, when a cube of 1 cm edge is subdivided into cubes of 100 nm edge there is a 10^5 increase in surface area and associated free energy. This free energy will be decreased if the particles aggregate or coalesce because of the reduction in interfacial area that accompanies such aggregation. Since any system will tend to react spontaneously to decrease its free energy to a minimum it follows that disperse systems are often unstable, the particles aggregating rather than remaining in contact with the dispersion medium. Dispersions that exhibit this behaviour are termed *lyophobic*, or solvent hating, dispersions. In other systems known as *lyophilic*, solvent loving, dispersions an affinity exists between the dispersed particles and the dispersion medium and this contributes to the stability of these systems. The terms *hydrophobic* and *hydrophilic* may be used when the dispersion medium is water.

Whilst the majority of dispersions used in pharmacy are aqueous they are by no means limited to water, thus dispersions of solids in oils include suspensions for injection and oral use and suspensions of solids in aerosol propellants.

This chapter is an attempt to describe colloidal systems and to show how their properties may be applied to the study of coarse dispersions of pharmaceutical interest.

COLLOID SCIENCE

Colloid science concerns systems in which one or more of the components has at least one dimension within the range of about 1 nm to 1 μm and thus includes shapes such as spheres, cubes, ellipsoids, rods, discs and random coils, where other dimensions may be significantly larger than 1 μm. As indicated, some colloids can be broadly classified as those that are lyophobic, these dispersions or *sols* are thermodynamically unstable and the particles tend to aggregate to lower the surface free energy of the system. They are irreversible systems in the sense that they are not easily reconstituted after phase separation. Water-insoluble drugs and clays such as kaolin and bentonite and oils form lyophobic dispersions. On the other hand macromolecular material such as the proteins, tragacanth and methylcellulose form lyophilic sols which, as true solutions, are thermodynamically stable. These are reversible systems because, after separation of· solute from solvent, they are easily reconstituted. Surfactant molecules, because of their affinity for water and their tendency to form micelles which are of colloidal dimensions, form hydrophilic colloidal dispersions in water but are usually classified separately as *association colloids*, the older term being colloidal electrolyte.

It has been suggested that the efficiency of certain substances, used in pharmaceutical preparations, may be increased if colloidal forms are used since these have large surface areas. Thus, for example, the adsorption of toxins from the gastrointestinal tract by kaolin, and the rate of neutralization of excess acid in the stomach by aluminium hydroxide, may be increased if these compounds are used in colloidal form.

In the purification of proteins, use is made of the changes in solubility of colloidal material with alteration of pH and addition of electrolyte.

The protective ability, or, as it is now known, the *steric stabilization* effect of hydrophilic colloids is used to prevent the coagulation of hydrophobic particles in the presence of electrolytes. Thus hydrophobic sols for injection, such as colloidal gold (^{198}Au) injection, must be sterically stabilized in this case by gelatin. Hydrophilic sols are viscous and use is made of this property in retarding the sedimentation of particles in pharmaceutical suspensions.

Blood plasma substitutes such as dextran, polyvinylpyrrolidone and gelatin aré hydrophilic colloids which exert an osmotic pressure similar to that of plasma and are thus used to restore or maintain blood volume.

Iron–dextran complexes form non-ionic hydrophilic sols suitable for injection for the treatment of anaemia.

Preparation of colloids

Lyophilic colloids

The affinity of lyophilic colloids for the dispersion medium leads to the spontaneous formation of colloidal dispersions. For example, acacia, tragacanth, methylcellulose and certain other cellulose derivatives disperse in water. This simple method of dispersion is a general one for the formation of lyophilic colloids.

Lyophobic colloids

The preparative methods for lyophobic colloids may be divided into those methods that involve the breakdown of larger particles into particles of colloidal dimensions (dispersion methods) and those in which the colloidal particles are formed by aggregation of smaller particles such as molecules (condensation methods).

Dispersion methods

The breakdown of coarse material may be effected by the use of a colloid mill or ultrasonics.

Colloid mills These mills cause the dispersion of coarse material by shearing in a narrow gap between a static cone (the stator) and a rapidly rotating cone (the rotor).

Ultrasonic treatment The passage of ultrasonic waves through a dispersion medium produces alternating regions of cavitation and compression in the medium. The cavities collapse with great force and cause the breakdown of coarse particles dispersed in the liquid.

With both these methods the particles will tend to reunite unless a stabilizing agent such as a surface-active agent is added.

Condensation methods

These involve the rapid production of supersaturated solutions of the colloidal material under conditions in which it is deposited in the dispersion medium as colloidal particles and not as a precipitate. The supersaturation is often obtained by means of a chemical reaction that results in the formation of the colloidal material. For example, colloidal silver iodide may be obtained by reacting together dilute solutions of silver nitrate and potassium iodide, sulphur from sodium thiosulphate and hydrochloric acid solutions, and ferric chloride boiled with excess of water produces colloidal hydrated ferric oxide.

A change in solvent may also cause the production of colloidal particles by condensation methods. If a saturated solution of sulphur in acetone is poured slowly into hot water, the acetone vaporizes leaving a colloidal dispersion of sulphur. A similar dispersion may be obtained when a solution of a resin, such as benzoin in alcohol, is poured into water.

Dialysis

Colloidal particles are not retained by conventional filter papers but are too large to diffuse through the pores of membranes such as those made from regenerated cellulose products, e.g. collodion (cellulose nitrate evaporated from a solution in alcohol and ether) and cellophane. The smaller particles in solution are able to pass through these membranes. Use is made of this difference in diffusibility to separate micromolecular impurities from colloidal dispersions. The process is known as dialysis. The process of dialysis may be hastened by stirring so as to maintain a high concentration gradient of diffusible molecules across the membrane and by renewing the outer liquid from time to time.

Ultrafiltration By applying pressure (or suction) the solvent and small particles may be forced across a membrane whilst the larger colloidal particles are retained. The process is referred to as ultrafiltration. It is possible to prepare membrane filters with known pore size and use of these allows the particle size of a colloid to be determined. However, particle size and pore size cannot be properly correlated because the membrane permeability is affected by factors such as electrical repulsion, when both the membrane and particle carry the same charge, and particle adsorption which can lead to blocking of the pores.

Electrodialysis An electric potential may be used to increase the rate of movement of ionic impurities through a dialysing membrane and so provide a more rapid means of purification. The concentration of charged colloidal particles at one side and at the base of the membrane is termed electrodecantation.

Pharmaceutical applications of dialysis These include the use of membrane filters, artificial membranes as models for the diffusion of drugs through natural membranes, in the study of drug/protein binding and as the principle of haemodialysis where small molecular weight impurities from the body are removed by passage through a membrane.

Properties of colloids

Kinetic properties

In this section several properties of colloidal systems, which relate to the motion of particles with respect to the dispersion medium, will be considered. Thermal motion manifests itself in the form of Brownian motion, diffusion and osmosis. Gravity (or a centrifugal field) leads to sedimentation. Viscous flow is the result of an externally applied force. Measurement of these properties enables molecular weights or particle size to be determined.

Brownian motion

Colloidal particles are subject to random collisions with the molecules of the dispersion medium with the result that each particle pursues an irregular and complicated zig-zag path. If the particles (up to about 2 μm diameter) are observed under a microscope or the light scattered by colloidal particles is viewed using an ultramicroscope, the erratic motion seen is referred to as Brownian motion after Robert Brown (1827) who first observed this phenomenon with pollen grains suspended in water.

Diffusion

As a result of Brownian motion colloidal particles spontaneously diffuse from a region of higher concentration to one of lower concentration. The rate of diffusion is expressed by Fick's first law

$$\frac{dm}{dt} = -DA \frac{dC}{dx} \tag{6.1}$$

where dm is the mass of substance diffusing in time dt across an area A under the influence of a concentration gradient dC/dx. (The minus sign denotes that diffusion takes place in the direction of decreasing concentration.) D is the diffusion coefficient and has the dimensions of area per unit time. The diffusion coefficient of a dispersed material is related to the frictional coefficient of the particles by Einstein's law of diffusion

$$Df = kT \tag{6.2}$$

where k is the Boltzmann constant and T temperature.

Therefore as the frictional coefficient f is given by Stokes

$$f = 6\pi\eta a \tag{6.3}$$

where η is the viscosity of the medium and a the radius of the particle, as a sphere

$$D = \frac{kT}{6\pi\eta a} = \frac{RT}{6\pi\eta a N} \tag{6.4}$$

where N is the Avogadro number and R is the universal gas constant. The diffusion coefficient may be obtained by an experiment measuring the change in concentration, via refractive index gradients, of the free boundary which is formed when the solvent and solution are brought together and allowed to diffuse. The diffusion coefficient can be used to obtain the molecular weight of an approximately spherical particle, such as egg albumin and haemoglobin, by using Eqn 6.4 in the form

$$D = \frac{RT}{6\pi\eta N} \cdot \sqrt[3]{\frac{4\pi N}{3M\bar{v}}} \tag{6.5}$$

where M is the molecular weight and $\bar{v}$ the partial specific volume of the colloidal material.

Sedimentation

Consider a spherical particle of radius a and density σ falling in a liquid of density ρ and viscosity η. The velocity v of sedimentation is given by Stokes' law

$$v = \frac{2a^2 g(\sigma - \rho)}{9\eta} \tag{6.6}$$

where g is acceleration due to gravity.

If the particles are only subjected to the force of gravity then, due to Brownian motion, the lower size limit of particles obeying Eqn 6.6 is about 0.5 μm. A stronger force than gravity is therefore needed for colloidal particles to sediment and use is made of a high speed centrifuge, usually termed an ultracentrifuge, which can produce a force of about $10^6 g$. In a centrifuge, g is replaced by $\omega^2 x$, where ω is the angular velocity and x the distance of the particle from the centre of rotation and Eqn 6.6 becomes

$$v = \frac{2a^2 (\sigma - \rho) \omega^2 x}{9\eta} \tag{6.7}$$

Modification of the sedimentation method using the ultracentrifuge is used in two distinct ways in investigating colloidal material.

In the sedimentation velocity method a high centrifugal field is applied — up to about $4 \times 10^5 g$ — and the movement of the particles, monitored by changes in concentration, is measured from time to time.

In the sedimentation equilibrium method, the colloidal material is subjected to a much lower centrifugal field until sedimentation and diffusion tendencies balance one another, and an equilibrium distribution of particles throughout the sample is attained.

Sedimentation velocity   The velocity dx/dt of a particle in a unit centrifugal force can be expressed in terms of the Svedberg coefficient s,

$$s = \frac{dx/dt}{\omega^2 x} \qquad (6.8)$$

Under the influence of the centrifugal force particles pass from position x_1 at time t_1 to position x_2 at time t_2 — the differences in concentration with time can be measured using changes in refractive index and the application of the schlieren optical arrangement whereby photographs can be taken showing these concentrations as peaks. Integration of Eqn 6.8 using the above limits gives

$$s = \frac{\ln x_2/x_1}{\omega^2 (t_2 - t_1)} \qquad (6.9)$$

By suitable manipulation of Eqns 6.7, 6.8 and 6.9 an expression giving molecular weight M can be obtained

$$M = \frac{RTs}{D(1 - \bar{v}\rho)} = \frac{RT \ln x_2/x_1}{D(1 - \bar{v}\rho)(t_2 - t_1)\omega^2} \qquad (6.10)$$

where $\bar{v}$ is the specific volume of the particle.

Sedimentation equilibrium   Equilibrium is established when sedimentation and diffusional forces balance. Combination of sedimentation and diffusion equations is made in the analysis and

$$M = \frac{2RT \ln C_2/C_1}{\omega^2 (1 - \bar{v}\rho)(x_2^2 - x_1^2)} \qquad (6.11)$$

where C_1 and C_2 are the sedimentation equilibrium concentrations at distances x_1 and x_2 from the axis of rotation.

Unfortunately in order to obtain equilibrium the centrifuge has to be run for about a week, with consequent experimental difficulties. A technique has therefore been developed which allows analysis to be made at intervals during the early stages of the experiment. Mathematical treatment of the results can then be used to obtain the molecular weight.

Osmotic pressure

The determination of molecular weights of dissolved substances from colligative properties is standard procedure but of these, osmotic pressure is the only one with a practical value in the study of colloidal particles. For example, consider a solution of 1 g of macromolecular material of molecular weight 70 000 dissolved in 100 cm³ of water. Assuming ideal behaviour, the depression of the freezing point is 0.0026 K and the osmotic pressure at 20 °C, 350 N m⁻² or about 35 mm of water. The above freezing point depression is far too small to be measured with sufficient accuracy by conventional methods and, of rather greater importance, the presence of about 1 mg of impurity of molecular weight 50 would more than double the above value. Not only does the osmotic pressure provide an effect which is measurable, but also the effect of any low molecular weight material, which can pass through the membrane is virtually eliminated.

However, the usefulness of osmotic pressure measurement is limited to a molecular weight range of about 10^4 to 10^6; below 10^4 the membrane may be permeable to the molecules under consideration and above 10^6 the osmotic pressure will be too small to permit accurate measurement.

If a solution and solvent are separated by a semipermeable membrane the tendency to equalize chemical potentials (and hence concentrations) on either side of the membrane results in a net diffusion of solvent across the membrane. The pressure necessary to balance this osmotic flow is termed the osmotic pressure.

For a colloidal solution the osmotic pressure π can be described by

$$\pi/C = RT/M + BC \qquad (6.12)$$

where C is the concentration of the solution, M the molecular weight of the solute and B a constant depending on the degree of interaction between the solvent and solute molecules.

Thus a plot of π/C verses C is linear with the value of the intercept as $C \to 0$ giving RT/M enabling the molecular weight of the colloid to be calculated.

The Donnan membrane effect

The diffusion of small ions through a membrane will be affected by the presence of a charged macromolecule that is unable to penetrate the membrane because of its size. At equilibrium the distribution of the diffusible ions is unequal, being greater on the side of the membrane containing the non-diffusible ions. This is known as the Donnan membrane effect. For a full discussion, the reader is referred to Shaw (1980).

Application of this principle suggests that co-administration of a large concentration of an anionic macromolecule, e.g. sodium carboxymethylcellu-lose, with a diffusible anion, e.g. potassium benzylpenicillin, should enhance the diffusion of the benzylpenicillin anion across body membranes.

Viscosity

Viscosity is an expression of the resistance to flow of a system under an applied stress and these properties are discussed in detail in Chapter 2. Some of those relationships are repeated here.

Einstein developed an equation of flow applicable to colloidal dispersions of spherical particles,

$$\eta = \eta_o (1 + 2.5 \, \phi) \qquad (6.13)$$

where η_o is the viscosity of the dispersion medium and η the viscosity of the dispersion when the volume fraction of colloidal particles present is ϕ.

A number of viscosity coefficients may be defined with respect to Eqn 6.13. These include *relative viscosity*

$$\eta_{rel} = \eta/\eta_o = 1 + 2.5 \, \phi \qquad (6.14)$$

specify viscosity

$$\eta_{sp} = \eta/\eta_o - 1 = (\eta - \eta_o)/\eta_o = 2.5 \, \phi$$

or $$\eta_{sp}/\phi = 2.5 \qquad (6.15)$$

Since volume fraction is directly related to concentration Eqn 6.15 may be written as

$$\eta_{sp}/C = K \qquad (6.16)$$

where C is the concentration expressed as grams of colloidal particles per 100 ml of total dispersion. If η is determined for a number of concentrations of macromolecular material in solution, η_{sp}/C plotted versus C and the line obtained extrapolated to infinite dilution the constant obtained is $[\eta]$ known as the *intrinsic viscosity*.

This constant may be used to calculate the molecular weight of the macromolecular material by making use of the Mark–Houwink equation

$$[\eta] = KM^\propto \qquad (6.17)$$

where K and $\propto$ are constants characteristic of the particular polymer–solvent system. These constants are obtained initially by determining $[\eta]$ for a polymer fraction whose molecular weight has been determined by another method such as sedimentation, osmotic pressure or light scattering. The molecular weight of the unknown polymer fraction may then be calculated. This method is suitable for use with polymers like the dextrans used as blood plasma substitutes.

Optical properties

Light scattering

When a beam of light is directed at a colloidal sol some of the light may be absorbed (when light of certain wavelengths is selectively absorbed a colour is produced), some is scattered and the remainder transmitted undisturbed through the sample. Due to the light scattered the sol appears turbid; this is known as the Tyndall effect. The turbidity of a sol is given by the expression

$$I = I_o \exp^{-\tau l} \qquad (6.18)$$

where I_o is the intensity of the incident beam, I that of the transmitted light beam, l the length of the sample and τ the turbidity.

Light scattering measurements are of great value for estimating particle size, shape and interactions, particularly of dissolved macromolecular materials, as the turbidity depends on the size (molecular weight) of the colloidal material involved. Measurements are simple in principle but experimentally difficult because of the need to keep the sample free from dust, the particles of which would scatter light strongly and introduce large errors.

As most colloids show very low turbidities, instead of measuring the transmitted light (which may differ only marginally from the incident beam), it is more convenient and accurate to measure the scattered light, at an angle — usually 90° — relative to the incident beam.

The turbidity can then be calculated from the intensity of the scattered light, provided the dimensions of the particle are small compared to the wavelength of the light used, by the expression

$$\tau = \frac{16\pi}{3} R_{90^\circ} \qquad (6.19)$$

R_{90° is given by $I_\theta r^2/I_\theta$ known as the Rayleigh ratio — where I_θ is the intensity of the scattered and I_θ the incident, light; r is the distance from the scattering particle to the point of observation. By use of the so-called fluctuation theory of statistical mechanics whereby light scattering is treated as a consequence of random non-uniformities of concentration, and hence refractive index, arising from random molecular movement the following relationship between turbidity and molecular weight was derived by Debye in 1947:

$$HC/\tau = 1/M + 2BC \qquad (6.20)$$

C is the concentration of the solute and B an interaction constant allowing for non-ideality. H is an optical constant for a particular system depending on refractive index changes with concentration and the wavelength of light used. A plot of HC/τ against concentration results in a straight line of slope $2B$. The intercept on the HC/τ axis is $1/M$ allowing the molecular weight to be calculated.

Light scattering measurements are particularly suitable for finding the size of association colloids and the number of molecules of surface-active agent forming them and for the study of proteins and natural and synthetic polymers.

It can be shown that the intensity of the scattered light is inversely proportional to the wavelength λ of the light used; so that blue light ($\lambda \approx 450$ nm) is scattered much more than red light ($\lambda \approx 650$ nm). With incident white light, a scattering material will, therefore, tend to be blue when viewed at right angles to the incident beam and red when viewed from end on — evident in the blue colour of the sky, tobacco smoke etc., and the yellowish-red of the rising and setting sun.

Ultramicroscope

Colloidal particles are too small to be seen with an optical microscope. Light scattering is made use of in the ultramicroscope first developed by Zsigmondy, in which a cell containing the colloid is viewed against a dark background at right angles to an intense beam of incident light. The particles, which exhibit Brownian motion, appear as spots of light against the dark background. The ultramicroscope is used in the technique of microelectrophoresis for measuring particle charge.

Electron microscope

The electron microscope, capable of giving actual pictures of the particles, is used to observe the size, shape and structure of colloidal particles. The success of the electron microscope is due to its high resolving power, defined in terms of d, the smallest distance by which two objects are separated yet remain distinguishable. The smaller the wavelength of the radiation used the smaller is d and the greater the resolving power. An optical microscope, using visible light as its radiation source, gives a d of about 0.2 μm. The radiation source of the electron microscope is a beam of high energy electrons having wavelengths in the region of 0.01 nm, d is thus about 0.5 nm. The electron beams are focused using electromagnets and the whole system is under a high vacuum of about 10^{-5} to 10^{-6} mmHg to give the electrons a free path. With wavelengths of the order indicated the image cannot be viewed direct, so use is made of a fluorescent screen.

One big disadvantage of the electron microscope for viewing colloidal particles is that only dried samples can be examined. Consequently it gives no information on solvation or configuration in solution and the particles may be affected by sample preparation.

Electrical properties

Electrical properties of interfaces

Most surfaces acquire a surface electric charge when brought into contact with an aqueous medium, the principal charging mechanisms being as follows.

Ion dissolution   Ionic substances can acquire a surface charge by virtue of unequal dissolution of the oppositely charged ions of which they are composed, for example, silver iodide in a solution with excess $[I^-]$ the particles will carry a negative charge, but the charge will be positive if excess $[Ag^+]$ is present. Since the concentrations of Ag^+ and I^- determine the electric potential at the particle surface, they are termed potential determining ions. In a similar way H^+ and OH^- are potential determining ions for metal oxides and hydroxides such as magnesium and aluminium hydroxides.

Ionization   Here the charge is controlled by the ionization of surface groupings, examples include the model system of polystyrene latex which frequently has carboxylic acid groupings at the surface which ionize to give negatively charged particles. In a similar way acidic drugs such as ibuprofen and nalidixic acid also acquire a negative charge.

Amino acids and proteins acquire their charge mainly through the ionization of carboxyl and amino groups to give $-COO^-$ and NH_3^+ ions. The ionization of these groups and so the net molecular charge depends on the pH of the system. At low pH the protein will be positively charged $-NH_2 \rightarrow NH_3^+$ and at high pH, negatively charged, $-COOH \rightarrow COO^-$. At a certain definite pH, specific for each individual protein, the total number of positive charges will equal the total number of negative charges and the net charge will be zero. This pH is termed the isoelectric point of the protein. The protein is probably ionized at the isoelectric point, existing in the zwitterion form but the apparent charge is zero. This may be represented as follows:

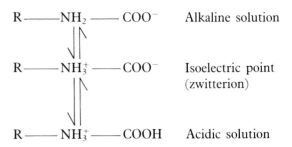

A protein is least soluble (the colloidal sol is least stable) at its isoelectric point and is readily desolvated by very water-soluble salts such as ammonium sulphate. Thus insulin may be precipitated from aqueous alcohol at pH 5.2.

Erythrocytes and bacteria usually acquire their charge by ionization of surface chemical groups such as sialic acid.

Ion adsorption   A net surface charge can be acquired by the unequal adsorption of oppositely charged ions. Surfaces in water are more often negatively charged than positively charged, because cations are generally more hydrated than anions and so the former have the greater tendency to reside in the bulk aqueous medium whereas the smaller, less hydrated and more polarizing anions have the greater tendency to reside at the particle surface. Surface-active agents, strongly adsorbed by the hydrophobic effect, will usually determine the surface charge when adsorbed.

The electrical double layer

Consider a solid charged surface in contact with an aqueous solution containing positive and negative ions. The surface charge influences the distribution of ions in the aqueous medium; ions, of opposite charge to that of the surface, termed counter ions, are attracted towards the surface, ions of like charge, termed co-ions, are repelled away from the surface. However, the distribution of the ions will also be affected by thermal agitation which will tend to redisperse the ions in solution. The result is the formation of an electric double layer made up of the charged surface and a neutralizing excess of counter ions over co-ions (the system must be electrically neutral) distribution in a diffuse manner in the aqueous medium.

The theory of the electrical double layer deals with this distribution of ions and hence with the magnitude of the electric potentials which occur in the locality of the charged surface. For a fuller explanation of what is a rather complicated mathematical approach the reader is referred to a textbook of colloid science (e.g. Shaw, 1980). A somewhat simplified picture of what pertains from the theories of Gouy, Chapman and Stern follows.

The double layer is divided into two parts (see Fig. 6.1(a)), the inner, which may include adsorbed ions, and the diffuse part where ions are distributed as influenced by electrical forces and random thermal motion. The two parts of the double layer are separated by a plane, the Stern plane, at about a hydrated ion radius from the surface, thus counter ions may be held at the surface by electrostatic attraction and the centre of these hydrated ions forms the Stern plane.

The potential changes linearly from ψ_0 (the surface potential) to ψ_δ (the Stern potential) in the Stern layer and decays exponentially from ψ_δ to zero in the diffuse double layer (Fig. 6.1(b)). A

plane of shear is also indicated in Fig. 6.1(a) and (b). In addition to ions in the Stern layer a certain amount of solvent will be bound to the ions and the charged surface. This solvating layer is held to the surface and the edge of the layer, termed the surface or plane of shear, represents the boundary of relative movement between the solid (and attached material) and the liquid. The potential at the plane of shear is termed the zeta, ζ, or electrokinetic, potential and its magnitude may be measured using microelectrophoresis or any other of the electrokinetic phenomena. The thickness of the solvating layer is ill-defined and the zeta potential therefore represents a potential at an unknown distance from the particle surface; its value, however, is usually taken as being slightly less than that of the Stern potential.

In the discussion above it was stated that the Stern plane existed at an hydrated ion radius from the particle surface; the hydrated ions are electrostatically attracted to the particle surface. It is possible for ions/molecules to be more strongly adsorbed at the surface — termed specific adsorption — than simple electrostatic attraction. In fact the specifically adsorbed ion/molecule may be uncharged as in the case with non-ionic surface-active agents. Surface-active ions specifically

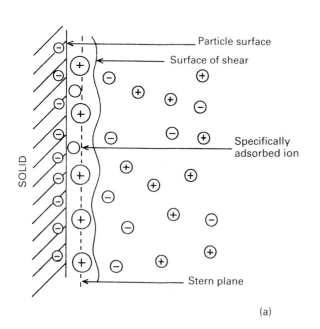

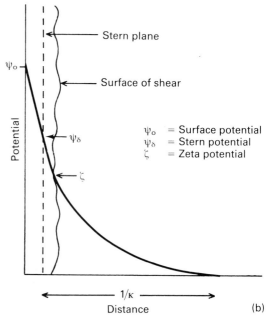

Fig. 6.1 The electric double layer: (a) schematic representation (b) changes in potential with distance from particle surface

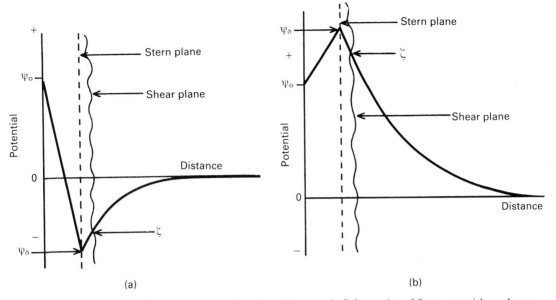

Fig. 6.2 Changes in potential with distance from solid surface: (a) reversal of charge sign of Stern potential ψ_δ, due to adsorption of surface-active or polyvalent counter ion, (b) increase in magnitude of Stern potential ψ_δ, due to adsorption of surface active co-ions

adsorb by the hydrophobic effect and can have a significant effect on the Stern potential causing ψ_0 and ψ_δ to have opposite signs as in Fig. 6.2(a) or for ψ_δ to have the same sign as ψ_0 but be greater in magnitude Fig. 6.2(b).

In Fig. 6.1(b) it is shown that the potential decays exponentially to zero with distance from the Stern plane, and the distance over which this occurs is $1/\kappa$, the Debye–Huckel length parameter known as the thickness of the electrical double layer. The parameter κ is dependent on the electrolyte concentration of the aqueous media (see Shaw, 1980 for details).

Increasing the electrolyte concentration means therefore that one is increasing the value of κ and consequently decreasing the value of $1/\kappa$, the thickness of the double layer, or as it is said one is 'compressing the double layer'; or the distance over which the potential decays exponentially is reduced. As ψ_δ stays constant this means that the zeta potential will be lowered.

As indicated earlier the effect of specifically adsorbed ions may be to lower the Stern potential and hence the zeta potential without compressing the double layer. Thus the zeta potential may be reduced by additives to the aqueous system in either (or both) of two different ways.

Electrokinetic phenomena

This is the general description applied to the phenomena which arise when attempts are made to shear off the mobile part of the electrical double layer from a charged surface. There are four such phenomena, namely, electrophoresis, sedimentation potential, streaming potential and electroosmosis. All of these electrokinetic phenomena may be used to measure the zeta potential but electrophoresis is the easiest to use and has the greatest pharmaceutical application.

Electrophoresis The movement of a charged particle (plus attached ions) relative to a stationary liquid under the influence of an applied electric field is termed electrophoresis. When the movement of the particles is observed with a microscope, or the movement of light spots scattered by particles too small to be observed with the microscope is observed using an ultramicroscope, this constitutes microelectrophoresis.

A microscope equipped with an eye piece graticule is used and the speed of movement of the particle under the influence of a known electric field is measured. This is the electrophoretic velocity, v, and the electrophoretic mobility, u, is given by

$$u = v/E \qquad (6.21)$$

where v is measured in m s^{-1}, and E, the applied field strength in V m^{-1}, so that u has the dimensions of m^2 s^{-1} V^{-1}. Typically a stable lyophobic colloidal particle may have an electrophoretic mobility of 4×10^{-8} m^2 s^{-1} V^{-1}. The equation used for converting the electrophoretic mobility, u, into the zeta potential depends on the value of κa (κ is the Debye–Huckel reciprocal length parameter described previously and a the particle radius). For values of $\kappa a > 100$ (as is the case for particles of radius 1 μm dispersed in 10^{-3} mol dm^{-3} sodium chloride solution) the Smoluchowski equation can be used:

$$u = \varepsilon \zeta/\eta \qquad (6.22)$$

Where ε is the permittivity and η the viscosity of the liquid used. For particles in water at 25 °C, $\zeta = 12.85 \times 10^{-5}\ u$ volts. So that for the mobility given above a zeta potential of 0.0514 volts or 51.4 millivolts is obtained. For values of $\kappa a < 100$ as complicated relationship which is a function of κa and the zeta potential is used (Wiersema et al., 1966).

The technique of microelectrophoresis finds application in the measurement of zeta potentials, of model systems (like polystyrene latex dispersions) to test colloid stability theory, of course dispersions (like suspensions and emulsions) to assess their stability, and in identification of charge groups and other surface characteristics of water-insoluble drugs and cells such as blood and bacteria.

Other electrokinetic phenomena The other electrokinetic phenomena are as follows: *sedimentation potential*, the reverse of electrophoresis, is the electric field created when particles sediment; *streaming potential*, the electric field created when liquid is made to flow along a stationary charged surface, e.g. a glass tube or a packed powder bed; and *electro-osmosis*, the opposite of streaming potential, the movement of liquid relative to a stationary charged surface, e.g. a glass tube, by an applied electric field.

Physical stability of colloidal systems

In colloidal dispersions, frequent encounters between the particles occur due to Brownian movement. Whether these collisions result in permanent contact of the particles (coagulation), when eventually the colloidal system will be destroyed as the large aggregates formed sediment out, or temporary contact (flocculation), or whether the particles rebound and remain freely dispersed (a stable colloidal system) depends on the forces of interaction between the particles. These forces can be divided into three groups: electrical forces of repulsion, forces of attraction and forces arising from solvation. An understanding of the first two explains the stability of lyophobic systems and all three lyophilic dispersions. Before considering the interaction of these forces it is necessary to define the terms *aggregation*, *coagulation* and *flocculation* as used in colloid science.

Aggregation is a general term signifying the collection of particles into groups.

Coagulation, from the latin coagulare, meaning to drive together, to compact, signifies that the particles are closely aggregated and difficult to redisperse — a primary minimum phenomenon of the DLVO theory of colloid stability (see next section).

Flocculation comes from the latin flocculare, meaning loose and woolly. Aggregates have an open structure in which the particles remain a small distance apart from one another. This may be a secondary minimum phenomenon (see the DLVO theory) or due to bridging by a polymer or polyelectrolyte as explained later in this section.

As a preliminary to discussion on the stability of colloidal dispersions a comparison of the general properties of lyophobic and lyophilic sols is given in Table 6.2.

Stability of lyophobic systems

DLVO theory In considering the interaction between two colloidal particles Derjaguin and Landau and independently, Verwey and Overbeek, in the 1940s produced a quantitative approach to the stability of hydrophobic sols. In what has come to be known as the *DLVO theory of colloid stability* they assumed that the only interactions involved are electrical repulsion, V_R, and van der Waals attraction, V_A, and that these parameters are additive. Therefore the total poten-

Table 6.2 Comparison of properties of lyophobic and lyophilic sols

Property	Lyophobic	Lyophilic
Effect of electrolytes	Very sensitive to added electrolyte leading to aggregation in an irreversible manner. Depends on: (a) type and valency of counter ion of electrolyte, e.g. with a negatively charged sol, $La^{3+} > Ba^{2+} > Na^+$. (b) Concentration of electrolyte. At a particular concentration sol passes from disperse to aggregated state. For the electrolyte types in (a) the concentrations are about 10^{-4}; 10^{-3}; 10^{-1} mol dm^{-3} respectively. These generalizations, (a) and (b), form what is known as the Schulze–Hardy rule	Dispersions are stable generally in the presence of electrolytes. May be salted out by high concentrations of very soluble electrolytes. Effect is due to desolvation of the lyophilic molecules and depends on the tendency of the electrolyte ions to become hydrated. Proteins more sensitive to electrolytes at their isoelectric points. Lyophilic colloids when salted out may appear as amorphous droplets known as a coacervate
Stability	Controlled by charge on particles	Controlled by charge and solvation of particles
Formation of dispersion	Dispersions usually of metals, inorganic crystals etc., with a high interfacial surface-free energy due to large increase in surface area on formation. A positive ΔG of formation, dispersion will never form spontaneously and is thermodynamically unstable. Particles of sol remain dispersed due to electrical repulsion	Generally proteins, macromolecules etc., which disperse spontaneously in a solvent. Interfacial free energy is low. There is a large increase in entropy when rigidly held chains of a polymer in the dry state unfold in solution. The free energy of formation is negative, a stable thermodynamic system.
Viscosity	Sols of low viscosity, particles unsolvated and usually symmetrical	Usually high, at sufficiently high concentration of disperse phase a gel may be formed. Particles solvated and usually asymmetric

tial energy of interaction V_T (expressed schematically in the curve shown in Fig. 6.3) is given by

$$V_T = V_A + V_R \qquad (6.23)$$

Repulsive forces between particles Repulsion between particles arises due to the osmotic effect produced by the increase in the number of charged species on overlap of the diffuse parts of

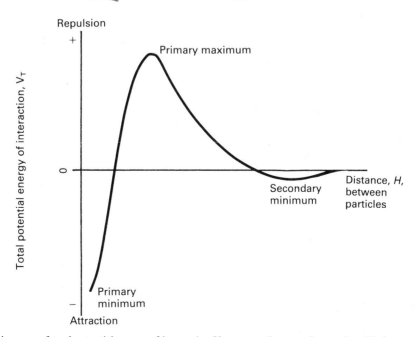

Fig. 6.3 Schematic curve of total potential energy of interaction V_T, versus distance of separation, H, for two particles. $V_T = V_R + V_A$

the electrical double layer. No simple equations can be given for repulsive interactions; however, it can be shown that the repulsive energy that exists between two spheres of equal but small surface potential is given by:

$$V_R = \frac{\varepsilon a \psi_0^2 \ln(1 + \exp^{-\kappa H})}{2} \qquad (6.24)$$

where ε is the permittivity of the polar liquid, a the radius of the spherical particle of surface potential ψ_0, κ is the Debye–Huckel reciprocal length parameter and H the distance between particles. An estimation of the surface potential can be obtained from zeta potential measurements. As can be seen the repulsion energy is an exponential function of the distance between the particles and has a range of the order of the thickness of the double layer.

Attractive forces between particles   The energy of attraction, V_A, arises from van der Waals universal forces of attraction, the so-called dispersion forces, the major contribution to which are the electromagnetic attractions described by London in 1930. For an assembly of molecules dispersion forces are additive summation leading to long range attraction between colloidal particles. As a result of the work of de Boer and Hamaker in 1936 it can be shown that the attractive interaction between spheres of the same radius, a, is given by:

$$V_A = \frac{-Aa}{12\,H} \qquad (6.25)$$

where A is the Hamaker constant for the particular material derived from London dispersion forces. The energy of attraction varies as the inverse of the distance between particles.

Total potential energy of interaction   Consideration of the curve, total potential energy of interaction V_T, versus distance between particles, H, Fig. 6.3, shows that attraction predominates at small distances, hence the very deep primary minimum, and at large interparticle distances. Here the secondary minimum arises because the fall off in repulsive energy with distance is more rapid than that of attractive energy. At intermediate distances double layer repulsion may predominate giving a primary maximum in the curve, if this maximum is large compared with the

thermal energy kT of the particles the colloidal system should be stable, i.e. the particles stay dispersed. Otherwise the interacting particles will reach the energy depth of the primary minimum and irreversible aggregation, i.e., coagulation occurs. If the secondary minimum is smaller than kT the particles will not aggregate but will always repel one another, but if significantly larger than kT a loose assemblage of particles will form which can be easily redispersed by shaking, i.e. flocculation occurs.

The depth of the secondary minimum depends on particle size and particles may need to be of radius 1 μm or greater before the attractive force is sufficiently great for flocculation to occur.

The height of the primary maximum energy barrier to coagulation depends upon the magnitude of V_R, which is dependent on ψ_0 and hence the zeta potential and in addition on electrolyte concentration via κ, the Debye–Huckel reciprocal length parameter. Addition of electrolyte compresses the double layer and reduces the zeta potential: this has the effect of lowering the primary maximum and deepening the secondary minimum (see Fig. 6.4). This latter means that there will be an increased tendency for particles to flocculate in the secondary minimum and is the principle of the *controlled flocculation* approach to pharmaceutical suspension formulation described later.

The primary maximum may also be lowered (and the secondary minimum deepened) by adding substances, such as ionic surface-active agents, which are specifically adsorbed within the Stern layer. Here ψ_δ is reduced and hence the zeta potential; the double layer is usually not compressed.

Stability of lyophilic systems

Solutions of macromolecules, lyophilic colloidal sols, are stabilized by a combination of electrical double layer interaction and solvation and both of these stabilizing factors must be sufficiently weakened before attraction predominates and the colloidal particles coagulate. For example gelatin has a sufficiently strong affinity for water to be soluble even at its isoelectric pH where there is no double layer interaction.

Hydrophilic colloids are unaffected by the small

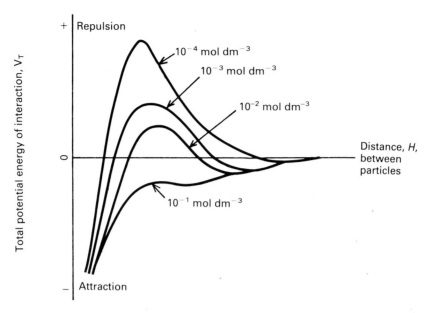

Fig. 6.4 Schematic curves of total potential energy of interaction V_T, versus distance of separation, H, showing the effect of adding electrolyte at constant surface potential

amounts of added electrolyte which cause hydrophobic sols to coagulate; however, when the concentration of electrolyte is high, particularly with an electrolyte whose ions become strongly hydrated, the colloidal material loses its water of solvation to these ions and coagulates, i.e. a 'salting out' effect occurs.

Variation in the degree of solvation of different hydrophilic colloids affects the concentration of soluble electrolyte required to produce their coagulation and precipitation. The components of a mixture of hydrophilic colloids can therefore be separated by a process of fractional precipitation, which involves the 'salting' out of the various components at different concentrations of electrolyte. This technique is used in the purification of antitoxins.

Lyophilic colloids can be considered to become lyophobic by the addition of solvents such as acetone and alcohol. The particles become desolvated and are then very sensitive to precipitation by added electrolyte.

Coacervation and microencapsulation Coacervation is the separation from a lyophilic sol, on addition of another substance, of a colloid-rich layer present in the form of an amorphous liquid. This constitutes the coacervate.

Simple coacervation may be brought about by a 'salting out' effect on addition of electrolyte or addition of a non-solvent. Complex coacervation occurs when two oppositely charged lyophilic colloids are mixed, e.g. gelatin and acacia. Gelatin at a pH below its isoelectric point is positively charged, acacia above about pH 3 negatively charged; a combination of solutions at about pH 4 results in coacervation. Any large ions of opposite charge, for example cationic surface-active agents (positively charged) and dyes used for colouring aqueous mixtures (negatively charged), may react in a similar way.

If the coacervate is formed in a stirred suspension of an insoluble solid the macromolecular material will surround the solid particles. The coated particles can be separated and dried and this technique forms the basic of one method of microencapsulation. A number of drugs including aspirin have been coated in this manner. The coating protects the drug from chemical attack and microcapsules may be given orally to prolong the action of the medicament.

Effect of addition of macromolecular material to lyophobic colloidal sols When added in small amounts many polyelectrolyte and polymer molecules (lyophilic colloids) can adsorb simul-

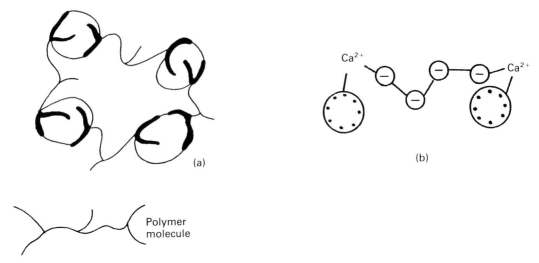

Fig. 6.5 Diagram of flocs formed (a) by polymer bridging and (b) polyelectrolyte bridging in the presence of divalent ions of opposite charge

taneously on to two particles and are long enough to bridge across the energy barrier between the particles. This can even occur with neutral polymers when the lyophobic particles have a high zeta potential (and would thus be considered a stable sol). A structured floc results (Fig. 6.5(a)).

With polyelectrolytes, where the particles and polyelectrolyte have the same sign, flocculation can often occur when divalent and trivalent ions are added to the system (Fig. 6.5(b)). These complete the 'bridge' and only very low concentrations of these ions are needed. Use is made of this property of small quantities of polyelectrolytes and polymers in removing colloidal material, resulting from sewage, in water purification.

On the other hand if larger amounts of polymer are added, sufficient to cover the surface of the particles, then a lyophobic sol may be stabilized to coagulation by added electrolyte — the so-called steric stabilization or protective colloid effect.

Steric stabilization (protective colloid action)

It has been known for a long time that non-ionic polymeric material such as gums, non-ionic surface-active agents and methylcellulose adsorbed at the particle surface can stabilize a lyophobic sol to coagulation even in the absence of a significant zeta potential. The approach of two particles, with adsorbed polymer layers, results in a steric interaction when the layers overlap leading to repulsion. In general the particles do not approach each other closer than about twice the thickness of the adsorbed layer and hence passage into the primary minimum is inhibited. An additional term has thus to be included in the potential energy of interaction for what is called steric stabilization, V_S, the older term being protective colloid action:

$$V_T = V_A + V_R + V_S \qquad (6.26)$$

The effect of V_S on the potential energy against distance between particles curve is seen in Fig. 6.6, showing that repulsion is generally seen at all shorter distances provided that the adsorbed polymeric material does not move from the particle surface.

One can explain steric repulsion by reference to the free energy changes which take place when two polymer covered particles interact. Free energy, enthalpy and entropy changes are related according to the Gibbs–Helmholtz equation:

$$\Delta G = \Delta H - T\Delta S \qquad (6.27)$$

The second law of thermodynamic implies that a positive value of ΔG is necessary for dispersion stability, a negative value indicating that the particles have aggregated.

A positive value of ΔG can arise in a number of ways, as when ΔH and ΔS are both negative

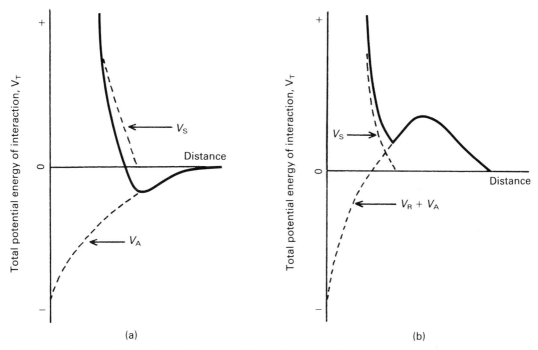

Fig. 6.6 Schematic curves of the total potential energy of interaction versus distance for two particles, showing the effect of the steric stabilization term V_S: (a) in the absence of electrostatic repulsion, the solid line representing $V_T = V_A + V_S$, (b) in the presence of electrostatic repulsion, the solid line representing $V_T = V_R + V_A + V_s$

but $T\Delta S > \Delta H$. Here the effect of the entropy change opposes aggregation and outweighs the enthalpy term; this is termed *entropic stabilization*. Interpenetration and compression of the polymer chains decreases the entropy as these chains become more ordered. Such a process is not spontaneous: 'work' must be expended to interpenetrate and compress any polymer chains existing between the colloidal particles and this work is a reflection of the repulsive potential energy. The enthalpy of mixing of these polymer chains will also be negative. Stabilization by these effects occurs in non-aqueous dispersions.

Again, a positive ΔG occurs if both ΔH and ΔS are positive but $\Delta H > T\Delta S$. Here enthalpy aids stabilization, entropy aids aggregation. Consequently this effect is termed enthalpic stabilization and is common with aqueous dispersions, particularly where the stabilizing polymer has polyoxyethylene chains. Such chains are hydrated in aqueous solution due to H-bonding between water molecules and the 'ether oxygens' of the ethylene oxide groups. The water molecules have thus become more structured and

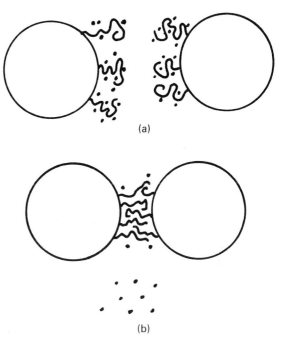

Fig. 6.7 Enthalpic stabilization: (a) particles with stabilizing polyoxyethylene chains and H-bonded water molecules, (b) stabilizing chains overlap, water molecules released $\rightarrow + \Delta H$

lost degrees of freedom. When interpenetration and compression of ethylene oxide chains occurs there is an increased probability of contact between ethylene oxide groups resulting in some of the bound water molecules being released (see Fig. 6.7). The released water molecules have greater degrees of freedom than those in the bound state. For this to occur they must be supplied with energy, obtained from heat absorption, i.e. there is a positive enthalpy change. Although there is a decrease in entropy in the interaction zone as with entropic stabilization this is over-ridden by the increase in the configurational entropy of the released water molecules.

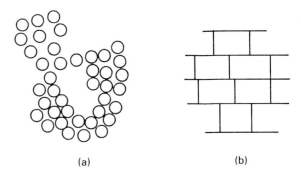

Fig. 6.8 Gel structure: (a) flocculated lyophobic sol, e.g. aluminium hydroxide, (b) 'card house' floc of clays, e.g. bentonite

GELS

The majority of gels are formed by aggregation of colloidal sol particles, the solid or semisolid system so formed being interpenetrated by a liquid. The particles link together to form an interlaced network thus imparting rigidity to the structure, the continuous phase is held within the meshes. This type of structure is supported by the fact that only a small percentage of disperse phase is required to impart rigidity, for example 1% of agar in water produces a firm gel. Further, diffusion of non-electrolytes in, and the electrical conductivity of, dilute gels are the same as the continous phase.

A gel rich in liquid may be called a jelly; if the liquid is removed and only the gel framework remains this is termed a xerogel. Sheet gelatin, acacia tears and tragacanth flakes are all xerogels.

Types of gel

Gels may be flocculated lyophobic sols where the gel can be looked upon as a continuous floccule (Fig. 6.8(a)). Examples are aluminium hydroxide and magnesium hydroxide gels.

Clays such as bentonite, aluminium magnesium silicate (Veegum) and to some extent kaolin form gels by flocculation in a special manner. Only a simplified general explanation of gel formation by clays can be given. They are hydrated aluminium (aluminium/magnesium) silicates whose crystal structure is such that they exist as flat plates, the flat part or 'face' of the particle carries a negative charge due to O^- atoms and the edge of the plate a positive charge due to Al^{3+}/Mg^{2+} atoms. As a result of electrostatic attraction between the face and edge of different particles a gel structure is built up, forming what is usually known as a 'card house floc' (Fig. 6.8(b)).

The forces holding the particles together in this type of gel are relatively weak — van der Waals forces in the secondary minimum flocculation of aluminium hydroxide, electrostatic attraction in the case of the clays — because of this these gels show the phenomenon of *thixotropy*, a non-chemical isothermal gel–sol–gel transformation. If a thixotropic gel is sheared (for example by simple shaking) these weak bonds are broken and a lyophobic sol is formed. On standing the particles collide, flocculation occurs and the gel is reformed. Flocculation in gels is the reason for their anomalous rheological properties (Chapter 2). This phenomenon of thixotropy is made use of in formulation of pharmaceutical suspensions, e.g. bentonite in calamine lotion and in the paint industry.

On the other hand lyophilic sols form gels in a different manner. The macromolecules may form a network simply by entanglement. e.g. tragacanth and methylcellulose, or by attraction between molecules such as hydrogen bonds or van der Waal's forces. An increase in temperature often breaks these weak bonds causing liquefaction of the gel. Systems that exhibit this type of transition such as agar and gelatin gels, are termed thermal gels. Gels often contract spontaneously and exude some of the fluid medium. This effect is known as *syneresis* and is thought to be due to an increase in the number of bonding points, resulting in a coarsening of the matrix structure and consequent expression of liquid from the gel.

The cross-binding of macromolecules by primary valency bonds provides a further mechanism for the formation of a gel network and here the gelling process is irreversible. This behaviour is exhibited by silica gel where silicic acid molecules are linked into a three-dimensional network by Si–O bonds. Silica gel has a great affinity for water and is used as a drying agent.

Applications

Mineral oils may be gelled by warming with the insoluble soap aluminium monostearate. Heat energy appears necessary for the molecules to orientate themselves into a gel structure. Such gels are used to suspend medicaments in oily injections. Liquid paraffin gelled similarly with polythene forms a proprietary ointment base. Other organic liquids may be gelled with aluminium monostearate and this forms the basis of a method of preparation of a slow release medicament. Particles of drug are suspended in a volatile solvent, aluminium monostearate is added and the mixture warmed to produce a gel the matrix of which enmeshes the drug particles. The solvent is then evaporated and the dry gel broken up into granules which contain particles of the drug suitable for tablet making. The gel particles provide water resistant barriers on exposure to the fluid of the gastrointestinal tract and hence slow the release of the drug.

SURFACE-ACTIVE AGENTS

Surface-active agents, or surfactants, are substances that alter the conditions prevailing at an interface, causing, for example, a marked decrease in the surface tension of water. These substances are of importance in a wide variety of fields as emulsifying agents, detergents, solubilizing agents, wetting agents, foaming and antifoaming agents, flocculants and deflocculants, and in drug stability and drug absorption.

All surfactants are characterized by having two regions in their molecular structure:

1 a lyophobic (or hydrophobic) group, such as a hydrocarbon chain, that has no affinity for aqueous solvents, and
2 a lyophilic (or hydrophilic) group that has an affinity for water.

To have such an affinity the group must possess an appreciable polar character, e.g. an ion or group with a large permanent dipole. A molecule or ion that possesses this type of structure is termed amphipathic.

Surface-active agents may be classified according to the nature of the ionic type of the hydrophilic group and various examples of the different classes are shown in Table 6.3.

A wide variety of drugs have also been reported to be surface active, this surface activity being a consequence of the amphipathic nature of the drugs. The hydrophobic portions of the drug molecules are usually more complex than those of the surface-active agents described being composed of aromatic or heterocyclic ring systems. Examples include drugs such as chlorpromazine and imipramine which have tricyclic ring systems; diphenhydramine and orphenadrine which are based on a diphenylmethane group; and tetrocaine and mepyramine which have a hydrophobic group composed of a single phenyl ring.

The dual nature of the structure possessed by surfactants is responsible for their characteristic properties. Thus in dilute aqueous solution the molecules tend to orientate themselves at the air/water interface in such a way as to remove the hydrophobic group from the aqueous phase, and hence achieve a minimum free energy state. However, at certain well defined concentrations, specific for any surfactant and depending on structural characteristics, relatively sharp changes occur in the physical properties of these solutions. These changes are attributed to the association of the amphipathic molecules into aggregates of colloidal dimensions known as micelles.

Ionic and non-ionic substances that exhibit this

Table 6.3 Classification of surface-active agents

	Hydrophobic	Hydrophilic
Anionic		
Sodium dodecanoate	$CH_3(CH_2)_{10}$———COO^-Na^+	
Sodium dodecyl (lauryl) sulphate	$CH_3(CH_2)_{11}$———$SO_4^-Na^+$	
Sodium dioctyl sulphosuccinate	$CH_3(CH_2)_7.OOC.CHSO_3^-Na^+$	
	$CH_3(CH_2)_7.OOC.CH_2$	
Cationic		
Hexadecyl trimethyl ammonium bromide (Cetrimide)	$CH_3(CH_2)_{15}$—N^+-CH_3Br^-	
Dodecyl pyridinium iodide	$CH_3(CH_2)_{11}$——— N^+Br^-	
Non-ionic		
Hexaoxyethylene monohexadecyl ether	$CH_3(CH_2)_{15}$———$(OCH_2CH_2)_6OH$	
Polyoxyethylene sorbitan mono-oleate (polysorbate 80)	$C_{17}H_{33}$———COO-CH_2	
	$HO(OCH_2CH_2)_n$ $(CH_2CH_2O)_nOH$	
	$(CH_2CH_2O)_nOH$	
Sorbitan mono-oleate	$C_{17}H_{33}$———$COOCH_2$	
Ampholytic		
N-dodecyl alanine	$CH_3(CH_2)_{11}$———$\overset{+}{N}H_2.CH_2.CH_2.COO^-$	
Lecithin	$C_{17}H_{35}$—$COO.CH_2$	
	$C_{17}H_{35}$—$COO.CH$	
	CH_2-O-$\overset{\bar{O}}{\underset{O}{P}}$.$(CH_2)_3.\overset{+}{N}(CH_3)_3$	

type of behaviour are referred to collectively as *association colloids*. Although the older term 'colloidal electrolyte' is strictly applicable to all ionized colloidal materials it is usually reserved for ionic association colloids. Since the early work in this field was carried out solely on ionic association colloids the term 'colloidal electrolyte' is still sometimes used erroneously as a synonym for all association colloids.

Micellization

As mentioned earlier surfactants in dilute aqueous solution orientate themselves at the air/water interface but, as the concentration of surfactant increases the molecules also aggregate together to form micelles. The primary reason that this occurs is the attainment of a state of minimum free energy. The free energy, enthalpy and entropy changes in a system are related by

$$\Delta G = \Delta H - T\Delta S$$

and, for surfactant solution systems, the entropy term is by far the most important in determining free energy changes.

The explanation most generally accepted for the entropy change is concerned with the structure of water. Water possesses a relatively high degree of structure due to hydrogen bonding between adjacent molecules. If an ionic or strongly polar solute is added to water it will disrupt this structure but the solute molecules can form hydrogen bonds with the water molecules which more than compensates for the disruption or distortion of the bonds existing in pure water. Ionic and polar materials thus tend to be easily soluble in water. No such compensation occurs with non-polar groups and their solution in water is accordingly resisted, the water molecules forming extra structured clusters around the non-polar region. This increase in structure of the water molecules leads to a negative entropy change and results in the withdrawal of the hydrophobic groups from the water. Surface-active agents, because of their dual hydrophilic/hydrophobic structure, should and do have a measurable solubility in water depending on whether or not the polar group with its hydrogen bonding to the water molecules is sufficient to overcome the repulsive effect of the water molecules around the hydrophobic group.

From a thermodynamic point of view, however, the outstanding feature of the process of dissolving a surface-active agent in water is this large negative entropy change which is intimately related to the structuring of water around the hydrophobic portion of the molecule. To counteract this, and achieve a state of minimum free energy, the hydrophobic groups tend to withdraw from the aqueous phase. This may occur by the molecules orientating themselves at the interface with the hydrocarbon chain away from the aqueous phase, i.e., the molecules collect at air/water, oil/water and solid/water interfaces. However, as the concentration is increased, this method of free energy reduction becomes inadequate, and at a certain concentration, the *critical micelle concentration* (abbreviated CMC), the surfactant molecules may also achieve segregation of their hydrophobic portions from the solvent by self-aggregation. These aggregates are *micelles*. When the hydrophobic part of the surface-active agent is a hydrocarbon chain the micelles will consist of a hydrocarbon core with polar groups at the surface serving to maintain solubility in water.

This tendency for hydrophobic materials to be removed from water due to the strong attraction of water molecules for each other and not for the hydrophobic solute, has been termed hydrophobic bonding. However, because there is in fact no

actual bonding between the hydrophobic groups the phenomenon is best described as the hydrophobic effect.

As the hydrophobic effect is due to the entropy changes associated with the structuring of water molecules around the hydrophobic group of the surface-active molecule it follows that as the length of this group increases there will be a greater entropy increase when it leaves the aqueous phase, i.e. the longer the hydrocarbon chain of a surfactant the more energetically favourable it is for such a molecule to be adsorbed at an interface or form a micelle.

There will be a similar entropy increase when a hydrocarbon chain is adsorbed at a solid hydrophobic surface, such as is present with many drugs. The same occurs at cell membranes, and it is not difficult to appreciate that surfactants can alter the characteristics of such membranes as bacterial cell walls or that of the gastrointestinal tract. Further, for exactly the same reasons, phospholipid molecules form themselves into layered structures, larger than micelles, termed liposomes.

Liposomes are liquid crystalline spherules formed when phospholipids are allowed to swell in aqueous media. They consist of concentric lipid bilayers alternating with aqueous compartments. The hydrocarbon chains are directed inwards in the structure away from the water for the same reason that micelles form. Lipid- and water-soluble substances can be trapped within the lipid or aqueous phase of the liposome respectively and give this structure possibilities as a drug delivery system.

An alternative explanation for the free energy decrease associated with micellization considers the increase in freedom of movement of the hydrocarbon chains, which occurs when these chains are transferred from the aqueous environment (where their movement is restrained by the structured water molecules) to the interior of the micelle, to be the important factor.

It should be emphasized that micelles are in dynamic equilibrium with monomer molecules in solution, continuously breaking down and reforming. It is this factor that distinguishes micelles from other colloidal particles and the reason why they are called association colloids.

The formation of micelles was originally

suggested by McBain in 1913 to explain the apparently anomalous changes in osmotic properties and electrical conductivity with concentration in solutions of potassium stearate. The osmotic activity and conductance were lower than expected as a certain concentration was reached. McBain's interpretation was for association of the molecules into large units called micelles but he postulated the existence of two types of micelle, one ionized and one neutral, to allow for the fall in conductivity.

Later, Hartley (1935) suggested that the experimental facts could be explained on the basis of a single type of spherical micelle composed of 50–100 units (see Fig. 6.9). Some counter ions will be attracted close to the micelle thus reducing the overall charge. The radius of the micelle will be slightly less than that of the extended hydrocarbon chain with the interior core of the micelle having the properties of a liquid hydrocarbon. He also postulated that once the CMC is reached further addition of material all goes to form micelles, that is, the concentration of monomeric surface-active agent remains constant above the CMC.

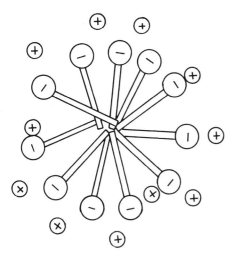

Fig. 6.9 Schematic diagram of the Hartley spherical micelle

The spherical micelle is now accepted as the most probable form existing in solutions above the CMC. However, as concentration is increased physical measurements, e.g. X-ray diffraction, viscosity, proton and deuterium magnetic resonance studies, indicate association of molecules in different ways forming cylindrical, lamellar and other structures.

With ionic surface-active agents repulsion between adjacent charged head groups tends to oppose micelle formation. It is for this reason that non-ionic surfactants form micelles at considerably lower concentrations.

Physical properties of surface-active agent solutions

Surface properties

Surface-active molecules in aqueous solution orientate themselves at the surface in such a way as to remove the hydrophobic group from the aqueous phase and hence achieve a minimum free energy state. As a result some of the water molecules at the surface are replaced by non-polar groups. The attractive forces between these groups and the water molecules, or between the groups themselves, are less than those existing between water molecules. The contracting power of the surface is thus reduced and so therefore is the surface tension. The adsorbed molecules can be looked upon as forming a bridge between the phases. The surface tension versus concentration curve for an aqueous solution of a surface-active agent thus shows a progressive decrease in surface tension until the CMC is reached. At this stage any additional surfactant goes to form micelles and the surface tension remains approximately constant beyond the CMC (Fig. 6.10). A minimum is frequently observed in the surface tension curve shown by the dotted curve in Fig. 6.10. Such minima are caused by the presence of surface-active impurities in the system, e.g. dodecanol present in sodium dodecyl (lauryl) sulphate. The initial adsorption into the surface layers of the surface-active agent of the impurity results in the lowering of the surface tension to a greater degree than that given by the pure surface-active agent. At the CMC the impurity is *solubilized* (see later in this chapter) by the micelles so that the surface tension rises to that of the pure surface-active agent beyond its CMC.

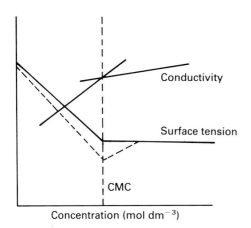

Fig. 6.10 Diagram of variation of conductivity and surface tension with concentration of an ionic surface-active agent such as sodium dodecyl sulphate

Electrical conductivity

The effect of micelle formation on the electrical conductivity of solutions of surface-active agents is also shown in Fig. 6.10. A number of factors contribute to the changes found.

The movement of ions towards an electrode is retarded by the viscous drag exerted on the charged particle by the solvent. There is actually a reduction in this viscous drag on micellization, e.g. a micelle formed of 100 monomers experiences less viscous drag than the total drag experienced by 100 individual monomers. The total charge on the micelle is the same as that of the constituent monomers so that this reduction in viscous drag should lead to increased conductance.

This, however, ignores the effect of the counter ions. First, the ionic atmosphere of opposite charge to the micelle exerts a braking effect due to relaxation (attraction between the charged micelle and the oppositely charged ions when these charged species move in opposite directions) and retardation (the counter ions, as they move, carry water molecules with them so that there is fluid flow counter to the movement of the micelle) effects. Second, due to the high charge and size of the micelle, some of the counter ions are bound to it, and move with it, thus travelling in a direction opposite to their normal direction of movement. These bound counter ions also reduce the effective charge on the micelle.

The counter ion effects cause a reduction in conductance and outweigh the reduction in viscous drag giving an overall fall of conductance on micellization. However, if a very high field strength is applied these counter ion effects can be removed and the expected increase in conductance occurs (the Wien effect).

Solubility; the Krafft point

The solubility behaviour of surface-active agents is anomalous in that as the temperature is increased a value is reached at which the material becomes highly soluble. If the CMC values for different temperatures are plotted on the same graph, it can be seen that at a particular temperature the solubility and CMC curves intersect. This temperature is the Krafft point and is characteristic for any particular surface-active agent. At temperatures below the Krafft point micelles will not form. It is therefore often necessary to use heat to get a surface-active agent into solution (the Krafft point for hexadecyltrimethyl ammonium bromide (cetrimide) is about 30 °C). Once the surface-active agent is in solution it may normally be cooled to room temperature without precipitation occurring.

Light scattering

The scattering of light by solutions of surface-active agents is increased by the aggregation of molecules into micelles. The slope of the graph of turbidity versus concentration therefore shows an abrupt increase at the CMC (Fig. 6.11(a)).

By use of Eqn 6.20 it is possible to obtain the micellar molecular weight and thus the number of monomer units forming the micelle.

Reference to Fig. 6.11(a) shows that the scattering due to micelles is $\tau - \tau_o$ whilst the concentration of surfactant present as micelles is $C - C_o$. Eqn 6.20 thus becomes

$$\frac{H(C - C_o)}{\tau - \tau_o} = 1/M_{\text{micelle}} + 2B(C - C_o) \qquad (6.28)$$

A plot of this equation (Fig. 6.11(b)) enables the micellar molecular weight to be evaluated.

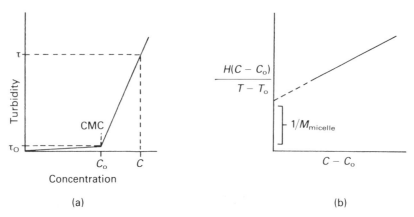

Fig. 6.11 Light scattering by solutions of surface-active agents: (a) turbidity versus concentration, (b) plot of the modified Debye equation for estimation of micellar size

Other methods of determining CMCs

Most physical properties change at the CMC and may be used to measure the magnitude of this concentration. At least 30 have been listed including, as well as those detailed above, all colligative properties, refractive index, viscosity and dye solubilization. In the latter case use is made of a solid dyestuff that is virtually insoluble in water, such as Orange OT. The amount of dyestuff in solution remains reasonably constant until the CMC is reached and then increases rapidly.

Solubilization

As mentioned previously the interior core of a micelle can be considered as having the properties of a liquid hydrocarbon and is thus capable of dissolving materials that are soluble in such liquids. This process whereby water-insoluble or partly soluble substances are brought into aqueous solution in quite high concentration is termed solubilization.

It was recognized early that the phenomenon of solubilization is connected in some way with the existence of micelles as solubilization does not occur until micelles are formed. Above the CMC the amount of substance solubilized (the solubilizate) increases as surfactant concentration increases, i.e. as the number of micelles increased.

The site of incorporation of the solubilizate is believed to be closely related to its chemical nature. Thus, it is generally accepted that non-polar solubilizates, e.g. aliphatic hydrocarbons, are dissolved in the hydrocarbon core of the micelle ((i) in Fig. 6.12(a)). Solubility of such a solubilizate should increase as the concentration of surface-active agent increases so that Hartley found that the solubility of *trans* azobenzene in the hydrocarbon interior of micelles of cetyl (hexadecyl) pyridinium chloride was quite close to its solubility in *n*-hexadecane. Water-insoluble compounds containing polar groups are orientated with the polar group at the surface of the ionic micelle amongst the micellar head groups and the hydrophobic group inside the hydrocarbon core of the micelle, the position of the molecule depending on the strength of the polar group, e.g. salicylic acid and naphthalene ((ii) and (iii) respectively in Fig. 6.12(a).

Solubilization in non-ionic polyoxyethylated surface-active agents can occur in the ethylene oxide shell which surrounds the core; thus *p*-hydroxy benzoic acid is entirely within this region hydrogen bonded to the ethylene oxide groups ((iv) in Fig. 6.12(b)) whilst esters such as the parabens are located at the shell core junction ((v) in Fig. 6.12(b)). Spectroscopic evidence for such orientations has been found by a number of research workers.

One method of determining the amount of solubilizate that will dissolve in a surface-active agent is to prepare a series of tubes of fixed concentration. Increasing amounts of solubilizate are added to the tubes which are then shaken to

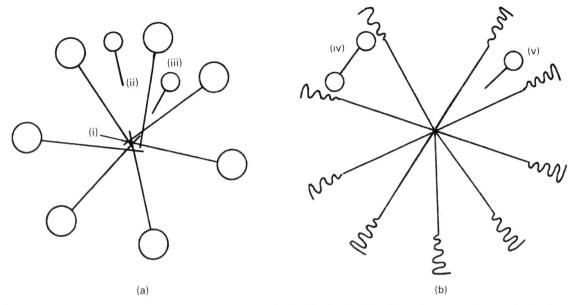

Fig. 6.12 Solubilization in micelles of (a) ionic and (b) non-ionic polyethoxylated surface active agents. See text for details

equilibrate. The maximum concentration of solubilizate forming a clear solution can then be determined visually or from turbidity measurements on the solutions.

Solubility data are expressed as solubility curves or, preferably, as ternary phase diagrams, the latter completely describing the effect of varying the composition of any of the three components of the system. The use of ternary diagrams is described briefly in Chapter 14. For a detailed explanation of the use of such diagrams and of the phenomenon of solubilization the reader is referred to the review by Elworthy *et al.* (1968).

Applications of solubilization

The principle of solubilization is used in the formulation of a large number of drugs. This is discussed in Chapter 14.

Whilst solubilization is an excellent means of producing an aqueous solution of a water-insoluble drug, it should be realized that it may well have effects on the drug's activity and absorption characteristics. As a generalization it may be said that low concentrations of surface-active agents increase absorption, possibly due to enhanced contact of the drug with the absorbing membrane, whilst concentrations above the CMC either produce no additional effect or cause decreased absorption. In the latter case the drug may be held within the micelles so that the concentration available for absorption is reduced. For a survey of this rather complex topic the review by Elworthy *et al.* (1968) should be consulted.

Solubilization and drug stability

Solubilization has been shown to have a modifying effect on the rate of hydrolysis of drugs. Nonpolar compounds solubilized deep in the hydrocarbon core of a micelle are likely to be better protected against attack by hydrolysing species than more polar compounds located closer to be micellar surface. Thus, Sheth and Parrott (1967) found that the alkaline hydrolysis of benzocaine and homatropine in the presence of several nonionic surfactants was retarded. The less polar benzocaine showed a greater increase in stability, compared to homatropine, because of its deeper penetration into the micelle.

An important factor in considering the breakdown of a drug located close to the micellar surface is the ionic nature of the surface-active agent. For base-catalysed hydrolysis anionic micelles should give an enhanced protection due to repulsion of the attacking OH^- group. For cationic micelles there should be the converse effect. Whilst this pattern has been found, enhanced protection by cationic micelles also occurs, suggesting that in these cases the positively charged polar head groups hold the OH^- groups and thus block their penetration into the micelle.

Protection from oxidative degradation has also been found with solubilized systems.

As indicated earlier drugs may be surface active. Such drugs form micelles and this self-association has been found to increase the drug's stability. Thus micellar solutions of penicillin G have been reported to be 2.5 times as stable as monomeric solutions under conditions of constant pH and ionic strength.

Detergency

Detergency is a complex process whereby surfactants are used for the removal of foreign matter from solid surfaces, be it removal of dirt from clothes or cleansing of body surfaces. The process includes many of the actions characteristic of specific surfactants. Thus the surfactant must have good wetting characteristics so that the detergent can come into intimate contact with the surface to be cleaned. The detergent must have the ability to remove the dirt into the bulk of the liquid; the dirt/water and solid/water interfacial tensions are lowered and thus the work of adhesion between the dirt and solid is reduced, so that the dirt particle may be easily detached. Once removed, the surfactant can be adsorbed at the particle surface creating charge and hydration barriers which prevent deposition. If the dirt is oily it may be emulsified or solubilized.

COARSE DISPERSE SYSTEMS
SUSPENSIONS

A pharmaceutical suspension is a coarse dispersion in which insoluble particles, generally greater than 1 μm in diameter, are dispersed in a liquid medium, usually aqueous.

An aqueous suspension is a useful formulation system for administering an insoluble or poorly soluble drug. The large surface area of dispersed drug ensures a high availability for dissolution and hence absorption. Aqueous suspensions may also be used for parenteral and ophthalmic use and provide a suitable form for the applications of dermatological materials to the skin. Suspensions are used similarly in veterinary practice and a closely allied field is that of pest control. Pesticides are frequently presented as suspensions for use as fungicides, insecticides, ascaricides and herbicides.

An acceptable suspension possesses certain desirable qualities among which are the following: the suspended material should not settle too rapidly; the particles which do settle to the bottom of the container must not form a hard mass but should be readily dispersed into a uniform mixture when the container is shaken; and the suspension must not be too viscous to pour freely from the orifice of the bottle or to flow through a syringe needle.

Physical stability of a pharmaceutical suspension may be defined as the condition in which the particles do not aggregate and in which they remain uniformly distributed throughout the dispersion. Since this ideal situation is seldom realized it is appropriate to add that if the particles do settle they should be easily resuspended by a moderate amount of agitation.

The major difference between a pharmaceutical suspension and a colloidal dispersion is one of size of dispersed particles, with the relatively large particles of a suspension liable to sedimentation due to gravitational forces. Apart from this, suspensions show most of the properties of colloidal systems. The reader is referred to Chapter 15 for a detailed account of the formulation of suspensions.

The controlled flocculation approach to suspension formulation

A pharmaceutical suspension which would be thought of as a stable dispersion if considered in terms of the DLVO theory of colloid stability will be deflocculated (the individual solid particles will remain discrete) but will sediment due to the size of the particles. The electrical repulsive forces between the particles will enable them to slip past one another to form a close packed arrangement at the bottom of the container with the small particles filling the voids between the larger ones. The supernatant liquid may remain cloudy after sedimentation due to the presence of colloidal particles which will remain dispersed. Those particles lowermost in the sediment are gradually pressed together by the weight of the ones above. The repulsive barrier is thus overcome, allowing the particles to pass into close contact with each other. Physical bonding leading to 'cake' or 'clay' formation may then occur due to the formation of bridges between the particles resulting from crystal growth and hydration effects, forces greater than agitation usually being required to disperse the sediment.

Coagulation in the primary minimum, resulting from a reduction in the zeta potential to a point where attractive forces predominate, produces coarse compact masses with a 'curdled' appearance, which may not be readily dispersed.

On the other hand particles flocculated in the secondary minimum form a loosely bonded structure, and, although sedimentation is fairly rapid, a loosely packed high volume sediment is obtained in which the flocs retain their structure and the particles are easily resuspended. The supernatant liquid is clear as the colloidal particles are trapped within the flocs and sediment with them. Thus secondary minimum flocculation is a desirable state for a pharmaceutical suspension. Unfortunately much of the work reported on suspensions in the literature describes aggregation of particles as flocculation and it is not always possible to decide whether it is coagulation or secondary minimum flocculation that has actually occurred.

Particles greater than 1 μm radius should, unless highly charged, show a sufficiently deep secondary minimum for flocculation to occur as the attractive force between particles, V_A, depends on particles size. Other contributing factors to secondary minimum flocculation are shape (asymmetric particles, especially those that are elongated, being more satisfactory than spherical ones) and concentration. The rate of flocculation depends on the number of particles present, so that the greater the number of particles the more collisions there will be and flocculation is more likely to occur. However, it may be necessary, as with highly charged particles, to control the depth of the secondary minimum to induce a satisfactory flocculation state. This can be achieved by addition of electrolytes or ionic surface-active agents which reduce the zeta potential and hence V_R, resulting in the displacement of the whole of the DLVO plot to give a satisfactory secondary minimum as indicated in Fig. 6.4. It will be noted that with a secondary minimum produced in this manner, the distance between the particles is decreased. Hence a more satisfactory compact floc may be produced the particles of which are still easily dispersed. The production of a satisfactory secondary minimum leading to floc formation in this manner is termed *controlled flocculation*.

A convenient parameter for assessing a suspension is the sedimentation volume ratio, F, which is defined as the ratio of the ultimate settled volume V_u to the original volume V_o. F may be expressed as a percentage:

$$F = V_u/V_o \qquad (6.29)$$

The ratio F gives a measure of the aggregated-deflocculated state of a suspension and may usefully be plotted, together with the measured zeta potential, against concentration of additive, enabling an assessment of the state of the dispersion to be made in terms of the DLVO theory. The appearance of the supernatant liquid should be noted and the redispersibility of the suspensions evaluated. For further discussion the reader is referred to the research papers of Kayes (1977a, b) and Rawlins and Kayes (1983).

It should be pointed out that in using the controlled flocculation approach to suspension formulation it is important to work at a constant, or narrow, pH range as the magnitude of the charge on the drug particle can vary greatly with pH (Kayes, 1977b).

Other additives such as flavouring agents may also affect particle charge.

The effect of adsorbed polymer layers on the physical stability of suspensions

As described earlier in this chapter, colloidal particles may be stabilized against coagulation in the absence of a charge on the particles by the use of non-ionic polymeric material, the concept of steric stabilization or protective colloid action.

This concept may be applied to pharmaceutical suspensions where naturally occurring gums such as tragacanth and synthetic materials like non-ionic surfactants and cellulose polymers may be used to produce satisfactory suspensions. These materials may increase the viscosity of the aqueous vehicle and thus slow the rate of sedimentation of the particles but they will also form adsorbed layers around the particles so that the approach of their surfaces and aggregation to the coagulated state is hindered.

Attractive forces exist, of course, between the particles but the tendency now is to look upon attraction as between the polymer layers themselves rather than a modified attraction between uncoated particles (Evans and Napper, 1973). As the two adsorbed layers interpenetrate, however, a repulsion arises — as explained previously, this is enthalpic in origin due to release of water of solvation from the polymer chains with entropy effects due to movement restriction — with the result that, in general, the particles will not approach one another closer than twice the thickness of the adsorbed layer.

However, as indicated above in the discussion on controlled flocculation, from a pharmaceutical point of view an easily dispersed aggregated system is desirable. To produce this state, a balance between attractive and repulsive forces is required. This is not achieved by all polymeric materials, as the equivalent of deflocculated and caked, and coagulated, systems may be produced. The balance of forces appears to depend both on the thickness and the concentration of the polymer in the adsorbed layer. These parameters determine the Hamaker constant and hence the attractive force which must be large enough to cause aggregation of the particles comparable to flocculation. The steric repulsive force, which depends on the concentration and degree of solvation of the polymer chains, must be of sufficient magnitude to prevent close approach of the uncoated particles, but low enough so that the attractive force is dominant leading to aggregation at about twice the adsorbed layer thickness. Thus it has been found that adsorbed layers of certain members of the range of surfactants which are polyoxyethylene–polyoxypropylene block copolymers will produce satisfactory flocculated systems, whilst

examples of a nonyl phenyl ethoxylate range will not. With both types of surfactant the molecular moieties producing steric repulsion are hydrated ethylene oxide chains, but the concentration of these in the adsorbed layers varies giving the results indicated above (Rawlins and Kayes, 1980).

Stability of non-aqueous dispersions

A number of non-aqueous dispersions are used in pharmacy. These include oily suspensions such as propyliodine oily injection and phenoxymethyl-penicillin mixture, and suspensions of solids in aerosol propellants (these are largely halogenated hydrocarbons such as dichlorodifluoromethane).

As regards the stability of this type of preparation a question that has to be asked is, do the same mechanisms apply as for aqueous systems? Although relatively little work has been carried out in this area, in answering this question it can be said that it is now generally accepted that in rigorously dried material of low polarity (the dielectric constant for water is 80.4 and olive oil 3.1 at 20 °C) the stabilization of dispersions by surface charge mechanisms only plays a minor role, if any, compared to contributions by steric stabilization. The steric stabilizing mechanism is entropic in origin as described earlier in this chapter. However, the stabilizing agents may be different to those used for aqueous systems. Fatty acids and derivatives and polymers based on methacrylates have been used for colloidal dispersions (Vincent, 1973).

With pharmaceutical aerosols there is evidence of steric stabilization of particles dispersed in halogenated hydrocarbons by surface-active agents of low HLB number (see later in this chapter), such as sorbitan trioleate.

Wetting agents

One of the problems encountered in dispersing solid materials in water is that the powder may not be readily wetted (see Chapter 4). This may be due to entrapped air or to the fact that the solid surface is hydrophobic. The wettability of a powder may be described in terms of the contact angle, θ, which the powder makes with the surface of the liquid. This is shown by Eqn 4.14

$$\gamma_{S/V} = \gamma_{S/L} + \gamma_{L/V} \cos \theta$$

where $\gamma_{S/V}$, $\gamma_{S/L}$ and $\gamma_{L/V}$ are the respective interfacial tensions.

Equation 4.14 may be rearranged to give

$$\cos \theta = \frac{\gamma_{S/V} - \gamma_{S/L}}{\gamma_{L/V}} \qquad (6.30)$$

For a liquid to wet a powder the contact angle must approach zero, or $\cos \theta \to 1$. In most cases where water is involved this may only be achieved by reducing the magnitude of $\gamma_{L/V}$ and $\gamma_{S/L}$ by use of a wetting agent. Wetting agent are surfactants that are adsorbed at the liquid/vapour and solid/liquid interfaces thus reducing the relevant interfacial tension.

It must be noted that addition of such a surfactant will, as it is adsorbed at the particle surface, also affect the charge characteristics of the solid particle as described under controlled flocculation.

Rheological properties of suspensions

These properties are discussed in more detail in Chapter 2. Flocculated suspensions tend to exhibit plastic or pseudoplastic flow, depending on concentration, while concentrated deflocculated dispersions tend to be dilatant. This means that the apparent viscosity of flocculated suspensions is relatively high when the applied shearing stress is low but it decreases as the applied stress increases and the attractive forces producing the flocculation are overcome. Conversely the apparent viscosity of a concentrated deflocculated suspension is low at low shearing stress but increases as the applied stress increases. This is due to the electrical repulsion which occurs when the charged particles are forced close together — see the DLVO plot of potential energy of interaction between particles (Fig. 6.3) — causing the particles to rebound leaving voids into which the liquid flows, leaving other parts of the dispersion dry.

In addition to the rheological problems associated with particle charge effects the sedimentation behaviour is influenced by the rheological properties of the liquid continuous phase and for this, and other problems encountered with the formulation of suspensions, the reader is referred to the relevant sections of Chapters 2 and 15, respectively.

EMULSIONS

An emulsion is a system consisting of two immiscible liquid phases, one of which, in fine droplets, is dispersed throughout the other. Such an emulsion is thermodynamically unstable and it is usually necessary to add a third component, the emulsifying agent.

The phase which is present as fine droplets is called the disperse phase and the phase in which the droplets are suspended the continuous phase. Most emulsions will have droplets with diameters of 0.1–100 μm; smaller globules exhibit colloidal behaviour and the stability of a hydrophobic colloidal dispersion.

Pharmaceutical emulsions usually consist of water and an oil. Two types of emulsion can exist, oil in water (o/w) and water in oil (w/o) depending upon whether the continuous phase is aqueous or oily. More complicated emulsion systems may exist; for example, an oil droplet enclosing a water droplet may be suspended in water to form a water in oil in water emulsion (w/o/w). Such as system or its o/w/o counterpart — termed *multiple emulsions* — may occur particularly in the neighbourhood of the emulsion inversion point. These multiple emulsions are of interest as delayed action drug delivery systems. Traditionally emulsions have been used to render oily substances such as castor oil and liquid paraffin in a more palatable form. It is possible to formulate together oil-soluble and water-soluble medicaments and drugs may be more easily absorbed owing to the finely divided condition of emulsified substances. Thus there is enhanced absorption of griseofulvin when presented suspended in oil in an o/w emulsion (Carrigan and Bates, 1973). Details of the formulation of emulsions is given in Chapter 16.

A large number of bases used for topical preparations are emulsions, water miscible being o/w type and greasy bases w/o. The administration of oils and fats by intravenous infusion, as part of a total parenteral nutrition programme, has been made possible by the use of suitable non-toxic emulsifying agents like lecithin. Here, the control of particle size of emulsion droplets is of paramount importance in the prevention of formation of emboli.

Microemulsions

As shown previously oils can be brought into solution by solubilization. It is difficult to make a sharp distinction between emulsification and solubilization since there is a gradual transition from one form into the other as the relative proportion of oil to surface-active agent is altered, a high proportion of surfactant being required for solubilization, lower for emulsification.

At the transition stage swollen micellar systems or *microemulsions* are likely to occur. An apparently isotropic system is obtained containing a high percentage of both oil and water and a high concentration of surfactant. These are essentially swollen micellar systems but it is difficult to assess the difference between a swollen micelle and a small emulsion droplet.

Theory of emulsion stabilization

Interfacial free energy and emulsification

When two immiscible liquids, e.g. liquid paraffin and water, are shaken together a temporary emulsion will be formed. The subdivision of one of the phases into small globules results in a large increase in surface area and thus interfacial free energy of the system. The system is thus thermodynamically unstable which results, in the first place, in the dispersed phase being in the form of spherical droplets (the shape of minimum surface area for a given volume) and secondly in coalescence of these droplets, causing phase separation, the state of minimum surface free energy.

The adsorption of a surface-active agent at the globule interface will lower the o/w interfacial tension, the process of emulsification will be made easier and the stability may be enhanced. However, if a surface-active agent such as sodium dodecyl sulphate is used, the emulsion, on standing for a short while, will still separate out into its constituent phases. On the other hand, substances like acacia, which are only slightly surface active, produce stable emulsions. Acacia forms a strong viscous interfacial film around the globules and it

is considered that the characteristics of the interfacial film, are most important in considering the stability of emulsions.

Whether or not a surface-active agent will stabilize an emulsion will depend on the type of film formed at the o/w interface (for a discussion on monolayer film characteristics the reader should refer to a publication such as that by Adam, 1970). Sodium dodecyl sulphate forms what is termed a gaseous film at the o/w interface. One of the properties of this type of film is that the molecules forming it are separate and free to move in the interface. As one film-covered droplet approaches another the charged head groups of the sodium dodecyl sulphate repel each other. If the charged groups were fixed at the interface this repulsion would confer stability on the emulsion droplets, but as they are not, surfactant molecules move away from corresponding areas of the droplets, allowing them to coalesce. On the other hand, a surface-active agent which forms a more condensed type film, such as sodium oleate, where the molecules are not free to move in the interface, produces a stable emulsion.

Interfacial complexes

Applying knowledge gained by studying monolayers at the air/water interface Schulman and Cockbain (1940) found that a mixture of an oil-soluble alcohol such as cholesterol and a surface-active agent such as sodium cetyl (hexadecyl) sulphate was able to form a stable complex condensed film at the oil/water interface. This film was of high viscosity, flexible, permitting distortion of the droplets, resisted rupture and gave an interfacial tension lower than that produced by either component alone, of extremely low value. The emulsion produced was stable, the charge arising from the sodium cetyl sulphate contributing to the stability as described for lyophobic colloidal dispersions.

For complex formation at the interface the correct 'shape' of molecule is necessary, thus Schulman and Cockbain found that sodium cetyl sulphate stabilized an emulsion of liquid paraffin when elaidyl alcohol (the *trans* isomer) was the oil-soluble component but not when the *cis* isomer, oleyl alcohol, was used.

In practice, applying the findings of Schulman and Cockbain, the oil-soluble and water-soluble components are dissolved in the appropriate phases; on mixing the two phases the complex is formed at the interface. Alternatively, an emulsifying wax may be used which consists of both components blended together. The wax is dispersed in the oil phase and the aqueous phase added at the same temperature. Examples of such mixtures are given in Table 6.4.

Table 6.4 Emulsifying waxes

Product	Oil-soluble component	Water-soluble component
Emulsifying wax (anionic)	Cetostearyl alcohol	Sodium lauryl (dodecyl) sulphate
Cetrimide emulsifying wax (cationic)	Cetostearyl alcohol	Cetrimide (hexadecyl trimethyl ammonium bromide)
Cetomacrogol emulsifying wax (non-ionic)	Cetostearyl alcohol	Cetomacrogol (polyoxyethylene monohexadecyl ether)

This principle is also applied with the non-ionic emulsifying agents which are sorbitan esters, for example sorbitan mono-oleate and polyoxyethylene sorbitan esters (e.g. polysorbate 80), mixtures of the two types giving the best results. These emulsifying agents are not charged and there is no electrical repulsive force contributing to stability. It is likely, however, that these substances, and the cetomacrogol emulsifying wax as mentioned above, sterically stabilize the emulsions as mentioned in the next section.

Emulsion stabilization by non-ionic surfactants

Non-ionic surfactants are widely used in the production of stable emulsions. They are generally less toxic than ionic surfactants and are less sensitive to electrolytes and pH variation. Examples include sorbitan esters, polysorbates and straight chain compounds such as the polyoxyethylene glycol monoethers of *n*-alkanols of which cetomacrogol is an example.

These surfactants form interfacial films at the o/w interface in the same way as discussed in the previous section, but, as the molecules are not charged, there is no electrostatic repulsive contribution to stability. However, the polar groups of the surfactant molecules consist largely of hydrated ethylene oxide chains and these bring about a steric repulsion in exactly the same way as discussed under suspensions.

For a comprehensive review of this subject readers should consult the review by Florence and Rogers (1971).

Hydrophilic colloids as emulsion stabilizers

A number of hydrophilic colloids are used as emulsifying agents in pharmacy. These include proteins (gelatin, casein) and polysaccharides (acacia, cellulose derivatives and alginates).

These materials, which generally exhibit little surface activity, adsorb at the oil/water interface and form multilayers. Thus Shotton and White (1963) demonstrated films of acacia of thickness of the order of 0.25 μm. Such multilayers have viscoelastic properties, resist rupture and presumably form mechanical barriers to coalescence. However, some of these substance have chemical groups which ionize, e.g. acacia consists of salts of arabic acid, proteins contain both amino and carboxylic acid groupings, thus providing electrostatic repulsion as an additional barrier to coalescence.

Most cellulose derivatives are not charged. There is evidence, however, from studies on solid suspensions, that these substances sterically stabilize and it would appear probable that there will be a similar effect with emulsions (Law and Kayes, 1983).

Solid particles in emulsion stabilization

Emulsions may be stabilized by finely divided solid particles if they are preferentially wetted by one phase and possess sufficient adhesion for one another so that they form a film around the dispersed droplets.

Solid particles will remain at the interface as long as a stable contact angle, θ, is formed by the liquid/liquid interface and the solid surface. The particles must also be of sufficiently low mass for gravitational forces not to affect the equilibrium.

Then Eqn 4.14 for two liquids A and B and a solid S becomes

$$\gamma_{B/S} = \gamma_{A/S} + \gamma_{A/B} \cos \theta$$

If a contact angle is not formed then the particle remains entirely in one of the liquid phases, and if $\gamma_{B/S} > \gamma_{A/S} + \gamma_{A/B}$ the particle will be totally immersed in liquid A and if $\gamma_{A/S} > \gamma_{B/S} + \gamma_{A/B}$ the particle will be totally immersed in liquid B. The liquid which preferentially wets the solid, that is the one whose angle of contact measured through that liquid is less than 90°, will form the continuous phase. Under these circumstances a curved surface is best for the particles to form a close packed layer at the interface with the major part of the solid in the continuous phase and the liquid least effective in wetting the solid forming the disperse phase.

Aluminium and magnesium hydroxides and clays such as bentonite are preferentially wetted by water and thus stabilize o/w emulsions, e.g. liquid paraffin and magnesium hydroxide emulsion.

Carbon black and talc are more readily wetted by oils and stabilize w/o emulsions.

For details of methods of preparation of emulsions and formulation aspects the reader is referred to Carter (1975) and Chapter 16 of this publication.

Emulsion type

When an oil, water and an emulsifying agent are shaken together, what decides whether an o/w or w/o emulsion will be produced? A number of simultaneous processes have to be considered, for example droplet formation, aggregation and coalescence of droplets, and interfacial film formation. On shaking together oil and water both phases initially form droplets. The phase that persists in droplet form for a longer period of time should become the disperse phase and it should be surrounded by the continuous phase formed from the more rapidly coalescing droplets. The phase volumes and interfacial tensions will determine the relative number of droplets produced and hence the probability of collision, i.e. the greater the number of droplets the higher the chance of collision, so that the phase present in greater amount should finally become the continuous phase. However, emulsions containing well over 50% of disperse phase are common.

A more important consideration is the interfacial film produced by the adsorption of emulsifier at the o/w interface. Such films significantly alter the rates of coalescence by acting as physical and chemical barriers to coalescence. As indicated in the previous section the barrier at the surface of an oil droplet may arise because of electrically charged groups producing repulsion between approaching droplets or because of the steric repulsion, enthalpic in origin, from hydrated polymer chains. The greater the number of charged molecules present, or the greater the number of hydrated polymer chains, at the interface the greater will be the tendency to reduce oil droplet coalescence. On the other hand the interfacial barrier for approaching water droplets arises primarily because of the non-polar or hydrocarbon portion of the interfacial film. The longer the hydrocarbon chain length and the greater the number of molecules present per unit area of film, the greater is the tendency for water droplets to be prevented from coalescing. Thus it may be said generally that it is the dominance of the polar or non-polar characteristics of the emulsifying agent which plays a major contribution to the type of emulsion produced. For a more complete discussion of this concept the reader is referred to the text by Davies and Rideal (1963).

It would appear then, that the type of emulsion formed, depending as it does on the polar/non-polar characteristics of the emulsifying agent, is a function of the relative solubility of the emulsifying agent, the phase in which it is more soluble being the continuous phase. This is a statement of what is termed the Bancroft rule, an empirical observation made in 1913.

The foregoing helps to explain why charged surface-active agents such as sodium and potassium oleates which are highly ionized and possess strong polar groups favour o/w emulsions, whereas calcium and magnesium soaps which are little dissociated tend to produce w/o emulsions. Similarly, non-ionic sorbitan esters favour w/o emulsions whilst o/w emulsions are produced by the more hydrophilic polyoxyethylene sorbitan esters.

By reason of the stabilizing mechanism involved, polar groups are far better barriers to coalescence than their non-polar counterparts. It is thus possible to see why o/w emulsions can be made with greater than 50% disperse phase and why w/o emulsions are limited in this respect and will easily invert (change type) if the amount of water present is significant.

Pharmaceutical preferences for o/w or w/o are discussed in Chapter 16.

Hydrophile–lipophile balance (HLB)

The fact that a more hydrophilic interfacial barrier favours o/w emulsions whilst a more non-polar barrier favours w/o emulsions is made use of in the hydrophile–lipophile balance (HLB) system for assessing surfactants and emulsifying agents, which was introduced by Griffin in 1949. Here an HLB number is assigned to an emulsifying agent which is characteristic of its relative polarity. Although originally conceived for non-ionic emulsifying agents with polyoxyethylene hydrophilic groups (where the precentage weight of the hydrophilic group is divided by 5 to give the HLB number), it has since been applied with varying success to other surfactant groups, both ionic and non-ionic.

By means of this number system an HLB range of optimum efficiency for each class of surfactant is established as seen in Fig. 6.13. This approach is empirical but it does allow comparison between different chemical types of emulsifying agent. Comparison of properties like solubility, interfacial tension and CMC have also been used to compare a surfactant with one of known HLB value.

Typical HLB values for some pharmaceutical surfactants are given in Table 16.2.

In addition it has been suggested that certain emulsifying agents of a given HLB value appear to work best with a particular oil phase and this has given rise to the concept of a required HLB value for any oil or combination of oils, this value may be ascertained by observing emulsion stability.

For reasons mentioned earlier, when discussing interfacial films, mixtures of surface active agents give more stable emulsions than when used singly. The HLB of a mixture of surfactants, consisting of fraction x of A and $(1 - x)$ of B, is assumed to be an algebraic mean of the two HLB numbers.

$$\text{HLB}_{\text{Mixture}} = x \, \text{HLB}_{\text{A}} + (1 - x) \, \text{HLB}_{\text{B}}$$

It has been found that, at the optimum HLB for a particular emulsion, the mean particle size of the emulsion is at a minimum and this factor contributes to the stability of the emulsion system. The use of HLB values in the formulation of emulsions is discussed in Chapter 16.

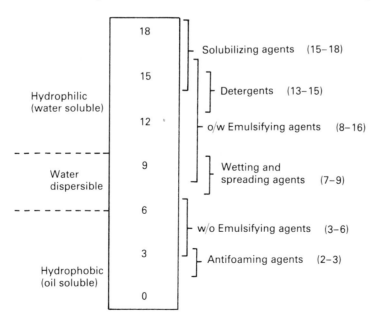

Fig. 6.13 HLB scale showing classification of surfactant function

Phase viscosity

The emulsification process and the type of emulsion formed are influenced to some extent by the viscosity of the two phases. Viscosity can be expected to affect interfacial film formation as the migration of molecules of emulsifying agent to the oil/water interface is diffusion controlled. Droplet movement prior to coalescence is also affected by the viscosity of the medium in which the droplets are dispersed.

Determination of emulsion type

Several tests are available to distinguish between o/w and w/o emulsions (see Chapter 16).

Stability of emulsions

A stable emulsion may be defined as a system in which the globules retain their initial character and remain uniformly distributed throughout the continuous phase. The function of the emulsifying agent is to form an interfacial film around the dispersed droplets; the physical nature of this barrier controls whether or not the droplets will coalesce as they approach one another. If the film is electrically charged then repulsive forces will contribute to stability.

Separation of an emulsion into its constituent phases is termed *cracking* or *breaking*.

It follows that any agent that will destroy the interfacial film will crack the emulsion. Some of the factors that cause an emulsion to crack are

1 the addition of a chemical that is incompatible with the emulsifying agent, thus destroying its emulsifying ability. Examples include surface-active agents of opposite ionic charge, e.g. the addition of cetrimide (cationic) to an emulsion stabilized with sodium oleate (anionic); addition of large ions of opposite charge, e.g. neomycin sulphate (cationic) to aqueous cream (anionic); addition of electrolytes such as calcium and magnesium salts to emulsion stabilized with anionic surface-active agents;
2 bacterial growth — protein materials and non-ionic surface-active agents are excellent media for bacterial growth;
3 temperature change — protein emulsifying

agents may be denatured and the solubility characteristics of non-ionic emulsifying agents change with a rise in temperature, heating above 70 °C destroys most emulsions. Freezing will also crack an emulsion; this may be due to the ice formed disrupting the interfacial film around the droplets.

Other ways in which an emulsion may show instability are as follows.

Flocculation

Even though a satisfactory interfacial film is present around the oil droplets, secondary minimum flocculation, as described earlier in this chapter under the discussion on the DLVO theory of colloid stability, is likely to occur with most pharmaceutical emulsions. The globules do not coalesce and may be redispersed by shaking. However, due to the closeness of approach of droplets in the floccule, if any weaknesses in the interfacial films occurs then coalescence may follow. Flocculation should not be confused with creaming (see below). The former is due to the interaction of attractive and repulsive forces and the latter due to density differences in the two phases, both may occur.

Phase inversion

As indicated under the section on emulsion type, phase volume ratio is a contributory factor to the type of emulsion formed. Although it was stated there that stable emulsions containing more than 50% of disperse phase are common, attempts to incorporate excessive amounts of disperse phase may cause cracking of the emulsion or phase inversion (conversion of an o/w emulsion to w/o or vice versa). It can be shown that uniform spheres arranged in the closest packing will occupy 74.02% of the total volume irrespective of their size. Thus Ostwald suggested that an emulsion which resembles such an arrangement of spheres would have a maximum disperse phase concentration of the same order. Although it is possible to obtain more concentrated emulsions than this, because of the non-uniformity of size of the globules and the possibility of deformation of shape of the globules, there is a tendency for emulsions containing more than about 70% disperse phase to crack or invert.

Further, any additive that alters the hydrophile–lipophile balance of an emulsifying agent may alter the emulsion type, thus addition of a magnesium salt to an emulsion stabilized with sodium oleate will cause the emulsion to crack or invert.

The addition of an electrolyte to anionic and cationic surfactants may suppress their ionization due to the common ion effect and thus a w/o emulsion may result even though normally an o/w emulsion would be produced, e.g. White Liniment BP is formed from turpentine oil, ammonium oleate, ammonium chloride and water. With ammonium oleate as emulsifying agent an o/w emulsion would be expected, but the suppression of ionization of the ammonium oleate by the ammonium chloride (the common ion effect) and a relatively large volume of turpentine oil, produce a w/o emulsion.

Emulsions stabilized with non-ionic emulsifying agents such as the polysorbates may invert on heating. This is due to the breaking of the H-bonds responsible for the hydrophilic characteristics of the polysorbate; its HLB value is thus altered and the emulsion inverts.

Creaming

Many emulsions cream on standing. The disperse phase, according to its density relative to that of the continuous phase, rises to the top or sinks to the bottom of the emulsion forming a layer of more concentrated emulsion. A common example is milk, an o/w emulsion, with cream rising to the top of the emulsion.

As mentioned earlier flocculation may occur as well as creaming but not necessarily so. Droplets of the creamed layer do not coalesce as may be found by gentle shaking which redistributes the droplets throughout the continuous phase. Although not so serious an instability factor as cracking, creaming is undesirable from a pharmaceutical point of view because a creamed emulsion is inelegant in appearance, provides the possibility of inaccurate dosage, and increases the likelihood of coalescence since the globules are close together in the cream.

Those factors which influence the rate of creaming are similar to those involved in the sedimentation rate of suspension particles and are indicated by Stokes' law (Eqn 6.6) as follows:

$$v = \frac{2a^2g(\sigma - \rho)}{9\eta}$$

here v is the velocity of creaming, a the globule radius, $\sigma - \rho$ the densities of disperse phase and dispersion medium respectively and η the viscosity of the dispersion medium. A consideration of this equation shows that the rate of creaming will be decreased:

1 by reduction in the globule size,
2 a decrease in the density difference between the two phases, and
3 an increase in the viscosity of the continuous phase.

This may be achieved by homogenizing the emulsion to reduce the globule size and increasing the viscosity of the continuous phase η by the use of thickening agents such as tragacanth or methylcellulose. It is seldom possible to satisfactorily adjust the densities of the two phases.

Assessment of emulsion stability

Approximate assessments of the relative stabilities of a series of emulsions may be obtained from estimations of the degree of separation of the disperse phase as a distinct layer, or from the degree of creaming. Whilst separation of the emulsion into two layers, i.e. cracking, indicates gross instability, a stable emulsion may cream, creaming being simply due to density differences and easily reversed by shaking. Some coalescence may, however, take place due to the close proximity of the globules in the cream, similar problems occur with flocculation.

However, instability in an emulsion results from any process which causes a progressive increase in particle size and a broadening of the particle size distribution, so that eventually the dispersed particles become so large that they separate out as free liquid. Accordingly, a more precise method for assessing emulsion stability is to follow the globule size distribution with time. An emulsion approaching the unstable state is characterized by the appearance of large globules as a result of the coalescence of others. Methods for determining particle size distribution have been reviewed by Sherman (1968).

Phase inversion temperature

One of the methods for predicting emulsion stability is the phase inversion temperature (PIT) technique of Parkinson and Sherman (1972). He has shown that the kinetics of globule coalescence in w/o and o/w emulsions stabilized by non-ionic emulsifying agents are influenced by the HLB values of the emulsifiers, i.e. as indicated earlier there is an optimum HLB value giving greatest stability for a particular emulsion system. Now the solubility of non-ionic surfactants, and hence the HLB, change when the temperature is raised, due to breaking of H-bonds, so that as mentioned previously the emulsion can invert. Sherman found a relationship between the PIT of o/w emulsions stabilized by non-ionic emulsifying agents and the rate of globule coalescence so that it should be possible to evaluate emulsion stability from PIT determinations, as the phase inversion temperature increases so globule coalescence decreases, i.e., the more stable the emulsion.

FOAMS

A foam is a coarse dispersion of a gas in a liquid which is present as thin films or lamellae of colloidal dimensions between the gas bubbles.

Foams find application in pharmacy as aqueous and non-aqueous spray preparations for topical, rectal and vaginal medication and for burn dressings. Equally important, however, is the destruction of foams and the use of antifoaming agents. These are not only of importance in manufacturing processes, preventing foam in for example liquid preparations, but foam inhibitors like the silicones are used in the treatment of flatulence, for the elimination of gas, air or foam from the gastrointestinal tract prior to radiography and for the relief of abdominal distension and dyspepsia.

Due to their high interfacial area (and surface-free energy) all foams are unstable in the thermodynamic sense. Their stability depends on two major factors — the tendency for the liquid films to drain and become thinner and their tendency to rupture due to random disturbances such as vibration, heat and diffusion of gas from small bubbles to large bubbles. Gas diffuses from the small bubbles to the large because the pressure in the former is greater, this is a phenomenon of curved interfaces and is described by the Kelvin equation (see Eqn 4.1 and Shaw, 1980 for a fuller description). The holes thus gradually merge to become larger and the foam gradually collapses.

Pure liquids do not foam. Transient or unstable foams are obtained with solutes such as short chain acids and alcohols which are mildly surface active. However, persistent foams are formed by solutions of surfactants. The film in such foams consists of two monolayers of adsorbed surface-active molecules separated by an aqueous core. The surfactants stabilize the film by means of electrical double layer repulsion or steric stabilization as described for colloidal dispersions.

Foams are often troublesome and knowledge of the action of substances that cause their destruction is useful. There are two types of antifoaming agent:

1 *foam breakers* such as ether and *n*-octanol. These substances are highly surface active and are thought to act by lowering the surface tension over small regions of the liquid film. These regions are rapidly pulled out by surrounding regions of higher tension, small areas of film are therefore thinned out and left without the properties to resist rupture.
2 *foam inhibitors*, such as polyamides and silicones. It is thought that these are adsorbed at the air/water interface in preference to the foaming agent, but they do not have the requisite ability to form a stable foam. They have a low interfacial tension in the pure state and may be effective by virtue of rapid adsorption.

AEROSOLS

Aerosols are colloidal dispersions of liquids or solids in gases. In general mists and fogs possess liquid disperse phases whilst smoke is a dispersion of solid particles in gases. However, no sharp distinction can be made between the two kinds because liquid is often associated with the solid particles. A *mist* consists of fine droplets of liquid which may or may not contain dissolved or suspended material. If the concentration of droplets becomes high it may be called a *fog*.

While all the disperse systems mentioned above are less stable than colloids which have a liquid as dispersion medium they have many properties in common with the latter and can be investigated in the same way. Particle size is usually within the colloidal range but if larger than 1 μm the life of an aerosol is short because the particles settle out too quickly.

Preparation of aerosols

In common with other colloidal dispersions aerosols may be prepared by either dispersion or condensation methods. The latter involve the initial production of supersaturated vapour of the material that is to be dispersed. This may be achieved by supercooling the vapour. The supersaturation eventually leads to the formation of nuclei, which grow into particles of colloidal dimensions. The preparation of aerosols by dispersion methods is of greater interest in pharmacy and may be achieved by the use of pressur-

ized containers with, for example, liquefied gases such as halogenated hydrocarbons as the propellants. If a solution or suspension of active ingredients is contained in the liquid propellant or in a mixture of this liquid and an additional solvent, then when the valve on the container is opened the vapour pressure of the propellant forces the mixture out of the container. The large expansion of the propellant at room temperature and atmospheric pressure produces a dispersion of the active ingredients in air. Although the particles in such dispersions are often larger than those in colloidal systems, the term aerosols is still generally applied to them.

Applications of aerosols in pharmacy

The use of aerosols as a dosage form is particularly important in the administration of drugs via the respiratory system. In addition to local effects, systemic effects may be obtained if the drug is absorbed into the blood stream from the lungs. Topical preparations are also well suited for presentation as aerosols. In the closely allied field of pesticides, insecticide aerosol preparations are widely used.

For a fuller account of the subject of therapeutic aerosols the reader is referred to Chapter 20.

REFERENCES

Adam, N. K. (1970) *The Physics and Chemistry of Surfaces*, Dover Edition, London.

Carrigan, P. G. and Bates, T. R. (1973) Biopharmaceutics of drugs administered in lipid containing dosage forms I. GI adsorption of griseofulvin from an o/w emulsion to the rat. *J. Pharm. Sci.*, **62**, 1476–1479.

Carter, S. J. (1975) *Dispensing for Pharmaceutical Students*, Pitman, London.

Davies, J. T. and Rideal, E. K. (1963) *Interfacial Phenomena*, 2nd edn, Academic Press, London.

Elworthy, P. H., Florence, A. T. and Macfarlane, C. B. (1968) *Solubilization by Surface Active Agents*, Chapman and Hall, London.

Evans, R. and Napper, D. H. (1973) Steric stabilization II Generalization of Fischers' solvency theory. *Kolloid. Z.u.Z. Polymere*, **251**, 329–336.

Florence, A. T. and Rogers, J. A. (1971) Emulsion stabilization by nonionic surfactants: experiment and theory. *J. Pharm. Pharmacol.*, **23**, 153–169.

Kayes, J. B. (1977a) Pharmaceutical suspensions: relation between zeta potential, sedimentation volume and suspension stability. *J. Pharm. Pharmacol.*, **29**, 199–204.

Kayes, J. B. (1977b) Pharmaceutical suspensions: micro electrophoretic properties. *J. Pharm. Pharmacol.*, **29**, 163–168.

Law, S. L. and Kayes, J. B. (1983) Adsorption of nonionic water soluble cellulose polymers at the solid water interface and their effect on suspension stability. *Int. J. Pharmaceut.*, **15**, 251–260.

Parkinson, C. and Sherman, P. (1972) Phase inversion temperature as an accelerated method for evaluating emulsion stability. *J. Colloid interface Sci.*, **41**, 328–330.

Rawlins, D. A. and Kayes, J. B. (1980) Steric stabilization of suspensions drug. *Dev. ind. Pharm.*, **6**(5), 427–440.

Rawlins, D. A. and Kayes, J. B. (1983) Pharmaceutical suspensions III. The redispersibility of suspensions. *Int. J. Pharmaceut.*, **13**, 171–181.

Schulman, J. H. and Cockbain, E. G. (1940) Molecular interactions at oil–water interfaces I. Molecular complex formation and the stability of oil-in-water emulsions. *Trans. Faraday. Soc.*, **36**, 651–660.

Shaw, D. J. (1980) *Introduction to Colloid and Surface Chemistry*, 3rd edn, Butterworths, London.

Sherman, P. (1968) *Emulsion Science*, Academic Press, London.

Sheth, P. B. and Parrot, E. L. (1967) Hydrolysis of solubilized esters. *J. Pharm. Sci.*, **56**, 983–986.

Shotton, E. and White, R. (1963) In *Rheology of Emulsions* (Ed. P. Sherman), Pergamon Press, Oxford.

Vincent, B. (1973) Non-aqueous systems. In: *Colloid Science*, Vol. I Chapter 7, The Chemical Society, London.

Wiersema, P. H., Loeb, A. L. and Overbeek, J. Th. G. (1966) Calculation of electrophoretic mobility of a spherical colloid particle. *J. Colloid interface Sci.*, **22**, 78–99.

BIBLIOGRAPHY

Ackers, R. J. (Ed.) (1976) *Foams*, Academic Press, London.

Adam, N. K. (1970) *The Physics and Chemistry of Surfaces*, Dover Edition, London.

Adamson, A. W. (1982) *Physical Chemistry of Surfaces*, 4th edn, Wiley, New York.

Davies, J. T. and Rideal, E. K. (1963) *Interfacial Phenomena*, 2nd edn, Academic Press, London.

Elworthy, P. H., Florence, A. T. and Macfarlane, C. B. (1968) *Solubilization by Surface Active Agents*, Chapman and Hall, London.

Florence, A. T. and Attwood, D. (1981) *Physicochemical Principles of Pharmacy*, Macmillan, London.

Kruyt, H. R. (Ed.) *Colloid Science*. Vol. I *Irreversible Systems* (1952), Vol. II *Reversible Systems* (1949), Elsevier, Amsterdam.

M.T.P. International Review of Science (1972) Physical Chemistry, Series One. Vol. 7 *Surface Chemistry and Colloids*, M. Kerker (Ed.), Chapter 4, Aggregation in Surfactant Systems, Butterworths, London.

Ottewill, R. H. (1973) Steric stabilization. In: *Colloid Science*, Vol. I, Chapter 5 Particulate Dispersions, The Chemical Society, London.

Parfitt, G. D. (1973) *Dispersions of Powders in Liquids*, 2nd edn, Applied Science.

Shaw, D. G. (1980) *Introduction to Colloid and Surface Chemistry*, 3rd edn, Butterworths, London.

Sherman, P. (1968) *Emulsion Science*, Academic Press, London.

Smith, A. L. (Ed.) (1976) *Theory and Practice of Emulsion Technology*, Academic Press, London.

Tanford, C. (1980) *The Hydrophobic Effect. Formation of Micelles and Biological Membranes*, 2nd edn, wiley, New York.

Van Olphen, H. (1977) *An Introduction to Clay Colloid Chemistry*, 2nd edn, Wiley, New York.

Kinetics and stability testing

Investigations into the rates at which changes occur in a particular system and the factors that influence such rates are known as kinetic studies. They are useful in providing information that:

1 gives an insight into the mechanism of the change involved, and
2 allows prediction of the degree of change that will occur after a given time has elapsed.

In general, the theories and laws of chemical kinetics are well proven and provide a sound basis for the application of such studies to pharmaceutical problems that involve chemical reactions: e.g. the decomposition of medicinal compounds.

The theoretical basis of drug kinetics is, however, often less well-founded than that of chemical kinetics. Nevertheless, the application of knowledge derived from these studies allows a more rational approach to be made towards the synthesis of medicinal compounds with particular activities and to the effects of formulation on these activities.

This chapter will explain briefly the laws governing the rates at which medicinal products degrade and the methods used in an industrial environment during product development to assess instability. Readers requiring more detailed information on the pharmaceutical applications of kinetics are referred to the review articles by Carstensen (1972, 1977, 1981), Connors *et al.* (1980), Fung (1979), Grimm and Schepky (1980) and Rhodes (1984).

It is not the intention of this chapter to discuss in detail the chemistry of instability and methods of prolongation of the effective life of a medicine. These are dealt with in other texts (see Bibliography). A useful source of information is a special edition of *Drug Development and Industrial*

Pharmacy (Volume 10, numbers 8 & 9, 1984). This source can be used by the reader who wishes to discover more about solid state reactions, stability of solids and disperse systems, stability of parenterals, stability aspects of preformulation, formulation and clinical trials, and stability testing of marketed products.

CHEMICAL KINETICS

Extent of reaction

Consider the formation of a compound B from the reaction between two molecules of a compound A; e.g. a dimerization. This reaction may be described by Eqn 7.1:

$$2A = B \qquad (7.1)$$

The extent to which this reaction has proceeded may be defined in terms of the change in either the amount of product B or the amount of reactant A.

The change in the amount of B is the difference between the amount of B produced (n_B) and the amount of B present at the starting point ($n_{B.0}$). (The starting point is usually the beginning of the reaction where $n_{B.0} = 0$.) Thus, the extent of reaction (ξ) defined in terms of the change in amount of substance B is given by Eqn (7.2).

$$\xi = n_B - n_{B.0} \qquad (7.2)$$

The change in the amount of A is the difference between the amount present at the starting point ($n_{A.0}$) and the amount that remains (n_A). However, two molecules of A are involved in the balanced Eqn 7.1 and the extent of reaction (ξ) defined in terms of the change in the amount of reactant A is given by Eqn 7.3:

$$\xi = \frac{n_{A.0} - n_A}{2} \qquad (7.3)$$

It is obvious from Eqn 7.1 that Eqns 7.2 and 7.3 will give the same value of ξ. It is therefore convenient to write a general equation for the definition of extent of reaction. This is represented by Eqn 7.4,

$$\xi = \frac{n_X - n_{X.0}}{v_X} \qquad (7.4)$$

where n_X and $n_{X.0}$ are the actual and initial amounts of a substance X that is involved in a reaction as a reactant or a product. v_X is called the stoichiometric number of X and it indicates the number of molecules (or atoms, or radicals, or ions) of X that are involved in the balanced equation, which describes the reaction under consideration. When X is a product the difference ($n_X - n_{X.0}$) is positive because the amount of product increases as the reaction proceeds; (i.e. $n_X > n_{X.0}$). However, if X is a reactant, ($n_X - n_{X.0}$) is negative because the amount of X will decrease as reaction proceeds (i.e. $n_X < n_{X.0}$). This variation in the sign of ($n_X - n_{X.0}$) is overcome by using the convention that the stoichiometric number v_X is positive for a product and negative for a reactant, so that the right-hand side of Eqn 7.4 is always positive.

It can be seen from Eqn (7.4) that the dimension of extent of reaction, ξ, will be amount of substance and, therefore, the units of ξ will be the same as those of n_X, for which the basic SI unit is the mole.

The change in extent of reaction ($d\xi$) with increasing change in amount of substance X (dn_X) may be expressed by Eqn 7.5, where v_X is defined as before.

$$dn_X = v_X d\xi \qquad (7.5)$$

Rate of reaction ($\dot{\xi}$)

This may be defined as the rate of increase of the extent of reaction (i.e. $d\xi/dt$) as is shown by Eqn 7.6:

$$\dot{\xi} = d\xi/dt \qquad (7.6)$$

The dimensions of $\dot{\xi}$ will be amount of substance per unit time and its basic SI unit will be moles per second (mol s^{-1}). From Eqns 7.5 and 7.6 it can be seen that

$$\dot{\xi} = \frac{d\xi}{dt} = \frac{1}{v_X}\frac{dn_X}{dt} \qquad (7.7)$$

where dn_X/dt may be called the rate of formation of X if X is a product, or the rate of disappearance of X if X is a reactant.

Equations 7.6 and 7.7 are general ones for the

definition of rate of reaction and they are independent of the conditions under which a reaction is carried out. For example, they are valid for reactions in which the volume varies with time or where the reaction occurs in more than one phase.

When discussing chemical kinetics it is convenient to divide reactions into two classes; homogeneous and heterogeneous reactions. The former occur in one phase, e.g. in solution, while the latter occur at the interface between two phases, e.g. at solid–gas or solid–liquid interfaces.

Homogeneous reactions

These reactions are usually classified on the basis of the effect of the concentration of reactants on the rates of increase in concentration of products or decrease in concentration of reactants. To convert Eqn 7.7 to concentration terms it is necessary to divide by the volume, V, of the homogeneous system, when Eqn 7.8 is obtained.

$$\frac{1}{V}\frac{d\xi}{dt} = \frac{1}{Vv_X}\frac{dn_X}{dt} \qquad (7.8)$$

If the volume, V, of the phase does not vary with time during the reaction then Eqn 7.8 may be written in the form of Eqn 7.9,

$$\frac{1}{V}\frac{d\xi}{dt} = \frac{1}{v_X}\frac{d(n_X/V)}{dt} \qquad (7.9)$$

However, the term n_X/V represents the concentration of substance X and may be replaced by a single term; e.g. C_X or [X], and Eqn 7.9 may be rewritten as,

$$\frac{1}{V}\frac{d\xi}{dt} = \frac{1}{v_X}\frac{dC_X}{dt} = \frac{1}{v_X}\frac{d[X]}{dt} \qquad (7.10)$$

If X is a product the rate at which its concentration increases is represented by the symbol r_X and is equal to the term dC_X/dt in Eqn 7.10. If X is a reactant, then r_X represents its rate of disappearance, given by $r_X = -dC_X/dt$. The minus sign is necessary in this latter case because the concentration of a reactant decreases with time. Thus, the term $-dC_X/dt$ is positive because dC_X is negative.

Order of reaction

Experiments show that the rates of change in the concentrations of products or reactants usually depend on the concentrations of the reactants. This dependence is indicated by Eqn 7.11:

$$r \propto [A]^a[B]^b \text{ or } r = k[A]^a[B]^b \qquad (7.11)$$

where [A] and [B] are the concentrations of reactants A and B respectively, a and b are some powers of these concentrations, and k is a proportionality constant known as the *rate constant* of the reaction at a particular temperature.

Classification of reactions may be achieved by division into various orders, where the order of a reaction is given by the sum of the powers of the concentration terms involved in equations, such as that represented by Eqn 7.11. For example, in this particular case the order of reaction is given by $(a + b)$. In fact, this represents the overall order of the reaction. It is also possible to refer to the order of a reaction with respect to a particular reactant. Thus, the above reaction is of order a with respect to A, and of order b with respect to B.

Homogeneous reactions are usually interpreted in terms of simple orders of reaction, which are discussed below.

First order reactions   The rate of change in the concentrations of products and reactants in this type of reaction is proportional to the first power of the concentration (C_X) of a single reactant (X) and is independent of the concentration of any other substance that may be present.

The rate of formation of a product Y is therefore given by Eqn 7.12 and the rate of disappearance of reactant X is given by Eqn 7.13:

$$r_Y = \frac{dC_Y}{dt} = kC_X \qquad (7.12)$$

$$r_X = -\frac{dC_X}{dt} = kC_X \qquad (7.13)$$

where k is the rate constant.

If the concentration of reactant X at the beginning of a reaction when time $t = 0$ is denoted by a, and the amount that has reacted after time t is denoted by x, then the amount of X that remains at this time is given by $(a - x)$. Equation 7.13

may therefore be rewritten in the form shown by Eqn 7.14

$$-\frac{dC_X}{dt} = k(a - x) \quad \text{or} \quad \frac{dC_X}{a - x} = -k \, dt \quad (7.14)$$

where $-dC_X/dt$ represents the rate of decrease in the concentration of X. Integration of Eqn 7.14 between the time limits of 0 and t gives

$$\int_a^{(a-x)} \frac{dC_X}{a - x} = -k \int_0^t dt$$

$$\therefore \ln (a - x) - \ln a = -kt$$

Converting from natural logarithms gives

$$\log (a - x) - \log a = -\frac{kt}{2.303}$$

or

$$\log (a - x) = \log a - \frac{kt}{2.303} \quad (7.15)$$

It can be seen that Eqn 7.15 is representative of a linear relation (i.e. $y = c + mx$) and the variables are $(a - x)$ and t. If the first order law is obeyed, then a graph of $\log (a - x)$ versus t will give a straight line with a slope of $-k/2.303$ and an intercept at $t = 0$ of $\log a$.

The rate constant k may therefore be calculated from the slope of such a graph. It may also be obtained by substitution of experimental values into Eqn 7.16 which is a rearranged form of Eqn 7.15.

$$k = \frac{2.303}{t} \log \frac{a}{a - x} \quad (7.16)$$

It can be seen that the dimension of k for a first order reaction it reciprocal time and the basic SI unit is the reciprocal second (s^{-1}).

Second order reactions   The rate of change in the concentrations of products and reactants in this type of reaction is proportional either to the second power of the concentration of a single reactant, or to the first powers of the concentrations of two reactants. These two possibilities are illustrated by Eqns 7.17 and 7.18, which refer to the rate of decrease in the concentration of reactant X:

(i) $r_X = -dC_X/dt = k[X][Y]$ (7.17)
(ii) $r_X = -dC_X/dt = k[X]^2$ (7.18)

where the rates of concentration change are dependent on the concentrations of reactants X and Y, or X only. In the first type of second order reaction given above the rate of decrease in concentration of reactant Y will be equal to that of X (i.e. $r_Y = r_X$). If the concentrations of reactants X and Y at time $t = 0$ are given by a and b respectively, and the concentration of each substance that has reacted after time t is equal to x, then the concentrations of X and Y that remain after this time are given by $(a - x)$ and $(b - x)$ respectively. Equation 7.17 may therefore be rewritten as

$$-\frac{dx}{dt} = k(a - x)(b - x) \quad (7.19)$$

where $-dx/dt$ represents the rate of decrease in the concentration of X (or Y). Integration of Eqn 7.19 yields Eqn 7.20:

$$kt = \frac{2.303}{(a - b)} \log \frac{b(a - x)}{a(b - x)} \quad (7.20)$$

where k is the rate constant.

Rearrangement of Eqn 7.20 yields

$$\log \frac{a - x}{b - x} = \frac{(a - b)kt}{2.303} + \log \frac{a}{b} \quad (7.21)$$

and if the second order law is obeyed, then a graph of the left hand side of Eqn 7.21 against time t should produce a straight line with a slope equal to $(a - b)k/2.303$, and an intercept at $t = 0$ of $\log(a/b)$.

When the initial concentrations of reactants X and Y are equal (i.e. $a = b$) or when the second power of a single reactant determines the rate of concentration change, then the integrated form of the rate equation is given by Eqn 7.22:

$$kt = \frac{x}{a(a - x)} \quad (7.22)$$

Rearrangement of Eqn 7.22 yields

$$\frac{1}{(a - x)} - \frac{1}{a} = kt \quad (7.23)$$

and if the second law is obeyed then a graph of $1/(a - x)$ against time should produce a straight line with a slope of k and an intercept of $1/a$ at $t = 0$,

It can be shown from the previous equations that the rate constant for a second order reaction has the dimensions of concentration^{-1} time^{-1} and the SI unit is m^3 mol^{-1} s^{-1}.

Pseudo first order reactions If a large excess of one of the reactants in a second order reaction is present throughout the reaction, then its concentration remains virtually constant and the rate of concentration change follows the first order law. Hydrolysis reactions in dilute aqueous solution are common examples of this type of reaction, which is known as a pseudo first order reaction.

However, it should be borne in mind that a decrease in the concentration of water, e.g. caused by a change in the composition of the solvent, may lead to a reaction that follows second order kinetics.

Reactions of third and higher orders The rates of change in concentrations in this type of reaction are proportional to three concentration terms. However, such reactions are rare and their analysis is complex. Reactions of even higher orders are unlikely to occur.

Zero order reactions The rates of change in the concentrations of reactants and products in reactions of this type are dependent on some factor other than the concentration of a reactant. They include photochemical reactions that depend on the absorption of light and heterogeneous reactions that depend on the area of the interface at which reaction occurs.

The rate of change in concentration of a reactant X is constant in a zero order reaction as indicated by Eqn 7.24, where k is the rate constant, which has the same dimensions as r_X; i.e. mol m^{-3} s^{-1}.

$$r_X = -\frac{dC_X}{dt} = k \qquad (7.24)$$

If the amount of X that reacts in time t is denoted by x then the integrated form of the equation for a zero order reaction is given by

$$x = kt \qquad (7.25)$$

Half-life $(t_{\frac{1}{2}})$

The half-life of a reaction is the time required for the concentration of a reactant to decrease to half its original value; i.e. when $x = a/2$ in the previous equations. The expressions of half-life in terms of the rate constant (k) for the disappearance of reactant are shown in Table 7.1 for simple orders of reaction. It can be seen from these expressions that half-life can be defined in terms of Eqn 7.26 for the simple orders given in Table 7.1.

$$t_{\frac{1}{2}} \propto \frac{1}{a^{(n-1)}} \qquad (7.26)$$

The half-life of a reaction provides a convenient means of expressing the rate of concentration change of a reactant and is particularly useful because the time taken for complete reaction is theoretically infinite except in zero order reactions.

Methods of determining the order of a reaction

Graphical method A straight line is obtained when the data from kinetic experiments are plotted in the form that is relevant to the order of a particular reaction. The ordinates and abscissae of graphs for simple orders are summarised in Table 7.1, together with the values of the slopes and intercepts of these graphs.

Substitution method The order of a reaction is indicated by the particular integrated rate equation that gives a constant value of k for data

Table 7.1 Summary of information on reactions of simple orders

Order	Integrated rate equation	Half-life equation	Linear graph			
			Ordinate	Abscissa	Slope	Intercept
Zero	$x = kt$	$t_{\frac{1}{2}} = \dfrac{a}{2k}$	x	t	k	0
First	$\log \dfrac{a}{(a-x)} = \dfrac{kt}{2.303}$	$t_{\frac{1}{2}} = \dfrac{0.693}{k}$	$\log(a-x)$	t	$-\dfrac{k}{2.303}$	$\log a$
Second $(a = b)$	$\dfrac{x}{a(a-x)} = kt$	$t_{\frac{1}{2}} = \dfrac{1}{ak}$	$\dfrac{1}{a-x}$	t	k	$\dfrac{1}{a}$

obtained from a kinetic experiment. The integrated equations are given in Table 7.1 for simple orders of reaction.

Half-life method   Consider a reaction in which the initial concentration of the reactant is a_1 and the concentration at a later time is a_2. These concentrations may be regarded as the starting points of two separate reactions, and the corresponding half-lives may be represented by $t_{\frac{1}{2}(1)}$ and $t_{\frac{1}{2}(2)}$, respectively. From Eqn 7.26 it is possible to write that

$$t_{\frac{1}{2}(1)} \propto \frac{1}{a_2^{(n-1)}}$$

and

$$t_{\frac{1}{2}(2)} \propto \frac{1}{a_2^{(n-1)}}$$

$$\therefore \frac{t_{\frac{1}{2}(1)}}{t_{\frac{1}{2}(2)}} = \frac{a_2^{(n-1)}}{a_1^{(n-1)}}$$

$$\therefore \log \frac{t_{\frac{1}{2}(1)}}{t_{\frac{1}{2}(2)}} = (n-1) \log \frac{a_2}{a_1}$$

$$\therefore n = \frac{\log (t_{\frac{1}{2}(1)}/t_{\frac{1}{2}(2)})}{\log (a_2/a_1)} + 1 \tag{7.27}$$

Effect of temperature on reaction rate

The effect of temperature on a rate constant, k, is indicated by the Arrhenius equation, Eqn 7.28.

$$k = Ae^{-E_aRT} \tag{7.28}$$

or

$$\log k = \log A - \frac{E_a}{2.303RT} \tag{7.29}$$

where A is a constant that is termed the frequency factor, E_a is the energy of activation, R is the gas constant, and T is the thermodynamic temperature.

Different interpretations of the constant A are given by the collision theory and the transition state theory of reaction rates. In addition, there is a slight difference in the interpretation of the constant E_a, and the student is recommended to read accounts of these theories given in the books listed at the end of this chapter.

It can be seen from Eqn 7.29 that a straight line will be obtained from a graph of $\log k$ against $1/T$ as shown in Fig. 7.1. The constants E_a and A may

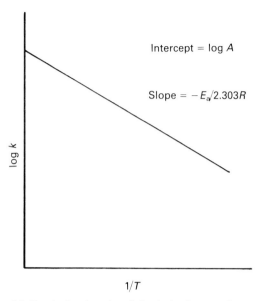

Fig. 7.1 Graph showing plot of the Arrhenius equation

be determined from the slope and intercept of this line, which are equal to $-E_a/2.303R$ and $\log A$, respectively. It should be borne in mind that temperature is decreasing when $1/T$ is increasing so that the higher temperatures lie towards the left hand side of the horizontal axis of the graph.

ACCELERATED STABILITY TESTING

Instabilities in modern formulations are often detectable only after considerable storage periods under normal conditions. To assess the stability of a formulated product it is usual to expose it to high stress conditions to enhance its deterioration and therefore reduce the time required for testing. This enables more data to be gathered in a shorter time which, in turn, will allow unsatisfactory formulations to be eliminated early within a study and will also reduce the time for a successful product to reach the market. It must be emphasized that extrapolations to 'normal' storage conditions must be made with care and that the formulator must be sure that such extrapolations are valid. It is advisable therefore to run concurrently a batch under expected normal conditions to confirm later that these assumptions are valid.

The objectives of such accelerated tests may be defined as:

1 the rapid detection of deterioration in different initial formulations of the same product — this is of use in selecting the best formulation from a series of possible choices;

2 the prediction of shelf-life, which is the time a product will remain satisfactory when stored under expected or directed storage conditions; and

3 the provision of a rapid means of quality control, which ensures that no unexpected change has occurred in the stored product.

All these objectives are based on obtaining a more rapid rate of decomposition by applying to the product a storage condition that places a higher stress or challenge to it when compared with normal storage conditions. However, the use of this basic method depends on the particular objective required. For example, in the first objective the best formulation from a series of possible choices is the one that exhibits the least amount of decomposition in a given time under the influence of a reasonably high stress. The results of such a test are illustrated in Fig. 7.2(a).

The second objective is achieved by using the results obtained from an accelerated test to predict the amount of decomposition in a product after a longer period of storage under normal conditions.

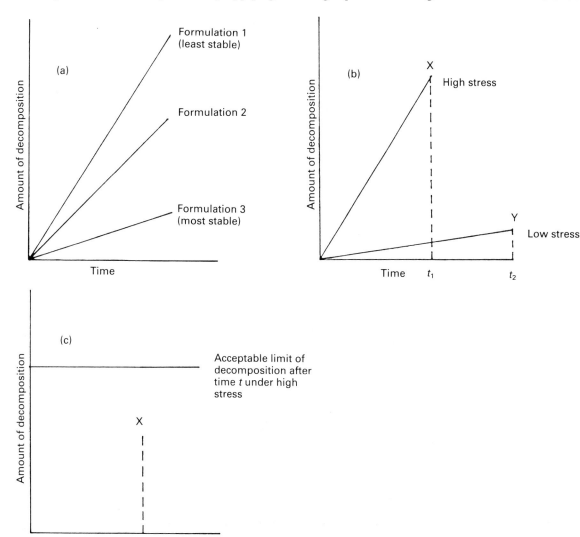

Fig. 7.2 The various aspects of accelerated stability testing

This is illustrated in Fig. 7.2(b) where the amount of decomposition X obtained after the short time t_1 is used to predict the value of Y after time t_2.

The use of accelerated tests in achieving the third objective is illustrated by Fig. 7.2(c) which shows that a single measurement taken after a given time t should fall below an acceptable limit of decomposition for a product subjected to the challenge involved in the test.

Common high stresses or challenges

Temperature

An increase in temperature causes an increase in the rate of chemical reactions. The products are therefore stored at temperatures greater than room temperature. The nature of the product often determines the range covered in the accelerated test. Samples are removed at various time intervals and the extent of decomposition is determined by analysis. Sensitive analytical methods should be used in all stability tests of this nature since small changes may be detected after very short storage periods.

The effects caused by high temperatures should not be confused with those that arise from the effect of low humidity. Such confusion is possible because the relative humidity inside a high temperature storage cabinet will be lower than that in the room. This low humidity causes loss of moisture, which may lead to apparent increases in the concentration of ingredients. If these concentration changes are not allowed for in subsequent analyses decomposition may be unsuspected.

Humidity

Storage of the product in atmospheres of high humidity will accelerate decompositions that result from hydrolysis. Marked acceleration will be obtained if the 'naked' product (i.e. not enclosed in a container) is subjected to these tests, which usually indicate the minimum humidity tolerated by the product without undue decomposition, and are therefore useful in determining the degree of protection that should be afforded by a container.

Light

A source of artificial light is used to accelerate the effects of sunlight or sky light. The source should emit a similar distribution of radiant energy to that in sunlight because photochemical reactions involve the absorption of light of definite wavelengths. Daylight fluorescent lamps provide a satisfactory source, and banks of such lamps may be used to accelerate the effects of light. However, although these lamps do not have a marked heating effect the use of glass plates to reduce such an effect is recommended, otherwise it is difficult to separate the accelerated decomposition caused by light from that caused by increased temperatures.

Stability testing protocols

Accelerated stability testing requires the careful design of protocols which must define clearly the following:

1 the temperature and humidity for storage,
2 storage time before sampling,
3 the number of batches to be sampled,
4 the number of replicates within each batch,
5 a suitable light challenge,
6 details of assay.

Although all pharmaceutical products have to satisfy governmental regulatory authorities, surprisingly there are no nationally or internationally standardized storage conditions. Storage conditions during stability testing vary from company to company and even within a single company. Often different types of products are given different challenges. A typical protocol may be as shown in Table 7.2. At least two, possibly three, batches are stored as indicated and subsequently tested in duplicate. Products are usually stored in their final container. If at this stage the final pack has not been confirmed, a range of packs and pack materials must be tested. For example, tablets may be stored in glass bottles, HDPE containers, aluminium foil and PVC or PVC/PVDC blisters (see Chapter 44). Some batches of liquid products may be stored in an inverted position to check for interaction between ingredients and the liner of the cap.

It is important that stability studies are performed at all stages of product development.

Table 7.2 A typical storage and testing protocol for accelerated stability assessment of pharmaceutical products.

Time of sampling	Storage temperature (°C) and humidity (%RH)						
	4	RT★	30	37	37/75%	50	75
6 weeks	S	S		T	T	T	T
3 months	S	S	T	T	T	T	T
6 months	S	S	T	T	T	T	
12 months	S	S	T	T			
18 months	S	S	T	T			
2 years	S	S	T	T			
3 years	S	S	T				
4 years	S	S	T				
5 years	T	T	T				

Notes

Apart from one, or rarely two, high humidity challenges, the remaining storage temperatures are at ambient humidities.

★RT (room temperature): often an uncontrolled cabinet in which the temperature can be between 15 and 25 °C.

S: the 4 °C and 25 °C samples are often retained as spares in the event of any problems with the analysis of any of the other samples.

T: testing is performed on these samples. To give an example — in the case of tablets these tests may consist of: assay for active ingredient(s) by h.p.l.c.; assay for degradation product(s) by t.l.c.; an assessment of appearance; tablet weight; tablet thickness; friability; crushing strength; moisture content; disintegration; dissolution.

The products may also be exposed to an additional light challenge. This may be in the form of a standard, fluorescent-tube light cabinet or, more simply, a south facing window.

Stability testing during preformulation is discussed in Chapter 13 of this book and by Monkhouse (1984). Stability programmes for formulation studies have been discussed by Dukes (1984) and during clinical trials and scale-up by Lantz (1984). Stability programmes for marketed batches are described by Kaminski (1984) and Thompson (1984).

The prediction of shelf life

This is the second of the objectives that were listed previously and it is based on the application of the Arrhenius equation, Eqn 7.29, which indicates the effect of temperature on the rate constant, k, of a chemical reaction. Figure 7.1 shows that a graph of log k versus the reciprocal of thermodynamic temperature, $1/T$, is a straight line. If the slope of this line is determined from the results of accelerated tests at high temperatures it is possible to determine the value of the rate constant at other temperatures (e.g. normal room temperature) by extrapolation. Substitution of this value of k into the appropriate order of reaction (i.e. the rate equation that applies to the reaction involved in the particular decomposition) allows the amount of decomposition after a given time to be calculated. As pointed out, this approach involves a knowledge of the order of the reaction involved and preliminary experiments are therefore necessary to determine this order.

Several difficulties and limitations are involved in this aspect of accelerated stability testing. First, as in all accelerated tests, there is the possibility that the application of high stresses may cause reactions that would not take place under the lower stresses associated with normal storage conditions. Secondly, the uncertain conditions defined by the term 'normal storage conditions' introduce a difficulty when attempting to forecast the shelf life of a product. Unless the storage conditions are defined precisely on the container, then allowance should be made for variations in the conditions likely to be encountered under normal storage. Attempts to allow for such a contingency often involve accepting the shortest shelf life for the range of conditions likely to be encountered. The climate of the country in which a product is to be marketed is particularly important in defining this range.

Decompositions in formulated products often proceed via a complex reaction series and may involve simultaneous, consecutive or chain reactions, because the formulated products themselves are complex systems. In addition, the order of a reaction may change after a certain time. Predictions of the extent of decomposition at future times are then impracticable and prolonged tests under normal storage conditions must be carried out.

In spite of these difficulties the application of accelerated testing to pharmaceutical products is often useful, and predicted shelf lives are sufficiently accurate. Statistical methods of designing such tests have therefore been reported, which allow the selection of the number of replicates, sampling times and other factors involved in the tests to be made on a logical basis for attaining the required degree of accuracy without wasting time on unnecessary experimentation (Boudreau and Harrison, 1980).

REFERENCES

Boudreau, C. F. and Harrison, D. J. (1980) *Drug Devel. Ind. Pharm.* **6**, 539 (1980).

Carstensen, J. T. (1972) *Theory of Pharmaceutical Systems*, Volumes I and II, Academic Press, New York.

Carstensen, J. T. (1977) *Pharmaceutics of Solids and Solid Dosage Forms*, John Wiley and Sons, New York.

Carstensen J. T. (1981) *Solid Pharmaceutics: Mechanical Properties and Rate Phenomena*, pp. 243–244 Academic Press, New York.

Connors, K. A., Amion, G. L. and Kennon, L. (1980) *Chemical Stability of Pharmaceuticals: A Handbook for Pharmacists*, Wiley–Interscience, New York.

Dukes, G. R. (1984) Stability programs for formulation studies. *Drug Devel. Ind. Pharm.* **10**(8 & 9), 1413–1424.

Fung, H. L. (1979) *Modern Pharmaceutics*, Chapter 7 *Ed. G. S. Baker and C. T. Rhodes*, Dekker, New York.

Grimm, W. and Schepky, G. (1980) *Stabilitatsprungen in der Pharmazie*, Edito Caritor Aulendof, Ravensburg.

Kaminski, E. E. (1984) Stability program for marketed batches. *Drug Devel. Ind. Pharm.* **10**(8 & 9), 1433–1448.

Lantz, R. J. Jr (1984) Stability aspects of clinical supplies and scale-up studies. *Drug Devel. Ind. Pharm.* **10**(8 & 9), 1425–1432.

Monkhouse, D. C. (1984) Stability aspects of preformulation and formulation of solid pharmaceuticals. *Drug Devel. Ind. Pharm.* **10**(8 & 9), 1373–1412.

Rhodes, C. T. (1984) An overview of kinetics for the evaluation of the stability of pharmaceuticals. *Drug Devel. Ind. Pharm.* **10**(8 & 9), 1163–1174.

Thompson, K. Gang stability programs for marketed batches. *Drug Devel. Ind. Pharm.* **10**(8 & 9), 1449–1462.

BIBLIOGRAPHY

Carstensen, J. T. (1972) *Theory of Pharmaceutical Systems*, Volume I. Academic Press, New York.

Carstensen, J. T. (1977) *Pharmaceutics of Solids and Solid Dosage Forms*, John Wiley and Sons, New York.

Drug Development and Industrial Pharmacy (1984). **10**(8 & 9) A special issue on expiration dating for pharmaceuticals.

Florence, A. T. and Attwood, D. (1981) *Physicochemical Principles of Pharmacy* The Macmillan Press Ltd, London.

Wallwork, S. C. and Grant, D. J. W. (1977) *Physical Chemistry for Students of Pharmacy and Biology*, 3rd edn, Longman, London.

PART TWO

Biopharmaceutics

Introduction to biopharmaceutics

The concept of bioavailability
The concept of biopharmaceutics

Before the reader can appreciate the meaning and clinical significance of *biopharmaceutics*, it is necessary to introduce the concept of drug bioavailability.

The concept of bioavailability

The therapeutic response of a drug is normally dependent on an adequate concentration of the drug being achieved and then maintained at the site or sites of action of the drug. In the case of systemically acting drugs (i.e. drugs that reach these sites via the systemic circulation) it is generally accepted for clinical purposes that a dynamic equilibrium exists between the concentration of drug at its site(s) of action and the concentration of drug in blood plasma. An important consequence of this dynamic equilibrium is that it permits a therapeutically effective concentration of drug to be achieved at its site(s) of action by adjustment of the concentration of drug in blood plasma. Strictly speaking, the concentration of drug in plasma water (i.e. protein-free plasma) is a more accurate index of drug concentration at the site(s) of action than is the concentration of drug in whole plasma since a drug may often bind in a reversible manner to plasma protein. Only drug which is unbound (i.e. dissolved in plasma water) can pass out of the plasma through the capillary endothelium and reach other body fluids and tissues and hence its site(s) of action. Drug concentration in whole blood is also not considered to be an accurate indirect index of the concentration of drug at its site(s) of action since drug can bind to and enter blood cells. However, to measure the concentration of an unbound drug in plasma water requires more complex and sensitive assay methods than to measure the total concentration of both unbound and bound drug in total plasma. Thus, for clinical purposes, drug concentration in blood plasma is usually measured and is regarded as an index of drug concentration at the site(s) of action of the drug and of the clinical effects of the drug. However, it should be realized that this is a simplification and may not always be valid. Indeed one should not draw inferences about the clinical effects of a drug from its plasma concentration until it has been established that the two are consistently correlated. For simplicity, in the remainder of this chapter, it has been assumed that the plasma drug concentration is directly proportional to the clinical effect of that drug.

The concentration of drug in blood plasma depends on numerous factors. These include the relative amount of an administered dose that enters the systemic circulation, the rate at which this occurs, the rate and extent of distribution of the drug between the systemic circulation and other tissues and fluids and the rate of elimination of the drug from the body.

A schematic representation of some of the factors which can influence the concentration of

a drug in the blood plasma and also at its site(s) of action is shown in Fig. 8.1.

Apart from the intravenous route of drug administration, where a drug is introduced directly into the blood circulation, all other routes of administering systemically acting drugs involve the absorption of drug from the place of administration into the blood. Drug must be absorbed in a sufficient quantity and at a sufficient rate in order to achieve a certain blood plasma concentration which, in turn, will produce an appropriate concentration of drug at its site(s) of action to elicit the desired therapeutic response.

It follows that there are two aspects of drug absorption which are important in clinical practice, namely, the rate and the extent to which the administered dose is absorbed. Simply because a certain dose of a drug is administered to a patient, there is no guarantee (except for intravenous administration) that all of that dose will reach the systemic circulation. The fraction of an administered dose of drug that reaches the systemic circulation in unchanged form is known as the *bioavailable dose*. The relative amount of an administered dose of a particular drug which reaches the systemic circulation intact and the rate

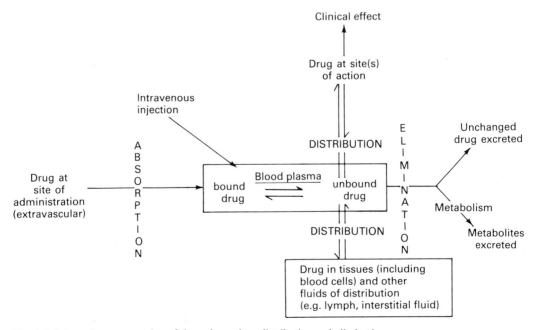

Fig. 8.1 Schematic representation of drug absorption, distribution and elimination

at which this occurs is known as the *bioavailability* of that drug. Bioavailability is thus concerned with the quantity and rate at which the *intact* form of a particular drug appears in the systemic circulation following administration of that drug. The bioavailability exhibited by a drug is thus very important in determining whether a therapeutically effective concentration is achieved at the site(s) of action of the drug.

In defining bioavailability in these terms it is assumed that intact drug is the therapeutically active form of the drug. This definition of bioavailability would not be valid in the case of a pro-drug, whose therapeutic action normally depends on it being converted into its therapeutically active form prior to or on reaching the systemic circulation. It should also be noted that in the context of bioavailability, the term systemic circulation refers primarily to venous blood (excluding the hepatic portal blood during the absorption phase) and arterial blood which carries the intact drug to the tissues.

Hence according to the definition of bioavailability an administered dose of a particular drug in an oral dosage form will be 100% bioavailable only if the drug is completely released from the dosage form into solution in the gastrointestinal fluids. The released drug must also be completely stable in solution in the gastrointestinal fluids and all of the drug must pass through the gastrointestinal barrier into the mesenteric circulation without being metabolized. Finally, all of the absorbed drug must pass into the systemic circulation without being metabolized on passing through the liver. Thus any factor which adversely effects either the release of the drug from the dosage form, its dissolution in the gastrointestinal fluids, its stability in the gastrointestinal fluids, its permeation through and stability in the gastrointestinal barrier or its stability in the hepatic portal circulation will influence the bioavailability exhibited by that drug from the dosage form in which it was administered.

The concept of biopharmaceutics

Many factors have been found to influence the time course of a drug in the plasma and hence at its site(s) of action. These include the foods eaten by the patient, the effect of the disease state on drug absorption, the age of the patient, the site(s) of absorption of the administered drug, the co-administration of other drugs, the physical and chemical properties of the administered drug, the type of dosage form, the composition and method of manufacture of the dosage form and the size of dose and frequency of administration of the dosage form. Thus, a given drug may exhibit differences in its bioavailability if it is administered in the same type of dosage form by different routes of administration, e.g. an aqueous solution of a given drug administered by the oral and intramuscular routes of administration. A given drug may also show differences in its bioavailability from one type of dosage form to another when given by the same route, e.g. a tablet, a hard gelatin capsule and an aqueous suspension administered by the peroral route. A given drug might show different bioavailabilities from different formulations of the same type of dosage form given by the same route of administration, e.g. different formulations of an aqueous suspension of a given drug administered by the peroral route. Variability in the bioavailability exhibited by a given drug from different formulations of the same type of dosage form or from different types of dosage froms etc., can cause patients to be under- or overmedicated. The result may be therapeutic failure or serious adverse effects particularly in the case of drugs which have a narrow therapeutic range (see Chapter 10).

The entry of a drug into the systemic circulation following the administration of a drug product usually involves

1 the release of the drug from its dosage form into solution in the biological fluids at the absorption site, and
2 the movement of the dissolved drug across biological membranes into the systemic circulation.

The study of the various factors which can affect these processes and the application of this knowledge to obtain the expected therapeutic effect from a drug product when it is used by a patient is known as *biopharmaceutics*.

BIBLIOGRAPHY

Cadwallader, D. E. (1973) *Biopharmaceutics and Drug Interactions*, F. Hoffman-La Roche, Basel.

Eadie, M. J., Tyrer, J. H. and Bochner, F. (1981) *Introduction to Clinical Pharmacology*, MTP Press Ltd, Lancaster.

Gibaldi, M. (1984) *Biopharmaceutics and Clinical Pharmacokinetics*, 3rd edn, Lea and Febiger, Philadelphia.

Notari, R. E. (1980) *Biopharmaceutics and Clinical Pharmacokinetics. An Introduction*, 3rd edn, Marcel Dekker Inc., New York.

Wagner, J. G. (1971) *Biopharmaceutics and Relevant Pharmacokinetics*, 1st edn, Drug Intelligence Publications, Hamilton, Illinois.

World Health Organisation (1974) *Bioavailability of Drugs: Principles and Problems*. Report of a WHO Scientific Group. Wld. Hlth. Org. Techn. Rep. Ser., 1974, No. 536. HMSO, London

Factors influencing bioavailability: factors influencing drug absorption from the gastrointestinal tract

DRUG ABSORPTION FROM THE GASTROINTESTINAL TRACT

The various factors which can influence drug release from dosage forms and absorption into the systemic circulation will be considered in this chapter by reference to the peroral (i.e. gastrointestinal) route of administration. This route is chosen as the example, since the majority of drugs are administered orally and the vast majority of orally administered drugs are intended to be absorbed from the gastrointestinal tract. Thus, a detailed consideration of the factors which can influence the absorption of drugs from this region is warranted.

In order that the reader may gain an insight into the numerous factors which can potentially influence the rate and extent of appearance of intact drug into the systemic circulation, a schematic illustration of the steps involved in the release and gastrointestinal absorption of a drug from a tablet is presented in Fig. 9.1. It is evident from this diagram that the rate and extent of appearance of intact drug into the systemic circulation depends

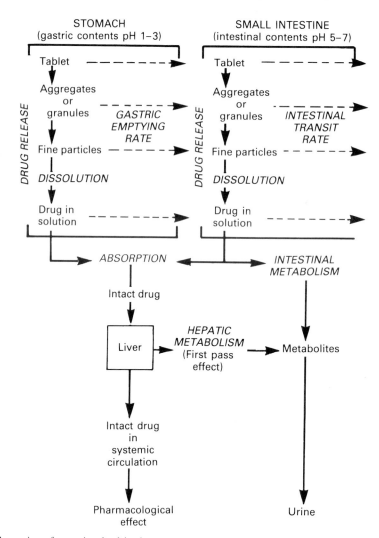

Fig. 9.1 Schematic illustration of steps involved in the appearance of intact drug in the systemic circulation following peroral administration of a tablet. Potential rate-limiting steps with respect to drug bioavailability are shown in italic capitals. (After Barr, 1972)

on a succession of rate (kinetic) processes. The slowest step in this series of rate processes, which is known as the rate-limiting step, will control the overall rate and extent of appearance of intact drug in the systemic circulation. The particular rate-limiting step may vary from drug to drug. Thus for a drug which exhibits a very poor aqueous solubility, the rate at which the drug dissolves in the gastrointestinal fluids is often the slowest step and therefore exhibits a rate-limiting effect on a drug bioavailability. In contrast, for a drug which has a high aqueous solubility, its dissolution rate will be rapid and the rate at which the drug crosses the gastrointestinal membrane may be the rate-limiting step. Other potential rate-limiting steps include the rate of release of the drug from the dosage form (especially important in the case of controlled released dosage forms), the rate at which the stomach empties the drug into the small intestine, the rate at which drug is metabolized by enzymes in the intestinal mucosal cells during its passage into the mesenteric blood vessels and the rate of metabolism of drug during its initial passage through the liver, i.e. the 'first pass' effect.

Structure of the gastrointestinal tract

The gastrointestinal tract consists of three major anatomical regions: the stomach, the small intestine and the large intestine (colon). The small intestine includes the duodenum, jejenum and ileum. As a drug descends through these regions of the gastrointestinal tract, it encounters different environments whth respect to pH, enzymes, electrolytes, fluidity and surface features, all of which can influence drug absorption (see later in this chapter).

The gastrointestinal tract is basically a hollow muscular tube composed of four concentric layers of tissue named from the innermost to the outermost as the mucosa (or mucous membrane), the submucosa, the muscularis externa and the serosa. These are shown diagrammatically in Fig. 9.2. Of these four layers, the mucosa is the most important with respect to the absorption of drugs

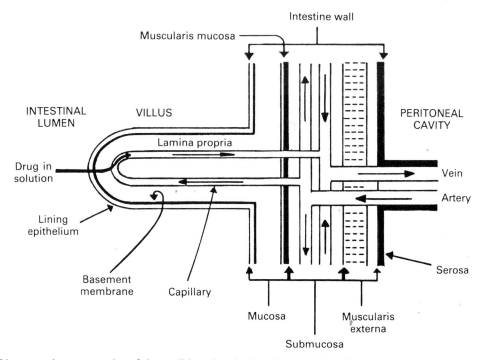

Fig. 9.2 Diagrammatic representation of the small intestine showing the absorption of a drug from the intestinal lumen into a blood capillary. (After Smith 1964)

from the lumen of the gastrointestinal tract. The mucosa contains the cellular membranes and regions through which a drug must pass in order to reach the blood (or lymph). Figure 9.2 shows that the mucosa, itself, consists of three layers: the lining epithelium, the lamina propria and the muscularis mucosa. The epithelium lining the lumen of the gastrointestinal tract comprises a single layer of columnar and some specialized secretory cells (e.g. mucus secreting goblet cells). Of these cells only the columnar cells are concerned with absorption. The layer underlying the epithelium is the lamina propria which contains connective tissue, blood and lymph vessels. The final layer comprising the mucosa is the muscularis mucosa which is a relatively thin layer of muscle fibres.

In *the stomach* the mucosa contains many folds which increase the total surface area over that afforded by a flat smooth lining. Although the stomach does not function primarily as an absorption organ, its excellent blood supply and the fact that a drug can potentially reside in the stomach for 30 minutes up to several hours in contact with a reasonably large epithelial surface, provide conditions which are conducive to the absorption of certain drugs, e.g. weak acidic drugs.

The *small intestine* is *the most important site* for drug absorption in the gastrointestinal tract. The outstanding anatomical feature of the small intestine is the tremendously large epithelial surface area through which drug absorption can take place. This large epithelial surface area results from the existence of (a) folds in the intestinal mucosa known as the folds of Kerckring, (b) villi and (c) microvilli. Villi are finger-like projections which arise from the entire mucosal surface (including the folds of Kerckring) of the small intestine. Villi range in length from 0.5 to 1.5 mm and there are estimated to be 10–40 villi per mm^2 of intestinal mucosa. Figure 9.2 shows that each villus is covered by a single continuous layer of epithelium (i.e. the epithelial lining of the intestinal mucosa) which is made up primarily of the columnar absorption cells and the mucus-secreting goblet cells. In terms of drug absorption from the small intestine the columnar cells are extremely important since it is the anatomical structure of the apical surface of each columnar cell (i.e. the cell surface facing the intestinal lumen) which further increases the epithelial surface area of the small intestine that is available for drug absorption. Figure 9.3 shows that the apical surface of each cell consists of numerous minute slender projections, approximately 1 μm long, known as microvilli. Microvilli appear to be microtubular projections of the apical cell membrane of each columnar cell. The microvilli (between 700 and 1000 per columnar cell), together with the villi and folds of Kerckring, are estimated to increase the surface area available for absorption by 600 times that which would be available if the inner surface of the small intestine was flat.

Intimately associated with the microvilli is a coating of fine filamentous material composed of mucopolysaccharides. This coating is known as the glycocalyx. In addition to the glycocalyx there are two further layers of material between the microvilli and the luminal contents of the small intestine, i.e. a layer of protective mucus secreted by the goblet cells and the so-called 'unstirred aqueous layer'. Figures 9.2 and 9.3 show that the absorption of a drug from the lumen of the intestine into the blood draining the villi involves the passage of drug through several barriers and regions. Thus drug molecules in the lumen of the small intestine must first diffuse through the unstirred aqueous layer, the mucous layer and the glycocalyx in order to reach the microvilli, i.e. the apical cell membrane of the columnar cell. The apical cell membrane of each epthelial cell lining the gastrointestinal tract appears to be tightly bound to that of adjacent epithelial cells. This so-called 'tight junction' between the cell membranes of adjacent epithelial cells (see Fig. 9.3) is thought to act as a barrier to the intercellular passage of drug molecules from the intestinal lumen to the lamina propria. Thus a drug molecule must cross the apical cell membrane into the interior of a columnar cell. After diffusing through the fluids within this cell, a drug molecule must cross the basal cell membrane of the columnar cell. On emerging from the columnar cell the molecule must cross the underlying basement membrane into the lamina propria. Finally, after diffusing through the tissue region of the lamina propria, drug molecules must cross the endothelium of one of the blood capillaries present in this region.

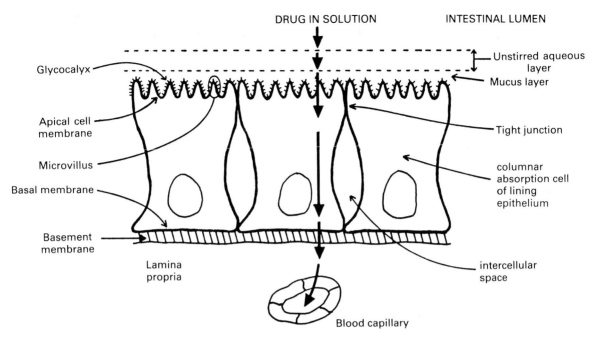

Fig. 9.3 Diagrammatic representation of intestinal columnar absorption cells in the lining epithelium showing a pathway of drug absorption from the intestinal lumen to a blood capillary lying in the lamina propria

Drug molecules would then be carried away in the blood to the systemic circulation via the liver. Most drugs reach the systemic circulation via the blood stream of the capillary metwork in the villi. However, it is possible that the absorption of highly lipid-soluble drugs, particularly if administered in an oily vehicle, may occur via fat absorption pathways. In such cases, drug removal from the villi would involve the central lacteals and the lymphatic circulation.

Although the above description of drug absorption refers specifically to the small intestine, absorption from other areas of the gastrointestinal tract would also involve the passage of drug through similar barriers and regions. Thus the term gastrointestinal absorption will be used in this chapter to encompass the separate processes by which drug passes from the lumen of the gastrointestinal tract into columnar absorption cells and its movement through and out of these cells into the blood vessels via the lamina propria.

The *large intestine* like the stomach lacks villi (and microvilli). However, the large intestine serves as a site for the absorption of drug which has not been completely absorbed in the more proximal regions of the gastrointestinal tract, i.e.

the stomach and small intestine. Incomplete drug absorption in the more proximal regions may be due to the physicochemical properties of the drug itself (e.g. very low aqueous solubility and dissolution rate) or as a result of the intended slow release of drug from a prolonged/sustained/controlled release dosage form. In general if a large proportion of an orally administered dose of drug reaches the large intestine, it is likely that the drug will exhibit poor bioavailability (Gibaldi, 1984).

Mechanisms of drug transport across the gastrointestinal/blood barrier

It is apparent from the previous section that absorption of a drug from the lumen of the gastrointestinal tract into the blood involves the passage of drug molecules across several cellular membranes and fluid regions within the mucosa, i.e. the gastrointestinal/blood barrier. The epithelium lining the gastrointestinal tract is considered to constitute the main cellular barrier to the absorption of drugs from the gastrointestinal tract (Blanchard, 1975). The permeability characteristics of this epithelial layer appear to be directly related to the properties of the apical cell membrane of the columnar absorption cell and thus gastrointestinal absorption becomes a special case of the general biological phenomenon of membrane transport (Levine, 1971). The apical cell membrane exhibits the characteristic trilaminar membrane structure upon electron microscopic examination and is composed largely of protein and lipid. Although the precise molecular structure of a cell membrane is not known, the apical cell membrane of the columnar absorption cell appears to behave, with respect to the absorption of drugs and nutrients, as a 'lipoidal' membrane penetrated periodically by submicroscopic aqueous filled channels or pores. Water-soluble substances of small molecular size (radius less than 0.4 nm), such as urea, are absorbed by simple diffusion through the water filled channels. Most drug molecules, however, are too large to pass through these channels and the apical cell membrane (and hence the gastrointestinal/blood barrier) behaves like a 'lipoidal sieve' with respect to the absorption of drugs. Thus the barrier allows the passage of lipid-soluble drugs in preference to lipid-insoluble drugs. The majority of drugs appear to cross the apical cell membrane of the lining epithelium (and other cell membranes within the gastrointestinal/blood barrier) by the mechanism known as passive diffusion. This and other mechanisms by which some drugs are absorbed will be considered.

Passive diffusion

In this process the apical cell membrane of a columnar absorption cell plays a passive role and does not participate actively in the transport process. The rate of drug transport is determined by the physicochemical properties of the drug, the nature of the membrane and the concentration gradient of drug across the membrane. The process of passive diffusion, shown in Fig. 9.4, initially involves partition of a drug between the aqueous fluid in the gastrointestinal tract and the lipoidal-like cell membrane of the lining epithelium. The drug in solution in the membrane then diffuses across the membrane followed by a second partition of drug between the membrane and the aqueous fluids within the columnar absorption cells. The drug would cross the other cell membranes in the gastrointestinal/blood barrier by this sequence of steps and thus would eventually enter the blood of the capillary network in the lamina propria. If we considered that the cell membranes and fluid regions making up the gastrointestinal/blood barrier could be represented by a single 'membrane', the gastrointestinal membrane, separating the aqueous gastrointestinal fluid from the capillary blood supply in the lamina propria, then the stages involved in the gastrointestinal absorption of a drug by passive diffusion could be represented by the model shown in Fig. 9.4.

Passive diffusion of drugs across the gastro-

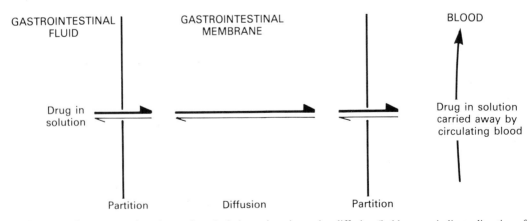

Fig. 9.4 Diagrammatic representation of gastrointestinal absorption via passive diffusion (bold arrows indicate direction of net movement of drug)

intestinal/blood barrier can often be described mathematically by Fick's first law of diffusion. Accordingly the rate of appearance of drug in the blood at the site of absorption is given by

$$\frac{\mathrm{d}m}{\mathrm{d}t} = \frac{D\,A\,(K_1 C_{\mathrm{g}} - K_2 C_{\mathrm{b}})}{h} \qquad (9.1)$$

where $\mathrm{d}m/\mathrm{d}t$ is the rate of appearance of drug in the blood at the site of absorption, D is the effective diffusion coefficient of the drug in the gastrointestinal (g.i.) 'membrane', A is the surface area of the gastrointestinal 'membrane' available for absorption by passive diffusion, K_1 is the apparent partition coefficient of the drug between the gastrointestinal 'membrane' and the gastrointestinal fluid i.e.

$$K_1 = \frac{\begin{array}{c}\text{concentration of drug inside 'membrane' at}\\ \text{g.i. fluid/membrane interface}\end{array}}{\text{concentration of drug in g.i. fluid}}$$

C_{g} is the concentration of drug in solution in the gastrointestinal fluid at the site of absorption, K_2 is the apparent partition coefficient of the drug between the gastrointestinal 'membrane' and the blood, C_{b} is the concentration of drug in the blood at the site of absorption, and h is the thickness of the gastrointestinal 'membrane'.

Hence $K_1 C_{\mathrm{g}}$ and $K_2 C_{\mathrm{b}}$ represent the concentrations of drug inside the gastrointestinal membrane at the g.i. fluid/membrane interface and g.i. membrane/blood interface respectively. The expression

$$\frac{(K_1 C_{\mathrm{g}} - K_2 C_{\mathrm{b}})}{h}$$

represents the concentration gradient of drug across the 'membrane'.

Eqn 9.1 indicates that the rate of gastrointestinal absorption of a drug by passive diffusion depends on the surface area of the 'membrane' that is available for drug absorption. This is compatible with the observation that the small intestine, particularly the duodenum, is the major site for drug absorption due principally to the presence of villi and microvilli which provide an enormous surface area for absorption. Eqn 9.1 also indicates that the rate of drug absorption depends on a large concentration gradient of drug existing across the gastrointestinal 'membrane'. It is of interest to note that the concentration gradient of drug across the membrane is influenced by the apparent partition coefficients exhibited by the drug with respect to the g.i. 'membrane'/g.i. fluid interface and the g.i. 'membrane'/blood interface. It is important that the drug has sufficient affinity (solubility) for the 'membrane' phase that it can partition readily into the gastrointestinal 'membrane', i.e. K_1 should exceed unity. In addition, after diffusing across the 'membrane' the drug should exhibit sufficient solubility for the blood such that it can partition readily out of the 'membrane' phase into the blood, i.e. K_2 should be less than 1. Drug on entering the blood in the capillary network in the lamina propria will be carried away from the site of absorption by the rapidly circulating gastrointestnal blood supply and will become diluted by

1 distribution in a large volume of blood, i.e. the systemic circulation,
2 distribution into body tissue and other fluids of distribution, and
3 by metabolism and excretion.

In addition, proteins in the blood may bind drug molecules and thereby further lower the concentration of 'free' (diffusible) drug in the blood. Consequently the blood acts as a 'sink' for absorbed drug and ensures that the concentration of drug in the blood at the site of absorption is low in relation to the concentration of drug in solution in the gastrointestinal fluids at the site of absorption, i.e. $C_{\mathrm{g}} \gg C_{\mathrm{b}}$. The 'sink' conditions provided by the systemic circulation ensures that a large concentration gradient is maintained across the gastrointestinal 'membrane' during the absorption process. The passive absorption process is driven solely by the concentration gradient of the diffusible species of the drug which exists across the gastrointestinal/blood barrier. Under such conditions that $K_1 C_{\mathrm{g}} \gg K_2 C_{\mathrm{b}}$ and thus $(K_1 C_{\mathrm{g}} - K_2 C_{\mathrm{b}})$ approximates to $K_1 C_{\mathrm{g}}$, Eqn 9.1 may be rewritten in the form

$$\frac{\mathrm{d}m}{\mathrm{d}t} = \frac{D\,A\,K_1 C_{\mathrm{g}}}{h} \qquad (9.2)$$

For a given drug and 'membrane' under specified conditions, D, A, K_1 and h may be regarded as constants which can be incorporated into a combined constant known as the permeability constant, P. Hence Eqn 9.2 becomes

$$\frac{dm}{dt} = P\,C_g \qquad (9.3)$$

where

$$P = \frac{D\,A\,K_1}{h}$$

Eqn 9.3 is an expression for a first order kinetic process and indicates that the rate of passive drug absorption will be proportional to the concentration of absorbable drug in solution in the gastrointestinal fluids at the site of absorption. In practice, the gastrointestinal absorption of most drugs by passive diffusion follows first order kinetics.

It has been assumed that the drug in aqueous solution on each side of the gastrointestinal/blood barrier (see Fig. 9.4) existed entirely in the form of a single absorbable (via passive diffusion) species which exhibited definite partition coefficients for distribution between

1 the aqueous gastrointestinal fluids and the lipoidal 'membrane', and
2 the blood and the lipoidal 'membrane'.

However, many drugs are weak electrolytes which exist in aqueous solution as two species, namely the unionized and ionized species. Since it is the unionized form of a weak electrolyte drug which exhibits greater lipid solubility compared to the corresponding ionized form, the gastrointestinal 'membrane' (like other membranes) is permeable preferentially to the unionized species. Thus the rate of passive absorption of weak electrolyte drugs is related to the fraction of total drug that exists in the unionized form in solution in the gastrointestinal fluids at the site of absorption. This fraction is determined by the dissociation constant of the drug (i.e. its pK_a value) and by the pH of its aqueous environment in accordance with the Henderson–Hasselbalch equations for weak acids and bases. The gastrointestinal absorption of a weak electrolyte drug is enhanced when the pH at the site of absorption favours the formation of a large fraction of the drug in aqueous solution that is unionized. These observations form the basis of the pH–partition hypothesis (see later in this chapter).

Carrier-mediated transport

Active transport Most drugs are absorbed from the gastrointestinal tract by passive diffusion. However, a few lipid-insoluble drugs (such as 5-fluorouracil) and many substances of nutritional interest are absorbed by active transport mechanisms. In contrast to passive diffusion, active transport involves active participation by the apical cell membrane of the columnar absorption cell (and presumably also by the other cell membranes constituting the gastrointestinal/blood barrier) in the gastrointestinal absorption of a drug. A 'carrier' which may be an enzyme or some other component of the cell membrane is responsible for effecting the transfer of drug by a process which is represented in Fig. 9.5.

Figure 9.5 shows that the drug molecule or ion forms a complex with the 'carrier' in the surface of the apical cell membrane of a columnar absorption cell involved in the active transport of the particular drug. The 'drug–carrier' complex then moves across the membrane and liberates the drug on the other side of the membrane. The carrier (now free) returns to its initial position in the surface of the cell membrane adjacent to the lumen of the gastrointestinal tract to await the arrival of another drug molecule or ion.

Active transport is a process whereby materials can be transported against a concentration gradient across a cell membrane, i.e. transport can occur from a region of lower concentration to one of higher concentration. Therefore active transport is an energy consuming absorption process. In the case of the gastrointestinal absorption of drugs by active transport, transfer of drug occurs in the direction of the gastrointestinal lumen to the blood and not normally in the reverse direction, i.e. drug absorption by active transport across the gastrointestinal/blood barrier does not normally occur against a concentration gradient of the drug. The carrier system is generally a 'one-way' transport system.

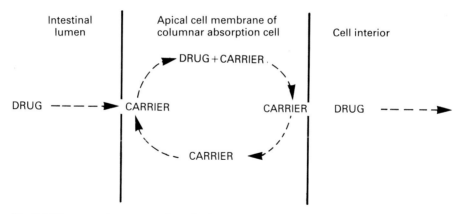

Fig. 9.5 Diagrammatic representation of active transport of a drug across a cell membrane

There appear to be several carrier-mediated active transport systems in the small intestine. Each carrier appears to be highly selective with respect to the chemical structure of the substance which it will transport. Thus if a drug structurally resembles a natural substance which is actively transported then that drug is also likely to be transported by the same carrier mechanism. For instance the drug levodopa, which is structurally related to the amino acids tyrosine and phenylalanine, is absorbed by the same active transport system that is used to transport these amino acids from the lumen of the small intestine into the blood. Each carrier system is generally concentrated in a specific segment of the gastrointestinal tract. The substance which is transported by that carrier will thus be absorbed preferentially in the location of highest carrier density. For instance, more riboflavin is absorbed from the proximal portion of the small intestine than from the large or upper intestine.

Unlike passive absorption, where the rate of absorption is directly proportional to the concentration of the absorbable species of the drug at the absorption site, active transport proceeds at a rate which is proportional to the drug concentration only at low concentrations. At higher concentrations the carrier mechanism becomes saturated and further increases in drug concentration will not increase the rate of absorption, i.e. the rate of absorption remains constant.

Many body nutrients such as sugars and L-amino acids are transported across the gastrointestinal 'membrane' by active transport processes.

Vitamins such as thiamine, nicotinic acid, riboflavin and B_6 require an active transport system. The anticancer drug 5-fluorouracil, methyldopa and nicotinamide are absorbed by active transport. Active transport also plays an important role in the renal and biliary excretion of many drugs and metabolites.

Facilitated diffusion or transport This is also a carrier-mediated transport system which differs from active transport in that it cannot transport a substance against a concentration gradient of that substance. Therefore facilitated diffusion does not require an energy input but it does require a concentration gradient for its driving force (as does passive diffusion). In terms of drug absorption, facilitated diffusion seems to play a very minor role.

Ion-pair absorption

This mechanism of absorption has been proposed to explain how certain drugs such as quaternary ammonium compounds and tetracyclines, which are ionized over the entire gastrointestinal pH range, are absorbed from the gastrointestinal tract. Such drug ions are considered to be too lipid insoluble to partition directly into the lipoidal apical cell membrane of the columnar absorption cells lining the gastrointestinal tract. In addition, these water-soluble drug ions are too large to pass through the aqueous filled pores or channels which are considered to exist in the cell membrane lining the gastrointestinal tract. However, the interaction of such drug ions with endogenous organic ions of opposite charge to form an absorbable neutral species (i.e. an ion-pair) is a possible explanation of their mechanism of absorption. Since the charges are 'buried' in the ion-pair, the latter can now partition into the lipoidal cell membrane lining the gastrointestinal tract and be absorbed by passive diffusion.

Convective absorption (pore transport)

Very small molecules such as water, urea and low molecular weight sugars and organic electrolytes are able to cross cell membranes as if the membrane contained aqueous filled channels or pores. The effective radius of these channels has been estimated to be of the order of 0.4 nm. As a result of molecular size limitations, this mechanism of absorption appears to be of minor importance with respect to the gastrointestinal absorption of large water-soluble drug molecules or ions. However, convective absorption is involved in the renal excretion of drugs and the uptake of drugs into the liver.

Pinocytosis

Pinocytosis is the only mechanism of absorption in which the material does not have to be in aqueous solution in order to be absorbed. The mechanism is comparable to phagocytosis and involves invagination of the material by the apical cell membrane of the columnar absorption cells lining the gastrointestinal tract to form vacuoles containing the material. These vacuoles then cross the columnar absorption cells. This mechanism of absorption appears to be of little importance for drugs but is important for the absorption of macromolecules such as proteins.

PHYSIOLOGICAL FACTORS INFLUENCING DRUG ABSORPTION FROM THE GASTROINTESTINAL TRACT

In discussing how various physiological properties of the gastrointestinal tract may influence drug absorption, it should be noted that it is assumed (unless otherwise stated) that the drug is in solution in the appropriate gastrointestinal fluid.

Where appropriate, consideration will be given also to the influence that physiological factors can have on the release and dissolution of a drug from a dosage form. A drug must be in solution before it can be absorbed and the rate of drug release/dissolution can under certain conditions be the rate-controlling step in the appearance of a drug in the systemic circulation (see later in this chapter).

Surface area of the gastrointestinal absorption sites

The biological environments and the areas of membrane available for absorption in the stomach, the small intestine and the large intestine are quite different and these differences give rise to variations in the rate and extent of absorption of a drug from these anatomical regions.

As previously discussed, the presence of (a) folds in the mucosa, (b) villi and (c) microvilli is responsible for the small intestine having the largest effective surface area available for absorption. Consequently the small intestine is the region of maximum absorption for the majority of drugs even though the pH of the intestinal fluid does not provide optimum conditions for the absorption of all drugs, e.g. weak acidic drugs. In addition to its large absorptive surface area the small intestine is the most important region for carrier-mediated drug absorption, i.e. the small intestine is the location of highest 'carrier' density.

In contrast to the small intestine, the absorptive surface areas of the stomach and the large intestine are relatively small since neither of these regions possess villi or microvilli. Despite the relatively small absorptive surface area available in the stomach, certain drugs (e.g. weak acidic drugs in solution which are unionized) are absorbed in this region. It should be noted that following oral ingestion of a drug in solution a major part of the stomach's absorptive area will be immediately in contact with dissolved drug and, providing that the intrinsic physicochemical properties of the drug permit permeation of the gastrointestinal/blood barrier, good absorption may occur. However, because the absorptive surface area in the stomach is so small compared to that in the small intestine, the rate and extent of absorption of a given drug from the stomach will, in most cases, be less than from the small intestine. The large intestine functions as an absorptive site for drugs that are so slowly absorbed that a significant portion of the administered dose passes through the stomach and small intestine. In addition, the large intestine is important for the absorption of some drugs such as sulphasalazine which must be degraded by the bacterial flora in this region before absorption can occur.

pH of gastrointestinal fluids

The pH of the fluids varies considerably along the length of the gastrointestinal tract. Gastric fluid is highly acidic, exhibiting a pH within the range 1–3.5. The fluid in the small intestine is generally considered to have a pH in the range 5–8, generally from a pH range of 5–6 in the duodenum to about pH 8 in the lower ileum. The fluid in the large intestine is generally considered to have a pH of about 8. Considerable variations within the above pH ranges may occur in an individual. For instance, there appears to be a diurnal cycle of gastric acidity, the fluids becoming more acidic at night and fluctuating during the day primarily in response to food ingestion. Gastric fluid pH generally increases when food is ingested and then slowly decreases over the following few hours. There is also considerable intersubject variation in gastrointestinal pH depending on such factors as:

1 the general health of the individual,
2 the presence of localized disease conditions (e.g. gastric and duodenal ulcers) along the gastrointestinal tract,
3 the types and amounts of food ingested, and
4 drug therapy.

In the case of drug therapy, anticholinergic drugs inhibit or reduce gastric secretion and the oral administration of antacids usually elevates gastric pH for a short period of time.

Gastrointestinal pH may influence drug absorption in a variety of ways. The degree to which a given weak electrolyte drug ionizes in solution in the gastrointestinal fluids is a function of pH (and pK_a of the drug). In general the unionized form of a drug in solution will be absorbed faster than the ionized form of the same drug at any particular site along the gastrointestinal tract. Thus any change in pH of the gastric fluid (caused by any of the above variables), to a value which increases the extent to which a weak electrolyte drug in solution exists in its unionized form, will result in faster absorption from the stomach than was observed from this site at the original pH. However, most drugs in solution are absorbed more rapidly from the small intestine regardless of differences in pH between the stomach, small intestine and large intestine. This is a reflection of the over-riding influence of the available absorptive surface area on the rate of absorption of drugs in solution from these sites.

Since the aqueous solubility of a weak electrolyte drug is influenced by pH, the rate of dissolution of such a drug from a solid dosage form will be pH dependent. In the case of a poorly soluble weak electrolyte drug administered in a solid dosage form, the rate of drug dissolution in the gastrointestinal fluids may be the rate-limiting step for the absorption of such a drug. Hence gastrointestinal pH would be expected to exert a major influence on the dissolution rate and hence the overall absorption rate of such a drug administered in a solid dosage form such as a tablet or a hard gelatin capsule. Consequently a poorly soluble weak acidic drug, which only exhibits a high dissolution rate in an alkaline aqueous environment, will only be expected to be rapidly absorbed from a solid dosage form when the drug passes through the acid environment of the stomach and reaches the more alkaline intestinal fluids where rapid drug dissolution can occur. In contrast, a poorly aqueous-soluble weak basic drug, which only exhibits a high dissolution rate in an acidic aqueous environment, must first dissolve in the acidic gastric fluid before it reaches the small intestine in order to be rapidly absorbed from the small intestine. Any undissolved weak basic drug which reaches the small intestine would be expected to exhibit a relatively low absorption rate since its dissolution rate in the relatively alkaline intestinal fluids would be low (Mayersohn, 1979).

A further way by which gastrointestinal pH can influence drug absorption is in the case of drugs which exhibit limited chemical stability in either acidic or alkaline environments. The influence that the chemical stability exhibited by a drug in the gastrointestinal fluids can have on the absorption of such a drug from the gastrointestinal tract is discussed later in this chapter.

Gastric emptying rate

Most drugs are optimally absorbed from the small intestine following peroral administration. Hence any reduction in the rate at which a drug in solution leaves the stomach and enters the duodenum (i.e. the gastric emptying rate) is likely to reduce the overall rate of drug absorption and therefore delay the onset of the therapeutic response of the drug. In addition the intensity of the therapeutic response may be reduced. The rate of gastric emptying is also important for drugs which are prone to chemical degradation in the stomach by virtue of the low pH or enzyme activity associated with the gastric fluid. The longer the time that a susceptible drug spends in the stomach, the more likely the drug is to be degraded with an accompanying reduction in its effective concentration and hence bioavailability. Drugs contained in enteric-coated dosage forms, which are formulated so as to prevent drug release into gastric fluid but to allow release into the fluid in the duodenum, will show a delayed onset of therapeutic activity if the gastric emptying rate is suppressed.

The gastric emptying of fluids and small particles appears to be an exponential process (Bechgaard and Christensen, 1982). Standard low bulk meals and liquids are transferred from the stomach into the duodenum in an apparent first order rate process, i.e. the rate of gastric emptying is proportional to the volume of the material remaining in the stomach. Gastric emptying rate is influenced by a large number of factors. Factors promoting gastric emptying rate include hunger, anxiety, the patient's body position (i.e. lying on the right side), the intake of liquids and the antiemetic drug, metoclopramide (Gibaldi, 1984). Gastric emptying rate is retarded by factors such as fatty foods, a high bulk (viscous) diet, mental depression, gastric ulcers, pyloric stenosis, hypothyroidism, the patient's body position (lying on the left side) and drugs such as anticholinergics, tricyclic antidepressants, aluminuim hydroxide

and alcohol (Mayersohn, 1979). In view of these numerous factors which can influence gastric emptying rate, it is not surprising that this is a highly variable parameter both among different individuals and within any one individual at different times. It is likely that such variation in gastric emptying rate contributes to the intersubject and intrasubject variation observed in the bioavailability of a given drug.

The gastric emptying of solution-type dosage forms and suspensions of fine drug particles is generally much faster and less variable than that of solid, non-disintegrating unit dosage forms and lumpy masses of aggregrated particles. For instance the gastric emptying times of single non-disintegrating tablets (diameter 10–16 mm) range from 0.5 to 4.5 hours whereas dosage forms which disintegrate into small subunits (e.g. granules, pellets) are emptied gradually from the stomach with a mean time of 1.5 hours (Bechgaard and Christensen, 1982). It is thus not surprising to find that the gastric emptying times of enteric-coated tablets, which are designed to remain intact in the stomach, are very erratic and this contributes to the unusually large intersubject variability found in the absorption of drugs from this type of dosage form (Gibaldi, 1984).

In general, the presence of food in the stomach reduces the gastric emptying rate and thus can delay the absorption of drugs which are normally absorbed from the small intestine. Hence, unless a drug is irritating to the gastric mucosa, a drug should not be administered with or immediately after a bulky meal. In general a drug will reach the small intestine most rapidly if it is administered with water to a patient whose stomach is empty of food. However, effects of food on drug absorption from the gastrointestinal tract are quite variable and are considered in greater detail later in this chapter.

Whilst the above discussion suggests that a decrease in gastric emptying rate will be disadvantageous with respect to the overall rate of absorption of many drugs, the opposite may also be true. An example is the case of a solid dosage form containing a poorly soluble drug which must first dissolve in gastric fluid prior to being absorbed rapidly from the small intestine. Such would be the case for a poorly soluble weak basic drug since any of this drug which reached the small intestine in the undissolved state would be expected to dissolve (and hence be absorbed) slowly. This is a consequence of the reduced solubility exhibited by such drugs at intestinal pH conditions. Hence a decrease in gastric emptying rate would permit a longer time in which dissolution of such a drug could occur in the more favourable acidic pH conditions of the stomach. A greater proportion of the administered dose of drug would dissolve and thus be in an absorbable form when it passed into the duodenum. The enchanced bioavailability exhibited by the poorly soluble drug nitrofurantoin in the presence of food was considered to be a result of the accompanying decreased gastric emptying rate which permitted a greater proportion of the drug to dissolve in the gastric fluids before passing into the duodenum from where it is optimally absorbed (Rosenberg and Bates, 1976).

Intestinal motility

Once a drug empties from the stomach and enters the small intestine it will be exposed to an environment which is totally different from that of the stomach. Since the small intestine is the primary site of drug absorption, the longer the residence time in this region the greater is the potential for efficient drug absorption assuming that the drug is stable in the intestinal fluids and does not react with endogenous materials to form poorly absorbable 'complexes' (Mayersohn, 1979).

There are two types of intestinal movements, propulsive and mixing. The propulsive movements primarily determine the intestinal transit rate and thus the residence time of a drug or a dosage form in the small intestine. The greater the intestinal motility, the shorter the residence time and the less time there is for dissolution and absorption of drugs to occur. Under normal circumstances, peristaltic waves propel the intestinal contents relatively slowly, i.e. it takes 3–10 hours to move a meal in the form of chyme along the entire length of the small intestine (Mayersohn, 1979). The residence time in the small intestine, as determined by intestinal motility, may be an important factor with respect to drug bioavailability. The longer a drug is in contact with the

absorption site(s) the greater the amount of drug absorbed (Bates and Gibaldi, 1970). Intestinal residence time will thus be important for

1 dosage forms which release drug slowly (e.g. controlled/sustained/prolonged release dosage forms) as they pass along the entire length of the gastrointestinal tract,
2 enteric-coated dosage forms which release drug only when they reach the small intestine,
3 drugs which dissolve slowly in the intestinal fluids and
4 drugs which are absorbed by intestinal carrier-mediated transport systems.

Mixing movements of the small intestine bring drug which is in solution in the intestinal contents into intimate contact with the large epithelial absorptive surface area of the small intestine. The mixing movements thus increase the area of contact between drug in solution and the gastrointestinal 'membrane'. In addition, the mixing movements will also increase the dissolution rate of drugs from solid dosage forms and this will be particularly significant in the case of poorly soluble drugs which exhibit dissolution rate-limited absorption.

Drug stability in the gastrointestinal tract

Absorption is not the only process that can occur as a drug in solution passes along the gastrointestinal tract. A drug may be chemically degraded and/or metabolized in the gastrointestinal tract. The consequence of this is usually incomplete bioavailability since only a fraction of the administered dose reaches the systemic circulation in the form of intact drug. Chemical degradation, particularly pH-dependent reactions such as hydrolysis, can occur in the fluids of the gastrointestinal tract. For instance, erythromycin undergoes acid-catalysed hydrolysis in gastric fluid. Drugs which resemble nutrients such as polypeptides, nucleotides or fatty acids may be especially susceptible to enzymic hydrolysis in the gastrointestinal tract. In addition to enzymic metabolism in the gastrointestinal fluids, drugs may be metabolized by enzymes located in the intestinal mucosa. For instance, intestinal metabolism accounts for orally administered isoproterenol being 1000 times less active than intravenously administered isoproterenol (Gibaldi, 1984). Other drugs which appear to be metabolized in the gastrointestinal mucosa include chlorpromazine, L-dopa, stilboestrol, progesterone and testosterone. The metabolic potential of the gastrointestinal microflora is also now recognized (Mayersohn, 1979).

It would seem that metabolism and degradation of a drug in the gastrointestinal tract would serve primarily to reduce the extent of its bioavailability. However, in some instances these processes may be essential for drug absorption to occur. Many pro-drugs such as erythromycin stearate and chloramphenicol palmitate depend on degradation in the gastrointestinal tract in order to release the therapeutically active parent molecule.

Hepatic metabolism

All drugs that are absorbed from the stomach, small intestine and colon pass into the hepatic portal system and are presented to the liver before reaching the systemic circulation. The liver is the primary site of drug metabolism. Hence this first pass of absorbed drug through the liver may result in extensive metabolism of the drug and a significant proportion of the absorbed dose of intact drug may never reach the systemic circulation. This phenomenon is known as the *first pass effect* and results in a decrease in bioavailability of those drugs which are rapidly metabolised by the liver. The bioavailability of a susceptible drug may be reduced to such an extent so as to render the gastrointestinal route of administration ineffective (as in the case of lignocaine where 70% of the oral dose is metabolized by the intestinal wall and liver) or to necessitate an oral dose which is many times larger than the intravenous dose (e.g. propranolol). Other drugs which are subject to the first pass effect include alprenolol, pethidine, organic nitrates and propoxyphene.

Influence of food and diet

There is considerable evidence that the rate and/or extent of drug absorption can be influenced by the presence of food in the gastrointestinal tract (Welling, 1980). Food may influence drug bioavailability by means of the following mechanisms.

Alteration in the rate of gastric emptying

For instance, solid meals (particularly those which are hot and contain a high proportion of fat) tend to decrease gastric emptying rate and can thus delay the onset of therapeutic action of some drugs. Further information on the potential consequences of reduced gastric emptying rate on drug bioavailability has been given earlier in this chapter.

Stimulation of gastrointestinal secretions

Gastrointestinal secretions (e.g. gastric hydrochloric acid, pepsin) secreted in response to the presence of food may result in the degradation of drugs which are susceptible to chemical hydrolysis or enzymic metabolism. This would lead to a reduction in drug bioavailability. In the case of stable drugs, the stimulation of gastrointestinal secretions may increase bioavailability by assisting drug dissolution. The ingestion of food, especially fat, stimulates the secretion of bile. Bile salts are surface-active agents and can increase the dissolution of some poorly soluble drugs thereby enhancing their absorption. For instance the enhanced absorption exhibited by griseofulvin when fatty meals are ingested may be due to the solubilizing effect of bile salts secreted in response to the fatty components of the meal. However bile salts have been shown to form insoluble, nonabsorbable complexes with such drugs as neomycin, kanamycin and nystatin.

Competition between food components and drugs for specialized absorption mechanisms

In the case of those drugs which have a chemcial structure similar to nutrients required by the body for which specialized absorption mechanisms exist, there is the possibility of competitive inhibition of drug absorption. One example appears to be L-dopa whose absorption may be inhibited by certain amino acids resulting from the breakdown of ingested proteins.

Complexation of drugs with components in the diet

The gastrointestinal absorption of tetracyline is reduced by virtue of the formation of a non-absorbable complex with calcium present in dairy foods. Foods containing a high iron content also reduce the bioavailability of tetracycline due to complex formation. In general, complexation is only important (with respect to bioavailability) when an irreversible or an insoluble complex is formed. In such cases the fraction of the administered dose of drug which becomes complexed is unavailable for absorption. Consequently the effective concentration of drug in solution in the gastrointestinal fluids is reduced and both the rate and/or extent of drug absorption is reduced. If the complex formed is water soluble and readily dissociates to liberate the 'free' (absorbable) drug, then little or no effect of complexation on drug absorption is noted. The rate at which the complex dissociates determines whether drug absorption is as rapid and/or complete as in the absence of complex formation. Further information on the effects of complexation on drug absorption is given later in this chapter.

Increased viscosity of gastrointestinal contents

The presence of food in the gastrointestinal tract will provide a viscous environment which may result in a reduction in the rate of drug dissolution in the gastrointestinal contents. In addition, the rate of diffusion of a drug in solution from the lumen to the absorbing membrane lining the gastrointestinal tract may be reduced by an increase in viscosity. Both of these effects will tend to decrease the bioavailability of drug.

Food-induced changes in blood flow to the liver

Blood flow to the gastrointestinal tract and liver increases shortly after a meal. This increased blood flow to the liver will increase the rate at which drugs are presented to the liver. The metabolism of some drugs (e.g. propranolol, hydralazine, dextropropoxyphene) is sensitive to their rate of presentation to the liver. The greater the rate of presentation of such drugs to the liver, the larger the fraction of drug that escapes first pass metabolism. This is because the enzyme systems responsible for their metabolism become 'swamped' (i.e. saturated) by the increased rate of presentation of drug to the site of biotransformation. Under these circumstances food, by virtue of causing a transient increase in hepatic blood flow, can increase the amounts of such drugs that reach the systemic circulation intact.

It is thus evident that food can influence the absorption of drugs from the gastrointestinal tract by a variety of mechanisms. A summary of the influences that food may have on the absorption of a number of drugs is given in Table 9.1. Whilst food has been reported to increase or decrease the rate and/or extent of absorption of numerous drugs, it should be noted that the absorption of some drugs does not appear to be influenced by food ingestion. Drugs whose absorption is reported to be unaffected by food include chlorpropamide, oxazepam and prednisolone (Welling, 1980).

Miscellaneous physiological factors influencing gastrointestinal absorption

Disease states and physiological disorders associated with the gastrointestinal tract are likely to influence the absorption and hence bioavailabilities of drugs administered via this route. Local disease states can cause alterations in gastric pH. For instance, the pH of gastric fluid is elevated (up to pH 6.9) in patients with gastric cancer. The various ways by which alterations in gastric pH can influence drug bioavailability have been discussed earlier in this chapter. Gastric surgery can cause drugs to exhibit different bioavailabilities in such patients compared to normal individuals. Partial or total gastrectomy results in drugs reaching the duodenum more rapidly than in the case of normal individuals. This increased rate of presentation of drug to the small intestine may result in an increased overall rate of absorption of drugs which are best absorbed from this segment of the gastrointestinal tract. However, drugs

Table 9.1 The influence of food on the gastrointestinal absorption of some drugs (Mayersohn, 1979)

Drug	Influence of food on absorption	Comments
Aspirin	Reduction in rate but not in extent of absorption	Reduced rate of gastric emptying gives delayed onset of analgesia
Barbiturates	Reduction in rate but not in extent of absorption	Reduced rate of gastric emptying gives delayed hypnotic response
Cephalosporins	Reduction in rate but not in extent of absorption	Reduced rate of gastric emptying gives lower peak plasma concentrations
Griseofulvin	Absorption increased when fatty meal ingested	Solubilizing effect of bile salts secreted in response to fatty meal
Nitrofurantoin	Reduced rate but increased extent of absorption gives higher urinary concentrations	Prolonged residence in stomach gives improved dissolution in gastric fluids
Penicillins (benzylpenicillin, methicillin, oxacillin)	Rate and extent of absorption reduced	Prolonged residence in stomach causes increased loss of those penicillins which are sensitive to acid hydrolysis
Hydralazine	Extent of absorption increased	Reduction in first pass degradation
Tetracyclines (tetracycline, oxytetracycline)	Extent of absorption decreased	Formation of non-absorbable complex with calcium ions present in dairy products

which require a period of time in the stomach in order to facilitate their dissolution may show reduced bioavailabilities in such patients. Diarrhoeal conditions may reduce drug bioavailability by virtue of reducing the drug's residence time in the small intestine.

Other factors which may influence the bioavailabilities of drugs from the gastrointestinal tract include age (i.e. children, adults and elderly patients), stress (e.g. stress induced through illness) and whether a patient is bedridden or not.

PHYSICOCHEMICAL FACTORS INFLUENCING DRUG ABSORPTION FROM THE GASTROINTESTINAL TRACT

In the previous section, drug absorption has been shown to be influenced by many physiological factors. The absorption and hence the bioavailability of a drug is also influenced by many of its physicochemical properties, notably pK_a, lipid solubility, dissolution rate, chemical stability and complexation.

Drug dissociation constant and lipid solubility

The dissociation constant and lipid solubility of a drug and the pH at the absorption site often dictate the absorption characteristics of a drug throughout the gastrointestinal tract. The interrelationship between the degree of ionization of a weak electrolyte drug (which is determined by its dissociation constant and the pH at the absorption site) and the extent of drug absorption is embodied in the pH-partition hypothesis of drug absorption.

pH-partition hypothesis of drug absorption

According to this hypothesis, the gastrointestinal/blood barrier acts as a lipid barrier towards weak electrolyte drugs which are absorbed by passive diffusion. The gastrointestinal/blood barrier is thus impermeable to the ionized (i.e. poorly lipid-soluble) form of a weak acidic or basic drug but relatively permeable to the non-ionized (i.e. more lipid-soluble) form of such a drug. Consequently, according to the pH-partition hypothesis, the absorption of a weak electrolyte drug will be determined chiefly by the extent to which the drug exists in its unionized form at the site of absorption.

In order to illustrate the concept of the pH-partition hypothesis, let us consider the distribution of weak acidic and basic drugs across the gastrointestinal barrier between the gastric fluid and the blood. The extent to which a weak acidic or basic drug ionizes in solution in gastric fluid or blood may be calculated using the appropriate form of the Henderson–Hasselbalch equation (see Chapter 3). For a weak acidic drug having a single ionizable group (e.g. aspirin, phenylbutazone, salicylic acid) the equation takes the form of . . .

$$\log \frac{[A^-]}{[HA]} = pH - pK_a \qquad (9.4)$$

where pK_a is the negative logarithm of the acid dissociation constant of the drug, [HA] and [A$^-$] are the respective concentrations (mol dm^{-3}) of the unionized and ionized forms of the weak acidic drug, which are in equilibrium and in solution either the gastric fluid or the blood. pH refers to the pH of the environment of the ionized and unionized species of the weak acidic drug, i.e. gastric fluid or blood.

For a weak basic drug possessing a single ionizable group (e.g. chlorpromazine) the analogous equation is

$$\log \frac{[BH^+]}{[B]} = pK_a - pH \qquad (9.5)$$

where [BH$^+$] and [B] are the respective concentrations (mol dm^{-3}) of the ionized and unionized forms of the weak basic drug which are in equibilibrium and in solution in either the blood or gastric fluid.

Absorption of a weak acidic drug Consider the distribution of a weak acidic drug having a pK_a of 3.0 between the blood and gastric fluid. For the purposes of this calculation, assume that the pH of gastric fluid is 1.2 and the pH of blood is 7.4. Equation 9.4 may be used to calculate the ratios of the concentrations of the ionized form (A$^-$) and unionized form (HA$^-$) of the weak acidic drug which exist in equilibrium in solution in gastric fluid and blood, respectively. In gastric fluid, pH 1.2

$$\log \frac{[A^-]}{[HA]} = pH - pK_a$$
$$= 1.2 - 3.0 = -1.8$$

Therefore,

$$\frac{[A^-]}{[HA]} = antilog (-1.8) = 0.016$$

Thus the ratio of the concentrations of the ionized and unionized forms of the weak acidic drug ($pK_a = 3.0$) in solution in gastric fluid (pH 1.2) is 0.016 : 1, respectively. The vast majority (98.4%) of the drug in solution in gastric fluid exists therefore in the unionized (absorbable) form. Thus the vast majority of the drug in solution in gastric fluid will be absorbed passively through the gastrointestinal barrier and enter the blood. On partitioning into the blood, the drug will experience a pH of 7.4. The extent of ionization of the weak acidic drug ($pK_a = 3.0$) in the blood (pH 7.4) may be calculated using Eqn 9.4 as follows:

$$\log \frac{[A^-]}{[HA]} = pH - pK_a$$
$$= 7.4 - 3.0 = 4.4$$

Therefore,

$$\frac{[A^-]}{[HA]} = antilog (4.4)$$
$$= 25\ 119$$

Thus the ratio of the concentrations of the ionized and unionized forms of the weak acidic drug in solution in the blood is 25 119 : 1, respectively. It is evident that the weak acidic drug, once present in the blood, will exist almost entirely (99.996%) in its ionized form, A$^-$. Thus irrespective of the sink conditions provided by the systemic circulation to absorbed drug, there will be virtually no tendency for the weak acidic drug in the blood to be absorbed back into the stomach since only 0.004% of the drug in the blood exists in the absorbable, unionized form.

If the stomach and blood are considered to be two enclosed compartments separated by the gastrointestinal barrier, which is freely permeable to the unionized form of the weak acidic drug but impermeable to the ionized form of the drug, then the unionized form of the drug (HA) will distribute between the gastric fluid and the blood until equilibrium is reached, i.e. the concentrations of unionized drug on each side of the gastrointestinal barrier are equal. However, because the pH on each side of the gastrointestinal barrier is different and the barrier is assumed to be impermeable to the ionized form of the drug, the concentration of the ionized form on each side of the membrane when this equilibrium is attained, may not be equal. The equilibrium distribution of the weak acidic drug ($pK_a = 3.0$) between gastric fluid (pH 1.2) and blood (pH 7.4) may be represented as shown in Fig 9.6.

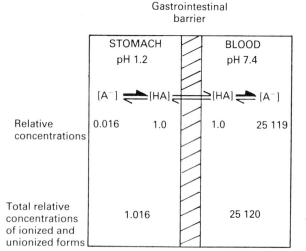

Fig. 9.6 Diagrammatic representation of the equilibrium distribution of a weak acidic drug (pK_a 3.0) between the stomach and the blood

For this particular example the total relative equilibrium concentrations of weak acidic drug in the stomach and the blood are in the ratio of 1.016 : 25 120 respectively. The total equilibrium concentration of weak acidic drug is thus approximately 25 000 times greater in the blood than in the stomach. Hence according to the pH-partition hypothesis drugs such as weak acidic drugs which exist predominantly in the unionized form at gastric pHs will be well absorbed from the stomach.

Absorption of a weak basic drug Let us now consider how a weak basic drug having a pK_a of 5.0 becomes distributed between the gastric fluid (pH = 1.2) and the blood (pH = 7.4). Eqn 9.5 may be used to calculate the ratios of the unionized (B) and ionized (BH⁺) forms of the drug which exist in equilibrium in solution in the gastric fluid and in the blood, respectively.

In gastric fluid, pH 1.2,

$$\log \frac{[BH^+]}{[B]} = pK_a - pH$$

$$= 5.0 - 1.2 = 3.8$$

Therefore,

$$\frac{[BH^+]}{[B]} = \text{antilog } (3.8)$$

$$= 6309.6$$

Hence, in gastric fluid (pH 1.2) the ratio of the equilibrium concentrations of the ionized and unionized forms of the weak basic drug ($pK_a = 5.0$) is 6309.6 : 1, respectively. The vast majority of the drug (i.e. 99.98%) in solution exists in the ionized, unabsorbable form.

In blood, pH 7.4,

$$\log \frac{[BH^+]}{[B]} = pK_a - pH$$

$$= 5.0 - 7.4 = -2.4$$

Therefore,

$$\frac{[BH^+]}{[B]} = \text{antilog } (-2.4)$$

$$= 0.004$$

Hence in blood (pH 7.4) the ratio of the equilibrium concentrations of the ionized and unionized forms of the weak basic drug ($pK_a = 5.0$) is 0.004 : 1, respectively. It is thus evident that any of the weak basic drug which is absorbed from the stomach into the blood will exist predominantly (i.e. 99.6%) in the unionized form. If we consider that the blood and stomach are enclosed compartments separated by the gastrointestinal barrier which is freely permeable to the unionized species (B) but impermeable to the ionized species (BH⁺) of the weak basic drug, then the unionized species will distribute between these two compartments until its concentration on each side of the barrier is equal. The equilibrium distribution of the weak basic drug ($pK_a = 5.0$) between the stomach and blood may be represented as shown in Fig. 9.7.

For this particular example, Fig. 9.7 shows that the total relative equilibrium concentrations of weak basic drug in solution in the gastric fluid and

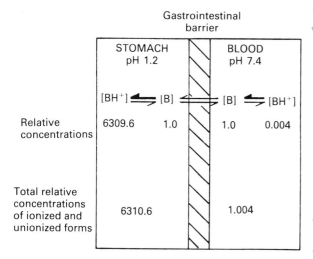

Gastrointestinal
barrier

STOMACH pH 1.2		BLOOD pH 7.4

Relative
concentrations

$[BH^+] \rightleftharpoons [B] \rightleftharpoons [B] \rightleftharpoons [BH^+]$

6309.6   1.0   1.0   0.004

Total relative
concentrations
of ionized and
unionized forms

6310.6   1.004

Fig. 9.7 Diagrammatic representation of the equilibrium distribution of a weak basic drug ($pK_a = 5.0$) between the stomach and the blood

the blood are in the ratio of 6310.6 : 1.004, respectively. At equilibrium the total concentration of the weak basic drug in the stomach is approximately 6300 times greater than that in the blood. Thus according to the pH-partition hypothesis, drugs such as weak basic drugs which are predominantly ionized at gastric pHs will be poorly absorbed from the stomach.

Limitations of the pH-partition hypothesis In calculating the distribution of a typical weak acidic drug and a typical weak basic drug between the stomach and blood, it has been assumed that an equilibrium distribution is attained. In practice such an equilibrium will rarely (if ever) be achieved since the stomach and the blood are not closed, static compartments. Drug is removed from the stomach into the intestine by the normal contractions of the stomach. Drug which enters the blood is removed from the site of absorption by circulation of the blood and is removed from the blood by distribution into tissues, by glomerular filtration and by metabolism. However, despite the above criticism, absorption from the stomach, as determined by direct measurements, generally conforms qualitatively to the pH-partition hypothesis. Weak organic acids are relatively well absorbed since they are all almost completely unionized at gastric pHs. Strong organic acids ($pK_a < 1$) which are ionized even in

the acid conditions of the stomach are not well absorbed. Weak bases, which are ionized at gastric pHs tend to be only absorbed negligibly but their absorption can be increased, as expected, by raising the pH of the gastric fluid. For more detailed informaiton concerning the influence of pK_a and pH on the gastric absorption of weak basic and acidic drugs the reader should refer to the work of Hogben *et al.* (1957), Schanker *et al.* (1957), Shore *et al.* (1957) and Brodie (1964).

The pH range of the small intestinal fluids is less acid than that of the stomach. Thus, in accordance with the pH-partition hypothesis, the absorption of weak bases generally tends to be favoured over weak acids since a larger fraction of a weak basic drug in solution will be in the unionized form. However, the extent to which a drug exists in the unionized form is not the sole criterion determining the extent of absorption of a drug form the small intestine. For instance, it is found that despite their high degree of ionization, weak acids are still quite well absorbed from the small intestine. In fact, the rate of intestinal absorption of a weak acid drug is often higher than its rate of absorption from the stomach even though the drug will be unionized in the stomach. The existence of an effective pH at the surface of the intestinal mucosa (the so-called 'virtual membrane pH' of about pH 5.3), which is lower than the bulk pH in the lumen of the small intestine, has been proposed to account for the unexpectedly high rate of absorption of weak acids from this segment of the gastrointestinal tract. However, it is likely that the larger mucosal surface area available for absorption in the small intestine more than compensates for the low degree of unionization of weak acidic drugs at intestinal pHs.

A further illustration that the absorption of a drug from the gastrointestinal tract is not soley dependent on the drug being unionized, is provided by the observation that a number of drugs are poorly absorbed from certain areas of the gastrointestinal tract despite the fact that their unionized forms predominate in such areas. For instance barbitone (pK_a 7.8), which is almost totally unionized at gastric pHs, is only poorly absorbed from the stomach. However thiopentone, which has a similar pK_a value (i.e. pK_a 7.6) is much better absorbed from the stomach than barbitone. The reason for this difference is that the absorption of drugs is also affected by the lipid solubility exhibited by the unionized form. Thus the unionized form of thiopentone, being more lipid soluble than the unionized form of barbitone, exhibits a greater affinity for the gastrointestinal 'membrane' and is thus better absorbed than barbitone from the stomach. The importance of lipid solubility to the gastrointestinal absorption of barbiturates has been demonstrated by Schanker (1960).

A further observation which cannot be explained by the pH-partition hypothesis is that certain drugs (e.g. quaternary ammonium compounds and tetracyclines) are absorbed readily despite being ionized over the enter pH range of the gastrointestinal tract. For more detailed discussions on the limitations of the pH-partition hypothesis of drug absorption, the reader is referred to articles by Benet (1973), Wagner and Sedman (1973) and Florence and Attwood (1981a).

To summarize, the gastrointestinal absorption characteristics of drugs which are weak electrolytes cannot be explained completely on the basis of their degree of ionization at any particular site of absorption. However, in general, the unionized form of drug in aqueous solution will be absorbed faster than the ionized form of the same drug at any particular site in the gastrointestinal tract. Since the absorptive surface area of the small intestine is so large in comparison to the stomach, this region is accepted as the major site of absorption for both weak acids and bases. Hence the rate of absorption of a given weak electrolyte drug from the small intestine will be greater than form the stomach even if the drug is ionized in the intestine and unionized in the stomach. Despite its limitations, the pH-partition hypothesis remains a useful guide in predicting general trends in drug absorption as a function of pH and pK_a within a specific region of the gastrointestinal tract.

Dissolution rate of drugs

Most drugs are absorbed and reach the systemic circulation by one of the following processes.

Absorption from solution or following rapid dissolution of solid drug particles

The drug is usually administered orally in the form of either a solution (e.g. an elixir) or a suspension, tablet or hard gelatin capsule from which rapid drug release/dissolution occurs. In such cases the bioavailability of a drug is influenced chiefly by:

1 how rapidly and how much of the drug in solution reaches the site(s) of absorption in an absorbable form,
2 the rate and extent of absorption across the gastrointestinal barrier, and
3 the extent to which the drug is metabolized during passage through the gastrointestinal barrier and/or the liver.

Absorption following the slow dissolution of solid drug particles

In those cases where a sparingly soluble drug* is administered in the form of a suspension, a tablet or a hard gelatin capsule, the rate at which the solid drug particles dissolve in the gastrointestinal fluids may be the slowest step in the sequence of events leading to the appearance of intact drug in the systemic circulation (refer back to Fig. 9.1). In such cases, drug absorption and hence bioavailability is dependent on how fast the drug dissolves in the gastrointestinal fluids, i.e. drug bioavailability is dissolution rate limited. Hence factors which influence the rate of dissolution of the drug in the gastrointestinal fluids will also influence the bioavailability of the drug.

Factors influencing the dissolution rates of drugs in the gastrointestinal tract

A schematic outline of the dissolution of a spherical drug particle in the gastrointestinal fluids is shown in Fig. 9.8.

* The term sparingly soluble refers to the solubility exhibited by a drug in the gastric and/or intestinal contents. A drug which was administered as an aqueous solution could still exhibit dissolution rate-limited absorption if the drug was precipitated by the conditions in the gastrointestinal tract and the dissolution rate exhibited by the precipitated drug was sufficiently low.

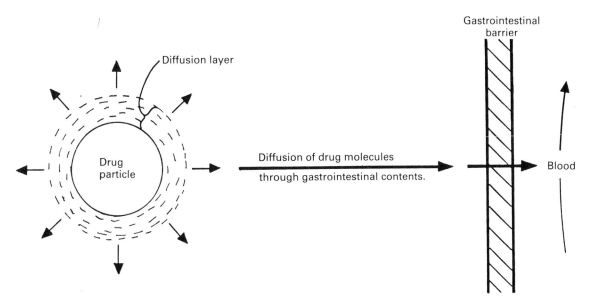

Fig. 9.8 Schematic representation of the dissolution of a drug particle in the gastrointestinal fluids

An equation which describes this process of dissolution is the Noyes–Whitney equation. This equation, which describes the rate of dissolution of spherical drug particles when the dissolution process is diffusion controlled and involves no chemical reaction, may be written

$$\frac{dm}{dt} = \frac{DA}{h}(C_s - C) \qquad (9.6)$$

where dm/dt is the rate of dissolution of the drug particles, D is the diffusion coefficient of the drug in solution in the gastrointestinal fluids, A is the effective surface area of the drug particles in contact with the gastrointestinal fluids, h is the thickness of the diffusion layer around each drug particle, C_s is the saturation solubility of the drug in the diffusion layer, and C is the concentration of drug in solution in the bulk of the gastrointestinal fluids.

The limitations of the Noyes–Whitney equation in describing the dissolution of drug particles are discussed in Chapter 5. Despite its limitations, the Noyes–Whitney equation serves to illustrate and explain how various physicochemical and physiological factors can influence the rate of dissolution of drugs in the gastrointestinal tract.

Physiological conditions   In this context, it is of interest to consider how certain parameters in the Noyes–Whitney equation (and hence the

dissolution rate of a drug) may be influenced by the physiological conditions in the gastrointestinal tract. For instance, the diffusion coefficient, D, of the drug in the gastrointestinal fluids may be decreased by the presence of substances which increase the viscosity of the fluids. Hence the presence of food in the gastrointestinal tract may cause a decrease in the dissolution rate of a drug by virtue of reducing the rate of diffusion of drug molecules away from the diffusion layer surrounding each undissolved drug particle. The thickness of the diffusion layer, h, will be influenced by the degree of agitation experienced by each drug particle in the gastrointestinal tract. Hence, an increase in gastric and/or intestinal motility may increase the dissolution rate of a sparingly soluble drug by virtue of decreasing the thickness of the diffusion layer around each drug particle. The concentration, C, of drug in solution in the bulk of the gastrointestinal fluids will be influenced by such factors as the rate of removal of dissolved drug by absorption through the gastrointestinal blood barrier and by the volume of fluid available for dissolution. In the stomach, the volume of fluid will be influenced by the intake of fluid in the diet. According to the Noyes–Whitney equation, a low value of C will favour rapid dissolution of the drug by virtue of increasing the value of the term $(C_s - C)$. In the case of drugs whose absorption is dissolution rate limited, the value of C is normally maintained at a very low value by virtue of absorption of the drug. Hence dissolution occurs under so-called 'sink' conditions, (see Chapter 5) i.e., under conditions such that the value of $(C_s - C)$ approximates to C_s. Thus for dissolution of a drug in the gastrointestinal fluids under sink conditions, the Noyes–Whitney equation may be expressed as

$$\frac{dm}{dt} = \frac{D\,A\,C_s}{h} \qquad (9.7)$$

Let us now consider how various physico-chemical properties exhibited by a drug can influence its rate of dissolution in the gastrointestinal fluids.

Particle size According to the Noyes–Whitney equation, an increase in the total effective surface area of drug in contact with the gastrointestinal fluids will cause an increase in dissolution rate. Provided that each particle of drug is intimately wetted by the gastrointestinal fluids, the effective surface area exhibited by the drug will be directly porportional to the particle size of the drug. Hence the smaller the particle size, the greater the effective surface area exhibited by a given mass of drug and the higher will be the dissolution rate. Particle size reduction is thus likely to result in increased bioavailability provided that absorption of the drug is dissolution rate limited.

A striking example of this effect is provided by griseofulvin. A reduction in particle size from about 10 μm (specific surface area = 0.4 m^2 g^{-1}) to 2.7 μm (specific surface area = 1.5 m^2 g^{-1}) was shown by Atkinson *et al.* (1962) to produce an approximate doubling in the amount of griseofulvin absorbed in humans. Duncan *et al.* (1962) also demonstrated that particle size reduction of griseofulvin permitted similar blood levels of this drug to be obtained in humans with half the original dose, i.e. a dose of 0.25 g instead of 0.5 g of griseofulvin.

Other drugs whose bioavailabilities have been enhanced by particle size reduction include sulphadiazine, phenothiazine, tolbutamide, spironolactone, aspirin, nitrofurantoin, digoxin and bishydroxycoumarin (Fincher, 1968; Shaw *et al.*, 1973; Florence *et al.*, 1974; Nash *et al.*, 1974/75). It is interesting to note that in the case of nitrofurantoin, the inclusion of small-sized particles of this drug in tablets gave an increased incidence of undesirable side effects. The enhanced bioavailability resulting from particle size reduction was believed to be responsible for these undesirable side effects. This is an example where improved bioavailability resulted in patients becoming overmedicated.

It is possible that particle size reduction may fail to increase the bioavailability exhibited by a drug. This would be the case for a drug whose absorption was not dissolution rate limited. In the case of a poorly soluble, hydrophobic drug, whose absorption is dissolution rate limited, extensive particle size reduction can increase the tendency of the particles to aggregate in the aqueous gastrointestinal fluids with a consequent reduction in effective surface area, dissolution rate and hence bioavailability. Certain drugs such as penicillin G and erythromycin are unstable in gastric fluids. Thus chemical degradation will be minimized if such a drug does not dissolve readily in gastric fluids. Hence particle size reduction would not only produce an increased rate of drug dissolution in gastric fluid but also an increase in the extent of drug degradation. This would result in a decrease in the amount of intact drug available for absorption from the small intestine.

Solid dispersions A unique approach to presenting a poorly soluble drug in an extremely fine state of subdivision to the gastrointestinal fluids, is the administration of the drug in the form of a solid eutectic mixture. Such a mixture consists of a microcrystalline dispersion of the poorly soluble drug (e.g. sulphathiazole) in a matrix consisting of a physiologically inert, readily water-soluble solid such as urea. The water-soluble solid is often referred to as the 'carrier'. Exposure of this type of solid dispersion system to the gastrointestinal fluids results in dissolution of the water-soluble matrix (carrier). As the matrix dissolves it exposes the dispersed poorly soluble drug, which is in an extremely fine state of subdivision, to the aqueous gastrointestinal fluids. Hence the poorly soluble drug is presented to the aqueous fluids in a form which facilitates its dissolution rate and bioavailability. It is interesting to note that the bioavailability of sulphathiazole was found to be increased when this drug was presented in the form of a solid eutectic mixture with urea (Sekiguchi and Obi, 1961). The formation of a solid solution of a poorly soluble drug in a water-soluble physiologically inert solid should offer a greater improvement in dissolution rate and bioavailability of the poorly soluble drug than would a eutectic mixture. In the case of a solid solution the poorly soluble drug would be dispersed as single molecules throughout the water-soluble solid (carrier), i.e. the dispersed drug is in the ultimate form of subdivision.

The advantages of the solid solution over the eutectic mixture has been discussed by Goldberg *et al.* (1965, 1966a, b, c). The increased dissolution rates and bioavailabilities exhibited by solid dispersions of griseofulvin in polyethylene glycols of high molecular weight were originally attributed to solid solution formation (Chiou and Riegelman, 1971). However, later work by Chiou (1977) and Kaur *et al.* (1980) suggested that griseofulvin had negligible or very limited solubility in polyethylene glycol dispersion systems. The marked enhancement of dissolution and absorption rate of griseofulvin dispersed in such systems seemed to be primarily the result of the reduced size of the griseofulvin crystals, i.e. griseofulvin was in the form of microcrystals. In addition to this reduction in crystal size, other factors may also contribute to the improved dissolution rate and bioavailability exhibited by a drug presented in the form of a solid dispersion system. These factors are:

1 an increase in aqueous solubility of the drug because of its extremely small particle size,
2 a possible solubilization effect on the drug by the 'carrier' in the diffusion layer surrounding each dissolving drug particle in the gastrointestinal fluids,
3 a reduction or absence of aggregation and agglomeration of the drug particles exposed to the gastrointestinal fluids,
4 excellent wettability and dispersibility of the exposed drug particles in the gastrointestinal fluids (factors 3 and 4 will ensure that the effective surface area of the drug in contact with the gastrointestinal fluids is very large), and
5 possible formation of metastable polymorphic forms (which are more soluble and rapidly

dissolving in the gastrointestinal fluids) of the drug during formation of the solid dispersion system (Chiou and Riegelman, 1971).

Crystal form

Polymorphism Many drugs can exist in more than one crystalline form, e.g. chloramphenicol palmitate, cortisone acetate, tetracyclines and sulphathiazole. This property is referred to as polymorphism and each crystalline form is known as a polymorph. As discussed in Chapter 5, a metastable polymorph usually exhibits a greater aqueous solubility and dissolution rate than the corresponding stable polymorph. Consequently the metastable polymorphic form of a poorly soluble drug may exhibit an increased bioavailability in comparison to the stable polymorphic form of that drug.

A classic example of the influence of polymorphism on drug bioavailability is provided by chloramphenicol palmitate. This drug exists in three crystalline forms designated A, B and C. At normal temperature and pressure, A is the stable polymorph, B is the metastable polymorph and C is the unstable polymorph. The unstable polymorphic form of chloramphenicol palmitate is too unstable to be included in a dosage form. However, the metastable form is sufficiently stable to permit its incorporation in a dosage form. The mean blood serum levels and urinary excretion rates of chloramphenicol from orally administered suspensions containing varying proportions of the polymorphic forms A and B of chloramphenicol palmitate were studied by Augiar *et al.* (1967). The extent of absorption of chloramphenicol increased as the proportion of polymorphic form B of chloramphenicol palmitate increased in each suspension. This was attributed to the more rapid *in vivo* rate of dissolution of the metastable polymorphic form, B, of chloramphenicol palmitate. Following dissolution, chloramphenicol palmitate is hydrolysed to give free chloramphenicol in solution which is then absorbed. The stable polymorphic form A of chloramphenicol palmitate dissolves so slowly and consequently is hydrolysed so slowly to chloramphenicol *in vivo* that this polymorph is virtually without biological activity. The importance of polymorphism to the gastrointestinal bioavailability of chloramphenicol palmitate is reflected by a limit being placed on the content of the inactive polymorphic form, A, in Chloramphenicol Palmitate Mixture BP.

Amorphous solids In addition to different polymorphic crystalline forms, a drug may exist in an amorphous form. Since the amorphous form is usually more soluble and rapidly dissolving than the corresponding crystalline form(s), the possibility exists that there will be significant differences in the bioavailabilities exhibited by the amorphous and crystalline form(s) of a given poorly soluble drug. A classic example of the influence of amorphous versus crystalline form of a drug on its gastrointestinal bioavailability is provided by the work of Mullins and Macek (1960) on the antibiotic drug, novobiocin. The more soluble and more rapidly dissolving amorphous form of novobiocin was readily absorbed following oral administration of an aqueous suspension to humans and dogs. However, the less soluble and slower dissolving crystalline form of novobiocin did not appear to be absorbed to any significant extent. The crystalline form was thus therapeutically ineffective. A further important observation was made in the case of aqueous suspensions of novobiocin. The amorphous form of novobiocin slowly converts to the more thermodynamically stable crystalline form with an accompanying loss of therapeutic effectiveness. Thus unless adequate precautions are taken to ensure the stability of the less stable, more therapeutically effective amorphous form of a drug in a dosage form, then unacceptable variations in therapeutic effectiveness may occur.

Solvates Another variation in the crystalline form of a drug can occur if the drug is able to associate with solvent molecules to produce crystalline forms known as solvates. When water is the solvent, the solvate formed is called a hydrate. Generally the greater the solvation in the crystal, the lower is the solubility and dissolution rate in a solvent identical to the solvation molecules. Since the solvated and non-solvated forms of a drug usually exhibit differences in solubility and dissolution rates, it is reasonable to expect that such forms may also exhibit differences in bioavailability particularly in the case of a poorly soluble drug which exhibits dissolution rate-limited bioavailability.

Poole *et al.* (1968) showed that the more aqueous soluble and rapidly dissolving anhydrous form of ampicillin was absorbed to a greater extent from hard gelatin capsule or aqueous suspension dosage forms administered to humans or dogs than was the less soluble, slower dissolving trihydrate form of ampicillin. However, it is possible that the observed difference may not have been due entirely to the state of solvation of ampicillin but also due to formulation differences within each type of dosage form tested.

Solubility of the drug in the diffusion layer (salt forms) According to the Noyes–Whitney equation (referred to earlier in this chapter) the dissolution rate of a drug in the gastrointestinal fluids is influenced by the solubility (C_s) that the drug exhibits in the diffusion layer surrounding each dissolving drug particle. In the case of drugs which are weak electrolytes, their overall aqueous solubilities are dependent on pH (see Chapter 5). Hence in the case of an orally administered solid dosage form containing a weak electrolyte drug, the dissolution rate of the drug will be influenced by its solubility and hence the pH in the diffusion layer surrounding each dissolving drug particle. It should be noted that the pH in the diffusion layer is not necessarily equal to the pH in the bulk of the gastrointestinal fluids. The dissolution rate of a weak acidic drug in gastric fluid (pH 1–3) will be relatively low. This is a consequence of the low solubility (C_s) exhibited by the drug in the diffusion layer because of the low pH in this layer. If the pH in the diffusion layer could be increased, then the solubility (C_s) exhibited by the weak acidic drug in this layer and hence the dissolution rate of the drug in the gastric fluids would be increased even though the bulk pH of the gastric fluids remained at the same low value. The pH of the diffusion layer would be increased if the chemical nature of the weak acidic drug was changed from that of the free acid to a strong alkali salt form of the free acid, e.g. the sodium or potassium salt form of the free acid. The pH in the diffusion layer surrounding each particle of the salt form would be higher (e.g. pH 5–6) than the low bulk pH (pH 1–3) of the gastric fluids because of the neutralizing action of the strong alkali cations (e.g. K^+ or Na^+ ions) present in the diffusion layer (see Fig. 9.9).

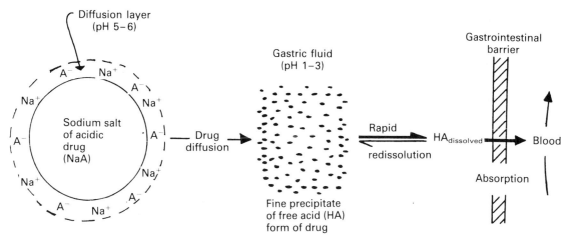

Fig. 9.9 Schematic representation of the dissolution process of a salt form of a weak acidic drug in gastric fluid. (After Cadwallader, 1973)

Since the salt form of the weak acidic drug has a relatively high solubility at the elevated pH in the diffusion layer, dissolution of the drug particles will take place at a faster rate. When dissolved drug diffuses out of the diffusion layer into the bulk of the gastric fluid where the pH is lower than that in the diffusion layer, precipitation of the free acid form of the drug is likely to occur. This will be a result of the lower overall solubility exhibited by the drug at the lower bulk pH. Thus the free acid form of the drug in solution, which is in excess of its solubility at the bulk pH of the gastric fluid, will precipitate out leaving a saturated (or near saturated) solution of free acid in the gastric fluid. It is considered that the precipitated free acid will be in the form of very fine, non-ionized, wetted drug particles which exhibit a very large total effective surface area in contact with the gastric fluids (much larger than would have been obtained if the free acid form of the drug had been administered). This large total effective surface area will facilitate rapid redissolution of the precipitated particles of free acid when additional gastric fluid becomes available as a consequence of either

1 dissolved drug being absorbed,
2 additional fluid accumulating in the stomach, or
3 the fine precipitated particles being emptied from the stomach into the intestine.

This rapid redissolution will ensure that the concentration of free acid in solution in the bulk

of the gastric fluids will be at or near to saturation (at the bulk pH conditions prevailing in the stomach).

Thus the oral administration of a solid dosage form containing a strong alkali salt of a weak acidic drug would be expected to give a more rapid rate of drug dissolution and (in the case of drugs exhibiting dissolution rate-limited absorption) a more rapid rate of drug absorption than if the free acid form of the drug itself had been included in the dosage form. This is well illustrated by the work of Nelson *et al* (1962) who showed that oral administration of a non-disintegrating disc of the more rapidly dissolving sodium salt of tolbutamide produced a very rapid decrease in blood sugar level (a consequence of the rapid rate of drug absorption) followed by a rapid recovery. In contrast, a non-disintegrating disc of the more slowly dissolving tolbutamide base produced a much slower rate of decrease of blood sugar level (a consequence of the slower rate of drug absorption) but the lower sugar level was maintained for a longer period of time. It is interesting to note that the gradual but prolonged decrease in blood sugar levels, and not the sharp dip and recovery is the preferred clinical response to oral hypoglycaemic drugs (Cadwallader, 1973).

An alternative method of increasing the dissolution rate of a weak acidic drug in gastric fluid is the inclusion of non-toxic basic substances in a solid dosage form containing the free acid form of the drug. The presence of the basic ingredients ensures that a relatively alkaline diffusion layer is formed around each dissolving drug particle. The inclusion of the basic ingredients aluminium dihydroxyaminoacetate and magnesium carbonate in acetylsalicylic acid tablets was found to increase the gastric dissolution rate and the bioavailability of this drug following oral administration (Cadwallader, 1973).

A similar scheme to that described and shown in Fig. 9.9 can also be used to explain why strongly acidic salt forms of weak basic drugs (e.g. chlorpromazine hydrochloride) dissolve more rapidly in gastric or intestinal fluids than do the corresponding free bases (e.g. chlorpromazine). The presence of strongly acidic cations (e.g. Cl^- ions) in the diffusion layer formed around each dissolving acidic salt particle of drug ensures that the pH in that layer is lower than the bulk pH in either gastric or intestinal fluid. This lower pH will increase the solubility of the drug (C_s) in the diffusion layer. The oral administration of a salt form of a weak basic drug in a solid dosage form generally ensures that dissolution of the drug occurs in the gastric fluid before the drug passes into the small intestine where the pH conditions are less favourable to the dissolution of weak bases. Hence the use of strong acidic salt forms of weak basic drugs generally ensures that stomach emptying (and not dissolution rate) is the rate-determining step for the absorption of such drugs from the small intestine (Notari, 1980).

For further information concerning the usefulness and limitations of salt forms of drugs, the reader is referred to the review by Berge *et al.* (1977).

Complexation The rate and extent of absorption of a drug depends on the effective concentration of that drug, i.e. the concentration of drug in solution in the gastrointestinal fluids which is in an absorbable form. Complexation is one of the principal types of physicochemical interactions which can influence the effective drug concentration in the gastrointestinal fluids. The other types of interaction are adsorption and micellar solubilization. Complexation of a drug may occur within the dosage form and/or in the gastrointestinal fluids.

An example of complexation between a drug and a normal component of the gastrointestinal tract is that between mucin and certain drugs. Mucin is a viscous mucopolysaccharide which lines the mucosal surfaces of the stomach and intestines. Streptomycin, dihydrostreptomycin, anticholinergic and hypotensive quaternary ammonium compounds bind strongly to mucin forming unabsorbable complexes. Thus complexation with mucin reduces the effective concentration and bioavailability of each of these drugs.

Another example of complexation occurring in the gastrointestinal fluids is that between certain drugs and dietary components. Tetracyclines form insoluble complexes with calcium ions and other polyvalent metal ions present in food (Remmers *et al.*, 1965). Since the complex formed is insoluble in the gastrointestinal fluids, that fraction of the antibiotic which has become complexed is unavailable for absorption. Consequently tetracyclines tend to show reduced absorption if taken with milk or dairy products which contain calcium ions. In addition antacids containing Ca^{2+}, Mg^{2+} or Al^{3+} ions and iron preparations (particularly those containing ferrous sulphate) also reduce the bioavailabilities exhibited by tetracyclines via the formation of insoluble complexes.

Tetracyclines also provide an example of drugs whose bioavailabilities are reduced by the formation of poorly soluble complexes with excipients present in dosage forms. The extent of absorption of tetracycline is reduced if dicalcium phosphate is included as a diluent in a tablet or hard gelatin capsule containing this antibiotic. Other examples of complexes which give reduced drug bioavailability are those between amphetamine and sodium carboxymethylcellulose and between phenobarbitone and polyethylene glycol 4000. Complexation between drugs and excipients such as cellulose derivatives, polyols, gums and surfactants probably occurs quite often in liquid dosage forms; complexation is sometimes used to increase drug stability or solubility.

In many cases the drug–excipient complexes are soluble in the gastrointestinal fluids and rapidly dissociate to liberate the 'free' drug. In such cases, little or no effect of complexation on drug absorption is noted. Hence the rate at which a complex dissociates will determine whether absorption of the drug is as rapid and/or complete as in the absence of complex formation.

It is also interesting to note that in a limited number of cases, complex formation has been found to improve drug absorption possibly as a consequence of increased drug solubility/dissolution rate and/or formation of well absorbed lipid-soluble complexes. The gastrointestinal absorption of ergotamine tartrate is increased by the simultaneous intake of caffeine (Schmidt and Fonchamps, 1974).

For additional information on complex formation, the reader is referred to Florence and Attwood (1981b).

Adsorption   The concurrent administration of drugs and medicinal products containing solid adsorbents (e.g. antidiarrhoeal mixtures) may result in the adsorbents interfering with the absorption of such drugs from the gastrointestinal tract. The adsorption of a drug onto solid adsorbents such as kaolin, attapulgite or charcoal may reduce the rate and/or extent of drug absorption from the gastrointestinal tract. A decrease in the effective concentration of drug in solution which is available for absorption will occur if a significant proportion of the administered dose of drug is adsorbed to the solid adsorbent at the site(s) of absorption of that drug. A consequence of the reduced concentration of 'free' (i.e. absorbable) drug in solution at the site(s) of absorption will be a reduction in the rate of drug absorption. Whether or not there will also be a reduction in the extent of drug absorption will depend on whether or not the drug–adsorbent interaction is readily reversible. If the adsorbed drug is not readily released from the solid adsorbent in order to replace that 'free' drug which has been absorbed from the gastrointestinal tract, then there will be a reduction in the extent of absorption of that drug.

Examples of drug–adsorbent interactions which give reduced extents of drug absorption are promazine/charcoal and lincomycin/kaopectate. In contrast the adsorption of promazine by the solid adsorbent, attapulgite, only produces a reduction in the rate but not extent of absorption of promazine in humans. This is because the adsorbed promazine is readily released from attapulgite in order to replace that 'free' promazine which has been absorbed from the gastrointestinal tract (Sorby, 1965).

Based on the above discussion, insoluble excipients included in dosage forms should exhibit little tendency to adsorb drugs present in the dosage form otherwise these so-called inert excipients could interfere with the absorption of drugs. Talc, which may be included in tablets as a glident is claimed to interfere with the absorption of cyancobalamin by virtue of its ability to adsorb this vitamin. For further details of the biopharmaceutical implications of adsorption, the reader is referred to Florence and Attwood (1981c).

Chemical stability of drugs in the gastrointestinal fluids

Poor bioavailability usually results if a drug undergoes extensive acid or enzyme hydrolysis in the gastrointestinal tract. For instance, both penicillin G and erythromycin are susceptible to acid-catalysed hydrolysis and the extent of absorption of these drugs is thus influenced by the time that they reside in the stomach and on the gastric pH. When a drug is unstable in gastric fluid, its extent of degradation would be minimized (and hence its bioavailability would be improved) if it exhibited minimal dissolution in gastric fluid and rapid dissolution in intestinal fluid. The concept of delaying the dissolution of a drug until it reaches the small intestine has been employed to improve the bioavailability exhibited by erythromycin from the gastrointestinal tract. Enteric coating of tablets containing the free base, erythromycin, is one method which has been used to protect this drug from gastric fluid. The enteric coating resists gastric fluid but disrupts or dissolves at the less acid pH range of the small intestine. Hence the drug is not liberated until the coated tablet reaches the small intestine (further details concerning enteric coating may be found later in this chapter and in Chapters 18 and 40). However, despite the protection offered to susceptible drugs from gastric fluid by enteric coating, the bioavailability exhibited by drugs from enteric-coated tablets is potentially more variable than from any other type of dosage form (see later in this chapter).

Pro-drugs   An alternative method of protecting a susceptible drug from gastric fluid, which has been employed in the case of erythromycin, is the administration of chemical derivations of the parent drugs. These derivatives (called pro-drugs) exhibit limited solubility (and hence minimal dissolution) in gastric fluid but, once in the small intestine, liberate the parent drug to be absorbed. For instance, erythromycin stearate after passing through the stomach undissolved, dissolves and dissociates in the intestinal fluid yeilding the free base, erythromycin, which is absorbed. In the case of erythromycin estolate, which is the lauryl sulphate salt of the ester erythromycin propionate, the improved bioavailability exhibited by this pro-drug is achieved in two ways. First, the poorly soluble lauryl sulphate salt remains undissolved and is thus not degraded during its passage through the stomach. Once in the small intestine, the lauryl sulphate salt dissolves and dissociates to give the ester, erythromycin propionate. Second, erythromycin propionate by virtue of its increased lipid solubility is better absorbed than the free base erythromycin. Once present in the blood, erythromycin propionate hydrolyses to liberate erythromycin, the active form of the antibiotic.

DOSAGE FORM FACTORS INFLUENCING DRUG ABSORPTION FROM THE GASTROINTESTINAL TRACT

The rate and/or extent of absorption of a drug from the gastrointestinal tract has been shown to be influenced by many physiological factors associated with this route of drug administration and by many physicochemical properties associated with the drug itself. The bioavailability of a drug administered in a dosage form can also be influenced by factors associated with the formulation and production of the dosage form. This aspect of biopharmaceutics will now be considered.

Influence of excipients

Drugs are almost never administered alone to patients but in the form of dosage forms. A dosage form generally consists of a drug (or drugs) together with a varying number of other substances (called excipients) that have been added to the formulation in order to facilitate the preparation, patient acceptability and functioning of the dosage form as a drug delivery system. Excipients include disintegrating agents, diluents, lubricants, suspending agents, emulsifying agents, flavouring agents, colouring agents, chemical stabilizers etc. Excipients are also referred to as adjuvants, additives or inert ingredients. Although excipients were considered to be inert in that they, themselves, should not exert any therapeutic or biological action or modify the biological action of the drug present in the dosage form, it is now recognized that excipients can potentially influence the rate and/or extent of absorption of the drug. For instance, the potential influence of excipients on drug bioavailability has already been implicated by virtue of the formation of poorly soluble, non-absorbable drug–excipients complexes between tetracyclines and dicalcium phosphate, amphetamine and sodium carboxymethylcellulose and phenobarbitone and polyethylene glycol 4000.

Diluents

A dramatic example of the influence that excipients employed as diluents can have on drug bioavailability is provided by the Australian outbreak of phenytoin intoxication which occurred in epileptic patients as a consequence of the diluent being changed in sodium phenytoin capsules (Tyler *et al.*, 1970). Many epileptic patients who had been previously stabilized with sodium phenytoin capsules containing calcium sulphate dihydrate as the diluent, developed clinical features of phenytoin overdosage when given sodium phenytoin capsules containing lactose as the diluent even though the quantity of drug in each capsule formulation was identical. It was later shown that the excipient calcium sulphate dihydrate had been responsible for decreasing the gastrointestinal absorption of phenytoin, possibly because part of the administered dose of drug formed a poorly absorbable calcium–phenytoin complex. Hence, although the size of dose and frequency of administration of the sodium phenytoin capsules containing calcium sulphate dihydrate gave therapeutic blood levels of phenytoin in epileptic patients, the efficiency of absorption of phenytoin has been lowered by the incorporation of this excipient in the hard gelatin capsules. Hence when the calcium sulphate dihydrate was replaced by lactose, without any alteration in the quantity of drug in each capsule or in the frequency of administration of such capsules, the accompanying improved bioavailability resulted in higher plasma levels of phenytoin. In many patients, the higher plasma levels exceeded the maximum safe concentration for phenytoin and produced toxic side effects. This case is also discussed in Chapter 19.

Surfactants

Surfactants are often employed as emulsifying agents, solubilizing agents, suspension stabilizers or as wetting agents in dosage forms. However, surfactants in general cannot be assumed to be 'inert' excipients since they have been shown to be capable of either increasing, decreasing or exerting no effect on the transfer of drugs across biological membranes. In addition, surfactants might also be able to produce significant changes in the biological activity of drugs by perhaps exerting an influence on drug metabolizing enzymes or on the binding of drugs to receptor proteins (Florence, 1981).

Many studies aimed at elucidating the mechanisms by which surfactants can influence drug absorption have involved simple animal models of drug absorption such as the gill membrane of the goldfish, the isolated rabbit gastric mucosa and the ligated gastric fundic pouch of the dog. Although it is not clear to what extent such animal studies can be extrapolated to humans, some potential ways in which surfactants might influence drug absorption from the gastrointestinal tract in humans are as follows. Surfactant monomers can potentially disrupt the integrity and function of a membrane. Hence, such a membrane-disrupting effect would tend to enhance drug penetration and hence absorption across the gastrointestinal barrier. Inhibition of drug absorption may occur as a consequence of a drug being incorporated into surfactant micelles. If such surfactant micelles are not absorbed, which appears to be usually the case, then solubilization of a drug may result in a reduction of the concentration of 'free' drug in solution in the gastrointestinal fluids which is available for absorption. Inhibition of drug absorption in the presence of micellar concen-

trations of surfactant would be expected to occur in the case of drugs which are normally soluble in the gastrointestinal fluids, i.e. in the absence of surfactant. However, in the case of poorly soluble drugs whose absorption is dissolution rate limited, the increase in saturation solubility of the drug by solubilization in surfactant micelles could result in more rapid rates of drug dissolution and hence absorption. Very high concentrations of surfactant in excess of that required to solubilize the drug could decrease drug absorption by decreasing the chemical potential of the drug.

Release of poorly soluble drugs from tablets and hard gelatin capsules may be increased by the inclusion of surfactants in their formulations. The ability of a surfactant to reduce the solid/liquid interfacial tension will permit the gastrointestinal fluids to wet more effectively and to come into more intimate contact with the solid dosage forms. This wetting effect may thus aid the penetration of gastrointestinal fluids into the mass of capsule contents which often remains when the hard gelatin shell has dissolved and/or reduce the tendency of poorly soluble drug particles to aggregate in the gastrointestinal fluids. In each case, the resulting increase in the total effective surface area of drug in contact with the gastrointestinal fluids would tend to increase the dissolution and absorption rates of the drugs.

It is interesting to note that the enhanced gastrointestinal absorption of phenacetin in humans resulting from the addition of polysorbate 80 to an aqueous suspension of this drug was attributed to the surfactant preventing aggregation and thus increasing the effective surface area and dissolution rate of the drug particles in the gastrointestinal fluids (Prescott *et al.*, 1970).

It is also possible that surfactants could influence drug absorption by exerting a physiological action of their own on the gastrointestinal tract, for instance by altering the gastric residence time of a drug.

The possible mechanisms by which surfactants can influence drug absorption are varied and it is likely that only rarely will a single mechanism operate in isolation. In most cases, the overall effect on drug absorption will probably involve a number of different actions of the surfactant (some of which will produce opposing effects on drug absorption) and the observed effect on drug absorption will depend on which of the different actions is the over-riding one. The ability of a surfactant to influence drug absorption will also depend on the physicochemical characteristics and concentration of the surfactant, the nature of the drug and on the type of biological membrane involved. Reviews on the effects of surfactants on drug absorption are provided by Gibaldi (1970), Gibaldi and Feldman (1970) and Florence (1981).

Viscosity-enhancing agents

Viscosity-enhancing agents are often employed in the formulation of liquid dosage forms for oral use in order to control such properties as palatability, ease of pouring and, in the case of suspensions, the rate of sedimentation of the dispersed particles. The viscosity-enhancing agent is often a hydrophilic polymer but many sugars serve the dual function of sweetening and viscosity-enhancing agents.

There are a number of mechanisms by which a viscosity-enhancing agent may produce a change in the gastrointestinal absorption of a drug. Complex formation between a drug and a hydrophilic polymer could reduce the concentration of drug in solution which is available for drug absorption (see earlier in this chapter). The administration of viscous solutions or suspensions may produce an increase in viscosity of the gastrointestinal contents. Such an increase in viscosity could lead to the following general effects:

1 a decrease in gastric emptying rate, i.e. an increase in gastric residence time,
2 a decrease in intestinal motility,
3 a decrease in dissolution rate of the drug, and
4 a decrease in the rate of movement of drug molecules to the absorbing membrane.

Normally, effect 3 would not be applicable to solution dosage forms unless dilution of the administerted solution in the gastrointestinal fluids caused precipitation of the drug. Levy and Jusko (1965) suggested that effects 1, 2 and 4 would lead to a decrease in the rates of absorption of drugs from viscous solutions. Studies in which increased viscosity was found to produce reduc-

tions in the rates of absorption of drugs from solutions include the effects of sucrose solutions on the induction time of phenobarbitone sodium (Malone *et al.*, 1960), methylcellulose on the absorption of solutions of sodium salicylate (Davison *et al.*, 1961) and salicylic acid (Levy and Jusko, 1965), different gums on the urinary excretion rate of sodium salicylate solution (Bachynsky *et al.*, 1976) and sodium alginate on the bioavailability of phenolsulphonphathalein (Ashley and Levy, 1973).

In the case of suspensions containing drugs with bioavailabilities that are dissolution rate dependent, an increase in viscosity could also lead to a decrease in the rate of dissolution of the drug in the gastrointestinal tract. Thus the observation by Seager (1968) that methylcellulose reduced the rate and extent of absorption of nitrofurantoin from aqueous suspensions of this drug could have been due to effects 1, 2, 3 and 4. In addition, nitrofurantoin may form complexes with methylcellulose which could also tend to reduce the absorption of this drug (Shah and Sheth, 1976).

The potential absorption-enhancing effects of increased viscosity have been considered by Barzegar-Jalali and Richards (1979). An extended gastric residence time, or a slower intestinal transit time produced by an increase in viscosity, would allow a longer period in which drug dissolution could occur in the gastrointestinal tract and this could lead to an increase in the extent of absorption of a drug from a suspension. In addition, the increase in gastric residence time caused by an increase in viscosity could also enhance the amount of absorption of drugs with pK_a values that permit absorption of those drugs from the stomach. Similarly an increase in intestinal transit time would favour an increase in the amount of absorption of the majority of drugs since the intestine is the optimal site of absorption of most drugs. The net effect of increased viscosity on the absorption of a particular drug from the gastrointestinal tract will thus depend on whether or not the absorption-enchancing effects outweigh the absorption-reducing effects of increased viscosity. It is interesting to note that the absorption-enhancing effects of increased viscosity appeared to outweigh the absorption-reducing effects in studies on the effects of various macromolecular suspending agents on the bioavailabilities of aspirin and salicylic acid in the rabbit (Barzegar-Jalali and Richards, 1979).

The above examples serve to illustrate that so-called 'inert' excipients can often markedly influence the bioavailabilities of drugs administered in dosage forms via the gastrointestinal route.

Influence of the type of dosage form

In addition to the amount and physicochemical nature of each so-called 'inert' excipient included in a formulation, the type of dosage form and its method of preparation or manufacture can influence bioavailability. Thus, whether a particular drug is incorporated and administered in the form of a suspension, a hard gelatin capsule or a tablet can influence the rate and/or extent of absorption of that drug from the gastrointestinal tract. The type of oral dosage form will influence the number of possible intervening steps between administration of the dosage form and the appearance of dissolved drug in the gastrointestinal fluids, i.e. the type of dosage form will influence the release of drug into solution in the gastrointestinal fluids. A simplified scheme depicting this is shown in Fig. 9.10.

In general, drugs must be in solution in the gastrointestinal fluids before absorption can occur. Thus the greater the number of intervening steps, the greater will be the number of potential obstacles to drug absorption and the greater will be the likelihood of that type of dosage form reducing the bioavailability exhibited by the drug. Hence the bioavailability of a given drug tends to decrease in the following order of types of dosage form: aqueous solutions > aqueous suspensions > hard gelatin capsules > uncoated tablets > coated tablets. Whilst the number of intervening steps between administration and the appearance of a drug in solution in the gastrointestinal fluids may be equal in the case of the hard gelatin capsule and tablet dosage forms (see Fig. 9.10), the fine particles of drug in a hard gelatin capsule are not normally subjected to high compression forces and the subsequent reduction in effective drug surface area as a consequence of the tablet manufacturing process and to the difficulty in regenerating well dispersed drug particles after administration. Hence, particularly in the case of a poorly soluble drug, the rate of appearance of a given drug in solution in the gastrointestinal fluids is likely to be slower from a tablet than from a hard gelatin capsule. Although the above

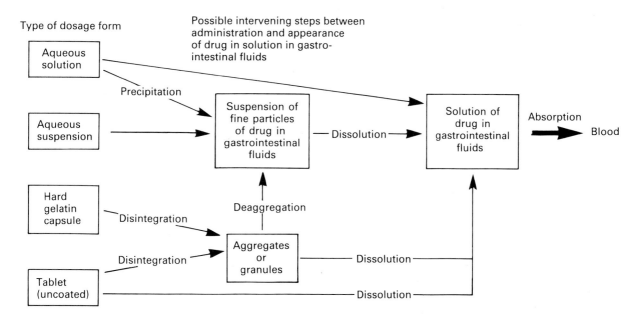

Fig. 9.10 Schematic outline of the influence of the dosage form on the appearance of a drug in solution in the gastrointestinal fluids

ranking of the types of oral dosage form is not universal, it does provide a useful guideline. In general solution and suspension dosage forms are most suitable for administering drugs intended to be rapidly absorbed. However, it should be noted that other factors (e.g. stability, patient acceptability etc.) can also influence the type of dosage form in which a drug is administered via the gastrointestinal route.

Aqueous solutions

For drugs which are water soluble and chemically stable in aqueous solution, formulation as a solution normally eliminates the *in vivo* dissolution step and presents the drug in the most readily available form for absorption (Rees, 1974). However, dilution of an aqueous solution of a poorly soluble drug (whose aqueous solubility has been increased by means of formulation techniques such as cosolvency, complex formation or solubilization) in the gastric fluids can result in precipitation of the drug. Similarly exposure of an aqueous solution of a salt of a weak acidic compound to gastric pH can also result in precipitation of the free acid form of the drug. However, in most cases, the extremely fine nature of the precipitate permits a more rapid rate of dissolution than if the drug had been administered in other types of oral dosage forms such as an aqueous suspension, a hard gelatin capsule or a tablet.

Factors associated with the formulation of aqueous solution dosage forms which can influence drug bioavailability include

1 the chemical stability exhibited by the drug in aqueous solution and the gastrointestinal fluids,
2 complexation, i.e. formation of a complex between the drug and an excipient included to increase the aqueous solubility, the chemical stability of the drug or the viscosity of the dosage form,
3 solubilization, i.e. the incorporation of the drug into micelles in order to increase the aqueous solubility of the drug and
4 the viscosity of solution dosage form, particularly if a viscosity-enhancing agent has been included.

Information concerning the potential influence of each of the above factors on drug bioavailability from the gastrointestinal tract is given in earlier sections of this chapter. Further details concerning the formulation of oral solution dosage forms are given in Chapter 14.

Aqueous suspensions

An aqueous suspension is a useful dosage form for administering an insoluble or poorly aqueous soluble drug. Usually the absorption of a drug from this type of dosage form is dissolution rate limited. Oral administration of a dose of an aqueous suspension results in a large total surface area of dispersed drug being immediately presented to the gastrointestinal fluids. This large surface area facilitates dissolution and hence absorption of the drug. In contrast to hard gelatin capsule and tablet dosage forms, dissolution of all drug particles commences immediately on dilution of the dose of suspension in the gastrointestinal fluids. A drug contained in a tablet or hard gelatin capsule may ultimately achieve the same state of dispersion in the gastrointestinal fluids but only after a time lag. Thus a well formulated, finely subdivided aqueous suspension is regarded as being an efficient oral drug delivery system, second in efficiency only to the solution-type dosage form (Gibaldi, 1984).

Factors associated with the formulation of aqueous suspension dosage forms which can influence the bioavailabilities of drugs from the gastrointestinal tract include:

1 the particle size and effective surface area of the dispersed drug,
2 the crystal form of the drug,
3 complexation, i.e. the formation of a non-absorbable complex between the drug and an excipient such as the suspending agent,
4 the inclusion of a surfactant as a wetting, flocculating or deflocculating agent and
5 the viscosity of the suspension.

Information concerning the potential influence of the above factors on drug bioavailability is given in earlier sections of this chapter. Further information concerning the formulation and uses of suspensions as dosage forms is given in Chapter 15.

Soft gelatin capsules

Soft gelatin capsules combine the convenience of a unit dosage form with the potentially rapid drug absorption associated with aqueous solution and suspension types of dosage forms (Rees, 1974). Drugs encapsulated in soft gelatin capsules for peroral administration are dissolved or dispersed in a non-toxic, non-aqueous vehicle. Such vehicles may be water immiscible (i.e. lipophilic) or water miscible (i.e. hydrophilic). Vegetable oils are popular water-immiscible vehicles whilst polyethylene glycols and certain non-ionic surfactants (e.g. polysorbate 80) are employed as water-miscible vehicles.

Release of the contents of a soft gelatin capsule is effected by dissolution and splitting of the flexible shell. Following release, a water-miscible vehicle disperses and/or dissolves readily in the gastrointestinal fluids liberating the drug, depending on its aqueous solubility, as a solution or a fine suspension in the gastrointestinal fluids. The drug is thus liberated in a form which is conducive to rapid absorption. Many poorly water-soluble drugs have been found to exhibit greater bioavailabilities from soft gelatin capsules containing water-miscible vehicles than from aqueous suspensions, hard gelatin capsules or tablets (Armstrong and James, 1980). In the case of soft gelatin capsules containing drugs in solution or suspension in water-immiscible vehicles, release of the contents will almost certainly be followed by dispersion in the gastrointestinal fluids. Dispersion will be facilitated by emulsifiers included in the vehicle and also by bile. If the lipophilic vehicle is a digestible oil and the drug is highly soluble in the oil, it is possible that the drug will remain in solution in the dispersed oil phase and be absorbed (along with the oil) by fat absorption processes (Armstrong and James, 1980). For a drug which is less lipophilic or is dissolved in a non-digestible oil, absorption probably occurs following partitioning of the drug from the oily vehicle into the aqueous gastrointestinal fluids. In this case, the rate of drug absorption appears to depend on the rate at which drug partitions from the dispersed oil phase. The increase in interfacial area of contact resulting from dispersion of the oily vehicle in the gastrointestinal fluids will facilitate partition of the drug across the oil/aqueous interface. For a drug which is suspended in an oily vehicle, drug release may involve dissolution in the vehicle, diffusion to the oil/aqueous interface, and partition across the interface. It is also possible that release could involve the passage of solid drug particles across the oil/aqueous interface followed by dissolution in the gastrointestinal fluids. This latter mechanism has been proposed by de Blaey and Polderman (1980) as a model for drug release from lipophilic suppository vehicles containing suspended drug.

Factors associated with the formulation of soft gelatin capsules which can influence the bioavailabilities of drugs from this type of dosage form include:

1 solubility of the drug in the vehicle (and gastrointestinal fluids),
2 particle size of the drug (if suspended in the vehicle),
3 nature of the vehicle, i.e. hydrophilic or lipophilic (and whether a lipophilic vehicle is a digestible or non-digestible oil),
4 inclusion of a surfactant as a wetting agent/emulsifying agent in a lipophilic vehicle or as the vehicle itself,
5 inclusion of a suspending agent (viscosity-enhancing agent) in the vehicle, and
6 complexation, i.e. formation of a non-absorbable complex between the drug and any excipient.

Additional information concerning soft gelatin capsules is given in Chapter 19.

Hard gelatin capsules

Generally the bioavailability of a drug from a well formulated hard gelatin capsule dosage form will be better than or at least equal to the bioavailability of the same drug from a compressed tablet. The small particles of drug in a capsule are not subjected to the same degree of compression and possible fusion which would reduce the effective surface area of the drug. Provided that the hard gelatin shell dissolves rapidly in the gastrointestinal fluids and the encapsulated mass disperses rapidly and efficiently, a relatively large effective surface area of drug will be exposed to the gastrointestinal fluids thereby facilitating drug dissolution. However, it is incorrect to assume that because a drug formulated as a hard gelatain capsule is in a finely divided form surrounded by a water-soluble shell, no bioavailability problems can occur (Rees, 1974). The overall rate of dissolution of drugs from capsules appears to be a complex function of the rates of different processes such as:

1 the dissolution rate of the gelatin shell,
2 the rate of penetration of the gastrointestinal fluids into the encapsulated mass,

3 the rate at which the mass deaggregates (i.e. disperses) in the gastrointestinal fluids, and
4 the rate of dissolution of the dispersed drug particles (Finholt, 1974).

The inclusion of excipients (e.g. diluents, lubricants and surfactants) in a capsule formulation can have a significant effect on the rate of dissolution of drugs, particularly those which are poorly soluble and hydrophobic. Figure 9.11 shows that a hydrophilic diluent (e.g. sorbitol, lactose) often serves to increase the rate of penetration of the aqueous gastrointestinal fluids into the contents of the capsule and to aid disper-

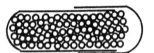

Hard gelatin capsule containing only hydrophobic drug particles

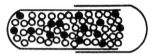

Hard gelatin capsule containing hydrophobic drug particles (o) and hydrophilic diluent particles (•)

In gastrointestinal fluids, hard gelatin capsule shell dissolves, thereby exposing contents to fluids

Contents remain as a capsule-shaped plug. Hydrophobic nature of contents impedes penetration of gastrointestinal fluids

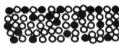

Particles of hydrophilic diluent dissolve in gastrointestinal fluids leaving a porous mass of drug

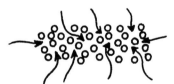

Gastrointestinal fluids can penetrate porous mass

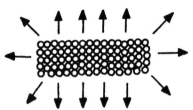

Dissolution of drug occurs only from surface of plug-shaped mass. Relatively low rate of dissolution

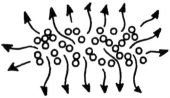

Effective surface area of drug and hence dissolution rate is increased

Fig. 9.11 Diagrammatic representation of how a hydrophilic diluent can increase the rate of dissolution of a poorly soluble, hydrophobic drug from a hard gelatin capsule

sion and subsequent dissolution of the drug in these fluids. However, the diluent should exhibit no tendency to adsorb or complex with the drug since either can impair absorption from the gastrointestinal tract. For instance, the bioavailability of tetracycline is reduced if dicalcium phosphate is included as the diluent in capsules of this antibiotic. A poorly soluble, non-absorbable calcium–tetracycline complex is formed as the contents of the capsule dissolve in the gastrointestinal fluids.

Magnesium stearate is commonly included as a lubricant for the capsule-filling operation. Its hydrophobic nature often retards liquid penetration so that a capsule-shaped plug often remains after the shell has dissolved in the gastrointestinal fluids, especially when the contents have been machine-filled as a consolidated plug (Rees, 1974). However, this effect can usually be overcome by the simultaneous addition of a wetting agent (i.e. a water-soluble surfactant) and a hydrophilic diluent to the contents.

Both the formulation and the type and conditions of the capsule-filling process can affect the packing density and liquid permeability of the capsule contents (Newton, 1972). In general, an increase in packing density (i.e. a decrease in porosity) of the encapsulated mass will probably result in a decrease in liquid permeability and dissolution rate particularly if the drug is hydrophobic or if a hydrophilic drug is mixed with a hydrophobic lubricant such as magnesium stearate. If the encapsulated mass is tightly packed and the drug is hydrophobic in nature, then a decrease in dissolution rate with a concomitant reduction in particle size would be expected unless a surfactant had been included to facilitate liquid penetration. Granulation can increase the dissolution rate of a micronized hydrophobic drug by increasing the liquid permeability of the encapsulated mass (Newton, 1972).

In summary, formulation factors which can influence the bioavailabilities of drugs from hard gelatin capsules include:

1 surface area and particle size of drug (particularly the effective surface area exhibited by the drug in the gastrointestinal fluids),
2 use of the salt form of a drug in preference to the parent weak acid or base,
3 crystal form of the drug,
4 the chemical stability of the drug (in the dosage form and gastrointestinal fluids),
5 the natures and quantities of the diluent, lubricant and wetting agent,
6 drug–excipient interactions (e.g. adsorption, complexation),
7 the type and conditions of the filling process,
8 the packing density of the capsule contents,
9 the composition and properties of the capsule shell (including enteric capsules), and
10 interactions between the capsule shell and contents.

Further information concerning the hard gelatin capsule as a dosage form is given in Chapter 19.

Tablets

Uncoated tablets When a drug is formulated as a compressed tablet, there is an enormous reduction in the effective surface area of the drug due to the granulation and compression processes involved in tablet making (see Chapters 37 and 39). These processes also necessitate the addition of excipients which themselves may alter the release of a drug from a tablet. Many bioavailability problems are associated with this reduction in effective surface area of drug and with the problems of generating a fine, well dispersed suspension of drug particles in the gastrointestinal fluids following administration of a tablet. Since the effective surface area of a poorly soluble drug is an important factor influencing its dissolution rate, it is especially important that tablets containing such drugs should disintegrate rapidly and completely in the gastrointestinal fluids if rapid drug release, dissolution and absorption is required. The overall rate of tablet disintegration is influenced by several interdependent factors which include the concentration and type of drug, diluent, binder, disintegrant, lubricant and wetting agent as well as the compaction pressure (see Chapter 18).

A diagrammatic representation of the disintegration and dissolution steps that normally occur with a tablet prior to drug absorption are shown in Fig. 18.1. The dissolution of a poorly soluble drug from an intact tablet is usually extremely limited because of the relatively small effective surface area of drug exposed to the gastrointestinal fluids. Disintegration of the tablet into granules causes a relatively large increase in effective surface area of drug and the drug dissolution rate may be likened to that of a coarse, aggregated suspension. Further disintegration into small, primary drug particles produces a further large increase in effective surface area and dissolution rate of the drug. The dissolution rate is probably comparable to that of a fine, well dispersed suspension of drug (Gibaldi 1984). Disintegration of a tablet into primary drug particles is thus important since it ensures that a large effective surface area of poorly soluble drug is generated in order to facilitate dissolution and subsequent absorption of the drug (Wells and Rubinstein, 1976).

However, simply because a tablet disintegrates rapidly does not necessarily guarantee that the liberated primary drug particles will dissolve rapidly in the gastrointestinal fluids and that the rate and extent of drug absorption will be adequate. In the case of poorly soluble drugs, the rate-controlling step for drug absorption is usually the overall rate of dissolution of the liberated drug particles in the gastrointestinal fluids. The overall dissolution rate and bioavailability of a poorly soluble drug from an uncoated conventional tablet is influenced by many factors associated with the formulation and manufacture of this type of dosage form (Finholt, 1974). These factors include:

1 the physicochemical properties of the liberated drug particles in the gastrointestinal fluids, e.g. wettability, effective surface area, crystal form, chemical stability,
2 the nature and quantity of the diluent, binder, disintegrant, lubricant and any wetting agent,
3 drug–excipient interactions (e.g. complexation) the size of the granules and their method of manufacture,
4 the compaction pressure and speed of compression used in tableting, and
5 the conditions of storage and age of the tablet.

Since drug absorption and hence bioavailability are dependent upon the drug being in the dissolved state, suitable dissolution characteristics can be an important property of a satisfactory tablet, particularly if it contains a poorly soluble drug. On this basis, specific *in vitro* dissolution test conditions and dissolution limits are included in the *British Pharmacopoeia* for tablets (and hard gelatin capsules) containing certain drugs, e.g. digoxin. That a particular drug product meets the requirements of a compendial dissolution standard provides a greater assurance that the drug will be released satisfactorily from the formulated dosage form *in vivo* and be absorbed adequately.

Further information on formulation and release of drugs from tablets is given in Chapter 18.

Coated tablets The most common of the various types of coated tablets are sugar-coated and film-coated tablets. The presence of a coating around a tablet presents a physical barrier between the tablet core and the gastrointestinal fluids. Hence coated tablets not only possess all the potential bioavailability problems associated with uncoated conventional tablets but are subject to the additional potential problem of being surrounded by a physical barrier. In the case of a coated tablet which is intended to disintegrate and release drug rapidly into solution in the gastrointestinal fluids, the coating must dissolve or disrupt before these processes can occur. The physicochemical nature and thickness of the coating can thus influence how quickly a drug is released from a tablet.

In the process of sugar coating, the tablet core is usually sealed with a thin continuous film of a poorly water-soluble polymer such as shellac or cellulose acetate phthalate (see Chapter 40). This sealing coat serves to protect the tablet core and its contents from the aqueous coating fluids used in the subsequent steps of the sugar-coating process. Hence the presence of this water-impermeable sealing coat can potentially retard drug release from sugar-coated tablets. In view of this potential problem, annealing agents such as polyethylene glycols or calcium carbonate which do not substantially reduce the water impermeability of the sealing coat during sugar coating but dissolve readily in gastric fluid, may be added to the sealer coat in order to reduce the 'barrier' effect of this coat to rapid drug release.

The coating of a tablet core by a thin film coat of a water-soluble polymer such as hydroxypropyl methylcellulose should have no significant effect on the rate of disintegration of the tablet core and subsequent drug dissolution provided that the film coat dissolves rapidly and independently of the pH of the gastrointestinal fluids. However, if hydrophobic water-insoluble film coating materials such as cellulose acetate phthalate, ethylcellulose or acrylic resins are used to coat tablet cores, the resulting film coat acts as a barrier which delays and/or reduces the rate of release of drugs from tablet cores. Thus these types of film coating materials form 'barriers' which can have a significant influence on the absorption of drugs from film-coated tablets. Whilst the formation of such 'barrier' coatings would be disadvantageous in the case of film-coated tablets intended to provide rapid rates of drug absorption, the concept of 'barrier' coating has been used (along with other techniques) to obtain more precise control over drug release than is possible with conventional uncoated tablets. In this context, film coating has been used to provide

1 limited control over the site at which a drug is released from a tablet into the gastrointestinal tract, and
2 a controlled continuous rate of drug release from a non-disintegrating (intact) tablet as it passes along the gastrointestinal tract.

In this latter case, 'barrier' coating is one of many formulation techniques which have been used to increase the duration of therapeutic action of a drug contained within a peroral dosage form. For information concerning controlled/sustained/ prolonged release peroral dosage forms, the reader should refer to the reviews by Ritschel (1973) and Hon-Leung Lee and Robinson (1978).

Enteric coated tablets The use of barrier coating in order to control the site of release of an orally administered drug is well illustrated by enteric-coated tablets. An enteric coat is designed to resist gastric fluids but to disrupt or dissolve when the coated tablet enters the duodenum. Polymers such as cellulose acetate phthalate, hydroxypropyl methylcellulose phthalate and polyvinyl acetate phthalate are used as enteric coatings. These materials dissolve slowly over the gastric pH range (i.e. pH 1–3) but dissolve rapidly at the less acid pH values associated with the small intestine.

Enteric coatings should preferably begin to dissolve at about pH 5 in order to ensure the availability of drugs which are absorbed primarily in the proximal region of the small intestine (Rees, 1974). Enteric coating thus provides a means of delaying the release of a drug until the dosage form reaches the small intestine. Such delayed release provides a means of protecting drugs which would otherwise be destroyed if released into gastric fluid (see earlier in this chapter). Hence enteric coating serves to improve the peroral bioavailability exhibited by such drugs from uncoated conventional tablets. Enteric coating also protects the stomach against drugs which can produce nausea or mucosal irritation if released at this site, e.g. phenylbutazone, aspirin.

In addition to the protection offered by enteric coating, the delayed release of drug also results in a significant delay in the onset of the therapeutic response of a drug. The onset of the therapeutic response is largely dependent on the residence time of the enteric-coated tablet in the stomach. Gastric emptying of such tablets is an all-or-nothing process, i.e. the tablet is either in the stomach or in the duodenum. Consequently drug is either not being released or being released. The residence time of an intact enteric-coated tablet in the stomach can vary within and between subjects from about 30 minutes to several hours (Bechgaard and Christensen, 1982). Hence there is considerable intrasubject and intersubject variation in the onset of therapeutic action exhibited by drugs administered as enteric-coated tablets.

The formulation of an enteric-coated product in the form of small individually enteric-coated granules or pellets contained in a rapidly dissolving hard gelatin capsule or a rapidly disintegrating tablet, would largely eliminate the dependency of this type of dosage form on the all-or-nothing gastric emptying process associated with the intact enteric-coated tablet. Provided that the coated granules or pellets were sufficiently small (less than 1 mm diameter), they would be able to pass the pylorus even when the sphincter was closed (Bechgaard and Christensen, 1982). Hence enteric-coated granules and pellets would exhibit a gradual but continual release from the stomach into the duodenum. This type of release would also avoid the complete dose of drug being released into the duodenum as occurs from an enteric-coated tablet. The intestinal mucosa would thus not be exposed locally to a potentially toxic concentration of drug (Taylor, 1982).

Further information on coated tablets is given in Chapters 18 and 40.

REFERENCES AND BIBLIOGRAPHY

Armstrong, N. A. and James, K. C. (1980) *Int. J. Pharm.*, **6**, 195–204.

Ashley, J. J. and Levy, G. (1973) *J. pharm. Sci.*, **62**, 688–690.

Atkinson, R. M., Bedford, C., Child, K. J. and Tomich, E. G. (1962) *Nature*, **193**, 588–589.

Augiar, A. J., Krc, J. Jnr., Krinkel, A. W. and Samyn, J. C. (1967) *J. pharm. Sci.*, **56**, 847–853.

Bachynsky, M. O., Bartilucci, A. J., Eisen, H. and Jarowski, C. I. (1976) *Drug Dev. Commun.*, **2**, 63–76.

Barr, W. H. (1972) *Pharmacology*, **8**, 55–101.

Barzegar-Jalali, M. and Richards, J. H. (1979) *Int. J. Pharm.*, **3**, 133–141.

Bates, T. R. and Gibaldi, M. (1970) In: *Current Concepts in the Pharmaceutical Sciences: Biopharmaceutics* (Ed. J. J. Swarbrick), pp. 57–99, Lea and Febiger, Philadelphia.

Bechgaard, H. and Christensen, F. N. (1982) *Pharm. J.*, **229**, 373–376.

Benet, L. Z. (1973) In: *Drug Design* (Ed. E. J. Ariens), Vol. IV, pp. 1–35, Academic Press, New York.

Berge, S. M., Bighley, L. D. and Monkhouse, D. C. (1977) *J. pharm. Sci.*, **66**, 1–19.

Blanchard, J. (1975) *Am. J. Pharm.*, **147**, 135–146.

Brodie, B. B. (1964) In: *Absorption and Distribution of Drugs* (Ed. T. B. Binns), pp. 16–48, E. and S. Livingstone Ltd, London.

Cadwallader, D. E. (1973) *Biopharmaceutics and Drug Interactions*, p. 58, F. Hoffman-La Roche and Co. Ltd, Basel.

Chiou, W. L. (1977) *J. pharm. Sci.*, **66**, 989–991.

Chiou, W. L. and Riegelman, S. (1971) *J. pharm. Sci.*, **60**, 1281–1302.

Davison, C., Guy, J. L., Levitt, M. and Smith, P. K. (1961) *J. Pharm. exp. Ther.*, **134**, 176–183.

de Blaey, C. J. and Polderman, J. (1980) In: *Drug Design* (Ed. E. J. Ariens), Vol. IX, pp. 237–266, Academic Press, London.

Duncan, W. A. M., Macdonald, G. and Thornton, M. J. (1962) *J. Pharm. Pharmacol.* **14**, 217–224.

Fincher, J. H. (1968) *J. pharm. Sci.*, **57**, 1825–1835.

Finholt, P. (1974) In: *Dissolution Techology* (Eds L. J. Leeson and J. T. Carstensen), pp. 106–146, Academy of Pharmaceutical Science, Washington.

Florence, A. T. (1981) *Pure appl. Chem.*, **53**, 2057–2068.

Florence, A. T. and Attwood, D. (1981a) *Physico-chemical Principles of Pharmacy*, pp. 337–342, The Macmillan Press Ltd, London.

Florence, A. T. and Attwood, D. (1981b) *Ibid.*, pp. 406–413.

Florence, A. T. and Attwood, D. (1981c) *Ibid.*, pp. 415–419.

Florence, A. T., Salole, E. G. and Stenlake, J. B. (1974) *J. Pharm. Pharmac.*, **26**, 479–480.

Gibaldi, M. (1970) *Fedn. Proc.*, **29**, 1343–1349.

Gibaldi, M. (1984) *Biopharmaceutics and Clinical Pharmacokinetics*, 3rd edn, Lea and Febiger, Philadelphia.

Gibaldi, M. and Feldman, S. (1970) *J. pharm. Sci.*, **59**, 579–589.

Goldberg, A. H., Gibaldi, M. and Kanig, J. L. (1965) *J. pharm. Sci.*, **54**, 1145–1148.

Goldberg, A. H., Gibaldi, M. and Kanig, J. L. (1966a) *Ibid.*, **55**, 482–487.

Goldberg, A. H., Gibaldi, M. and Kanig, J. L. (1966b) *Ibid.*, **55**, 487–492.

Goldberg, A. H., Gibaldi, M. and Kanig, J. L. (1966c) *Ibid.*, **55**, 581–583.

Hogben, C. A. M., Schanker, L. A., Tocco, D. J. and Brodie, B. B. (1957) *J. Pharm. exp. Ther.*, **120**, 540–545.

Hon-Leung Lee, V. and Robinson, J. R. (1978) In: *Drugs and the Pharmaceutical Sciences. Vol. I. Sustained and Controlled Release Drug Delivery Systems* (Ed. J. R. Robinson), pp. 123–209, Marcel Dekker, Inc., New York.

Kaur, R., Grant, D. J. W. and Eaves, T. (1980) *J. pharm. Sci.*, **69**, 1317–1321.

Levine, R. R. (1971) In: *Topics in Medicinal Chemistry, Vol. 4, Absorption Phenomena* (Eds J. L. Rabinowitz and R. M. Myerson), pp. 27–95, Wiley-Interscience, London.

Levy, G. and Jusko, W. (1965) *J. pharm. Sci.*, **54**, 219–225.

Malone, M. H., Gibson, R. D. and Miya, T. S. (1960) *J. pharm. Sci.*, **49**, 529–534.

Mayersohn, M. (1979) In: *Modern Pharmaceutics* (Eds G. S. Banker and C. T. Rhodes), pp. 23–85, Marcel Dekker Inc., New York.

Mullins, J. D. and Macek, T. J. (1960) *J. Am. Pharm.*, **49**, 245–248.

Nash, J. F., Childers, R. F., Lowary, L. R. and Rose, H. A. (1974/75) *Drug Dev. Commun.*, **1**, 459–470.

Nelson, E., Knoechel, E. L., Hamlin, W. E. and Wagner, J. G. (1962) *J. pharm. Sci.*, **51**, 509–514.

Newton, J. M. (1972) *Pharm. Weekblad.*, **107**, 485–498.

Notari, R. E. (1980) *Biopharmaceutics and Clinical Pharmacokinetics. An Introduction*, 3rd edn, pp. 107–172, Marcel Dekker Inc., New York.

Poole, J. W., Owen, G., Silverio, J., Freyhof, J. H. and Roseman, S. B. (1968) *Curr. ther. R.*, **10**, 292–303.

Prescott, L. F., Steel, R. F. and Ferrier, W. R. (1970) *Clin. Pharmac. Ther.*, **11**, 496–504.

Rees, J. E. (1974) *Pharm. J.*, **213**, 266–270.

Remmers, R. G., Barringer, W. C., Sieger, G. M., Anagnostakos, N., Corbett, J. C. and Doerschuk, A. P. (1965) *J. Pharm. Sci.*, **54**, 49–52.

Ritschel, W. A. (1973) In: *Drug Design* (Ed. E. J. Ariens), Vol. IV, pp. 37–73, Academic Press, New York.

Rosenberg, H. A. and Bates, T. R. (1976) *Clin. Pharmac. Ther.*, **20**, 227–231.

Schmidt, R. and Fonchamps, A. (1974) *Eur. J. clin. Pharmacol.*, **7**, 213–216.

Seager, H. (1968) *J. Pharm. Pharmac.*, **20**, 968–969.

Sekiguchi, K. and Obi, N. (1961) *Chem. Pharm. Bull.*, **9**, 866–872.

Shah, N. B. and Sheth, B. B. (1976) *J. Pharm. Sci.*, **65**, 1618–1623.

Schanker, L. S. (1960) *J. mednl Chem.*, **2**, 343–359.

Schanker, L. S., Shore, P. A., Brodie, B. B. and Hogben, C. A. M. (1957) *J. Pharm. exp. Ther.*, **120**, 528–539.

Shaw, T. R. D., Carless, J. E., Howard, M. R. and Raymond, K. (1973) *Lancet*, **ii**, 209–210.

Shore, P. A., Brodie, B. B. and Hogben, C. A. M. (1957) *J. Pharm. exp. Ther.*, **119**, 361–369.

Smith, D. H. (1964) In: *Absorption and Distribution of Drugs* (Ed. T. B. Binns), pp. 1–15, E. and S. Livingstone Ltd, London.

Sorby, D. L. (1965) *J. pharm. Sci.*, **54**, 677–683.

Taylor, D. C. (1982) *Pharm. J.*, **229**, 371–373.

Tyler, J. H., Eadie, M. J., Sutherland, J. M. and Hooper, W. D. (1970) *Br. med. J.*, **4**, 271–273.

Wagner, J. G. and Sedman, A. J. (1973) *J. Pharmacokin. Biopharm.*, **1**, 23–50.

Welling, P. G. (1980) *Pharm. Int.*, **1**, 14–18.

Wells, J. I. and Rubinstein, M. H. (1976) *Pharm. J.*, **217**, 629–631.

Assessment of bioavailability

ASSESSMENT OF BIOAVAILABILITY

In order to study the bioavailability of a drug from a dosage form it is necessary to have some means of assessing the extent and rate of absorption of the drug. Ideally one would like to measure the bioavailability of a drug from a dosage form in terms of the clinical response of a patient or in terms of the amount of drug available at the site(s) of action at suitable periods of time after administration. However, except for a few clinical responses (e.g. heart rate, blood pressure, electrocardiograms) accurate quantitative measurement of clinical responses is often not practical or possible. Similarly the measurement of drug concentration at its site(s) of action is not generally possible because either the precise site(s) of action is not known or, where this is known, it is impracticable to measure accurately the drug concentration at that point. The methods of bioavailability assessment which are used at present depend on the assumption that the measurement of the concentration of the drug in a suitable body fluid (usually blood plasma, urine or occasionally saliva) over a period of time after administration in its dosage form can be correlated with the clinical efficacy of the drug in treating a given disease condition.

REPRESENTATION OF BIOAVAILABILITY DATA

The most commonly used method of assessing the bioavailability of a drug involves the construction of a blood plasma concentration–time curve.

Plasma concentration–time curves

Let us consider that a single dose of a drug is administered orally to a patient (say in the form of a tablet) and serial blood samples are withdrawn and assayed for plasma concentration of the drug at specific periods of time after administration of the drug.

Figure 10.1 shows a typical plasma concentration versus time curve following the administration of an oral tablet.

At zero time when the drug is first administered, the concentration of drug in the plasma will be zero. As the tablet passes into the stomach and/or intestine it disintegrates, the drug dissolves and absorption ensues. Initially the concentration of drug in the plasma rises since the rate of absorption exceeds the rate at which the drug is being removed from the plasma by distribution and elimination. Drug concentrations in the plasma continue to rise until a maximum (or *peak*) concentration is attained. The peak concentration represents the highest concentration of drug achieved in the plasma following the adminis-

tration of a single dose. It is reached when the rate of appearance of drug in the plasma is equal to its rate of removal by distribution and elimination.

The ascending portion of the plasma concentration–time curve (i.e. that part of the curve to the left of the peak concentration) is sometimes called the *absorption phase* of the curve. Here the rate of absorption outweighs the rate of removal of drug by distribution and elimination. It should be noted that drug absorption usually does not abruptly stop at the time of the peak concentration but may continue for some time into the descending portion of the curve. The early descending portion of the curve can thus reflect the net result of drug absorption, distribution and elimination but in this phase the rate of drug removal from the blood exceeds the rate of drug absorption. Therefore the concentration of drug in the plasma declines.

Eventually drug absorption ceases when the bioavailable dose of drug has been absorbed and the concentration of drug in the plasma is now controlled only by its rate of elimination by metabolism and/or excretion. This is sometimes

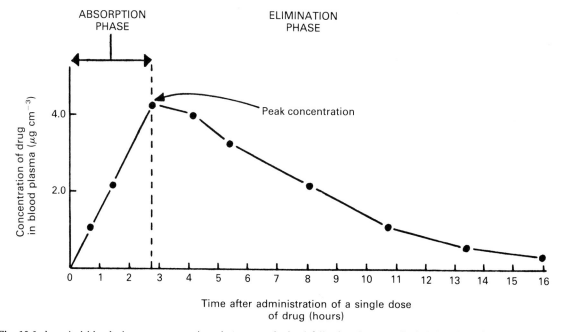

Fig. 10.1 A typical blood plasma concentration–time curve obtained following the peroral administration of a single dose of a drug in a tablet. (After Chodos and Di Santo, 1973)

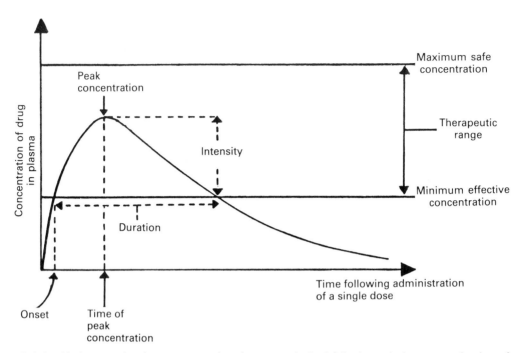

Fig. 10.2 Relationship between the plasma concentration–time curve obtained following a single extravascular dose of a drug and parameters associated with the therapeutic or pharmacological response

called the *elimination phase* of the curve. It should be appreciated, however, that elimination of a drug begins as soon as the drug appears in the plasma.

Let us now consider several parameters based on the plasma concentration–time curve which are important in bioavailability studies. These are shown in Fig. 10.2 and are discussed below.

Minimum effective (or therapeutic) plasma concentration

It is generally assumed that some minimum concentration of drug must be achieved in the plasma before the desired therapeutic or pharmacological effect is achieved. This concentration is called the *minimum effective* (or *therapeutic*) *plasma concentration*. Its value not only varies from drug to drug but also from individual to individual and with the type and severity of the disease state. In Fig. 10.2, the minimum effective concentration is indicated by the lower line.

Maximum safe concentration

The concentration of drug in the plasma above which side effects or toxic effects occur in a patient is known as the *maximum safe concentration*.

Therapeutic range

A range of plasma drug concentrations is also assumed to exist over which the desired response is obtained yet toxic effects are avoided. This range of plasma drug concentrations is called the *therapeutic range*. The intention in clinical practice is to maintain plasma drug concentrations within this range.

Onset

The *onset* may be defined as the time required to achieve the minimum effective plasma concentration following administration of the dosage form.

Duration

The *duration* of the therapeutic effect of the drug is the period during which the concentration of drug in the plasma exceeds the minimum effective plasma concentration.

Peak concentration

This represents the highest concentration of the drug achieved in the plasma.

Intensity

In general the difference between the minimum effective plasma concentration and the peak concentration is a relative measure of the intensity of the therapeutic response of the drug.

The time of the peak concentration

This is the period of time required to achieve the peak plasma concentration of drug after administration of a single dose of the drug. This parameter is related to the rate of absorption of the drug and can be used to assess that rate.

Area under the plasma concentration–time curve

This is related to the total amount of drug absorbed into the systemic circulation following the administration of a single dose of that drug. However, changes in the area under the plasma concentration–time curve need not necessarily reflect changes in the total amount of drug absorbed but can reflect modifications in the kinetics of distribution, metabolism and excretion of a drug.

The use of plasma concentration–time curves in bioavailability studies

In order to illustrate the usefulness of blood plasma concentration–time curves in bioavailability studies, let us consider the administration of single *equal* doses of three different formulations, A, B, and C of the *same* drug to the *same* healthy individual by the *same* route of administration on three separate occasions. Let us assume that sufficient time was allowed to elapse between the administration of each formulation such that the systemic circulation contained no residual concentration of drug and no residual effects from

any previous administrations of the drug. Let us also assume that the kinetics and pattern of distribution of the drug, its binding phenomena, the kinetics of elimination of the drug and the experimental conditions under which each plasma concentration–time curve was obtained, were the same on each occasion. Hence, it is reasonable to assume that the differences in plasma concentration–time curves of the three formulations, shown in Fig. 10.3, are due solely to differences in the rate and/or extent of absorption of the drug from each formulation.

Consideration of the three curves in Figure 10.3 show that each of the three formulations (A, B and C) of the same dose of the same drug results in a different peak plasma concentration. However, the areas under the curves for formulation A and B are similar and this indicates that the drug is absorbed to a similar extent from these two formulations. Consideration of the times at which the peak plasma concentrations occur for formulations A and B show that the drug is absorbed faster from formulation A than from formulation B. Figure 10.3 shows that the faster rate of absorption of drug from formulation A means that this formulation shows a fast onset of therapeutic action but since its peak plasma concentration exceeds the maximum safe concentration it is likely that this formulation of the drug will result in toxic side effects. Formulation B, which gives a slower rate of drug absorption than formulation A, shows a slower onset for its therapeutic action than formulation A but its peak plasma concentration lies within the therapeutic range. In addition the duration of action of the therapeutic effect obtained with formulation B is longer than that obtained with formulation A. Hence formulation B appears to be superior to formulation A from a clinical view point in that its peak plasma concentration lies within the therapeutic range of the drug and the duration of the therapeutic effect is longer.

Formulation C gives a much smaller area under the plasma concentration–time curve indicating that a lower proportion of the administered dose has been absorbed. This, together with the slower rate of absorption of drug from formulation C (the time of peak concentration is longer than for formulations A and B) results in the peak plasma

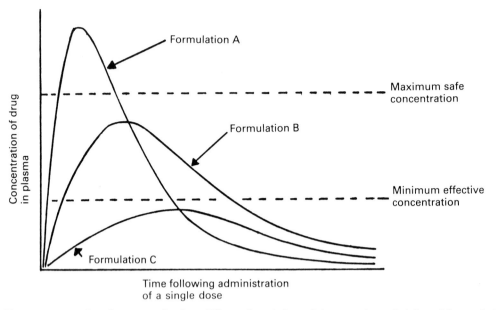

Fig. 10.3 Plasma concentration–time curves for three different formulations of the same drug administered in equal single doses by the same extravascular route

concentration not reaching the minimum effective concentration, i.e. formulation C does not produce a therapeutic effect, and consequently is clinically inefficacious as a single dose.

This simple hypothetical example illustrates how differences in bioavailability exhibited by a given drug from different formulations can result in a patient being either over-, under- or correctly medicated.

It is important to realize that the study of bioavailability based on drug concentration measurements in the plasma (or urine or saliva) is complicated by the fact that such drug concentration–time curves are affected by factors other than the biopharmaceutical factors of the drug product itself. Factors such as body weight, sex and age of the test subjects, disease states, genetic differences in drug metabolism, excretion and distribution, food and water intake, concomitant administration of other drugs, stress and time of administration of the drug are some of the variables which can complicate the interpretation of bioavailability studies. In so far as possible, bioavailability studies should be designed to control these factors. This aspect of bioavailability studies is considered later in this chapter.

Whilst plots such as Fig. 10.3 can be used to compare the relative bioavailability of a *given* drug from different formulations, such plots cannot be used indiscriminantly to compare *different* drugs. It is quite usual for different drugs to exhibit different rates of absorption, metabolism, excretion and distribution, different distribution patterns and differences in their binding phenomena, all of which would influence the drug concentration–time curve obtained for each drug. Hence it would be extremely difficult to attribute differences in the drug concentration–time curves obtained for different drugs presented in different formulations to differences in their bioavailabilities.

Cumulative urinary drug excretion curves

Measurement of the concentration of intact drug and/or its metabolite(s) in the urine can also be used to assess the bioavailability of a drug. Collection of urine samples is easier and less unpleasant for the test subject than is the collection of blood samples. In addition, the concentration of intact drug and/or its metabolites in the urine is often greater than that of intact drug in the blood and this, together with the presence of lower concentrations of protein and other endogenous materials, facilitates easier assay of the drug and/or its metabolites in urine.

When a suitable specific assay method is not available for the intact drug in the urine or the specific assay method available for the parent drug is not sufficiently sensitive, it may be necessary to assay the principal metabolite or intact drug plus its metabolite(s) in the urine to obtain an index of the bioavailability of a drug. Measurements involving metabolite levels in the urine for estimating the bioavailability of a drug are only valid when the drug in question is not subject to metabolism prior to reaching the systemic circulation. If an orally administered drug is subject to intestinal metabolism or first pass liver metabolism, then measurement of the principal metabolite or of intact drug plus metabolites in the urine would give an overestimate of the systemic availability of that drug. It should be remembered that the definition of bioavailability is in terms of the extent and the rate at which *intact* drug appears in the systemic circulation after administration of a known dose of the drug.

The assessment of bioavailability by urinary excretion is based on the assumption that the appearance of the drug and/or its metabolites in the urine is a function of the rate and extent of drug absorption. This assumption is only valid when a drug and/or its metabolites is extensively excreted in the urine and where the rate of urinary excretion is proportional to the concentration of the intact drug in the blood plasma. This proportionality does not hold if

1 the drug and/or its metabolites is excreted by an active transport process into the distal kidney tubule, or
2 the intact drug and/or its metabolites is weakly acidic or weakly basic (i.e. their rate of excretion is dependent on urine pH), or
3 the excretion rate depends on the rate of urine flow.

The important parameters in urinary excretion studies are the cumulative amount of intact drug and/or metabolites excreted and the rate at which this excretion takes place. A cumulative urinary excretion curve is obtained by collecting urine

samples (resulting from total emptying of the bladder) at known intervals of time after a single dose of the drug has been administered. Urine samples must be collected until all drug and/or its metabolites have been excreted (this is indicated by the cumulative urinary excretion curve becoming parallel to the abscissa) if a comparison of the extent of absorption of a given drug from different formulation or dosage forms is to be made. A typical cumulative urinary excretion curve and the corresponding plasma concentration–time curve obtained following the administration of a single dose of a given drug by the peroral route to a subject is shown in Fig. 10.4.

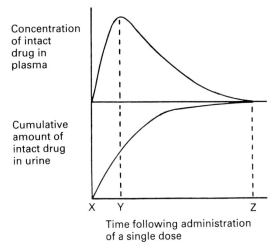

Fig. 10.4 Corresponding plots showing the plasma concentration–time curve (*upper curve*) and the cumulative urinary excretion curve (*lower curve*) obtained following the administration of a single dose of a drug by the peroral route

The initial segments (X–Y) of the curves reflect the 'absorption phase' (i.e. where absorption is the dominant process) and the slope of this segment of the urinary excretion curve is related to the rate of absorption of the drug into the blood. The total amount of intact drug (and/or its metabolite) excreted in the urine at point Z corresponds to the time at which the plasma concentration of intact drug is zero and essentially all the drug has been eliminated from the body. The total amount of drug excreted at point Z may be quite different in value to the total amount of drug administered (i.e. the dose) because of incomplete absorption of the drug and/or some of the drug being eliminated by processes other than urinary excretion.

The use of urinary drug excretion curves in bioavailability studies

In order to illustrate how cumulative urinary excretion curves can be used to compare the bioavailabilities of a given drug from different formulations, let us consider the urinary excretion data that would have been obtained following the administration of the single equal doses of the three different formulations, A, B and C of the same drug to the same healthy individual by the same extravascular route of administration on three different occasions and that gave the plasma concentration–time curves shown in Fig. 10.3. The corresponding cumulative urinary excretion curves are shown in Fig. 10.5.

The cumulative urinary excretion curves show that the rate at which drug appeared in the urine (i.e. the slope of the initial segment of each urinary excretion curve) from each formulation decreased in order A > B > C. Since the slope of the initial segment of the urinary excretion curve

is related to the rate of drug absorption, the cumulative urinary excretion curves indicate that the rates of absorption of drug from the three formulations decrease in the order A > B > C. Inspection of the corresponding plasma concentration–time curves in Fig. 10.3 shows that this is the case, i.e. peak concentration times (which are inversely related to the rate of drug absorption) for the three formulations increase in the order A < B < C. Although Fig. 10.5 shows that the rate of appearance of drug in the urine from formulation A is faster than from formulation B, the total amount of drug eventually excreted from these two formulations is the same, i.e. the cumulative urinary excretion curves for formulations A and B eventually meet and merge. Since the total amount of intact drug excreted is assumed to be related to the total amount of drug absorbed, the cumulative urinary excretion curves for formulations A and B indicate that the extent of drug absorption from these two formulations is the same. This is confirmed by the plasma concentration–time curves for formulations A and B in Fig. 10.3 which exhibit similar areas under their curves.

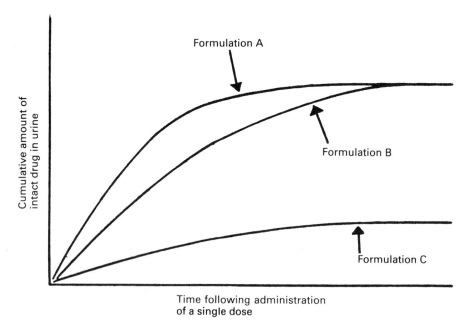

Fig. 10.5 Cumulative urinary excretion curves corresponding to the plasma concentration–time curves shown in Fig. 10.3 for three different formulations of the same drug administered in equal single doses by the same extravascular route

Thus both the plasma concentration–time curves and corresponding cumulative urinary excretion curves for formulations A and B show that the extent of drug absorption from these formulations is equal even though drug is absorbed at different rates from these formulations.

Consideration of the cumulative urinary excretion curve for formulation C shows that this formulation not only results in a slower rate of appearance of intact drug in the urine but also shows that the total amount of drug which is eventually excreted is much less than that from the other two formulations. Thus the cumulative urinary excretion curve suggests that both the rate and extent of drug absorption is reduced in the case of formulation C. This is confirmed by the plasma concentration–time curve shown in Fig. 10.3 for formulation C, i.e. formulation C exhibits a longer peak concentration time and a smaller area under its plasma concentration–time curve than do formulations A and B. Thus one can conclude that cumulative urinary excretion curves may be used to compare the rate and extent of absorption of a given drug presented in different formulations.

ABSOLUTE AND RELATIVE BIOAVAILABILITY

Absolute bioavailability

The absolute bioavailability of a given drug from a dosage form is the fraction (or percentage) of the administered dose which is absorbed intact into the systemic circulation. Absolute bioavailability may be measured by comparing the total amount of intact drug that reaches the systemic circulation after administration of a known dose of the dosage form via an absorption site with the total amount of intact drug that reaches the systemic circulation after administration of an equivalent dose of the drug in the form of an intravenous bolus injection. An intravenous bolus injection of the drug is used as a reference to compare the systemic availability of the drug administered via an absorption site since in the former case the entire administered dose of drug is introduced into the systemic

circulation and is considered to be totally bioavailable.

The absolute bioavailability of a given drug using blood plasma data may be calculated by comparing the total areas under the plasma concentration–time curves obtained following the administration of equivalent doses of the drug via an adsorption site and via the intravenous route to the same subject on different occasions. Typical plasma concentration–time curves obtained by administering equivalent doses of the same drug by the intravenous route (bolus injection) and the gastrointestinal route are shown in Fig. 10.6.

For equivalent doses of administered drug,

$$\text{absolute bioavailability} = \frac{(\text{AUC}_\text{T})_\text{abs}}{(\text{AUC}_\text{T})_\text{i.v.}}$$

where $(\text{AUC}_\text{T})_\text{abs}$ is the total area under the plasma concentration–time curve following administration of a single dose of drug via a given absorption site, and $(\text{AUC}_\text{T})_\text{i.v.}$ is the total area under the plasma concentration–time curve following administration of the drug by rapid intravenous injection.

If different doses of the drug are administered by both routes a correction for the sizes of the doses is made, as in the following equation:

$$\text{absolute bioavailability} = \frac{(\text{AUC}_\text{T})_\text{abs}/D_\text{abs}}{(\text{AUC}_\text{T})_\text{i.v.}/D_\text{i.v.}}$$

where D_abs is the size of the single dose drug administered via the absorption site, and $D_\text{i.v.}$ is the size of the dose of the drug administered as an intravenous bolus injection.

Absolute bioavailability using urinary excretion data may be determined by comparing the total cumulative amounts of unchanged drug ultimately excreted in the urine following administration of the drug via an absorption site and the intravenous route (bolus injection), respectively on different occasions to the same subject.

For equivalent doses of administered drug,

$$\text{absolute bioavailability} = \frac{(X_U^\infty)_\text{abs}}{(X_U^\infty)_\text{i.v.}}$$

where $(X_U^\infty)_\text{abs}$ and $(X_U^\infty)_\text{i.v.}$ are the total cumulative amounts of unchanged drug ultimately excreted in

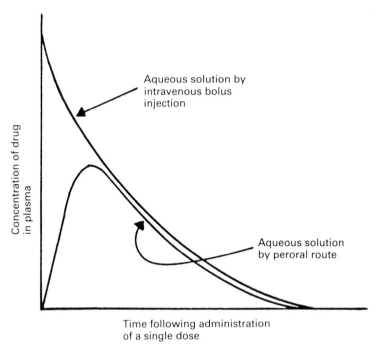

Fig. 10.6 Typical plasma concentration–time curves obtained by administering equivalent doses of the same drug by intravenous bolus injection and by the peroral route

the urine following administration of equivalent single doses of drug via an absorption site and as an intravenous bolus injection, respectively.

If different doses of drug are administered,

$$\text{absolute bioavailability} = \frac{(X^\infty_U)_{abs}/D_{abs}}{(X^\infty_U)_{i.v.}/D_{i.v.}}$$

The absolute bioavailability of a given drug from a particular type of dosage form may be expressed as a fraction or as a percentage.

Measurements of absolute bioavailability obtained by administering a given drug in the form of a simple aqueous solution by the peroral and intravenous routes, respectively, provide an insight into the effects that factors associated with the peroral route may have on the bioavailability of the drug, e.g. first pass metabolism by the liver, the formation of complexes between the drug and endogenous substances (e.g. mucin) at the site of absorption and drug stability in the gastrointestinal fluids.

It should be noted that the value calculated for the absolute bioavailability will only be valid if, for the drug being examined, the kinetics of elimination and distribution are independent of the route and time of drug administration, and also of the size of dose administered (if different doses are administered by the intravenous route and absorption site). If this is not the case, one cannot assume that the observed differences in the total areas under the plasma concentration–time curves or in the total cumulative amounts of unchanged drug ultimately excreted in the urine are due entirely to differences in bioavailability of the drug.

Relative bioavailability

In the case of drugs which cannot be administered in the form of an intravenous bolus injection, the relative (or comparative) bioavailability is determined rather than the absolute bioavailability. In the case of relative bioavailability, the bioavailability of a given drug from a 'test' dosage form is compared to the bioavailability of the same drug administered in a 'standard' dosage form which is either an orally administered solution of the drug (from which the drug is known to be well absorbed) or an established commercial preparation of proven clinical effectiveness. Hence relative bioavailability is a measure of the fraction (or percentage) of a given drug that is absorbed intact into the systemic circulation from a dosage form relative to a recognized (i.e. clinically proven) standard dosage form of that drug. The relative bioavailability of a given drug administered as equal doses of a test dosage form and a recognized standard dosage form, respectively, by the same route of administration to the same subject on different occasions may be calculated from the corresponding plasma concentration–time curves as follows.

For equivalent doses of administered drug,

$$\text{relative bioavailability} = \frac{(\text{AUC}_T)_{\text{test}}}{(\text{AUC}_T)_{\text{standard}}}$$

where $(\text{AUC}_T)_{\text{test}}$ and $(\text{AUC}_T)_{\text{standard}}$ are the total areas under the plasma concentration–time curves following administration of a single dose of the test dosage form and of the standard dosage form, respectively.

When different doses of the test and standard dosage forms are administered, a correction for the size of dose is made as follows:

$$\text{relative bioavailability} = \frac{(\text{AUC}_T)_{\text{test}}/D_{\text{test}}}{(\text{AUC}_T)_{\text{standard}}/D_{\text{standard}}}$$

where D_{test} and D_{standard} are the sizes of the single doses of the test and standard dosage forms administered, respectively.

Relative bioavailability, like absolute bioavailability may be expressed as a fraction or as a percentage.

Urinary excretion data may also be used to measure relative bioavailability. The relative bioavailability of a given drug following administration of equivalent doses of the test and standard dosage forms is given by

$$\text{relative bioavailability} = \frac{(X_U^\infty)_{\text{test}}}{(X_U^\infty)_{\text{standard}}}$$

where $(X_U^\infty)_{\text{test}}$ and $(X_U^\infty)_{\text{standard}}$ are the total cumulative amounts of unchanged drug ultimately excreted in the urine following administration of single doses of the test dosage form and standard dosage form, respectively.

If different doses of the test and standard dosage forms are administered on separate occasions, the total amounts of unchanged drug ultimately excreted in the urine per unit dose of drug must be used in the above equation.

It should be noted that measurements of relative and absolute bioavailability based on urinary excretion data may also be made in terms of either the total amounts of principal drug metabolite or of unchanged drug plus its metabolites ultimately excreted in the urine. However, the assessment of relative and absolute bioavailability in terms of urinary excretion data is based on the assumption that the the total amount of unchanged drug (and/or its metabolites) ultimately excreted in the urine is a reflection of the total amount of intact drug which enters the systemic circulation (refer back to the earlier section in this chapter on cumulative urinary excretion curves).

Relative bioavailability measurements are often used to determine the effects of dosage form differences on the systemic bioavailability of a given drug. Numerous factors associated with the dosage form in which a given drug is incorporated can influence the bioavailability of that drug. These factors include the type of dosage form (e.g. a tablet, a solution, a suspension, a hard gelatin capsule), differences in the formulation of a particular type of dosage form and manufacturing variables employed in the production of a particular type of dosage form. A more detailed account of the influence of these factors on the bioavailabilities of drugs from dosage forms is given in Chapter 9.

Bioequivalence

An extension of the concept of relative bioavailability, which essentially involves comparing the total amounts of a particular drug that are absorbed intact into the systemic circulation from a test and a recognized standard dosage form, is that of determining whether the test and standard dosage forms containing equal doses of the same drug are equivalent or not in terms of their rates and extents of drug absorption (i.e. systemic availabilities). This application of the concept of bioavailability is called *bioequivalence*.

Two or more chemically equivalent products

(i.e. products containing equal doses of the same therapeutically active ingredient(s) in identical types of dosage form, which meet all the existing physicochemical standards in official compendia) are said to be bioequivalent if they do not differ significantly in their bioavailability characteristics when administered in the same dose under similar experimental conditions. Hence in those cases where bioavailability is assessed in terms of plasma concentration–time curves, two or more chemically equivalent drug products may be considered bioequivalent if there is no significant difference between *any* of the following parameters: peak height concentrations, times of peak height concentration and areas under the plasma concentration–time curves. In those cases where the bioavailabilities of two or more chemically equivalent drug products have been measured in terms of cumulative urinary excretion curves, neither their rates of urinary excretion nor the total amounts of drug ultimately excreted in the urine must differ significantly for the drug products to be classified as being bioequivalent.

In conducting a bioequivalence study, it is usual that one of the chemically equivalent drug products under test is a clinically proven, therapeutically effective product which serves as a standard against which the other 'test' products may be compared with respect to their bioavailabilities. If a test product and this standard product are found to be bioequivalent then it is reasonable to expect that the test product will also be therapeutically effective, i.e. the test and the reference products are therapeutically equivalent. Hence bioequivalence studies are important in determining whether chemically equivalent drug products manufactured by different companies are therapeutically equivalent, i.e. produce identical therapeutic responses in patients.

If two chemically equivalent drug products were absolutely bioequivalent, their plasma concentration–time and/or cumulative urinary excretion curves would be superimposable. In such a case there would be no problem in concluding that these products were bioequivalent. Nor would there be a problem in concluding bioinequivalence if the parameters associated with the plasma concentration–time and/or cumulative urinary excretion curves for the test differed

from the standard product by, for instance, 50%. However, a problem arises in deciding whether the test and standard drug products are bioequivalent when such products show relatively small differences in their plasma concentration–time curves and/or cumulative urinary excretion curves. The problem is how much of a difference can be allowed between two chemically equivalent drug products and still permit them to be considered bioequivalent. Should this permitted difference be 10, 20, 30% or more? The magnitude of the difference that could be permitted will depend on the significance that such a difference has on the safety and therapeutic efficacy of the particular drug present in the test and standard drug products. This will depend on such factors as the toxicity, the therapeutic range and the therapeutic use of the drug. In the case of a drug that has a wide therapeutic range and toxic effects only occur at relatively high plasma concentrations of the drug, chemically equivalent products giving quite different plasma concentration–time curves (see Fig. 10.7) may still be considered satisfactory from a therapeutic point of view even though they are not bioequivalent.

Thus in the case of the hypothetical example shown in Fig. 10.7, providing that the observed difference in the rates of absorption (as assessed by the times of peak plasma concentration) and hence in the times of onset for formulations X and Y is not considered to be therapeutically significant, then formulations X and Y may be both considered to be therapeutically satisfactory. However, if the drug in question was a hypnotic drug, in which case the time of onset for the therapeutic response is important, then the observed difference in the rates of absorption would become more important. If the times of peak plasma concentration for formulations X and Y were 0.5 hour and 1.0 hour, respectively, it is likely that both formulations would still be deemed to be therapeutically satisfactory despite a 100% difference in their times of peak plasma concentration. However, if the times of peak plasma concentration for formulations X and Y were 2 and 4 hours, respectively, these formulations may no longer be regarded as being therapeutically equivalent even though the percentage difference in their times of peak plasma concentration is the

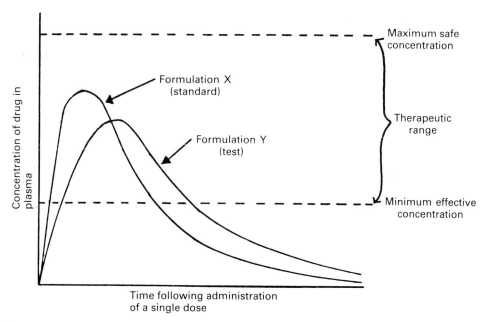

Fig. 10.7 Plasma concentration–time curves for two chemically equivalent drug products administered in equal single doses by the same extravascular route

same. Hence one can appreciate the problems in trying to quote a universally acceptable percentage difference that can be tolerated before two chemically equivalent drug products are regarded as being bioinequivalent and/or therapeutically inequivalent. In the case of chemically equivalent drug products containing a drug which exhibits a narrow range between its minimum effective plasma concentration and maximum safe plasma concentration (e.g. digoxin), the concept of bioequivalence is of fundamental importance since, in such cases, small differences in the plasma concentration–time curves of chemically equivalent drug products may result in patients being overmedicated (i.e. exhibiting toxic responses) or undermedicated (i.e. experiencing therapeutic failure). These two therapeutically unsatisfactory conditions are illustrated in Figs. 10.8(a) and 10.8(b), respectively.

Despite the problems of putting a value on the magnitude of the difference that can be tolerated before two chemically equivalent drug products are deemed to be bioinequivalent, a value of 20% for the tolerated difference has been suggested as a possible general 'rule of thumb' for determining bioequivalence. Thus if all the major parameters in either the plasma concentration–time or cumu-

lative urinary excretion curves for two or more chemically equivalent drug products differ from each other by less than 20%, then these products would be judged to be bioequivalent. However, if any one or more of these parameters differed by more than 20% then there may be a problem with the bioequivalence of the test product(s) with respect to the standard product.

A further crucial factor in determining bioequivalence or in determining the influence of the type of dosage form, the route of administration, etc., on the bioavailability exhibited by a given drug, is the proper design, control and interpretation of such studies.

CRITERIA FOR VALID *IN VIVO* BIOAVAILABILITY TESTING

The criteria for valid bioavailability testing may be illustrated by the design, control and interpretation of a study to compare the plasma concentration–time curves resulting from the peroral administration of single doses of two chemically equivalent drug products to selected human subjects. This type of comparative bioavailability study should be designed so as to reduce as many

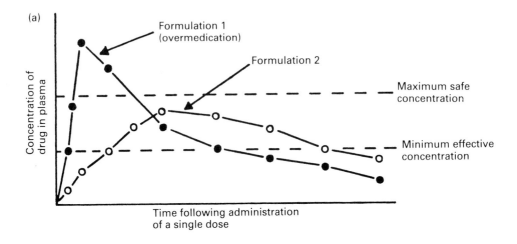

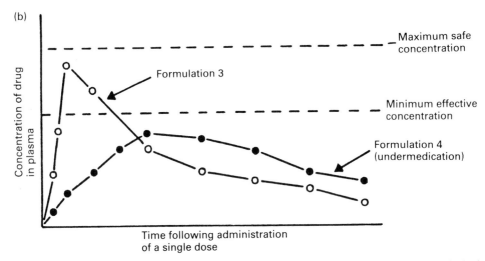

Fig. 10.8 Plasma concentration–time curves for chemically equivalent drug products administered in equal single doses by the same extravascular route showing potential consequences of bioinequivalence for a drug having a narrow therapeutic range, i.e. overmedication (a), undermedication (b). (After Chodos and Di Santo, 1973)

possible sources of variation which are not directly related to the drug products under test. Ideally the only potential source of variation in a bioequivalence study should be actual differences in the drug products. The conditions under which the study is performed, including the human subjects themselves, should be standardized as far as possible.

Subject to subject variation

When different individuals are given equal doses or even equal doses per kilogram of body weight of the same drug product, large variations in the corresponding plasma concentration–time curves

are often observed. This subject to subject variation in plasma drug levels must be minimized in a bioavailability study designed to determine the bioequivalence of two drug products. Proper selection of a group of subjects for such a study will assist in reducing subject to subject variation. Since factors such as disease, body weight, the ratio of fat:lean body tissues, age and sex can influence the plasma drug levels, the selected group of individuals should all be in a similar (usually normal) state of health and their ages, body weights and body build types should be within acceptable limits. A typical set of criteria for selecting individuals for a bioequivalence study could be that all are normal healthy male or female volunteers, between 20 and 50 years old, between 54 and 91 kilograms body weight and of normal body build. The number of males and females used in the study should be specified since sex factors may be quite influential in bioavailability studies involving drugs such as hormonal agents and steroids (Hem and Stoll, 1979). It is interesting to note that patients who would normally be treated with the drug under test are *not* usually preferred to normal healthy subjects unless the disease processes or other clinical variables alter the absorption, distribution and elimination of the drug such that bioavailability studies in normal healthy subjects are meaningless (Barr, 1972). According to Hem and Stoll (1979) some of the problems of carrying out bioavailability studies in patients suffering with a given disease are as follows.

1 Different patients are likely to show different severities of the given disease.
2 Different patients are unlikely to be at the same stage in the time course of the disease.
3 Patients may be already under treatment with a drug which is different to that to be tested. It is well known that drug interaction can influence blood level data obtained for drugs (Gibaldi, 1984).
4 There are ethical problems associated with using sick patients in order to evaluate test formulations of drug products which may not be therapeutically efficacous.

It is evident, particularly from points 1–3, that the use of patients suffering from a given disease in preference to normal healthy subjects would introduce a greater source of intersubject variation in a bioequivalence study.

No matter how much the designer of a comparative bioavailability study attempts to match individuals in terms of health, weight, age,

etc., considerable intersubject variation in plasma drug levels will still occur due to intersubject differences in gastrointestinal physiology and in the rates of distribution, excretion and metabolism of drugs. However, subject to subject variation in plasma drug levels may be kept to a minimum by ensuring that each individual in a bioequivalence study receives each drug product being tested once over a period of time. This permits each individual to act as his or her own control.

Crossover studies

A comparative bioavailability study which is designed on this basis is called a *complete crossover study*. A widely used type of complete crossover study is one in which each individual receives each drug product once in a sequence based on a latin square. A comparison of two chemically equivalent drug products, denoted A and B, according to a latin square complete crossover design is shown in Table 10.1. The 20 normal healthy volunteers selected for this bioequivalence study are randomly assigned into two equal size groups in order to ensure that uniformity exists between the two groups with respect to age, body weight, sex, etc. The first group (subjects 1–10) are given a specific dose of product A and the second group (subjects 11–20) are given the equivalent dose of product B. In a bioequivalence study, one of the products would be a recognized standard product of proven clinical efficacy. An appropriate number of blood samples are taken from each individual at predetermined time intervals over a suitable period of time (see later in this chapter). The initial period of dosing and sampling is called the *first stage* of the crossover study. Following this first stage, a period of time is allowed to elapse before each subject receives a single dose of the second product. This period, which is called the washout period, is of sufficient duration to permit

Table 10.1 Latin square complete crossover design used in a comparative bioavailability study of two chemically equivalent drug products. A and B (after Hem and Stoll, 1979)

| Subject group number | Patient number | Treatment in each stage of study | |
		Stage I	Stage II
1	1, 2, 3, 4, 5, 6, 7, 8, 9, 10	product A	product B
2	11, 12, 13, 14, 15, 16, 17, 18, 19, 20	product B	product A

complete elimination of the drug and its metabolites from the body of each subject. The normal duration of this period is at least 10 half-lives* of the particular drug being studied. Over such a period, at least 99.9% of the administered dose of the drug will be eliminated from the body of each subject. Thus the washout period ensures that there is minimal carryover of drug (or its metabolities from the first stage into the next stage of the crossover study. The actual duration of the washout period will vary depending on the value of the half-life of the drug under study.

Following the washout period, the *second stage* of the crossover study is initiated. The first group of subjects (1–10) now receive product B and the second group (subjects 11–20) receive product A. Thus all 20 subjects have now received each product in a crossover design. Blood samples should be removed from each subject at exactly the same predetermined times employed in the first stage of the study.

The total number of subjects selected for a latin square complete crossover bioequivalence study will depend on the variability observed both between subjects and in the method used to assay the drug in the blood. The more variability observed in these parameters, the larger will be the number of subjects required. A minimum of 10–20 subjects is desirable for studies involving two to four drug products under test (Hem and Stoll, 1979).

Further details regarding the design of latin square complete crossover studies to compare three and more drug products and also of alternative designs (e.g. randomized block and incomplete block designs) may be obtained by reference to Westlake (1973) and Hem and Stoll (1979).

Study conditions

It is essential that the conditions under which the drug products are tested in each group of subjects are kept identical before and during each stage of

the crossover study. For instance, the period of time before the commencement of the first stage of the crossover study during which no medicine may be taken by each subject should be stipulated. The period of fasting of each subject prior to and after administration of each drug product under test, the types of food and drink (if any) and the degree of physical activity permitted during the period for which blood samples are taken should be rigorously controlled. Such control of the study conditions is necessary since each of the above factors can potentially influence the plasma levels of drug obtained following oral administration of each drug product under test.

Frequency and duration of removing blood samples

The frequency of removing blood samples from the subjects and the period of time over which the variation of the concentration of drug in the plasma is followed, must be adequate to construct a representative plasma concentration–time curve for each drug product under test. Thus the frequency and duration of sampling should be such as to define the absorption phase, the peak concentration and the elimination phase of the plasma concentration–time curve for each drug product. According to Hem and Stoll (1979), at least two or three experimental points (excluding the zero time point) are required in each of the absorption and elimination phases and sampling should continue over a period of time corresponding to three to five half-lives of the drug under study. Thus sampling should continue until 87.5–96.9% of the administered dose of the drug has been eliminated or until the plasma drug levels fall to 5–10% of the peak concentration. It is also important to ensure that blood samples are removed from each subject at the same predetermined intervals of time of each product under test. This permits a proper statistical analysis (e.g. an analysis of variance) to be performed on the plasma levels of drug obtained for each product under test at each sampling time interval. Many designers of comparative bioavailability studies prefer that the administration of doses to and the subsequent blood sampling of the groups of subjects should not be carried out in a sequential

---

* The biological half-life of a particular drug, t, is a parameter used to quantify the persistence of that drug in the body. The half-life of a drug, based on blood level data, is defined as the time required for the body to eliminate one-half (50%) of the drug which it contained (Notari, 1980).

Table 10.2 Comparison of sequential and randomly assigned sequences of drug administration and blood sampling in a latin square complete crossover designed bioavailability study of two chemically equivalent drug products, A and B

Subject group number	Patient number	Treatment in each stage of study Stage I	Stage II	Order of dosing and blood sampling in each stage of study Sequential sequence	Randomly assigned sequence
1	1			1st	3rd
	2			2nd	20th
	3			3rd	8th
	4	product A	product B	4th	6th
	5			5th	11th
	6			6th	18th
	7			7th	16th
	8			8th	15th
	9			9th	12th
	10			10th	2nd
2	11			11th	5th
	12			12th	17th
	13			13th	4th
	14			14th	7th
	15			15th	9th
	16	product B	product A	16th	13th
	17			17th	10th
	18			18th	19th
	19			19th	14th
	20			20th	1st

sequence but according to a randomly assigned sequence. Table 10.2 shows that a *sequential sequence* of dose administration and blood sampling of two groups of subjects introduces a bias into the study since the first group of subjects are always dosed and sampled before the second group of subjects. However, the administration of doses and removal of blood samples from the two groups according to a *randomly assigned sequence* (see Table 10.2) removes this bias from the bioavailability study.

Assay procedure

All blood samples removed from each subject should be treated and stored under identical conditions and assayed by the same method. It is possible that if a given blood sample was divided into two aliquots and each assayed for drug content by two completely different methods (e.g. h.p.l.c. and radioimmunoassay) two different results would be obtained. This discrepancy is usually caused by differences in the specificity and

sensitivity of each assay method towards a given drug. Consequently different plasma concentration–time curves for two chemically equivalent drug products could be obtained if all the blood samples corresponding to one drug product were assayed by one method and all samples corresponding to the other product were assayed by another method irrespective of whether the drug products were bioequivalent or not.

Statistical analysis of plasma drug level data

The plasma drug level data should be analysed statistically in order to establish whether any differences between the plasma concentration–time curves for each drug product under test are simply due to biological and/or experimental variation or are due to actual bioavailability differences in the drug products. For details of the statistical treatment and the presentation of plasma drug level data obtained in a comparative bioavailability study, the reader is referred to articles by Westlake (1973) and Hem and Stoll (1979).

REFERENCES

Barr, W. H. (1972) The use of physical and animal models to assess bioavailability. *Pharmacology*, 8, 55–101.

Chodos, D. J. and DiSanto, A. R. (1973) *Basis of Bioavailability*, The Upjohn Company, Kalamazoo, Michigan.

Gibaldi, M. (1984) *Biopharmaceutics and Clinical Pharmacokinetics*, 3rd edn, Lea and Febiger, Philadelphia.

Hem, S. L. and Stoll, R. G. (1979) Appraisal of drug product quality and performance. In: *Modern Pharmaceutics*. (Eds G. S. Banker and C. T. Rhodes), pp. 649–710, Marcel Dekker Inc., New York.

Notari, R. E. (1980) *Biopharmaceutics and Clinical Pharmacokinetics. An Introduction*, 3rd edn, p. 52, Marcel Dekker Inc., New York.

Westlake, W. J. (1973) The design and analysis of comparative blood level trials. In: *Current Concepts in the Pharmaceuticals Sciences. Dosage Form Design and Bioavailability* (Ed. J. Swarbrick), pp. 149–179, Lea and Febiger, Philadelphia.

BIBLIOGRAPHY

American Pharmaceutical Association (1978) *The Bioavailability of Drug Products*, American Pharmaceutical Association, Washington.

Chodos, D. J. and DiSanto, A. R. (1973) *Basis of Bioavailability*, The Upjohn Company, Kalamazoo, Michigan.

Gibaldi, M. and Perrier, D. (1975) *Drugs and the Pharmaceutical Sciences. Volume 1. Pharmacokinetics* (Ed. J. Swarbrick), Marcel Dekker Inc., New York.

Shargel, L. and Yu, A. B. C. (1980) *Applied Biopharmaceutics and Pharmacokinetics*, Appleton-Century-Crofts, New York.

Dosage regimens: their influence on the concentration–time profile of a drug in the body

The influence that

1 physiological factors,
2 the physicochemical properties of a drug, and
3 dosage form factors

can have in determining whether a therapeutically effective concentration of a drug is achieved in the plasma (and hence at the site(s) of action of the drug) following peroral administration of a *single* dose of drug has been discussed previously in Chapters 8 and 9. Some drugs such as hypnotics, analgesics and antiemetics may provide effective treatment following the administration of a single dose. However, the duration of most illnesses is longer than the therapeutic effect produced by the administration of a single dose of a drug in a conventional dosage form, i.e. a dosage form which is formulated to give rapid and complete drug release. In such cases, doses of the drug are usually administered on a repetitive basis over a period of time determined by the nature of the illness. For instance, one 250 mg ampicillin capsule may be administered every 6 hours for a period of 5 days to treat a bacterial infection. Such a dosing regimen, in which the total dose of drug (i.e., 5 g) administered over 5 days is given in the form of multiple doses (i.e., 250 mg) at given intervals of time (i.e. every 6 hours) is known as a *multiple dosage regimen*. The proper selection of both the dose size and the frequency of administration are important factors which influence whether a satisfactory therapeutic plasma concentration is achieved and maintained over the prescribed course of drug treatment. Thus the design of a multiple dosage regimen is crucial to successful drug therapy.

ONE-COMPARTMENT OPEN MODEL OF DRUG DISPOSITION IN THE BODY

In order to understand how the design of a dosage regimen can influence the time course of a drug in the body, as measured by its plasma concentration–time curve, let us consider that the complex kinetic processes of drug input, output and distribution in the body may be represented by the pharmacokinetic model of drug disposition, the one-compartment open model, shown in Fig. 11.1.

In the case of a one-compartment open model, the drug is considered to be distributed instantly throughout the whole body following its release and absorption from the dosage form. Thus the body behaves as a single compartment in which absorbed drug is distributed so rapidly that a concentration equilibrium exists at any given time between the plasma, other body fluids and the tissues into which the drug has become distributed.

To assume that the body behaves as a one-compartment open model does not necessarily mean that the drug concentrations in all body tissues at any given time are equal. However, the model does assume that any changes which occur in the plasma reflect quantitatively changes occurring in the concentration of drug at the site(s) of action.

Rate of drug input versus rate of drug output

In a one-compartment open model, the overall kinetic processes of drug input and drug output are described by first order kinetics. In the case of a perorally administered dosage form, the process of drug input into the body compartment involves drug release from the dosage form and passage of drug across the cellular membranes constituting the gastrointestinal barrier. The rate of drug input or absorption represents the net result of all these processes. The rate of drug input (absorption) at any given time is proportional to the concentration of drug, which is in an absorbable form, in solution in the gastrointestinal fluids at the site(s) of absorption, i.e. the effective concentration, C_e, of drug at time, t. Hence,

$$\text{rate of drug input at time } t \propto C_e \qquad (11.1)$$

and

$$\text{rate of drug input at time } t = -k_a C_e \qquad (11.2)$$

where k_a is the apparent absorption rate constant.

The negative sign in Eqn 11.2 indicates that the effective concentration of drug at the absorption site(s) decreases with time. The apparent absorption rate constant gives the proportion (or fraction) of drug which enters the body compartment per unit time. Its units are time^{-1}, e.g. hours^{-1}. Unlike the rate of drug input into the body compartment, the apparent absorption rate constant, k_a, is independent of the effective concentration of drug at the absorption site(s). Since the rate of drug input is proportional to the effective drug concentration, the rate of drug input will be maximal following administration of a dose of drug contained in a peroral dosage form which gives rapid and complete drug release. The rate of drug input will decrease gradually with time as a consequence of the effective drug concentration at the absorption site(s) decreasing progressively with time, chiefly as a result of absorption into the body compartment. Other processes, such as chemical degradation and movement of drug away from the absorption site(s) will also contribute to the gradual decrease in the effective drug concentration with time.

In the case of a one-compartment open model, the rate of drug output or elimination is a first order process. Consequently, the magnitude of this parameter at any given time is dependent on the concentration of drug in the body compart-

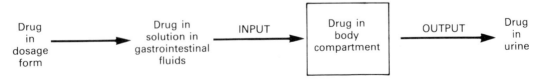

Fig. 11.1 One-compartment open model of drug disposition for a perorally administered drug

ment at that time. Immediately following administration of the first dose of a peroral dosage form, the rate of drug output from the body will be low since little of the drug will have been absorbed into the body compartment. However, as absorption proceeds, initially at a higher rate than the rate of drug output, the net concentration of drug in the body will increase with time. Likewise the rate of drug output from the body compartment will also increase with time. Since the rate of drug output is increasing with time whilst the rate of drug input into the body compartment is decreasing with time, the situation is eventually reached when the rate of drug output just exceeds the rate of drug input. Consequently, the net concentration of drug in the body compartment will reach a peak value and then begin to fall with time. The ensuing decreases in the net concentration of drug in the body will also cause the rate of drug output to decrease with time. These changes in the rates of drug input and output,

relative to each other, with time are responsible for the characteristic shape of the concentration time course of a drug in the body shown in Fig. 11.2 following peroral administration of a single dose of drug.

It is evident from the preceding discussion and Fig. 11.2, that the greater the rate of drug input relative to the rate of drug output from the body compartment over the net absorption phase, the higher will be the peak concentration achieved in the body or plasma following peroral administration of a single dose of drug. This explains why increases in dose size and formulation changes in dosage forms which produce increases in the effective concentration of drug at the absorption site(s), result in higher peak plasma and body concentrations being obtained for a given drug. It should also be noted that any unexpected decrease in the rate of drug output relative to the rate of drug input, which may occur as the result of renal impairment, is also likely to result in higher

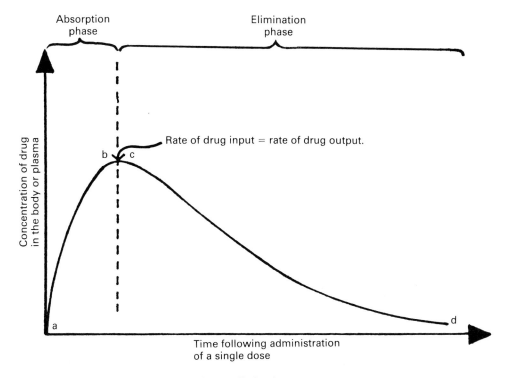

a−b rate of drug absorption > rate of drug elimination
c−d rate of drug elimination > rate of drug absorption

Fig. 11.2 Concentration–time course of a drug in the body following peroral administration of a single dose of drug which confers one-compartment open model characteristics on the body

plasma and body concentrations of drug than expected and the possibility of the patient exhibiting undesirable side effects of the drug. The adjustment of dosage regimens in cases of patients having severe renal impairment is considered later in this chapter.

For a more detailed mathematical account of the kinetics of drug input and output in a one-compartment open model and for details of other pharmacokinetic models of drug disposition in the body, the reader is referred to the bibliography at the end of this chapter.

The elimination rate constant and biological half-life of a drug

In the case of a one-compartment open model, the rate of elimination or output of a drug from the body compartment follows first order kinetics and is related to the concentration of drug, C_t, remaining in the body compartment at time t, by the following equation:

$$\text{rate of elimination at time } t = -k_e\, C_t \qquad (11.3)$$

where k_e is the apparent elimination rate constant. The negative sign in Eqn 11.3 indicates that elimination is removing drug from the body compartment.

The apparent elimination rate constant of a drug gives the proportion or fraction of that drug which is eliminated from the body per unit time. Its units are in terms of time^{-1}, e.g. hours^{-1}. The apparent elimination constant of a given drug thus provides a quantitative index of the persistence of that drug in the body. An alternative parameter used is the biological or elimination half-life of the drug, $t_{\frac{1}{2}}$. The biological half-life of a given drug is the time required for the body to eliminate 50% of the drug which it contained. Thus, the larger the biological half-life exhibited by a drug, the slower will be its elimination from the body or plasma. For a drug whose elimination follows first order kinetics, the value of its biological half-life is independent of the concentration of drug remaining in the body or plasma. Hence, if a single dose of a drug having a biological half-life of 4 hours was administered perorally, then after the peak plasma concentration had been reached, the plasma concentration of drug would fall by

50% every 4 hours until all the drug had been eliminated or a further dose was administered. The relationship between the numbers of half-lives elapsed and the percentage of drug eliminated from the body following administration of a single dose is given in Table 11.1. An appreciation of the relationship between the percentage of drug eliminated from the body and the number of biological half-lifes elapsed is useful when considering how much drug is eliminated from the body over the time interval between successive doses in a multiple dosage regimen.

Table 11.1

Number of half-lives elapsed	Percentage of drug eliminated
0.5	29.3
1.0	50.0
2.0	75.0
3.0	87.5
3.3	90.0
4.0	94.0
4.3	95.0
5.0	97.0
6.0	98.4
6.6	99.0
7.0	99.2

The biological half-life of a drug varies from drug to drug and, for a given drug, varies from patient to patient. Some biological half-lifes for various drugs are given in Table 11.2. For a drug whose elimination follows first order kinetics (see Chapter 7), the biological half-life of the drug, $t_{\frac{1}{2}}$, is related to the apparent elimination rate constant, k_e, of that drug according to the following equation

$$t_{\frac{1}{2}} = \frac{0.693}{k_e} \qquad (11.4)$$

This equation indicates that the biological half-life of a drug will be influenced by any factor which influences the apparent elimination rate constant of the drug. This explains why factors such as genetic differences between individuals, age and

Table 11.2

Drug	Biological half-life (hours)
Phenobarbitone	50 to 120
Digoxin	36 to 51
Theophylline	3 to 8

disease can affect the biological half-life exhibited by a given drug. The biological half-life of a drug is an important factor which influences the plasma concentration–time curve obtained following peroral administration of a multiple dosage regimen.

Concentration–time curve of a drug in the body following the peroral administration of equal doses of a drug at fixed intervals of time

In discussing how the design of a multiple peroral dosage regimen can influence the concentration-time course of a drug in the body, the following assumptions have been made.

1 The drug confers upon the body the characteristics of a one-compartment open model.
2 The values of the apparent absorption rate and apparent elimination rate constants for a given drug do not change during the period for which the dosage regimen is administered to a patient.
3 The fraction of each administered dose which is absorbed by the body compartment remains constant for a given drug.
4 The aim of drug therapy is to achieve promptly

and maintain a concentration of drug at the appropriate site(s) of action which is both clinically efficacious and safe for the desired duration of drug treatment. This is assumed to be achieved by the prompt attainment and maintenance of plasma concentrations of drug which lie within the therapeutic range of the drug.

If the time interval between each perorally administered dose is longer than the time required for complete elimination of the previous dose, then the plasma concentration time profile of a drug will exhibit a series of isolated single dose profiles as shown in Fig. 11.3.

Consideration of the plasma concentration–time profile shown in Fig. 11.3 in relation to the minimum effective and maximum safe plasma concentrations for the drug reveals that the design of this particular dosage regimen is unsatisfactory. The plasma concentration only lies within the therapeutic range of the drug for a relatively short period of time following the administration of each dose and the patient remains undermedicated for relatively long periods of time. If the dosing time

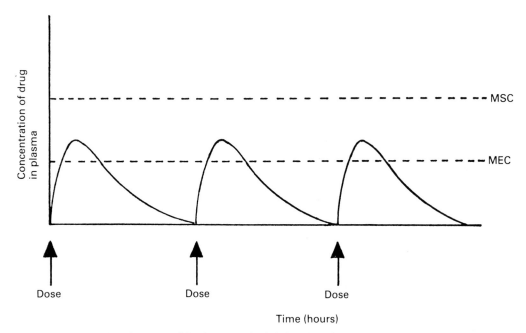

Fig. 11.3 Plasma concentration–time curve following peroral administration of equal doses of a drug at time intervals which allow complete elimination of the previous dose. (MSC is the maximum safe plasma concentration of the drug. MEC is the minimum effective plasma concentration of the drug. These terms are defined in Chapter 10.)

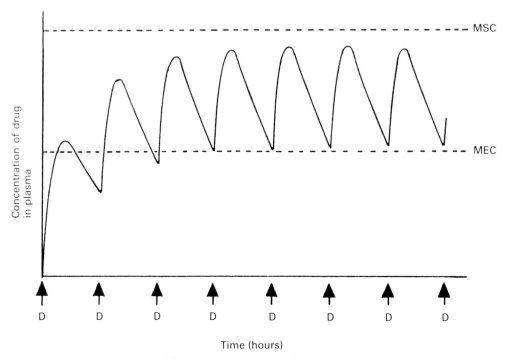

Fig. 11.4 Plasma concentration–time curve following peroral administration of equal doses, D, of a drug every 4 hours. (MSC is the maximum safe plasma concentration of the drug. MEC is the minimum effective plasma concentration of the drug)

interval is reduced such that it is now shorter than the time required for complete elimination of the previous dose, then the resulting plasma concentration–time curve exhibits the characteristic profile shown in Fig. 11.4.

Figure 11.4 shows that at the start of this multiple dosage regimen, the maximum and minimum plasma concentrations of drug observed during each dosing time interval tend to increase with successive doses. This is a consequence of the time interval between successive doses being less than that required for complete elimination of the previous absorbed dose. Consequently the total amount of the drug remaining in the body compartment at any time after a dose is equal to the sum of that remaining from the current dose and that remaining from all the previous doses. This accumulation of drug in the body and plasma with successively administered doses does not continue indefinitely. Providing drug elimination follows first order kinetics, the rate of drug elimination will increase as the average concentration of drug in the body (and plasma) rises. If the amount of drug supplied to the body compartment

per unit dosing time interval remains constant, then a situation is eventually reached when the overall rate of elimination of drug from the body over the dosing time interval becomes equal to the overall rate at which drug is being supplied to the body compartment over the dosing time interval. The overall rate of elimination has effectively caught up with the overall rate of supply of drug to the body compartment over each dosing time interval. When the overall rate of drug supply equals the overall rate of drug output from the body compartment, a *steady state* is reached with respect to the average concentration of drug remaining in the body over each dosing time interval. At steady state, the amount of drug eliminated from the body over each dosing time interval is equal to the amount of drug which was absorbed into the body compartment following administration of the previous dose. Figure 11.5 shows that the amount of drug in the body, as measured by the plasma concentration of drug, fluctuates between maximum and minimum values which remain more or less constant from dose to dose. At steady state the average concentration of

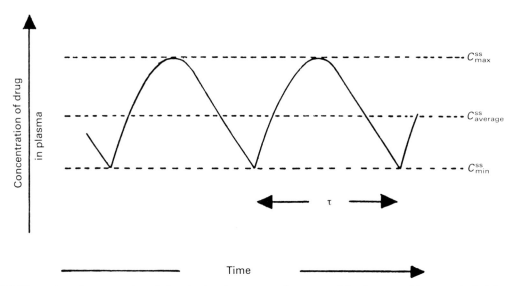

Fig. 11.5 Fluctuation of concentration of drug in the plasma at steady state resulting from repetitive peroral administration of equal doses, D, of drug at a fixed interval of time, τ. C_{max}^{ss}, C_{min}^{ss} and $C_{average}^{ss}$ represent the maximum, minimum and average plasma concentrations of drug, respectively, achieved at steady state.

drug in the plasma, $C_{average}^{ss}$, over successive dosing time intervals remains constant.

For a drug administered repetitively in equal doses and at equal time intervals, the time required for the average plasma concentration to attain the corresponding steady state value is a function only of the biological half-life of the drug and is independent of both the size of the dose administered and the length of the dosing time interval. The time required for the average plasma concentration to reach 95% of the steady state value corresponding to the particular multiple dosage regimen is 4.3 times the biological half-life of the drug. The corresponding figure for 99% is 6.6 times. Therefore, depending on the magnitude of the biological half-life of the drug being administered, the time taken to attain the average steady state plasma concentration may range from a few hours to several days. From a clinical viewpoint, the time required to reach steady state is important since for a properly designed multiple dosage regimen, the attainment of steady state corresponds to the achievement and maintenance of maximal clinical effectiveness of the drug in the patient.

It should be noted that for a drug, such as phenytoin, whose elimination is not described by first order kinetics, the peroral administration of equal doses at fixed intervals of time may not result in the attainment of steady state plasma levels of the drug. If the concentration of such a drug in the body rises sufficiently following repetitive administration, the pathway responsible for its elimination may become saturated with the drug. If this occurs the rate of elimination would become maximal and could not increase to cope with any further rises in the average concentration of drug in the body. Hence the overall rate of elimination would not become equal to the overall rate of supply of drug to the body over each dosing time interval and the condition necessary for the attainment of steady state would not be achieved. If repetitive administration of the drug continued at the same rate, the average concentration of drug in the body and plasma would tend to continue to accumulate rather than reach a plateau.

IMPORTANT FACTORS INFLUENCING STEADY-STATE PLASMA CONCENTRATIONS OF DRUG

Dose size and frequency of administration

In designing a multiple dosage regimen which balances patient convenience with achievement and maintenance of maximal clinical effectiveness, only two parameters can be adjusted for a given drug: the size of dose and the frequency of administration. Let us consider how the maximum, minimum and average steady state plasma concentrations of drug are influenced by these parameters.

Size of dose

Figure 11.6 illustrates the effects of changing the dose size on the level of drug in the plasma accompanying repetitive administration of peroral doses at equal intervals of time. As the size of the administered dose is increased, the higher are the corresponding maximum, minimum and average plasma drug levels, C_{max}^{ss}, C_{min}^{ss} and $C_{average}^{ss}$ respectively, achieved at steady state. What may not be so well appreciated is that the larger the size of dose administered, the larger is the fluctuation between C_{max}^{ss} and C_{min}^{ss} during each dosing time interval. Large fluctuations between C_{max}^{ss} and C_{min}^{ss} can be hazardous, particularly with a drug such as digoxin which has a narrow therapeutic range. In the case of such a drug, it is possible that C_{max}^{ss} could exceed the maximum safe plasma concentration of the drug. Figure 11.6 also illustrates

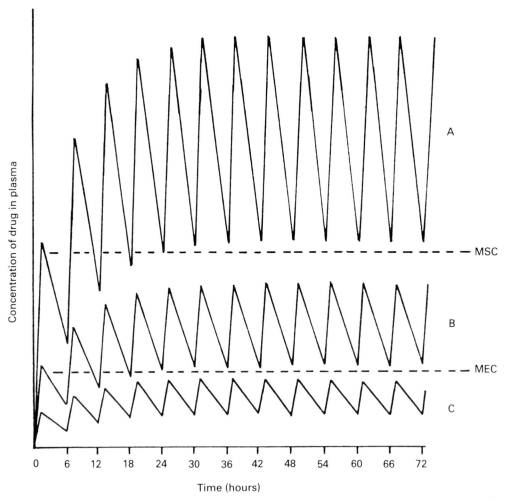

Fig. 11.6 Diagrammatic representation of the effect of dose size on the plasma concentration–time curve obtained following peroral administration of equal doses of a given drug at fixed intervals of time equal to the biological half-life of the drug. Curve A, dose = 250 mg. Curve B, dose = 100 mg. Curve C, dose = 40 mg

that the time required to attain steady state plasma levels of drug is independent of the size of the administered dose.

Interval of time between successive equal doses

Figure 11.7 illustrates the effects of constant doses administered at various dosing intervals which are multiples of the biological half-life of the drug, $t_{\frac{1}{2}}$. The uppermost plasma concentration–time curve in Fig. 11.7 shows that the repetitive administration of doses at a time interval which is less than the biological half-life of the drug results in higher steady state plasma drug concentrations being obtained. This is a consequence of the extent of elimination of the drug from the body over a dosing time interval equal to $0.5\ t_{\frac{1}{2}}$ being smaller than that which is eliminated when the

dosing time interval is equal to $t_{\frac{1}{2}}$. (see Table 11.1). Figure 11.7 also shows that repetitive administration of doses at time intervals greater than the biological half-life of the drug results in the lower steady state plasma drug concentrations being obtained. This is a consequence of a greater proportion of the drug being eliminated over a dosing time interval equal to $2t_{\frac{1}{2}}$ as compared to that which is eliminated when the dosing time interval is equal to $t_{\frac{1}{2}}$.

Summary of the effects of dose size and frequency of administration

Consideration of the effects of administered dose size and the dosage time interval on the levels of a given drug achieved in the body, as measured by the plasma concentration of drug, following

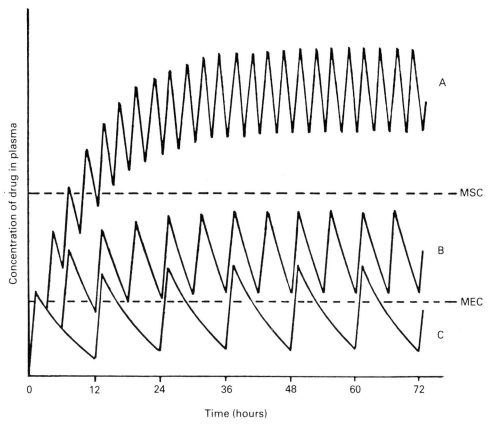

Fig. 11.7 Diagrammatic representation of the effect of changing the dosing time interval, τ, on the plasma concentration–time curve obtained following repetitive peroral administration of equal size doses of a given drug. Curve A, dosing time interval = 3 hours ($0.5\ t_{\frac{1}{2}}$). Curve B, dosing time interval = 6 hours ($t_{\frac{1}{2}}$). Curve C, dosing time interval = 12 hours ($2t_{\frac{1}{2}}$)

repetitive peroral administration of equal doses of the drug have revealed the following relationships.

1 The magnitude of the fluctuations between the maximum and minimum steady state levels of drug in the body is determined by the size of dose administered or, more accurately, by the amount of drug absorbed following each dose administered.

2 The magnitude of the fluctuations between the maximum and minimum steady state plasma concentrations of a drug are an important consideration for any drug which has a narrow therapeutic range, e.g. digoxin. The administration of smaller doses at more frequent intervals is a means of reducing the steady state fluctuations without altering the average steady state plasma concentration of the drug. For example, a 500 mg dose of drug given every 6 hours will provide the same $C^{ss}_{average}$ value as a 250 mg dose of the same drug given every 3 hours, whilst the C_{max} and C_{min} fluctuation for the latter dose will be decreased by one-half.

3 The average maximum and minimum levels of drug achieved in the body at steady state are influenced by either the dose size, the dosage time interval in relation to the biological half-life of the drug or both. The greater the dose size and the smaller the dosage time interval relative to the biological half-life of the drug, the greater are the average, maximum and minimum steady state levels of drug in the body.

4 For a given drug, the time taken to achieve steady state is independent of dose size and the dosage time interval.

5 If the maximum safe and minimum effective plasma concentrations are represented by the dashed lines shown in Fig. 11.6 and 11.7, respectively, then it is evident that the proper selection of dose size and dosage time interval are important with respect to achieving and maintaining steady state plasma levels which lie within the therapeutic range of the particular drug being administered.

It is evident from the preceding discussion that the proper selection of the dose size and the dosage time interval is crucial to ensure that a multiple dosage regimen provides steady state levels of drug in the body which are both clinically efficacious and safe. Mathematical relationships which predict the values of the various steady state parameters achieved in the body following repetitive administration of doses at constant intervals of time have been used to assist the design of clinically acceptable multiple dosage regimens. For example, a useful equation for predicting the average amount of drug achieved in the body at steady state, $D^{ss}_{average}$, following repetitive peroral administration of equal doses, D, at a fixed time interval, τ is given by:

$$D^{ss}_{average} = \frac{F \cdot D \cdot t_{\frac{1}{2}} \cdot 1.44}{\tau} \qquad (11.5)$$

where F is the fraction of drug absorbed following administration of a dose, D, of drug — thus $F \cdot D$ is the bioavailable dose of drug, and $t_{\frac{1}{2}}$ is the biological half-life of the drug. The average amount of a given drug in the body at steady state, $D^{ss}_{average}$, is related to the corresponding average plasma concentration of the drug by the factor known as the apparent volume of distribution of the drug, i.e.:

$$D^{ss}_{average} = V_d \, C^{ss}_{average} \qquad (11.6)$$

where V_d is the apparent volume of distribution of the drug and $C^{ss}_{average}$ is the average steady state plasma concentration of the drug. Eqn 11.5 can be rewritten in terms of the average steady state plasma concentration of the drug as follows:

$$C^{ss}_{average} = \frac{F \cdot D \cdot t_{\frac{1}{2}} \cdot 1.44}{\tau \cdot V_d} \qquad (11.7)$$

If the value of the average body amount or the average plasma concentration of a given drug at steady state which gives a satisfactory therapeutic response in a patient is known, then Eqn 11.5 or 11.7, respectively, can be used to estimate either the size of dose which should be administered repetitively at a preselected constant dosage time interval or the dosage time interval that a preselected dose should be administered repetitively. In order to illustrate a dosage regimen calculation, based on the average steady state plasma concentration of a drug, consider the following worked example.

An antibiotic is to be administered on a repetitive basis to a male patient weighing 76 kg. The antibiotic is commercially available in the form of tablets each containing 250 mg of the drug. The fraction of the drug which is absorbed following peroral administration of one 250 mg tablet is 0.9. The antibiotic has been found to exhibit a biological half-life of 3 hours and the patient has an apparent volume of distribution of 0.2 litre kg^{-1} of body weight. What dosage time interval should be selected to administer this drug on a repetitive basis in order that a therapeutic average steady state plasma concentration of 16 mg l^{-1} will be achieved?

Using Eqn 11.7,

$$C^{ss}_{average} = \frac{F \cdot D \cdot t_{\frac{1}{2}} \cdot 1.44}{\tau \cdot V_d}$$

where the average steady state plasma concentration of drug, $C^{ss}_{average} = 16$ mg l^{-1}, the fraction of each administered dose absorbed, $F = 0.9$, the side of administered dose, $D = 250$ mg, the biological half-life of the drug, $t_{\frac{1}{2}} = 3$ hours, the apparent volume of distribution, $V_d = 0.2$ litre kg^{-1} of patient's body weight.

Hence, for a patient weighing 76 kg, the value of·

$V_d = 0.2 \times 76$ litres

$= 15.2$ litres.

τ, the dosage time interval is to be calculated. Substituting the above values into Eqn 11.7 gives

$$16 = \frac{0.9 \times 250 \times 3 \times 1.44}{\tau \times 15.2}$$

$$\tau = \frac{0.9 \times 250 \times 3 \times 1.44}{16 \times 15.2}$$

$$= \frac{972.0}{243.2} \text{ hours}$$

$$= 4 \text{ hours}.$$

Thus one 250 mg tablet should be administered every 4 hours in order to achieve the required averaged average steady state plasma concentration.

Mathematical equations which predict the maximum or minimum steady state plasma concentrations of a drug achieved in the body followed by repetitive administration of equal doses at a fixed interval of time are also available for drugs whose time course in the body is described by the one-compartment open pharmacokinetic model. For information concerning dosage regimen calculations based on C^{ss}_{max} and C^{ss}_{min}, the reader is referred to the bibliography section at the end of this chapter.

The concept of 'loading doses'

As discussed earlier, the time required for a given drug to reach 95% of the average steady state plasma concentration is 4.3 biological half-lives, when equal doses of the drug are administered repetitively at equal intervals of time. Thus, for a drug with a long half-life of 24 hours it would take more than 4 days for the average drug concentration in the plasma to reach 95% of its steady state value. Since the attainment of steady state plasma concentrations is normally associated with the attainment of maximal clinical effectiveness of the drug, it is conceivable that a number of days could elapse before a patient experienced the full therapeutic benefit of a drug having a long half-life. To reduce the time required for onset of the full therapeutic effect of a drug, a large single dose of the drug may be administered initially in order to achieve a peak plasma concentration which lies within the therapeutic range of the drug and is approximately equal to the value of C^{ss}_{max} required. This initial dose is known as the 'loading dose' or 'priming dose'. Thereafter smaller, equal doses are administered repetitively at suitable fixed intervals of time in order to maintain the plasma concentrations of drug at maximum, minimum and average state levels which provide the patient with the full therapeutic benefit of the drug. These smaller, equal doses are known as 'maintenance doses'. As a general rule, the loading dose should be twice the size of the maintenance dose if the selected dosage time interval corresponds to the biological half-life of the drug. Figure 11.8 illustrates how rapidly therapeutic steady state plasma levels of drug are achieved when the dosage regimen consists of an initial loading dose followed by equal maintenance doses at fixed intervals of time in comparison to a 'simple' multiple dosage regimen consisting of doses that are equal in size and are administered at the same dosage time intervals as the maintenance doses. For details of methods of calculating

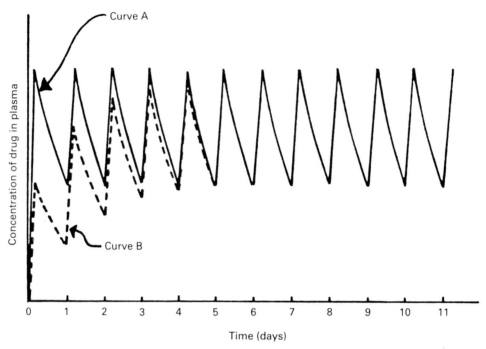

Fig. 11.8 Diagrammatic representation of how the initial administration of a loading dose following by equal maintenance doses at fixed intervals of time ensure rapid attainment of steady state plasma levels for a drug having a long biological half-line of 24 hours. Curve A represents the plasma concentration–time curve obtained following peroral administration of a loading dose of 500 mg followed by a maintenance dose of 250 mg every 24 hours. Curve B represents the plasma concentration–time curve obtained following peroral administration of a 250 mg dose every 24 hours

loading doses and maintenance dosage regimens, the reader is referred to the bibliography section at the end of this chapter.

Effect of changes in the apparent elimination rate constant of a drug: the problem of patients with renal impairment

Whilst the loading dose, maintenance dose and dosage time interval may be varied in order to design a clinically efficacious multiple dosage regimen, one factor cannot normally be adjusted. That factor is the apparent elimination rate constant exhibited by the particular drug being administered. However, the elimination rate constant of a given drug does vary from patient to patient and is influenced by whether the patient has normal or impaired renal function. Figure 11.9 indicates the effects produced by changes in the apparent elimination rate constant on the plasma concentration–time curve obtained following repetitive, peroral administration of equal doses of a given drug at equal intervals of time. Any reduc-

tion in the apparent elimination rate constant of a drug will produce a proportional increase in the biological half-life exhibited by that drug. This, in turn, will result in a greater degree of accumulation of the drug in the body following repetitive administration before steady state drug levels are achieved. The greater degree of drug accumulation is a consequence of a smaller proportion of the drug being eliminated from the body over each fixed dosage time interval when the biological half-life of the drug is increased. Patients who develop severe renal impairment normally exhibit smaller apparent elimination rate constants and consequently longer biological half-lives for drugs which are eliminated substantially by renal excretion than do patients with normal renal function. For instance, the average apparent elimination rate constant for digoxin may be reduced from 0.021 hour^{-1} in patients with normal renal function to 0.007 hour^{-1} in patients with severe renal impairement. Since the average steady state level of drug in the body is only achieved and maintained when the overall rate of drug supply

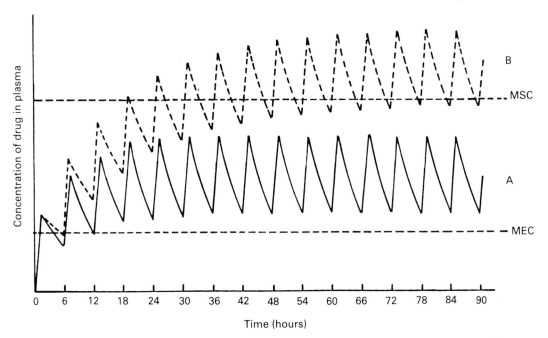

Fig. 11.9 Diagrammatic representation of the effect of changing the biological half-life of a given drug on the plasma concentration–time curve exhibited by the drug following peroral administration of one 250 mg dose every 6 hours. Curve A — biological half-life of drug = 6 hours. Curve B — biological half-life of drug = 12 hours

equals the overall rate of elimination of drug from the body over successive dosing time intervals, any reduction in the overall rate of elimination of a drug as a result of renal disease without a corresponding compensatory reduction in the overall rate of drug supply, will result in increased steady state levels of drug in the body. This, in turn, may lead to side effects and toxic effects if the increased steady state levels of drug exceed the maximum safe concentration of the drug. In order to illustrate this concept, let us consider that curves A and B in Fig. 11.9 correspond to the plasma concentration time curves obtained for a given drug in patients having normal renal function and severe renal impairment, respectively, and that the upper and lower dashed lines represent the maximum safe and minimum effective plasma concentrations, respectively. It is thus evident that administration of a drug according to a multiple dosage regimen which produces therapeutic steady state plasma levels of drug in patients with normal renal function, will give drug levels which exceed the maximum safe plasma concentration of the drug in patients with severe renal impairment. Hence adjustment of

multiple dosage regimens in terms of dose size, frequency of administration or both is necessaray if patients suffering with renal disease are to avoid the possibility of overmedication. For details of methods of calculating dosage regimens which are suitable for individual patients suffering with renal disease, the reader should refer to the bibliography section at the end of this chapter.

Influence of the 'overnight no dose period'

In our discussions so far, we have considered that multiple dosage regimens comprise of doses being administered at uniform time intervals around the clock. In practice, it is unusual to administer doses under such conditions. If a multiple dosage regimen requires a dose to be administered 'four times a day' it is unlikely that a dose will be administered at 6-hourly intervals around the clock. Instead the four doses are likely to be administered during the 'waking' hours of each day according to such time schedules as 10 a.m.–2 p.m.–6 p.m.–10 p.m.   or   9 a.m.– 1 p.m.–5 p.m.–9 p.m. (Niebergall et al., 1974). The significant feature of both these dosing schedules is that the patient will experience an overnight no dose period of 12 hours. Whilst overnight no dose periods undoubtedly give patients periods of undisturbed sleep, such periods may also cause problems in maintaining therapeutic steady state levels of drug in the body. It is conceivable that overnight no dose periods of 8–12 hours could result in substantial decreases occurring in the level of a drug in the plasma and body particularly for drugs having biological half-lives which are relatively short compared to the overnight no dose period. For instance, in the case of a drug having a biological half-life of 4 hours, an overnight no dose period of 12 hours would correspond to the elapse of three biological half-lives and consequently, a large reduction in the levels of drug in the body. The potential problems of overnight no dose periods with respect to maintaining therapeutic steady state drug levels in patients is illustrated in Fig. 11.10. This figure shows that for a drug having a biological half-life of 4 hours, a multiple dosage regimen comprising one 60 mg dose administered perorally four times each day according to the timetable, 9 a.m.–1 p.m.–5 p.m.–9 p.m., does not permit a true steady state to be attained. Thus the concentration of drug in the plasma does not fluctuate between constant maximum and minimum values over successive dosage time intervals as would occur if the doses were administered every

4 hours around the clock. Figure 11.11 also shows that even if a loading dose of 120 mg was included in the dosage regimen in order to ensure that a true steady state was obtained before the first overnight no dose period, the steady state would not be re-established after the first overnight no dose period. If the upper and lower dashed lines in Figs. 11.10 and 11.11 represent the therapeutic range of the drug, then the patient would experience periods during which the level of drug in the plasma and body would fall below that necessary to elicit the therapeutic effect of the drug. Hence unless the therapeutic range of the drug is sufficiently large to accommodate the fluctuations in drug level associated with overnight no dose periods, problems could arise with regard to maintaining therapeutic drug levels in patients. The potential problems associated with overnight no dose periods are even further complicated by patients who forget to take one of the daytime doses.

MAINTENANCE OF THERAPEUTIC DRUG LEVELS BY SUSTAINED/CONTROLLED RELEASE PERORAL DOSAGE FORMS

For many disease states, the ideal dosage regimen is that by which an acceptable therapeutic concentration of drug at the site(s) of action is attained

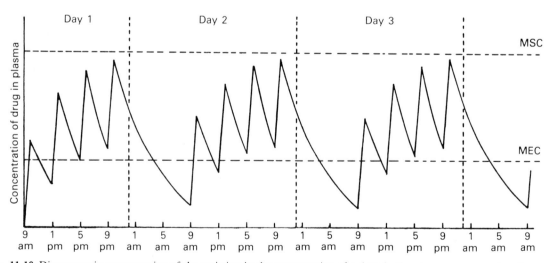

Fig. 11.10 Diagrammatic representation of the variation in the concentration of a drug in the plasma accompanying the peroral administration of a single dose of 60 mg four times a day according to the time schedule, 9 a.m.–1 p.m.–5 p.m.–9 p.m. The biological half-life of the drug is 4 hours

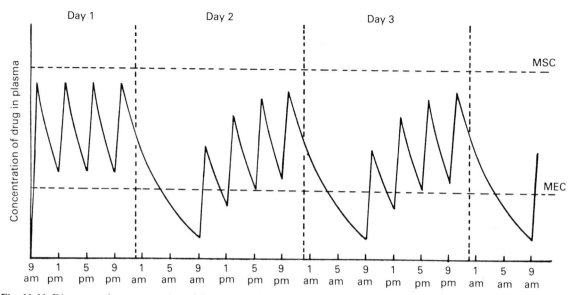

Fig. 11.11 Diagrammatic representation of the variation in the concentration of drug in the plasma accompanying the peroral administration of a loading dose of 120 mg followed by single maintenance doses of 60 mg four times a day according to the time schedule, 9 a.m.–1 p.m.–5 p.m.–9 p.m. The biological half-life of the drug is 4 hours

immediately and is then maintained constant for the desired duration of the treatment. It is evident from the preceding discussions that providing dose size and frequency of administration are correct, therapeutic 'steady state' levels of a drug can be achieved promptly and maintained by the repetitive administration of conventional* peroral dosage forms. However, there are a number of potential limitations associated with the repetitive administration of conventional dosage forms.

1 The concentration of drug in the plasma and hence at the site(s) of action of the drug fluctuates over successive dosing time intervals, even when the so-called 'steady state' condition is achieved. Hence it is not possible to maintain a therapeutic concentration of drug *which remains constant* at the site(s) of action for the duration of drug treatment. At best, the mean value of the maximum and minimum plasma

levels associated with each successive dose administered remains constant for the period of drug treatment.

2 The inevitable fluctuations in steady state concentrations of drug in the plasma and hence at the site(s) of action can lead to a patient being overmedicated or undermedicated for periods of time if the values of C_{max}^{ss} and C_{min}^{ss} rise or fall, respectively, beyond the therapeutic range of the drug.

3 For drugs with short biological half-lives, frequent administration of doses are required to maintain steady state plasma levels within the therapeutic range. For such drugs, the maintenance of therapeutic plasma levels is particularly susceptible to the consequence of forgotten doses and the overnight no dose period. Lack of patient compliance, which is more likely in the case of dosage regimens requiring *frequent* administration of conventional dosage forms, is often an important reason for therapeutic inefficiency or failure. Clearly, not even a peroral dosage regimen which has been designed to perfection can achieve and maintain clinically efficacious and concentrations of a drug at its site(s) of action if the patient does not comply with the regimen.

---

* In the context of this section, a 'conventional' peroral oral dosage form is assumed to be one which is designed to release rapidly the complete dose of drug contained therein immediately following administration. In addition, the released drug is assumed to be in a form which is therapeutically active and immediately available for absorption into the systemic circulation.

The potential limitations of drug therapy based on the repetitive administration of conventional single dose, peroral dosage forms, particularly those containing drugs with short biological half-lives, has led to the development of a more specialized group of peroral dosage forms. Such dosage forms are commonly referred to as sustained release dosage forms (as for example by the *British National Formulary*) but many other titles have been used to describe them over the years (see later). A sustained release dosage form is designed to release the drug contained therein at a *continuous* and *more controlled rate* for a longer period of time than can normally be achieved with its conventional 'non-sustained' counterpart. Consequently, peroral administration of a 'single dose' of a sustained release product increases the duration of therapeutic action of the drug contained therein beyond that achieved normally with a single dose of the corresponding non-sustained conventional counterpart.

Over the years, there has been a proliferation of terms used to describe those products which are collectively known as sustained release products. Terms such as long acting, gradual release, prolonged release, slow release, have been used (Ritschel, 1973). Although attempts have been made to distinguish between many of the above terms, there does not appear to be any universal accepted standard definition of each of the above terms. Consequently the term 'sustained release' will be used collectively to describe peroral dosage forms which continuously release drugs at rates which are sufficiently controlled to provide periods of prolonged therapeutic drug action following each administration of a 'single dose' of such products. Whilst all sustained release products could be described literally as controlled release systems, the term 'controlled release' will only be used in this chapter to describe a peroral sustained release product which is able to maintain a constant therapeutic steady state concentration of drug in the plasma, tissues or at the site of action of the drug. This use of the term 'controlled release' is in accordance with the proposals of Chien and Robinson (1982).

The degree of precision of control over the rate of drug release from a sustained release dosage form varies according to the particular formulation technique employed in that dosage form to control drug release. Consequently, depending on the degree of control over release (and consequently over drug absorption) that is achieved, peroral sustained release products are generally designed to provide either.

1 the prompt achievement of a plasma concentration of drug that remains essentially constant at a value within the therapeutic range of the drug for a satisfactory prolonged period of time, or

2 the prompt achievement of a plasma concentration of drug which, whilst not remaining constant, declines at such a sufficiently slow rate that the plasma concentration remains within the therapeutic range for a satisfactory prolonged period of time.

Typical drug concentration–time profiles corresponding to the above criteria for sustained drug release products are shown in Fig. 11.12.

Kinetic pattern of drug release required for the ideal sustained/controlled release peroral dosage form

If it is assumed that the drug which is to be incorporated into the ideal sustained release dosage form, confers upon the body the characteristics of a one-compartment open model, then the basic kinetic design of such a product may be represented diagrammatically as shown in Fig. 11.13.

To achieve a therapeutic concentration promptly in the body and then to sustain that concentration for a given period of time requires that the total drug in the dosage form consists of two portions — a portion which provides the *initial* priming/loading dose, D_i, and a portion which provides the *maintenance* or sustained dose, D_m.

The initial priming dose of drug, D_i, is released rapidly into the gastrointestinal fluids immediately following administration of the sustained release dosage form (see step 1 in Fig. 11.13). The released dose is required to be absorbed into the body compartment rapidly following a first order kinetic process that is characterized by the apparent absorption rate constant, k_a^1 (see step 2 in Fig. 11.13). The aim of this initial rapid release

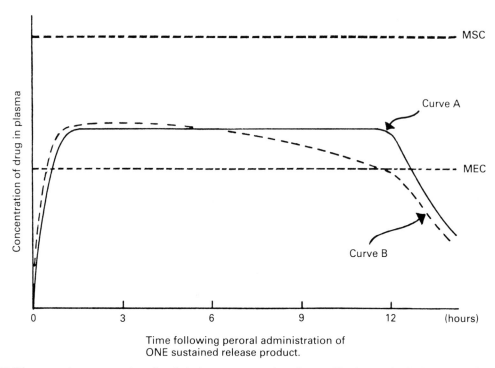

Fig. 11.12 Diagrammatic representation of typical plasma concentration–time profiles for sustained release peroral products which, following rapid attainment of a therapeutic plasma concentration of drug, provide a period of prolonged therapeutic drug action by either (a) maintaining a *constant* therapeutic plasma concentration of drug (curve A) or, (b) ensuring that the plasma concentration of drug remains within the therapeutic range for a satisfactory prolonged period of time (curve B)

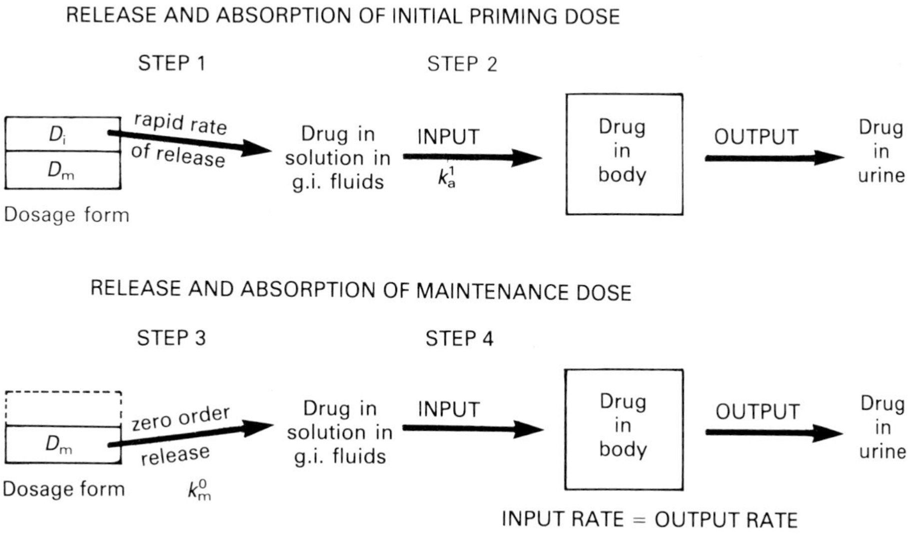

RELEASE AND ABSORPTION OF INITIAL PRIMING DOSE

| STEP 1 | | STEP 2 | |

| D_i | rapid rate of release | Drug in solution in g.i. fluids | INPUT k_a^1 | Drug in body | OUTPUT | Drug in urine |
| D_m | | | | | | |

Dosage form

RELEASE AND ABSORPTION OF MAINTENANCE DOSE

STEP 3   STEP 4

| D_m | zero order release k_m^0 | Drug in solution in g.i. fluids | INPUT | Drug in body | OUTPUT | Drug in urine |

Dosage form

INPUT RATE = OUTPUT RATE

Fig. 11.13 A one-compartment open model of drug disposition in which the source of drug input is an *ideal* sustained release peroral drug product. *Key*: D_i is the initial priming dose of drug in dosage form; D_m is the maintenance dose of drug in dosage form; k_a^1 is the first order apparent absorption rate constant of drug from the priming dose; k_m^0 is the zero order release rate constant of drug from the maintenance dose

and subsequent absorption of the initial priming dose of drug is the rapid attainment of a therapeutic concentration of drug in the body. This, in turn, provides a rapid onset of the desired therapeutic response of the drug in the patient. Following this period of rapid drug release, the portion, D_m, of drug remaining in the dosage form is released at a slow but controlled rate (see step 3 in Fig. 11.13). In order to maintain a constant plasma level of drug, the maintenance dose, D_m, must be released by the dosage form according to zero order kinetics. It thus follows that the rate of release of drug will remain constant and be independent of the amount of the maintenance dose remaining in the dosage form at any given time. The rate of release of the maintenance dose may be characterized by the zero order rate constant, k_m^0. Two further conditions must be fulfilled in order to ensure that the therapeutic concentration of drug in the body remains constant.

1 The zero order rate of release of drug from the maintenance dose must be rate determining with respect to the rate at which the released drug is absorbed subsequently into the body. The kinetics of absorption of the maintenance dose will thus be characterized by the same zero order release rate constant, k_m^0 (at step 3 in Fig. 11.13).
2 The rate at which the maintenance dose is released from the dosage form, and hence the rate of absorption (input) of drug into the body, must be equal to the rate of drug output from the body when the concentration of drug in the body is at the required therapeutic value (see step 4 in Fig. 11.13).

In practice, the design of an ideal sustained/controlled release product, which is capable of releasing the maintenance dose at a precise controlled rate that is in mass balance with the rate of drug elimination corresponding to the required therapeutic concentration of drug in the plasma, is difficult to achieve. There are problems in achieving and maintaining zero order release and absorption of the maintenance dose of drug in the presence of all the variable physiological conditions associated with the gastrointestinal tract (see Chapter 9). In addition, the apparent

elimination rate constant of a given drug varies from patient to patient depending on such factors as genetic differences, age differences and differences in the severity of disease. Consequently it is likely that most peroral sustained release products in current use will not fall into the category of ideal sustained/controlled release peroral dosage forms. However, such prescribed products may be referred to simply as sustained release products and may be differentiated from their ideal counterparts by the following definition. A sustained release product/dosage form is a system in which a portion (the initial priming dose) of the drug is released immediately in order to achieve the desired therapeutic response promptly. The remaining dose of drug (the 'maintenance' dose) is then released slowly thereby resulting in a therapeutic drug/tissue level which is prolonged but not maintained constant (after Chien and Robinson, 1982).

Formulation methods of achieving sustained drug release

It is evident from the preceding discussion that formulation techniques, which permit rapid release of the priming dose followed by slow release of the maintenance dose, are required in order to design peroral sustained release products. All sustained release formulations employ a chemical or physical 'barrier' to provide slow release of the maintenance dose. Many formulation techniques have been used to 'build' the barrier into the peroral dosage form. These techniques include the use of coatings, embedding the drug in a wax, fat or plastic matrix, microencapsulation, chemical binding to ion-exchange resins and incorporation in an osmotic pump. The initial rapidly releasing priming dose of drug may be provided by incorporating that portion of the drug in a separate rapidly releasing form in the dosage form, for instance, as uncoated, rapidly releasing granules or pellets along with coated, slowly releasing granules or pellets in a tablet or hard gelatin capsule dosage form. Alternatively, immediate and rapid release of the priming dose has been achieved by virtue of the position of that portion of the drug being at the surface of a porous wax or plastic matrix. The maintenance dose is provided by drug embedded deeper in the porous matrix. The drug at the surface dissolves quickly in the gastrointestinal fluids whilst the remainder of the drug is leached out slowly from within the matrix by the fluids. For further information concerning the different formulation techniques that have been used in the various types of proprietary sustained release products, the reader should consult the following references: the Consumer Association Report (1984), Kydonieus (1980), Notari (1980), Lee and Robinson (1978) and Garcia *et al.* (1978).

Potential advantages of sustained release drug therapy over conventional drug therapy

1 Improved control over the maintenance of therapeutic plasma levels of drugs permits

(a) improved treatment of many chronic illnesses where symptom breakthrough occurs if the plasma level of drug drops below the minimum effective level, e.g. asthma, depressive illnesses,

(b) maintenance of the therapeutic action of a drug during overnight no dose periods, e.g. overnight management of pain in terminally ill patients permits improved sleep,

(c) reduction in the incidence and severity of untoward systemic side effects related to high peak plasma drug concentrations,

(d) reduction in the total amount of drug administered over the period of drug treatment. This contributes to the reduced incidence of systemic and local side effects observed in the cases of many drugs administered in sustained release formulations.

2 Improved patient compliance resulting from the reduction in the number and frequency of doses required to maintain the desired therapeutic response, e.g. one peroral sustained release product every 12 hours, contributes to the improved control of therapeutic drug levels achieved with sustained release products.

3 There is a reduction in the incidence and severity of localized gastrointestinal side effects produced by 'dose dumping' of irritant drugs from conventional dosage forms, e.g. potassium chloride. The more controlled, slower release of

potasium chloride from its peroral sustained release formulations minimizes the buildup of localized irritant concentrations in the gastrointestinal tract. Consequently potassium chloride is now administered perorally almost exclusively in sustained release form.

4 Economic savings are claimed to be made from better disease management achieved with sustained release products. Patients miss fewer working days and make fewer visits to hospitals and medical practitioners.

Potential limitations of peroral sustained release dosage forms

1 Variable physiological factors such as gastrointestinal pH, enzyme activities, gastric and intestinal transit rates, food and severity of patient's disease, which often influence drug bioavailability from conventional peroral dosage forms, may also interfere with the precision of control of release and absorption of drugs from peroral sustained release dosage forms. The achievement and maintenance of prolonged drug action depends on such control.

2 The rate of transit of sustained release peroral products along the gastrointestinal tract limits the maximum period of time for which a therapeutic response can be maintained following administration of a 'single dose' to approximately 12 hours plus the length of time that absorbed drug continues to exert its therapeutic activity.

3 Sustained release products, which tend to remain intact, may become lodged at some site along the gastrointestinal tract. If this occurs, slow release of drug from the dosage form may produce a high localized concentration of drug which causes local irritation to the gastrointestinal mucosa. Sustained release products which are formulated to disperse in the gastrointestinal fluids are less likely to cause such problems.

4 There are constraints placed on the types of drugs which are suitable candidates for incorporation into peroral sustained release formulations. For instance, drugs having biological half-lives of 1 hour or less are difficult to formulate as sustained release formulations. The high rates of elimination of such drugs from the

body would mean that an extremely large maintenance dose would be required to provide 8–12 hours of continuous therapy following single administratioin of a sustained released product. Apart from the potential hazards of administering such a large dose, the physical size of the sustained release dosage form could make it difficult to swallow. Drugs having biological half-lives of between 4 and 6 hours make good candidates for inclusion in sustained release formulations. Factors other than the biological half-life can preclude a drug from being formulated as a sustained release product. Drugs which have specific requirements for their absorption from the gastrointestinal tract are poor candidates. In order to provide a satisfactory period of prolonged drug therapy, a drug is required to be well absorbed from all regions as the sustained release dosage form passes along the gastrointestinal tract.

5 Sustained release products normally contain a larger total amount of drug than the single dose normally administered in a conventional dosage form. There is the possibility of unsafe overdosage if a sustained release product is improperly made and the total drug contained therein is released at one time or over too short a time interval. Consequently, it may be unwise to include potent drugs in such formulations.

6 As a general rule, sustained release formulations cost more per unit dose than conventional dosage forms containing the same drug. However, fewer 'unit doses' of a sustained release formulation should be required.

REPEAT ACTION VERSUS SUSTAINED ACTION DRUG THERAPY

A repeat action tablet or hard gelatin capsule may be distinguished from its sustained released counterpart by the fact that the repeat action

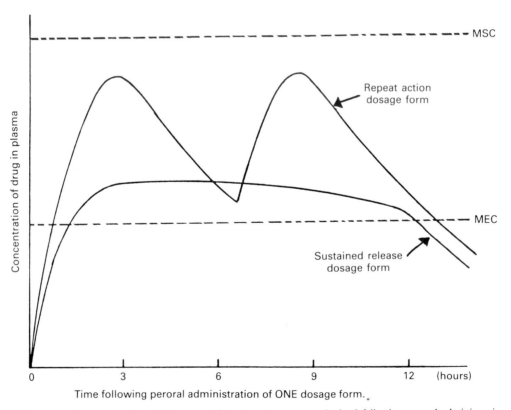

Fig. 11.14 Diagrammatic representation of plasma concentration–time curves obtained following peroral administration of (a) one repeat action dosage form containing two doses and (b) one sustained release dosage form containing the same drug

product does not release the drug contained therein in a slow controlled manner and consequently does not give a plasma concentration–time curve which resembles that of a sustained release product. A repeat action tablet usually contains two doses of drug, the first dose being released immediately following peroral administration in order to provide a rapid onset of the therapeutic response. The release of the second dose is delayed, usually by means of an enteric coat. Consequently when the enteric coat surrounding the second dose is breached by the intestinal fluids, the second dose is released immediately. Figure 11.14 shows that the plasma concentration–time curve obtained following the administration of one repeat action preparation exhibits the 'peak and valley' profile associated with the intermittent administration of conventional dosage forms. The primary advantage provided by a repeat action tablet over a conventional tablet is that of the administration of two (or occasionally three) doses without the necessity of taking more than one tablet.

REFERENCES

Chien, Y. W. and Robinson, J. R. (1982) Smart drug-delivery systems. *J. Parenteral Science and Technology*, **36**, 231.
Consumer Association (1984) Oral sustained release products: pro's and con's. *Drug. Ther. Bull.*, **22**, 57–60.
Garcia, C. R., Siqueiros, A. and Benet, L. Z. (1978) Oral controlled release preparations. *Pharm. Acta Helv.*, **53**, 99–109.
Kydonieus, A. (1980) Fundamental concepts of controlled release. In: *Controlled Release Technologies: Methods, Theory and Applications*. Vol. 1, pp. 1–19, CRC Press Inc., Boca Raton, Florida.
Lee, V. H. L. and Robinson, J. R. (1978) Methods to achieve sustained drug delivery — the physical approach: oral and parenteral dosage forms. In: *Drugs and the Pharmaceutical Sciences. Vol. 6. Sustained and Controlled Release Drug Delivery Systems* (Ed. J. R. Robinson), pp. 123–210, Marcel Dekker Inc., New York.
Niebergall, P. J., Sugita, E. T. and Schnaare, R. L. (1974) Potential dangers of common dosing regimens. *Am. J. hosp. Pharm.*, **31**, 53–58.
Notari, R. E. (1980) *Biopharmaceutics and Clinical Pharmacokinetics. An Introduction*, 3rd edn, pp. 155–162, Marcel Dekker Inc., New York.
Ritschel, W. A. (1973) Peroral solid dosage forms with prolonged action. In: *Drug Design* (Ed. E. J. Ariens), Vol. 4, pp. 38–73, Academic Press, New York.

Banker and C. T. Rhodes), pp. 87–142, Marcel Dekker Inc., New York.
Gibaldi, M. and Perrier, D. (1975) *Drugs and the Pharmaceutical Sciences. Vol. 1. Phaarmacokinetics* (Ed. J. Swarbrick), Marcel Dekker Inc., New York.
Levy, R. H. and Smith, G. H. (1973) Dosage regimens of antiarrhythmics. Part 1: pharmacokinetic properties. *Am. J. Hosp. Pharm.*, **30**, 398–404.
Mawer, G. E. (1982) Dosage adjustment in renal insufficiency. *Br. J. clin. Pharmacol.*, **13**, 145–153.
Notari, R. E. (1980) *Biopharmaceutics and Clinical Pharmacokinetics. An Introduction*, 3rd edn, Marcel Dekker Inc., New York.
Robinson, J. R. (1978) *Drugs and the Pharmaceutical Sciences. Vol. 6. Sustained and Controlled Release Drug Delivery Systems* (Ed. J. R. Robinson), Marcel Dekker Inc., New York.
Rowland, M. and Tozer, T. T. (1980) *Clinical Pharmacokinetics: Concepts and Applications*, Lea and Febiger, Philadelphia.
Schumacher, G. E. (1972) Practical pharmacokinetics techniques for drug consultation and evaluation. I: use of dosage regimen calculations. *Am. J. hosp. Pharm.*, **29**, 474–484.
Schumacker, G. E. (1973) Practical pharmacokinetic techniques for drug consultation and evaluation. II: a perspective on the renal impaired patient. *Am. J. hosp. Pharm.*, **30**, 824–830.
Schumacher, G. E. and Weiner, J. (1974) Practical pharmacokinetic techniques for drug consultation and evaluation. III: psychotherapeutic drugs as prototypes for illustrating some considerations in Pharmacist-generated dosage regimens. *Am. J. hosp. Pharam.*, **31**, 59–66.
Shargel, L. and Yu, A. D. C. (1980) *Applied Biopharmaceutics and Pharmacokinetics*, Appleton–Century–Crofts, New York.
Wagner, J. G. (1975). *Fundamentals of Clinical Pharmacokinetics*. Drug Intelligence Publications, Hamilton, Illinois.

BIBLIOGRAPHY

Calvert, R. T. (1975) Drug dosage regimen calculations. *J. Hosp. Pharm.*, **33**, 157–161.
Clark, B. and Smith, D. A. (1981). *An Introduction to Pharmacokinetics*, Blackwell Scientific Publications, London.
Dittert, L. W. and Bourne, D. W. A. (1979) Pharmacokinetics. In: *Modern Pharmaceutics* (Eds G. S.

PART THREE

Drug delivery systems

Packs for pharmaceutical products

The role of the pack

THE PACK AS A PROTECTION
Mechanical hazards
  Shock or impact damage
  Compression
  Vibration
  Abrasion
  Puncture
Climatic or environmental hazards
  Moisture
  Temperature
  Pressure
  Light
  Atmospheric gases
  Solid airborne contamination (particulates)
Biological hazards
  Microbiological
  Other forms of infestation
  Pilferage and adulteration risks
Chemical hazards

STAGES IN THE DEVELOPMENT OF A
  PACK–PRODUCT COMBINATION
Development stages
  Preformulation
  Product formulation
  Consideration of container materials
  Pack feasibility tests
  Formal stability tests
  Ongoing stability
  Complaints

PACK SELECTION
Factors influencing choice of pack
  The product
  The market

The distribution system
Manufacturing facilities
Summary

Packaging can be defined as an economical means of providing, presentation, protection, identification/information, containment, convenience and compliance for a product during storage, carriage, display and use until such time as the product is used or administered. This total time scale must be within the shelf life of the product which is controlled by the selection of the right combination of product and pack. In looking at the above definition emphasis on any one factor may change with time, advancements in science and technology or trends in product form. For instance there has been a distinct move from unpleasant oral liquids to the solid dose form which has more recently concentrated on delayed or sustained release products. Such changes can have a positive influence on the type of pack used as shown by the increasing applications of blister and strip packaging. Both sustained release and these unit type packs offer obvious patient convenience since a selected number of units can be readily detached and carried as a day's treatment possibly leading to improved compliance. However, packaging can offer convenience factors anywhere along its life cycle, e.g. reel fed materials used for the production of blisters and strips need relatively little storage space compared with any preformed bottle which literally wastes space by the storage of air prior to being filled. Further examples of packs offering patient convenience include a whole range of unit dose presentations which permit immediate disposal after use, metered dose aerosols and nasal sprays which combine convenience with dosage control, squeeze eye drop packs (when compared with the earlier bottle, dropper and teat assembly) etc.

The role of the pack

The role of the pack and the packaging operation needs emphasis since the shelf life of all pharmaceutical products, irrespective of whether they are ethicals, semi-ethicals or proprietaries (over-the-counter or OTC), is largely dependent on certain functions of the pack. The pack must be economical and therefore contribute to overall profitability, it must provide protection against climatic, biological, physical and chemical hazards, it must provide an acceptable presentation which will contribute to or enhance product confidence whilst at the same time maintaining adequate identification and information, and last and not least it must contribute in terms of convenience and compliance. Each of these aspects has to be considered against the total (shelf) life of the product which involves periods of storage (static), carriage (motion), possible display and finally use or administration directly by a patient or indirectly by a professional person. In certain cases the pack may form part of the administration system as seen by an aerosol, a metered dose nasal pump, a prefilled syringe, etc. As these total pack requirements become increasingly extensive and sometimes conflicting, it is not surprising to find that the final choice is inevitably a compromise, hence the question 'What is an ideal pack?' rarely has a simple answer. For example, the external image of the pack must not only compliment product confidence, provide clear and concise product identification, adequate information related to the contents (including legal requirements), the route of administration, storage conditions, batch number, expiry date, manufacturer's name and address, product licence number but also assist in patient compliance. Producing an aesthetically acceptable design is therefore only one stage where compromise has to be exercised.

In addition to this aesthetic requirement the majority of the remaining pack factors are associated with its function. The primary pack consists of those packaging components which form the part of the pack directly containing the product (i.e. bottle, cap, cap liner, label, etc). The main functions of the primary pack are to contain, and to restrict any chemical, climatic or biological or occasionally mechanical hazards which may cause or lead to product deterioration. Since the primary pack also represents the pack of 'use', it must also function in the hands of the user as a means of drug administration. The packaging external to the primary pack, known as the secondary packaging, mainly provides the additional physical protection necessary to ensure the safe warehousing and delivery of the product to the point where bulk quantities are broken down into individual units.

THE PACK AS A PROTECTION

Although each function of the pack has to assume a certain level of importance, protection is almost invariably the most critical factor since it controls the total shelf life of the product. Asking the question 'protection against what?' produces a whole list of possible hazards many of which are listed below. These are not identified in any particular order of importance as the hazards which are relevant to a specific product will vary in both number and criticality. They cover mechanical, climatic, biological and chemical factors.

Mechanical hazards

Physical or mechanical damage may occur due to the following.

Shock or impact damage

This phrase infers rough handling where rapid deceleration occurs (drops, impacts). Shock can normally be reduced or overcome by various forms of cushioning, restriction of movement, more careful handling, etc. However, it should be noted that damage can occur to the pack or packaging material before it reaches the stage of a packed product.

Compression

Top pressure or loading can distort and crush a pack and damage the product inside. The crushing of a carton can make a product unsaleable even though no damage has occurred to the contents. Although this is most likely to occur during stacking in the warehouse or in transit where vibration adds a further hazard, compression of the pack can occur in other situations (i.e. capping on a production line, when being carried home by the user, etc.).

Vibration

Vibration consists of two variables, frequency and amplitude. These can vary enormously, e.g. a load on a truck may bounce up and down say 0–50 mm, up to 120 times per minute, whereas vibration from aircraft/ships engines may have an extremely low amplitude but a very high frequency. Each extreme may produce different forms of damage to product and/or pack, i.e. components of product separate, screw caps may loosen, labels or decoration may abrade, etc.

Abrasion

Although this results from both regular and irregular forms of vibration it is listed separately since the visual appearance of the product or pack can be affected, e.g. a rectangular bottle in a carton will move up and down and from side to side. A round bottle in the same circumstances will suffer from an additional possibility of rotation. See below under Chemical hazards.

Puncture

Many materials can suffer penetration from sharp objects. Again this can happen at any stage from basic material supply to the finished pack. Adequate cushioning and/or resistance to penetration helps to reduce the risks. Poor control of fork lift trucks is an inherent puncture hazard.

Climatic or environmental hazards

These may be ever present hazards or hazards which are specific to a local environment. Although climatic conditions are covered by such phrases as arctic, antarctic, temperate, subtropical, tropical, severe conditions can occur elsewhere, i.e. in a deep freeze (-19 to -22 °C), in a bathroom or kitchen where conditions can be worse than many tropical areas, displayed under high wattage bulbs in a shop window, stored near pipes or heaters in a shop, warehouse, etc. Climatic hazards therefore include the following.

Moisture

Moisture as liquid or water vapour may cause physical changes (e.g. dulling, softening, hardening, etc.) or chemical change (hydrolysis, effervescence, etc.) It may also act as a carrier for other contaminants. Certain materials (including all plastics) are to some degree permeable to moisture and even screw closures which appear to make a good seal are likely to permit some passage of moisture depending on the sealing media, the torque, the evenness and shape of the sealing surface, the aperture size and circumferential area of the container, etc. It must be emphasized that either moisture loss or moisture gain may be critical to some products.

Temperature

Extremes of temperature (cold and hot) or cycling temperature can cause deterioration to product and/or pack. Although higher temperatures generally represent an acceleration effect occasions can be found where deterioration increases at lower temperatures (certain plastic will become more brittle and crack, for example). A high temperature coupled with a high RH will produce a shower effect if the temperature is lowered sufficiently to reach dew point. Contamination from liquid moisture can then encourage mould and bacterial growth.

Pressure

Air pressure differentials are frequently seen as a danger for materials sent by air using unpressurized aircraft. Pressurized aircraft are pressurized to the equivalent to about 3000 m above sea level; hence there is a -0.25 bar differential compared with takeoff. Goods filled in factories at sea level, and sent to mountainous areas or vice versa will suffer from similar patterns, i.e. goods packed in Johannesburg, South Africa, at 2000 m and then sent to Durban at sea level will be exposed both to a positive pressure and probably a temperature change.

Light

Light consists of wavelengths from the u.v. zone through the visible to infra red. Although u.v. is a potential source of photochemical change, such changes may not always be visible. Printed or decorated packaging materials may also suffer from discoloration (white may go yellow, deeper colours may fade) and this may be seen as inferring a change in product efficacy or strength. Although light can be excluded by using selected materials, tin plate, foil, etc., opacity and/or colour may reduce penetration or filter out selected wavelengths. The additional use of u.v. absorbers in plastics may also restrict light rays entering the pack. It should also be noted that many products are protected by a carton, outer, etc. for a larger proportion of their life. Protection may then only be necessary for a relatively short display or use period when exposure to light occurs.

Atmospheric gases

These include oxygen, carbon dioxide, nitrogen and any other airborne gases. Oxygen leading to oxidation is the more obvious hazard. Carbon dioxide, however, can cause a pH shift (unbuffered solution in plastic bottles particularly LDPE which is relatively permeable to CO_2), and/or lead to precipitation of some products. The permeation of the common gases through plastic is typically in the ratio of 1 : 4 : 20 for nitrogen, oxygen and carbon dioxide respectively, with the latter being the most permeable.

Odorous gases, or volatile ingredients associated with perfumes, flavours, product formulations, may also pass into or out of a pack. If a volatile ingredient is lost from a flavour, an unpleasant odour or taste may result.

Solid airborne contamination (particulates)

Particulates may be carried by or in the atmosphere. In the case of most plastic contamination may be increased by electrostatic attraction under dry conditions whereby particulates are drawn from the atmosphere by electrical charges. The presence of particulates will inevitably increase microbiological contamination risk.

Biological hazards

Microbiological

There is a general tendency towards improved microbial control for all products. This means that the packaging materials must be reasonably clean initially and when put together to form a finished pack restrict any further contamination as much as possible. In the case of sterile products the pack and its closure must maintain a 100% effective seal against microbiological ingress, i.e. bacteria, moulds, yeast. Ingress of yeasts is critical with sugar-based products, e.g. syrups, as fermentation may occur. Mould will also grow on cellulose-based materials, i.e. paper, board if these are kept under humid conditions.

Other forms of infestation

In common with foods, other sources of infestation which can contaminate pharmaceutical products include attack by insects, termites, vermin, rodents or any other bird- or animal-contaminating source. Although this is more likely to happen under poorly controlled conditions of hygiene and house keeping, such infestation can still occasionally cause problems even in the UK.

Pilferage and adulteration risks

Pilferage being a human failing is broadly another biological hazard. The example of the Tylenol poisonings in 1982 has placed greater emphasis on the need for tamper-resistant packs. Prior to this, various seals were used to indicate whether any product had been removed or replaced rather than as a means of protecting against deliberate adulteration. Security seals, a possibly preferred phrase to tamper evidence, are widely used for pharmaceutical products as a means of increasing and maintaining user confidence in the product and pack.

Chemical hazards

Since chemical interaction, if inherent to the formulation, cannot normally be reduced or avoided by pack selection (unless it is associated with exchange between the product and external atmosphere), the main risk must relate to interaction or incompatibility between product and pack. Compatibility investigations must basically cover any exchange which can occur between the product and the pack and vice versa. These may be associated with interaction or contamination covering migration, absorption, adsorption, extraction, corrosion, erosion, etc. whereby ingredients may be lost or gained. Such exchange may be identifiable as organoleptic changes, increase in toxicity/irritancy, degradation, loss or gain of microbial effectiveness, precipitation, haze, turbidity, colour change, pH shift, etc. Again other external influences may catalyse, induce, or even nullify chemical changes.

Some examples of chemical interaction between a product and its pack and the resulting contamination are described below.

1 Adsorption of chemical entities on to component surfaces occasionally occurs. Losses of EDTA and certain preservatives (e.g. benzalkonium chloride, thiomersal and other mercurials) have been observed.
2 The more volatile preservatives, e.g. chlorbutol, phenol, 2-phenylethanol, show fairly rapid loss through low density polythene by absorption and surface evaporation. If an external overwrap, which is not permeable to the preservative, is added, then loss can usually be restricted to relatively low levels, i.e. less than 10%.
3 Other surface-active ingredients which may be found in plastics may also enter the product by dissolution, surface abrasion, etc. These include antistatic additives, slip additives, antislip additives, mould release agents, antiblock agents, lubricants, etc.
4 Detachment of glass spicules may occur when alkaline solutions of citrates, tartrates, chlor-

ides, salicylates are stored in soda glass containers. This may occasionally occur when treated or even neutral glass is autoclaved in the presence of similar alkaline salts.
5 Organoleptic changes may occur, caused by permeation of volatile or odorous substances through plastic materials, e.g., solvents from printing inks.

STAGES IN THE DEVELOPMENT OF A PACK–PRODUCT COMBINATION

Development stages

To follow the theme that no pharmaceutical excipient, drug entity, intermediate or finished product can exist without a pack means that knowledge of the pack employed is relevant for all developmental stages of a dosage form, from preformulation studies right through to the finally chosen pack. The placing of formulations on test without reference to the packaging material, the closuring system, the torque to which a screw cap has to be closed etc. is condemned.

Attempts to accelerate deterioration by the use of excessively high temperatures should also not be employed. In the same way that products may change when exposed to accelerated conditions, packs, packaging materials, may similarly suffer changes, e.g. caps can tighten and crack (if plastic) or loosen and become ineffective as closures. It is therefore advised that packs generally should not be exposed to temperatures of more than 45 °C and even at this condition the time period should not exceed 12 months, with a maximum of 6 months being preferable.

With modern analytical techniques t.g.a., d.t.a., g.c., g.p.c., d.s.c., h.p.l.c., i.r., u.v., t.l.c., etc., changes in product or pack are becoming easier to detect and define in terms of actual change. It is also interesting to note the change in emphasis from identifying product purity to identification and quantification of impurity and degradation products which in earlier years would have remained unidentified. These can now be fully quantified by the analytical techniques available. However, the student is warned that total reliance on so-called scientific methods is not enough. Sensual observations related to feel, appearance, texture, colour, smell, taste (where safe) should also be used as these simple observations can occasionally detect change before any analytical procedure has been developed.

The stages broadly associated with packaging development are as follows.

Preformulation

All preformulation studies need some form of container. It is therefore important to understand the limitations associated with any packaging contact material used to contain or retain the material under test even in this very early stage of product development.

Product formulation

Formulations and any intermediates all require to be contained and stored. It is therefore necessary to make certain that all packaging contact materials are defined and that all pack parameters (torque, heat seal, etc) are identified, controlled and documented (all part of good laboratory practice (GLP) and good pharmaceutical manufacturing practice (GMP)) during formulation studies.

Consideration of container materials

It is important to have a basic knowledge of all packaging materials, their properties, characteristics, etc. and the processes by which they are fabricated/decorated as a packaging container or component with knowledge of how these and any subsequent processes may effect their properties, e.g. sterilization by ethylene oxide can lead to ethylene oxide and ethylene glycol residues. Gamma irradiation of low density polyethylene not only marginally reduces material flexibility due to molecular cross-linkage but can give rise to formic acid and formaldehyde residues.

Pack feasibility tests

This is the stage where a product (preferably the formulation selected for ultimate sale) is tested in

a range of possible packs, usually over a range of conditions from say $-20\,°C$ to $45\,°C$, together with some cycling conditions covering a temperature–humidity range. Note the weakness of testing under constant temperature conditions — when in actual practice all conditions are cycling and therefore variable. In addition to the storage tests indicated above immersion of pieces of pack or pack components, if plastic, in the product or a simulant, i.e. an extractive type test, may also be employed. Extractive tests are usually mandatory for plastics used for injectables and ophthalmic products. All materials used for these tests should be given a provisional specification and thoroughly checked (more rigorous quality control tests) prior to any use. Feasibility tests usually extend over 1–12 month test periods with 3–6 months normally being the minimum period of test before a decision to proceed with a certain pack is taken. However, decisions based on accelerated conditions are sometimes difficult to interpret as limited failure at say $45\,°C$ or severe cycling conditions, e.g. $15–37\,°C$, 50–90% relative humidity (RH) over 12 hourly cycles, does not necessarily mean a pack (or the product) will fail under more realistic climatic conditions.

Formal stability tests

Once sufficient confidence has been generated in the pack–product by the previously described tests, formal stability tests (see Chapter 7) on which the ultimate shelf life will be based, can proceed. At this stage, tests are normally carried out on three batches of product for each pack variant, each being stored at, for example $4\,°C$, $20\,°C$, $30\,°C$, $37\,°C$ and 75% RH for a period of 5 years with examination intervals at initial (0), 3, 6, 9, 12, 18, 24, 30, 36, 48 and 60 months. The resulting data can then be documented and sent out to regulatory authorities as part of a drug submission.

Ongoing stability

This consists of repeated stability on random batches from production in order to confirm that the shelf life does not change.

Complaints

This is the final means of monitoring the success of the product and pack. It is somewhat similar to the monitoring and recording of adverse reactions in that it is a safeguard to both the company producing the drug and the person receiving it.

In all the above tests analytical and packaging technological support is essential to check both the product and the pack. Some of the types of test employed are identified both in this chapter and in Chapter 44. The aims quoted earlier bear repeating as without them there is no assurance that a satisfactory product pack has been achieved, i.e.

1 a specifiable product,
2 a specifiable pack,
3 a specifiable series of processes controlling all operations from raw material to the assembly of the finished pack as this ultimately becomes the basis for the control of all future production.

To achieve these specifiable parameters requires the cooperation and coordination of virtually all company disciplines in order that the final aim of having a successful product which is effective, safe and makes a profit is met. The pack therefore must carry the product image literally from inception to disposal.

PACK SELECTION

Factors influencing choice of pack

Before a pack can be selected and the relevance of the various hazards considered, it is necessary to establish a thorough background brief which covers consideration of the product, the market, the distribution system, manufacturing facilities and other considerations. These are discussed below.

The product

Product detail must include chemical and physical characteristics of the drug entity, the excipients and the formulation. It must also cover any recognized routes of deterioration or degradation, the dosage and frequency of dosage, the mode of administration, type of patient (baby, child, teenager, adult, elderly, infirm, etc.) any of which could influence the product and pack style and any controlling legislative detail. Whether product is seasonal or has an all the year round use may be a further influence to pack selection.

The market

The eventual channels of sale should be considered, i.e. where, when, how and by whom it is to be used or administered (e.g. doctor, dentist, nurse, patient, etc.). Where the product may be used (i.e. clinic, home, hospital), whether for home trade and/or export, the quantity per pack and the predicted sales for initial launch and follow-up sales, must all be carefully considered during pack design and selection.

The distribution system

The distribution system should be carefully thought out, for example conventional wholesale/retail outlets or direct to selected outlets. How a product is to be distributed may be more relevant to export markets where less sophisticated transport systems (mules, donkeys, camels, etc.) may be used, and where climatic conditions may be more severe particularly if intermediate storage facilities are non-existent (e.g. no dock-side warehouses) whereby the consignment will be directly exposed to the atmosphere.

Manufacturing facilities

The suitability of the manufacturing facilities may have to be considered for a number of reasons, i.e. new pack, increased sales, improvements in GMP, revised product, new product, etc. For example, can the envisaged product be manufactured and packed with existing facilities or are new plant, equipment and buildings required? If the latter applies then the likely profit has to be equated against the likely cost of the venture. For example, an entirely new facility for the introduction of a packed product by an aseptic or a terminal autoclaving process would be more expensive than that required for a solid or liquid oral dosage form.

Details of industrial pack-filling techniques can be found in Chapter 44.

Summary

The above introduction to the packaging of pharmaceuticals should serve to establish the broad in-depth knowledge required by the packaging technologist. The fact that all products only have a shelf life when packed emphasizes the importance of what has frequently been seen as a minor role in the past. The success of any product depends on an effective marriage between both product and pack.

BIBLIOGRAPHY

Briston, J. H. (1983) *Plastics in Packaging. Properties and Applications*, IOP, Stanmore, Middlesex.

Briston, J. H. (1983) *Plastics in Packaging. Conversion Processes*, IOP, Stanmore, Middlesex.

BS 1133: 1961–. Covering the Packaging Code; series of booklets, published by British Standards Institute)

Cairns, J. A., Down and Paine, F. A. (1974) *Packaging for Climatic Protection*, Newnes Butterworth, London.

Griffin, R. C. and Sacharow, S. (1972) *Principles of Package Development*, Avi Publishing Company Inc., Westport.

Griffin, R. C. and Sacharow, S. (1973) *Plastics in Packaging*, Cahness Books, Boston.

Montresor, J. M., Mostyn, H. P. and Paine, F. A. (1983) *Packaging Evaluation*, IOP, Stanmore, Middlesex.

Moody, B. E. (1977) *Packaging in Glass*, Hutchinson, London.

Oswin, C. R. (1983) *Package Life*, Institute of Packaging (IOP), Stanmore, Middlesex.

Paine, F. A. (Ed.) (1967) *Packaging Materials and Containers*, Blackie and Son Ltd, Glasgow.

Paine, F. A. (Ed.) (1973) *Packaging and the Law*, Newnes Butterworth, London.

Paine, F. A. (Ed.) (1977) *The Packaging Media*, Blackie and Son Ltd, Glasgow.

Paine, F. A. (Ed.) (1981) *Fundamentals of Packaging*, Blackie and Son Ltd, Glasgow.

Paine, F. A. and Paine, H. Y. (1983) *A Handbook of Food Packaging*, Leonard Hill, Glasgow.

Sacharow, S. (1976) *Handbook of Packaging Materials*, Avi Publishing Company Inc., Westport.

Sacharow, S. (1978) *A Packaging Primer*, Book for Industry Division of Magazine for Industry, Inc., New York.

Sacharow, S. (1979) *Packaging Regulations*, Avi Publishing Co. Inc., Westport.

Swinbank, C. (1973) *Packaging of Chemicals*, C. Newnes Butterworth, London.

Swinbank, Colin (1983) *Intermediate Bulk Containers*, IOP, Stanmore, Middlesex.

Preformulation

THE CONCEPT OF PREFORMULATION

Almost all new drugs which are active orally are marketed as tablets, capsules or both (Table 13.1). Although only a few drug compounds are eventually marketed as an injection (25% of those drugs marketed as tablets), an injection, particularly by the intravenous route, is always required during early toxicity, metabolic, bioavailability and clinical studies in order to guarantee precise drug and dose deposition. Other dosage forms may be required (Table 13.1) but these are usually drug specific and often depend to a large extent on the successful development of tablets, capsules and injections.

Prior to the development of these three major dosage forms with a new drug candidate, it is essential that certain fundamental physical and chemical properties of the drug molecule and other derived properties of the drug powder are determined. This information will dictate many of the subsequent events and possible approaches in formulation development. This first learning phase is known as *preformulation*.

A suggested list of information required in preformulation is shown in Table 13.2. It is assembled in a logical order recognizing the relative importance of the data and probable existence of only limited quantities of bulk drug (mg rather than g) at this stage of its development. Investigators should also be pragmatic and only generate data which is of immediate relevance, especially if the likely dosage forms are known.

However, a knowledge of two fundamental properties is mandatory for a new compound:

1 intrinsic solubility (C_o),
2 dissociation constant (pK_a).

These will immediately determine (a) the need and (b) the possibility of making more soluble salts of the drug to eliminate solubility-related poor bioavailability, particularly from solid dosage forms.

Independent of this pharmaceutical profiling (Table 13.2), analysts will need to generate data (Table 13.3) to support the assay of existing and

Table 13.1 Frequency distribution of dosage form types manufactured in the UK (Data Sheet Compendium)

Dosage form	Frequency (%)
Tablets	45.8
Liquid oral	16.0
Injections	15.0
Capsules	13.0
Suppositories and pessaries	3.3
Topicals	3.0
Eye preparations	1.8
Aerosols (inhalation)	1.2
Others	0.3

Table 13.2 Preformulation drug characterization

Test	Method/function/characterization	References/Bibliography
1 Spectroscopy	Simple u.v. assay	Dalglish (1969)
2 Solubility	Phase solubility, purity	Mader (1954); Higuchi and Connors (1965)
aqueous	Intrinsic solubility, pH effects	
pK_a	Solubility control, salt formation	Albert and Serjeant (1984)
salts	Solubility, hygroscopicity, stability	Berge, et al. (1977)
solvents	Vehicles, extraction	Yalkowski and Roseman (1981)
partition coeff K_w^o	Lipophilicity, structure activity	Leo, et al. (1971)
dissolution	Biopharmacy	Swarbrick (1970)
3 Melting point	DSC — polymorphism, hydrates, solvates	Wendlandt (1974); Haleblian (1975), Haleblian and McCrone (1969)
4 Assay development	u.v., t.l.c., h.p.l.c.	Jaffe and Orchin (1962); Bristow (1976)
5 Stability (in solution and in solid state)	Thermal, hydrolysis, oxidation, photolysis, metal ions, pH	Mollica et al. (1978); Connors et al. (1979)
6 Microscopy	Morphology, particle size	McCrone et al. (1978)
7 Powder flow		
(a) bulk density	Tablet and capsule formulation	Neumann (1967)
(b) angle of repose	Tablet and capsule formulation	Neumann (1967)
8 Compression properties	Aids excipient choice	DeBoer et al. (1978); Jones (1981)
9 Excipient compatibility	Preliminary screening by DSC, confirmation by t.l.c.	Smith (1982)

Table 13.3 Analytical preformulation

Attribute	Test
Identity	Nuclear magnetic resonance (n.m.r.)
	Infra red spectroscopy (i.r.)
	Ultraviolet spectroscopy (u.v.)
	Thin layer chromatography (t.l.c.)
	Differential scanning calorimetry (DSC)
	Optical rotation, where applicable
Purity	Moisture (water and solvents)
	Inorganic elements
	Heavy metals
	Organic impurities
	Differential scanning calorimetry (DSC)
Assay	Titration
	Ultraviolet spectroscopy (u.v.)
	High performance liquid chromatography (h.p.l.c.)
Quality	Appearance
	Odour
	Solution colour
	pH of slurry (saturated solution)
	Melting point

new bulk material. Although their data meet a different need, it can often be used to complement and confirm pharmaceutical data. Their greater training and knowledge in analysis will assist, for example, in the identification of suitable stability-indicating assays by ultraviolet spectroscopy (u.v.) or high performance liquid chromatography (h.p.l.c.) and the screening of incompatibilities by thin layer chromatography (t.l.c.).

1 SPECTROSCOPY

The first step in preformulation is to establish a simple analytical method so that all future measurements can be quantitative. Most drugs absorb light in the ultraviolet wavelengths (190–390 nm) since they are generally aromatic and/or contain double bonds. Confirmation of synthetic structure is, of course, the responsibility of the synthetic chemist. The acidic or basic nature of the molecule can be predicted from the functional groups in its structure (Perrin *et al.*, 1981). This will indicate suitable solvents to ensure solution of either the ionized or undissociated species. This is important since the ionic status of a drug can alter the shape of the u.v. spectrum by increasing absorption or changing the wavelengths (bathochromic (red) or hypsochromic (blue) shifts) at which maxima, minima or both occur.

Once the u.v. spectrum of the new drug molecule is established, it is possible to choose an analytical wavelength (often λ_{max}) that is suitable to quantify the amount of drug in a particular solution. Excitation of the molecule in solution causes a loss in light energy and the net change from the intensity of the incident light (I_o) and the transmitted light (I) can be measured. The amount of light absorbed by a solution of drug is proportional to the concentration (C) and the path length of the solution (l) through which the light source has passed. Equation 13.1 is the well-known Beer–Lambert law where e is the molar extinction coefficient.

$$\text{Absorbance } (A) = \log_{10}(I_o/I) = eCl \quad (13.1)$$

However, it is usual in pharmacy to quote the *specific absorption coefficient* ($E^1_{1\,cm}$, or E^1_1 for short) where the pathlength is 1 cm and the solution concentration is 1% w/v (10 mg ml^{-1}) since doses and concentrations are generally in metric units.

2 SOLUBILITY

When a preformulation programme begins, the availability of drug is always limited and the preformulation scientist may only have 50 mg. Thus, it is important that the best use of this limited bulk is made to support the continuing efforts to the synthetic chemists and the biologists pursuing activity and toxicity screens. Furthermore, because the compound is new, the quality is invariably poor, so that a large number of impurities may be present and often the first crystals come down as a metastable polymorph (see Section 3 of this chapter and Chapter 5). Accordingly, if nothing else is measured, the solubility and pK_a must be determined. These control all future work. The solubility dictates the ease with which formulations for intravenous injection studies in animals are obtained. The pK_a allows the informed use of pH to maintain solubility and to choose salts should they be required to achieve good bioavailability from the solid state (Chapter 9) and improve stability (Chapter 7) and powder properties (Chapter 36).

Kaplan (1972) suggested that unless a compound has an aqueous solubility in excess of 1% (10 mg ml^{-1}) over the pH range 1–7 at 37 °C, then potential bioabsorption problems may occur. He also found that if the intrinsic dissolution rate was greater than 1 mg cm^{-2} min^{-1} then absorption was unimpeded. However, dissolution rates of less than 0.1 mg cm^{-2} min^{-1} were likely to give dissolution rate-limited absorption. This ten-fold difference in dissolution rate translates into a lower limit for solubility of 1 mg ml^{-1} since, under sink conditions, dissolution rate and solubilities are proportional (Hamlin *et al.*, 1965).

A solubility of less than 1 mg ml^{-1} indicates the need for a salt, particularly if the drug will be formulated as a tablet or capsule. In the range 1–10 mg ml^{-1} serious consideration should be given to salt formation. When the solubility of the drug cannot be manipulated in this way (as in the case of neutral molecules, glycosides, steroids, alcohols or where the pK_a is less than 3 for a base or greater than 10 for an acid) then liquid filling in soft gelatin capsules (in a solution in PEG 400, glyceryl triacetate or fractionated coconut oil) or as a paste or semisolid (dissolved in oil or triglyceride) in a hard gelatin capsule may be necessary.

Intrinsic solubility (C_o)

An increase in solubility of the new drug in an acidic solution compared with its aqueous solubility suggests a weak base, and an increase in alkali, a weak acid. In both cases a dissociation constant (pK_a) will be measurable and salts should form. An increase in both acidic and alkaline solubility suggests either amphoteric or zwitterion behaviour; in this case there will be two pK_as, one acidic and one basic. No change in solubility suggests a non-ionizable, neutral molecule with no measurable pK_a. Here solubility manipulations will require either solvents or complexation.

When the purity of the drug sample can be assured, the solubility value obtained in acid for a weak acid or alkali for a weak base can be assumed to be the intrinsic solubility (C_o). The solubility should ideally be measured at two temperatures: (a) 4 or 5 °C to ensure good physical stability and to extend short-term storage and chemical stability until more definitive data is available and (b) 37 °C to support biopharmaceutical evaluation.

However, since absolute purity is often in doubt for the first few batches of new drug, it is more accurate to determine this crucial solubility by use of a phase-solubility diagram (Fig. 13.1). The data are obtained from a series of experiments in which the ratio of the amount of drug to the amount of dissolving solvent is varied. Any deviation from the horizontal is indicative of impurities which a higher drug loading and its inherent impurities

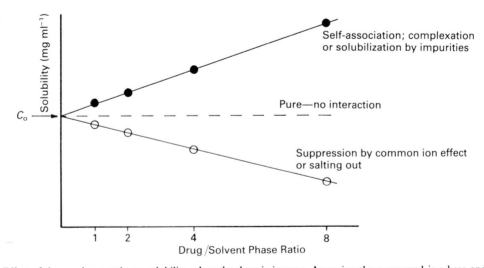

Fig. 13.1 Effect of drug: solvent ratio on solubility when the drug is impure. Assuming the compound is a base and the estimate of its solubility in 0.1 M NaOH was 1 mg ml^{-1}, four solutions of 3 ml should be set up containing 3, 6, 12 and 24 mg of drug. These give the phase ratios shown here. 3 ml is the smallest volume which can be manipulated for either centrifugation or filtration and dilution for u.v. analysis. The vials should be agitated continuously overnight and then the concentration in solution determined

Table 13.4 Potential pharmaceutical salts

	Basic drugs			Acidic drugs		
Anion	pK_a	% Usage★		Cation	pK_a	% Usage★
Hydrochloride	−6.10	43.0		Potassium	16.00	10.8
Sulphate	−3.00, +1.96	7.5		Sodium	14.77	62.0
Tosylate	−1.34	0.1		Lithium	13.82	1.6
Mesylate	−1.20	2.0		Calcium	12.90	10.5
Napsylate	0.17	0.3		Magnesium	11.42	1.3
Besylate	0.70	0.3		Diethanolamine	9.65	1.0
Maleate	1.92, 6.23	3.0		Zinc	8.96	3.0
Phosphate	2.15, 7.20, 12.38	3.2		Choline	8.90	0.3
Salicylate	3.00	0.9		Aluminium	5.00	0.7
Tartrate	3.00	3.5		Others		8.8
Lactate	3.10	0.8				
Citrate	3.13, 4.76, 6.40	3.0				
Benzoate	4.20	0.5				
Succinate	4.21, 5.64	0.4				
Acetate	4.76	1.3				
Others		30.2				

★ Martindale (1982), *The Extra Pharmacopoeia*, 28th edition. The Pharmaceutical Press, London.

either promotes or suppresses solubility. In the cases where the observed result changes with the amount of solvent, the line is extrapolated to zero phase ratio, where solubility will be independent of solvent level and a true estimate of the intrinsic solubility of the drug. The United States Pharmacopoeia uses this method to estimate the purity of mecamylamine hydrochloride.

pK_a from solubility data

Seventy-five per cent of all drugs are weak bases (20% are weak acids and the remaining 5% are non-ionic, amphoteric or alcohols). It is therefore appropriate to consider the Henderson–Hasselbalch equations for weak bases and acids. These have been discussed in Chapter 3 and their bioavailability consequences in Chapter 9.

For weak bases

$$pH = pK_a + \log_{10}([B] / [BH^+]) \quad (13.2)$$

and for weak acids

$$pH = pK_a + \log_{10}([A^-] / [HA]) \quad (13.3)$$

Equations (13.2) and (13.3) are used:

(a) to determine the pK_a by following changes in solubility,
(b) to allow the prediction of solubility at any pH provided that the intrinsic solubility (C_o) and pK_a are known, and
(c) to facilitate the selection of suitable salt-

forming compounds and predict the solubility and pH properties of the salts.

Albert and Serjeant (1984) give a detailed account of how to obtain precise pK_a values by potentiometry, spectroscopy and conductivity and there is further discussion in Chapter 3 of this book.

Salts

A major improvement in solubility can be achieved by selection of a salt. Acceptable pharmaceutical salts are shown in Table 13.4 which also includes their corresponding pK_a values (see Chapter 3 for further discussion). As an example, the consequences of changing chloridiazepoxide to various salt forms is shown in Table 13.5.

Table 13.5 Theoretical solubility and pH of salts of chlordiazepoxide

Salt	pK_a	Salt pH	Solubility ($mg\ ml^{-1}$)
Base	4.80	8.30	2.0
Hydrochloride	−6.10	2.53	<165[1]
Sulphate	−3.00	2.53	Freely soluble
Besylate	0.70	2.53	Freely soluble
Maleate	1.92	3.36	57.1
Tartrate	3.00	3.90	17.9
Benzoate	4.20	4.50	6.0
Acetate[2]	4.76	4.78	4.1

[1] Maximum solubility of chlordiazepoxide hydrochloride, achieved at pH 2.89, is governed by crystal lattice energy and common ions.
[2] Chlordiazepoxide acetate may not form; pK_a too high and close to drug.

In some cases, salts prepared from strong acids or bases are freely soluble but also very hygroscopic. This can lead to instability in tablet or capsule formulations since some drug will dissolve in its own adsorbed films of moisture (the usual prerequisite for breakdown) and in the case of a weak base, a strongly acid solution may be autocatalytic. Accordingly it is often better to use a weak acid or base to form the salt provided any solubility requirements are met. A salt which is less soluble will also be generally less hygroscopic and form less acidic or basic solutions (Table 13.5). This may also be important in physiological terms. Injections should lie in the pH range 3–9 to prevent vessel or tissue damage and pain at the injection site. Oral syrups should not be too acidic to enhance palatability. Packaging may also be susceptible; undue alkalinity will attack glass, and hydrochloride salts should not be used in aerosol cans since a propellant-acid reaction will corrode the canister.

It is also clear from Table 13.5 that not only does the intrinsic pH of the base solution, in this example chlordiazepoxide, fall significantly from pH 8.3 if salt forms are produced but, as a consequence, the solubility increases exponentially (Eqns 13.2 and 13.3). This has important implications in vivo. A weak base with an intrinsic solubility greater than 1 mg ml^{-1} will be freely soluble in the gastrointestinal tract, especially in the stomach. None the less it is usually better to formulate with a salt since it will control the pH of the diffusion layer (the saturated solution immediately adjacent to the dissolving surface). For example, although chlordiazepoxide base (C_s = 2 mg ml^{-1} at pH 8.3) meets the requirements for in vivo 'solubility' (Kaplan, 1972); commercial capsules contain chlordiazepoxide hydrochloride (C_s = 165 mg ml^{-1} at pH 2.53).

A weak base will have a high dissolution rate in the stomach, but as it moves down the gastrointestinal tract the pH rises and dissolution rate falls. Conversely a weak acid has minimal dissolution in the stomach but it becomes more soluble and its dissolution rate increases as it moves down the gut. Paradoxically as dissolution rate increases, so absorption falls because the drug is ionized.

The dissolution rate of a particular salt is usually much greater than the parent drug. Sodium and potassium salts of weak acids dissolve much more rapidly than the parent acid and some comparative data are shown in Table 13.6. On the basis of bulk pH these salts would be expected to have lower dissolution rates in the stomach. However, the pH of the diffusion layer (found by measuring the pH of a saturated bulk solution) is higher than the pH of gastric fluid (which is usually approximately pH 1.5) because of their buffering action. The pH approximates to a saturated unbuffered aqueous solution (calculated pH in Table 13.6) and the dissolution rate is governed by this pH and not the bulk media pH. In the intestine, the salt does not depress the pH, unlike the acid which is neutralized, and the diffusion layer pH is again raised to promote dissolution. Since solubility is exponentially dependent on pH (Eqns 13.2 and 13.3) there is a significant increase in dissolution rate over the free acid. Providing that the acid forming the salt is strong, the pH of the solution adjacent to the dissolving surface will be that of the salt, whereas for the dissolving free base, it will be the pH of the bulk dissolving media. With weak bases, their salts dissolve rapidly in the stomach but there is no absorption since the drug is ionized and absorption is delayed until the intestine. There, any undissolved drug, as salt, rapidly dissolves since the higher diffusion layer pH compensates for the higher bulk pH which would be extremely unfavourable to the free base. Data for chlordiazepoxide are shown in Table 13.5. The maleate

Table 13.6 Dissolution rates of weak acids and their sodium salts

Drug	pKa	pH (at C_S)	Dissolution rate (mg cm^{-2} min^{-1}) $\times$ 10^2	
			Dissolution media	
			0.1M HCl (pH 1.5)	phosphate (pH 6.8)
Salicylic acid	3.0	2.40	1.7	27
Sodium salicylate		8.78	1870	2500
Benzoic acid	4.2	2.88	2.1	14
Sodium benzoate		9.35	980	1770
Sulphathiazole	7.3	4.97	<0.1	0.5
Sodium sulphathiazole		10.75	550	810

Dissolution rate data from Nelson (1958).

salt has a predicted solubility of 57 mg ml^{-1} but more importantly reduces the pH by 5 units. By controlling diffusion layer pH, the dissolution rate can increase many fold, independently of its position in the gastrointestinal tract.

Miller and Holland (1960) stated that different salts of a drug rarely change its pharmacology, only its physical properties. Wagner (1961) qualified this statement to acknowledge that salts do effect the intensity of the response. The salt form does change the physicochemical properties of the drug. Changes in dissolution rate and solubility affect the rate and extent of absorption (bioavailability), and changes in hygroscopicity and stability influence formulation.

Consequently each new drug candidate must be examined extensively to choose the most suitable salt for formulation and because each potential salt will behave differently, each requires separate preformulation screening.

Solvents

As mentioned in the introduction, it is generally necessary to anticipate the formulation of an injection even if there is no intention of actually marketing such a product. The first choice for a solvent is obviously water. However, although the drug may be freely soluble, some are unstable in aqueous solution. Accordingly water-miscible solvents must be used (a) as cosolvents in formulations to improve solubility or stability and (b) in analysis to facilitate extraction and separation (e.g. in chromatography).

Oils are used in emulsions, topicals (creams and ointments), intramuscular injections and liquid-fill oral preparations (soft and hard gelatin capsules) when aqueous pH and cosolvent solubility and stability are unattainable. Table 13.7 shows a range of solvents to fulfil these needs. Aqueous methanol is widely used in h.p.l.c. and is the standard solvent in sample extraction during analysis and stability testing. It is often made acidic or alkaline to increase solvent power and ensure consistent ionic conditions for u.v. analysis. Other pharmaceutical solvents are available (see Spiegel and Noseworthy, 1963) but are generally only required in special cases. The most acceptable non-aqueous solvents pharmaceutically are glycerol, propylene glycol and ethanol. Generally for a lipophilic drug (i.e. one with a partition coefficient (log P) greater than 1), solubility doubles through this series.

Where bulk is limited and when the aqueous solubility is inadequate, it is useful to measure the solubility in aqueous cosolvent mixtures rather than in a pure organic solvent. Whereas solubilities at other levels and their mixtures can be predicted, the solubility in pure solvent is often inconsistent. Furthermore, formulations rarely demand pure non-aqueous solvent, particularly injections. For example, ethanol should only be used up to 10% in an injection to prevent haemolysis and pain at the injection site (Cadwallader, 1978).

The reader will find more details on the properties of solutions in Chapter 3 and on the formulation of solutions in Chapter 14.

Partition coefficient (K_w^o)

Partition coefficient (solvent:water quotient of drug distribution) has a number of applications which are relevant to preformulation.
(a) Solubility: both aqueous and in mixed solvents.

Table 13.7 Recommended solvents for preformulation screening

Solvent	Dielectric constant (ϵ)	Solubility parameter (δ)	Application
Water	80	24.4	All
Methanol	32	14.7	Extraction, separation
0.1 M HCl (pH 1.07)			Dissolution (gastric), basic extraction
0.1 M NaOH (pH 13.1)			Acidic extraction
Buffer (pH 7)			Dissolution (intestinal)
Ethanol	24	12.7	Formulation, extraction
Propylene glycol	32	12.6	Formulation
Glycerol	43	16.5	Formulation
PEG 300 or 400	35		Formulation

Solvents are considered further in the chapter on the formulation of solutions (Chapter 14).

(b) Drug absorption *in vivo*: applied to a homologous drug series for structure activity relationships (SAR).

(c) Partition chromatography: choice of column (h.p.l.c.) or plate (t.l.c.) and choice of mobile phase (eluant), see Section 4.

The measurement of K_w^o and its use in cosolvent solubility and structure activity relationships are pertinent here, while application in aqueous solubility prediction is discussed under melting point (Section 3) and in chromatography in Section 4.

Cosolvent solubility

The relative polarities of solvents have been scaled using dielectric constant (ϵ), solubility parameter (δ), interfacial tension (γ) and hydrophilic–lipophilic balance (HLB), the latter normally being applied to non-ionic surfactants in emulsion technology. The best solvent in any given situation is one whose polarity matches that of the solute; an ideal, fully compatible solution exists when $\delta_{solvent} = \delta_{solute}$. This can be ascertained by determining solubility maxima, using a substituent contribution approach (Fedors, 1974). An alternative measure is to evaluate the dielectic requirement of the system (Paruta & others, 1965).

However the most practically useful scale of polarity or lipophilicity for a solute is its K_w^o oil: water partition coefficient, since the other approaches do not allow easy estimates for the behaviour of crystalline solids (solutes).

For a wide range of drugs it is possible to relate solvent solubility and the partition coefficient ($\log K_w^o = \log P$). Yalkowsky and Roseman (1981) derived the following expression for 48 drugs in propylene glycol

$$\log C_s = \log C_w + f (0.89 \log P + 0.03) \quad (13.4)$$

Equation 13.4 can be applied more generally by introducing a factor ϕ to account for the relative solvent power of pharmaceutical solvents found in practice (Table 13.8), and predicted by comparison of interfacial tension against a liquid hydrocarbon, tetradecane (Yalkowsky *et al.*, 1975).

Equation 13.4 now becomes, for a wide range of solvents:

Table 13.8 Solvent power (ϕ) of some pharmaceutical solvents

Solvent	Relative solvent power
Glycerol	0.5
Propylene glycol (PEG 300 and 400)	1
Ethanol	2
DMA, DMF	4

$$\log C_s = \log C_o + f(\log \phi + 0.89 \log P + 0.03) \quad (13.5)$$

Methodology and structure activity prediction

Choice of non-aqueous solvent (oil) The oil: water partition (K_w^o) is a measure of the relative lipophilicity (oil-loving) nature of a compound, usually in the unionized state (HA or B), between an aqueous phase and an immiscible lipophilic solvent or oil. Many partition solvents have been used (Leo *et al.*, 1971), but the largest data base has been generated using *n*-octanol. This is, aside from any scientific argument, the major justification to continue its use in preformulation. The solubility parameter of octanol ($\delta = 10.24$) lies midway in the range for the majority of drugs (δ = between 8 and 12) although some non-polar ($\delta < 7$) and polar drugs ($\delta > 13$) are encountered. This allows more easily measurable results than in inert solvents (e.g. hydrocarbons) since it is convenient to partition between equal volumes of oil and aqueous phases.

A typical technique is the *shake flask method* whereby the drug, dissolved in one of the phases, is shaken with the other partitioning solvent for 30 minutes, allowed to stand for 5 minutes and then the majority of the lower aqueous phase (density of octanol = 0.8258 g ml^{-1}) is run off and centrifuged for 60 minutes at 2000 rpm. The aqueous phase is assayed before (ΣC) and after (C_w, aqueous solubility) partitioning to give $K_w^o = (\Sigma C - C_w)/C_w$.

Clearly if the transfer of solute to the oil phase is small, ΔC_w is small and any analytical error increases error in the estimate of K_w^o. Indeed to encourage greater aqueous loss ($>\Delta C_w$) a considerably more polar solvent, *n*-butanol, has been used. Where the partition coefficient is high, it is usual to reduce the ratio of the oil phase from 1:1 to 1:4 or 1:9 in order to increase the aqueous concentration (C_w) to a measurable level. For a 1:9 oil:water ratio $K_w^o = (10 \, \Sigma C - C_w)/C_w$.

The partition of a polar solute between an inert non-polar hydrocarbon e.g. hexane, heptane etc., is quite different to hydrogen bonding solvents like octanol (Hansch and Dunn, 1972). The behaviour of the weak acid phenol ($pK_a = 10$) and weak base nicotine ($pK_a = 3.1$) is worthy of note. For phenol, $K_w^{octanol} = 29.5$ whereas $K_w^{hexane} = 0.11$. The acidic solvent, chloroform, suppresses partition ($K_w^o = 2.239$) whereas although ethyl acetate and diethyl ether are more polar, the basic behaviour of the solvents give the highest K_w^o. With solvents capable of both hydrogen donation and acceptable (octanol, nitrobenzene and oleyl alcohol) K_w^o is intermediate. For nicotine, the behaviour is reversed and the hydrogen donor (acidic) solvent, chloroform, partitions most strongly ($K_w^o = 77.625$), even though the neutral solvent, nitrobenzene, which is marginally more lipophilic (log P = 1.87 against 1.96 for chloroform) gives similar values for both phenol and nicotine. Clearly solute and solvent characteristics are important.

In general, polar solvents are advocated to correlate biological activity with physicochemical properties (Hansch and Dunn, 1972). Solvents less polar than octanol, measured by water solvency, have been termed hyperdiscriminating by Rekker (1977) while those more polar, e.g. butanols and pentanols, as hypodiscriminating. This concept refers to the discriminating power of a partitioning solvent within a homologous series. With n-butanol, the values of log P tend to be too close while with heptane and other inert hydrocarbons, the differences in solute lipophilicities are exaggerated. n-Octanol generally gives a range consistent with other physicochemical properties when compared to drug absorption in the g.i. tract. Hyperdiscriminating solvents reflect more closely the transport across the blood–brain barrier, while hypodiscriminating solvents give values consistent with buccal absorption (Fig. 13.2).

Based on the assertion by Leo *et al.* (1971) in rationalizing the effects of different partitioning · solvents, a good correlation exists between the solvent water content at saturation (log [H_2O] mg/100 ml) and solvent lipophilicity. This relationship also indicates the lipophilicity of biological membranes and the relative discrimination power (Rekker, 1977) of the partitioning solvents.

Certainly within a laboratory it is imperative to standardize on methodology, especially the solvent. Where solubility constraints allow, this should invariably be n-octanol especially since the existing data bank is extensive (Hansch and Leo, 1979).

Structure-activity relationships Since the pioneering work of Meyer (1899) and Overton (1901) numerous studies on correlating molecular structure and biological activity have been reported (Tute, 1971). These structure–activity relationships (SAR) can rationalize drug activity and, particularly in modern medicinal chemistry, facilitate a scientific approach to the design of more effective, elegant structural analogues.

The application of SAR depends on a sound knowledge of the physicochemical properties of each new drug candidate in a therapeutic class, and therefore preformulation is a particularly useful information source.

It is assumed in SAR that (Collander, 1951):

$$\log K_w^o = a \times \log K_w^{octanol} + b \quad (13.6)$$

This relationship holds for for all polar and semi-polar solvents. However, correlations are poor with non-polar solvents (hexane, heptane, cyclohexane, carbon tetachloride and iso-octane) and again this seems to be related to water content. Given the obvious importance of water, it is imperative that the octanol is saturated with the aqueous phase and the aqueous phase with octanol prior to any determination; otherwise the partitioning behaviour of the drug will be complicated by the mutual partitioning of the two solvents.

While the aqueous phase is often simply water, it is better to measure log P under controlled pH using aqueous buffers. All drugs capable of ionization and with a measurable pK_a, whether weak acids or bases will have intrinsic buffer capacity affecting the aqueous pH. Depending on the degree of dissociation, this will lead to an apparent K_w^o rather than the true (absolute) value, when the

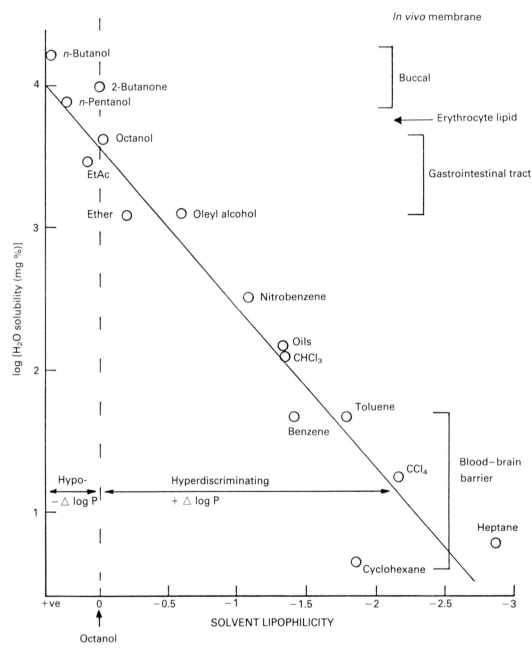

Fig. 13.2 Discriminating power of partitioning solvents as a function of their water capacity

drug is unionized. Since the ionized species will have greater aqueous solubility and lower lipophilicity to HA or BOH then the measured K_w^o (apparent) will be inevitably lower. Accordingly K_w^o (true) should be measured at >2 pH units away from the pK_a ($pK_a - 2$ (acid); $pK_a + 2$ (base)) and the aqueous phase should contain a suitable buffer. Given the importance of $\log P$ ($\log K_w^o$) in SAR, comparative data generated in a therapeutic class ($R_n.X$, where X is the therapeutic nucleus and n is a number of substituents R) should also be determined at a physiological pH of 7.4.

Quantitative SAR (QSAR) is based on the

premise that drug absorption is a multi-partitioning process (repeated adsorption and desorption) across cellular membranes and dependent on the lipophilicity of the drug, and the rate of penetration is proportional to the drug partition coefficient *in vitro*. Clearly the ionic condition *in vivo* will affect any correlation and accordingly for dissociating drugs, the *in vitro* conditions should be similar. The widespread use of octanol in these studies (Hansch & Dunn, 1972) and the existence of many excellent correlations *in vivo* is probably not entirely fortuitous. Octanol exhibits hydrogen bonding acceptor and donor properties typical of many biological macromolecules. Furthermore the partial polarity of octanol allows the inclusion of water, which is also a feature of biological lipid membranes. This leads to a more complex partitioning behaviour than a less polar, essentially anhydrous solvent.

The effect of salt formation on the measured log P is shown in Table 13.9. Generally the log P differs from between 3 and 4 (i.e. K_w^o ranges from 1000 to 10 000), and the lipophilicity falls by three to four orders of magnitude which accounts for the significant increase in solubility of the salt.

The physicochemical model for biological activity assumes that activity of a compound is related to these different factors associated with molecular structure:

(a) electronic (charge)
(b) steric (spatial size)
(c) hydrophobic effects (partitioning).

Table 13.9 The effect of salt formation on the log P of some weakly basic drugs

Free base and hydrochloride salt	log P	Δ log P
Chlorpromazine	5.35	3.84
Chlorpromazine HCl	1.51	
Promazine	4.49	3.58
Promazine HCl	0.91	
Trifluopromazine	5.19	4.28
Trifluopromazine HCl	1.78	
Trifluoperazine	5.01	3.34
Trifluoperazine HCl	1.69	
Diphenylhydramine	3.30	3.42
Diphenylhydramine HCl	−0.12	
Propranolol	3.18	3.63
Propranolol HCl	−0.45	
Phenylpropanolamine	1.83	2.92
Phenylpropanolamine HCl	−1.09	

Account must also be taken of structural and theoretical aspects so that:

$$\text{Biological Activity} = f[(\text{electronic}) + (\text{steric}) + (\text{hydrophobic}) + (\text{structural/theoretical})]$$

$$(13.7)$$

The electronic parameter above is quantified by the sigma (σ) substituent constant of Hammelt (1940) and reflects chemical reactivity in a homologous series. The substituent constant (σ) is positive for electron withdrawal (acids), while electron donor groups (bases) give a negative value. It can be used to predict pK_a (Perrin *et al.*, 1981).

Steric effects occur when there is a direct interaction between the substituent and the parent nucleus and is also related to substituent bulk. High positive values of the steric effect parameter, E_s, indicate significant steric effects with intra- and intermolecular hindrance to a reaction or binding at the active site.

The hydropholic component is measured by the partition or distribution behaviour of a compound between an aqueous phase and an immiscible lipid phase and parallels drug adsorption and distribution *in vivo*. Hansch and Fujita (1964) demonstrated a general relationship between the partition coefficient within a series by quantifying differences using an additive substituent constant (π). This constant is related almost completely to the effect of particular substituent and much less to the parent compound and this allows the prediction of the partition coefficient, log P, of a new derivative with reasonable accuracy. Additionally π can be related to biological effect since it is an additive component of the partition coefficient and has led to the wider application of SAR, which by other modifications, notably taking into account aromatic electron density and steric effects, to give *quantitative* SAR (i.e. QSAR) (see Davis and Higuchi, 1970 for application of QSAR equations).

While all these substituents are useful, log P remains the most useful physical parameter and undoubtedly the most reliable data and correlations still come from experimentally derived partition values for the analogues of a series.

Dissolution

The dissolution rate of a drug is only important where it is the rate-limiting step in the absorption process. Kaplan (1972) suggested that provided that the solubility of a drug exceeded 10 mg ml^{-1} at pH 7 then no bioavailability or dissolution related problems were to be expected. Below 1 mg ml^{-1}, such problems were quite possible and salt formation (see Section 2, Salts) could improve absorption and solubility by controlling the pH of the microenvironment independently of the drug and dosage forms position within the g.i. tract.

The equations controlling the rate of dissolution of solids are described in Chapter 5 and the biopharmaceutical consequences discussed in Chapter 9. The Nernst (1904) modification to the Noyes–Whitney (1897) equation can be applied generally to the dissolution of solids (see Chapter 5).

Intrinsic dissolution rate

When dissolution is solely controlled by diffusion (transport control) the rate of diffusion is directly proportional to the saturated concentration of the drug in solution (i.e. solubility). Under these conditions the rate constant K_1 is defined by (Levich, 1962):

$$K_1 = 0.62 \ D^{2/3} \ \nu^{1/6} \ \omega^{1/2} \qquad (13.8)$$

where ν is the kinematic viscosity and ω is the angular velocity of a rotating disc of drug. By maintaining the dissolution fluid viscosity and rotational speed of the sample constant, the dissolution rate (dm/dt) from a constant surface area (A) will be constant and related solely to solubility. Under sink conditions $(C_s >>> C)$ gives

$$dc/dt = \frac{A}{V} \ K_1 \ C_s \qquad (13.9)$$

and the intrinsic dissolution rate (IDR) is given by

$$IDR = K_1 \ C_s \ (\text{mg cm}^2 \ \text{min}^{-1}) \quad (13.10)$$

This constant rate differs from the dissolution from conventional dosage forms, which is known as total dissolution (mg min^{-1}), where the exposed surface area (A) is uncontrolled as disintegration, deaggregation and dissolution proceed. Accord-

ingly the IDR is independent of formulation effects and measures the intrinsic properties of the drug and salts as a function of dissolution media effects, e.g. pH, ionic strength and counter ions.

Measurement of intrinsic dissolution rate At the preformulation stage a compressed disc of the material can be made by slow compression of 200 mg of drug in a 13 mm i.r. disc punch and die set to a high compaction pressure greater than 350 MPa (to ensure zero porosity) and a long dwell time (to improve compaction).

The metal surfaces in contact should be prelubricated with, for example, stearic acid using a 5% w/v solution in chloroform. The compressed disc is fixed to the holder of the rotating basket apparatus BP using a low melting paraffin wax and successively dipped so that the top and sides of the disc are coated. The lower circular face should be cleared of residual wax using a scalpel and carefully scraped to remove any stearic acid transferred from the punch face.

The coated disc is rotated at 100 rpm, 20 mm from the bottom of a 1-litre flat bottomed dissolution flask containing 1 litre of fluid at 37 °C. The amount of drug release is then monitored, usually by u.v. spectrometry, with time. The slope of the line divided by the exposed surface area gives the IDR, for example, in mg cm^2 min^{-1}.

Each candidate should be measured in 0.05 M HCl (gastric : pH 1) and phosphate buffer pH 7 (intestinal), and distilled water especially if sink conditions are not possible for a weak base at pH 7 or a weak acid in 0.05 M HCl. Sink conditions maintain the bulk concentration (C) at a low level, otherwise the rate of dissolution is progressively reduced and the plot of concentration against time becomes non-linear. It is recommended that C should not exceed 0.1 C_s.

By comparing the IDR of a salt in water with that obtained in acid and alkali, or the free base with its salts in the same medium, a measure of the salt's ability to control its immediate microenvironment will emerge.

The equation derived from the Henderson–Hasselbalch equation (see Chapter 3)

$$IDR = k' \ (C_o(1 + \text{antilog} \ (pK_a - pH))) \quad (13.11)$$

shows that the rate of dissolution of a drug

candidate is clearly a function of its intrinsic solubility (C_o), its dissociation constant (pK_a) and either the pH of the bulk dissolution medium or microenvironment created by the dissolving salt. Using the measured rate of the free base at known bulk pH, expected rates in other media, using the experimental salts, can be calculated and compared with experimental values.

The importance of improvements in the IDR, due to microenvironmental pH control, lies in the likely improvement in *in vivo* performance of a salt over the parent drug. Where no increase is found, there is likely to be no advantage in using that particular salt. Improvements are obviously more likely if the salt former is strong. For a weak base, the hydrochloride $(pK_a = -6.10)$ offers the best advantage, but this may prove, in some instances, disappointing. Thus measurement of IDR can be useful diagnostically.

Common ion effect

A common interaction with solvent, which is often overlooked, is the common ion effect. The addition of a common ion often reduces the solubility of a slightly soluble electrolyte (Long & McDevitt, 1952). This 'salting out' results from the removal of water molecules as solvent due to the competing hydration of other ions. The reverse process, 'salting in', arises with larger anions, e.g. benzoate, salicylate, which open the water structure. These hydrotropes increase the solubility of poorly water-soluble compounds, e.g. diazepam.

Hydrochloride salts often exhibit suboptimal solubility in gastric juice due to the abundance of Cl^- ions. A number of examples from the pharmaceutical literature are shown in Table 13.10 for acidic hydrochloride solutions. Other counter ions, other than Cl^-, such as nitrate, sulphate and phosphate, have also been implicated.

To identify a common ion interaction, the IDR of the hydrochloride salt should be compared between:

(a) water and water containing 1.2% w/v NaCl,
(b) 0.05 M HCl and 0.9% w/v NaCl in 0.05 M HCl.

Both saline media contain 0.2 M Cl^-, which is typically encountered in fluids *in vivo*.

Table 13.10 Examples of weakly basic drugs which have decreased solubility in acidic (HCl) solution

Chlortetracycline
Demethylchlortetracycline
Methacycline
Demeclocycline
Papaverine
Trihexyphenidyl
Isoxsuprine
Phenazopyridine
Cyproheptadine
Bromhexine
Triamterene

A common ion effect with Cl^- will result in a significantly reduced IDR in the presence of sodium chloride. Other salt forms are then indicated, e.g. sulphate, tosylate, mesylate etc., but the parent molecule may well still remain sensitive to Cl^- and solubilities will be suppressed in the presence of saline although not to the same extent since Cl^- is not involved in the dissolving microenvironment. Any improvement with the new salt can be assessed by again measuring the IDR with and without saline. Since some compounds are sensitive to other counter ions, e.g. nitrate, sulphate and phosphate, this can be demonstrated by including the appropriate sodium salt in the dissolution medium. The phase solubility studies of Dittert *et al.* (1964) indicated that basic amine drugs were more soluble in organic acids than inorganic. Where a hydrochloride salt exhibits suboptimal solubility then the next logical choice is probably a salt of toluene sulphonic acid (tosylate: $pK_a - 1.34$). Mesylate, napsylate, besylate and maleate salts offer progressively more weaker acidic alternatives (Table 13.4). With low solubility amine drugs the salts of polyhydroxy acids, e.g. lactate, often give the greatest aqueous solubility due to their accessible hydroxy groupings (Senior, 1973; Agharkar *et al.*, 1976).

3 MELTING POINT

The melting point of a drug can be measured using three techniques:

(a) capillary melting
(b) hot stage microscopy
(c) differential scanning calorimetry thermal analysis.

Capillary melting

Capillary melting (the observation of melting in a capillary tube in contact with a heated metal block) gives information about the melting range but it is difficult to assign an accurate melting point.

Hot stage microscopy

This is the visual observation of melting under a microscope equipped with a heated and lagged sample stage. The heating rate is controllable and up to three transitions can be registered. It is more precise since the phase transitions (first melt, 50% melt and completion) can be registered on a recorder as the melting proceeds and, by virtue of high magnification, the values are more accurate.

Differential scanning calorimetry and differential thermal analysis

Neither of the previous methods is as versatile as either differential thermal analysis (DTA) or differential scanning calorimetry (DSC). An additional advantage is that the sample size required is only 2–5 mg.

DTA measures the temperature difference between the sample and a reference as a function of temperature or time when heating at a constant rate. DSC is similar to DTA except that the instrument measures the amount of energy required to keep the sample at the same temperature as the reference, i.e. it measures the enthalpy of transition.

When no physical or chemical change is occurring within the sample then there is neither a temperature change nor the need to input energy to maintain an isotherm. However, when phase changes occur then latent heat suppresses the temperature increase (or fall) and the change in temperature or isothermal energy required registers on a recorder as a result of an electrical signal generated by thermocouples. Crystalline transitions, fusion, evaporation and sublimation are obvious changes in state which can be quantified (Fig. 13.3).

The major concern in preformulation is polymorphism and the measurement of melting point and other phase changes are the primary diag-

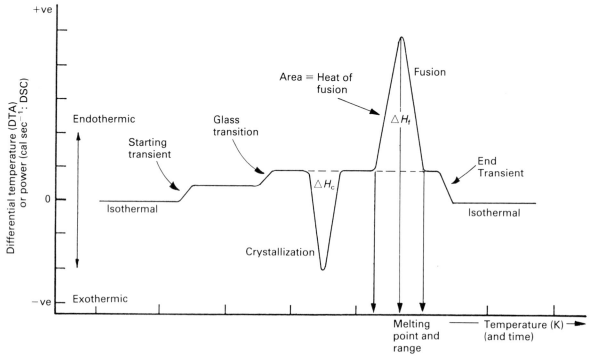

Fig. 13.3 Schematic differential scanning calorimeter thermogram

nostic tool. Confirmation by ion spectroscopy and X-ray diffraction are common.

Polymorphism

A polymorph is a solid material with at least two different molecular arrangements each of which gives a distinct crystal species. These differences disappear in the liquid or vapour state. Of concern are their relative stabilities and solubility. The lowest melting species is generally stable and other polymorphs are metastable and convert to the stable form. There are also large differences in their physical properties so that they behave as distinct chemical entities. Solubility (particularly important in suspensions and biopharmaceutically), melting point, density, crystal shape, optical and electrical properties and vapour pressure are often very different for each polymorph.

Polymorphism is remarkably common, particularly within certain structural groups: 63% of barbiturates, 67% of steroids and 40% of sulphonamides exhibit polymorphism (Kuhnert-Brandstatter, 1965).

The steroid, progesterone, has as many as five polymorphs, while the sulphonamide sulphabenz-amide has four polymorphs and three solvates. The importance of polymorphism is illustrated by the biopharmaceutical data for fluprednisolone (Fig. 13.4).

It is convention to number the polymorphs in order of stability at room temperature starting with Form I using Roman numerals. Form I usually has the highest melting point and lowest solubility; in suspension formulation it is essential to use the least soluble polymorph because of Ostwald ripening (Pearson & Varney, 1969).

Accordingly, in preformulation, the following should be investigated.

(a) How many polymorphs exist?
(b) How stable are the metastable forms?
(c) Is there an amorphous glass?
(d) Can the metastable forms be stabilized?
(e) What is the solubility of each form?
(f) Will a more soluble form survive processing and storage?

Pseudopolymorphism

Before this study begins, the presence of false polymorphs, or pseudopolymorphs, should be identified since most polymorphs can be obtained by changing the recrystallizing solvent. Typical

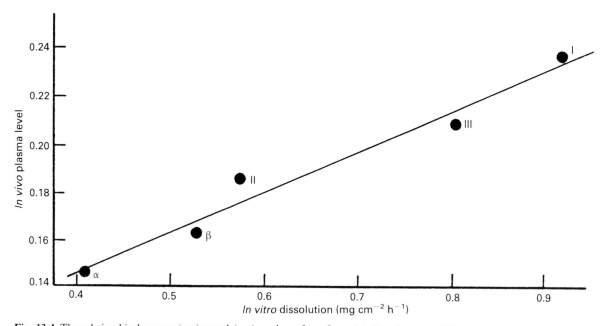

Fig. 13.4 The relationship between *in vitro* and *in vivo* release from fluprednisolone implants. (From the data of Haleblian and Biles, 1967)

solvents inducing polymorphic change are: water, methanol, ethanol, acetone and chloroform, *n*-propanol, isopropyl alcohol, *n*-butanol, *n*-pentanol, toluene and benzene. The presence of trace levels of solvent (either water or organic) is usual in early batches of new drug candidates, as residues from the precipitation process used in the final crystallization. These can become molecular additions to the crystal and change its habit. These hydrates (water) and solvates (e.g. methanolate, ethanolate) have been confused with true polymorphism and led to the term pseudopolymorphism. The distinction between these false forms and true polymorphs can be obtained by observing the melting behaviour of the compound dispersed in silicone oil using hot stage microscopy. Pseudopolymorphs will evolve a gas (steam or solvent vapour) causing bubbling of the oil. True polymorphs merely melt, forming a second globular phase. The temperature at which the solvent volatilizes will be close to the boiling point of the solvent and can be used for identification.

True polymorphism

After the study of pseudomorphism, the evaluation of true polymorphism can proceed unconfounded. Many polymorphs are obtained by solvent manipulation. Others can be produced without the presence of solvent by thermal techniques, notably sublimation and recrystallization from the melt. Supercooling of the melt is particularly useful in discovering unstable modifications.

The initial difficulty is to measure the melting point of the metastable form, and here heating rate, either by DSC or hot stage, is critical. Too rapid heating will obscure the endotherm, while too slow a heating rate may allow transition or encourage decomposition. Often therefore comparison at two rates, e.g. 2 and 20 °C min^{-1} is necessary.

The difference in melting point (Δm.p.) between polymorphs is a measure of the metastable polymorph stability. Where Δm.p. < 1 °C then neither is significantly more stable and either may be obtained upon conventional crystallization. If Δm.p. is 25–50 °C then the lower melting species will be difficult to crystallize and will revert rapidly. The closer the two melting

points (Δm.p. between 1 and 25 °C), then the unstable forms(s) can be obtained easily before a solid–solid transformation occurs. This can be suppressed by using small samples since individual crystals of even highly unstable forms can be melted.

If it appears that polymorphism is occurring, or is likely to occur, in the samples supplied for preformulation work then a cooperative study with the bulk chemists should determine the most stable form (chemically and physically). Differences in solubility and melting point must also be assessed and then a decision can be made to determine which form to progress through to the next stage of formulation. Small differences in stability but higher solubility of a relatively metastable form may lead to a preferential choice of a polymorph other than Form I.

Crystal purity

Thermal analysis has been widely used as a method of purity determination (Grady *et al.*, 1973) and the USP includes an appendix describing the method. This is particularly pertinent at the preformulation stage since early samples of a new drug are inevitably 'dirty' while improvements in synthetic route are made. Thermal analysis is rapid and will discriminate 0.002 mole % of impurity.

Solubility

Possibly the most important reason that melting point studies are performed during preformulation is that it reflects crystalline solubility. Such studies are particularly important at this stage because the scarcity of available powder often precludes accurate solubility determinations.

It has been found that melting point and solubility are related *via* the latent heat of fusion which is the amount of heat generated during melting or fusion. It is the amount of energy required to increase interatomic or intermolecular distances to facilitate an increase in disorder, to overcome crystal lattice energy and allow melting. A crystal with weak bonds has a low melting point and low heat of fusion. Conversely a strong crystal lattice leads to a high melting point and a high heat of fusion. Since solubility also requires the disruption of crystal structure to allow molecular dispersion in the solvent, it is also influenced by intermolecular forces.

Polymorphs differ in melting point and solubility. The existence of different crystal arrangements for the same compound inevitably leads to differences in crystal lattice energy since intermolecular distances will be different in the alternative forms. This effect is shown for riboflavine in Fig. 13.5.

The differences outlined above have led to differences *in vivo* in the blood level curves of some polymorphs. Some examples of this and the resulting biopharmaceutical consequences are discussed in Chapter 9 and the reader is referred to this for further information.

4 ASSAY DEVELOPMENT

In Section 1 of this chapter a simple u.v. assay was described which enabled the quantitative determination of drug in solution and could be used to generate the solubility data described in Section 2. However, the assumption that the drug is stable enough to survive these manipulations may not always be valid since drugs are notoriously unstable, particularly as hydrolysis is often the predominant cause (see Section 5). In order to

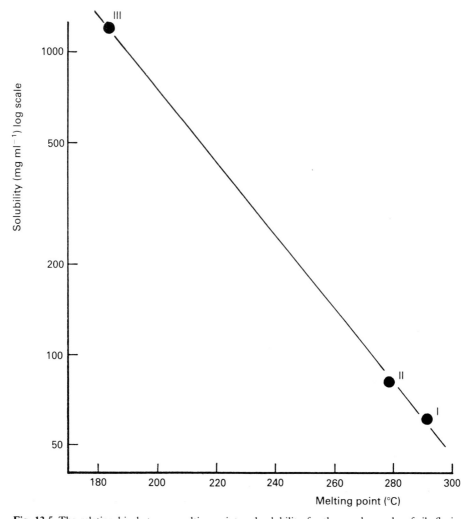

Fig. 13.5 The relationship between melting point and solubility for three polymorphs of riboflavine

follow drug stability, both in solution and in solid phase, it is necessary to have suitable stability indicating assays. In some cases u.v. spectroscopy can be used, but in general chromatography is required to separate the drug from its degradation products and interfering excipients. Thin layer chromatography (t.l.c.) is widely used in a semi-quantitative mode to estimate impurity levels, to establish the number of impurities and for collecting samples from the plate for subsequent injection into the column of h.p.l.c. (high performance (pressure) liquid chromatography) equipment. H.p.l.c. is now acknowledged as the most versatile and powerful technique in pharmaceutical analysis; it is the method of choice in preformulation stability assessment (Section 5).

U.v. spectroscopy

The principles of u.v. spectroscopy were enumerated in Section 1 and at that stage of preformulation will have served to quantify many of the subsequent physical constants and solubilities in Section 2. However, in general, u.v. analysis is not a potent and widely applicable method when stability is a concern or where other compounds (drugs or excipients) in the analytical sample absorb u.v. light. Consequently t.l.c. and particularly h.p.l.c. have largely superseded u.v. spectroscopy as a basic analytical tool in stability assessment, although of course u.v. detection is still a feature in both t.l.c. and h.p.l.c., once the components have been separated (resolved). None the less some compounds decompose to yield products which do not interfere, i.e. their chromophores or spectra do not overlap, and then u.v. analysis is perfectly acceptable and recourse to chromatography quite unnecessary.

Notwithstanding these reservations, certain u.v. techniques are worthy of discussion:

(a) solubility (section 2)
(b) molecular weight
(c) pK_a
(d) assay (potency: Section 1)
(e) mixtures
   (i) resolving compound products
   (ii) stability: hydrolysis, oxidation (coloured products).

First it is important to recognize the attributes of an acceptable assay and the dependence on adequate instrumentation, cells and solvents. This is dealt with in detail in analytical texts and will not be repeated here.

Molecular weight

To a first approximation, the molar extinction coefficient (e) of a chromophore (absorbing molecular group) is unaffected by distant substituent groups in the molecule, especially if they do not absorb in the vicinity of the main chromophore. If, therefore, e of a chromophore is known from another related compound in the series, the molecular weight (mol. wt) of the new derivative can be calculated from the absorbance of a solution of known concentration (Cunningham et al., 1951) since mol. wt = $10 \, e/E$.

pK_a

The determination of pK_a by spectroscopy is indicated when solubility is too low, or when the pK_a is particularly low (<2) or high (>11) for determination by potentiometry. The method depends upon determining the ratio of molecular species (neutral molecule at pH $< pK_a - 2$ (acid), pH $> pK_a + 2$ (base)) to the ionized species in a series of seven buffers (pH = $\pm 1 + pK_a$). The analytical wavelength (λ) is chosen where the greatest difference in absorbance exists between the molecular species and the pure ionized moiety at two pH units from the pK_a.

Mixtures

The lack of specificity of u.v. generally requires the separation of mixtures by h.p.l.c. before u.v. detection of the individual components. However, in some cases the breakdown products have sufficiently different chromophores and absorption spectra to enable differentiation of the main peak from the minor components even though their individual spectra significantly overlap, since the absorption of a mixture is the sum of the separate absorptions of the components.

Thin layer chromatography (t.l.c.)

All chromatographic procedures emanate from the work of the Russian botanist Tswett (1906) who separated plant pigments by pipetting solutions on to the top of glass tubes packed with alumina, silica, chalk and sucrose and eluting them with various solvents. This interest in colours led to the term chromatography. The term has been retained and is now applied to all chemical quantitative separations. Tswett's work led to the development of column chromatography and then, under pressure by pumping the eluant, to h.p.l.c. Other workers used paper as a support, and before the advent of h.p.l.c., paper chromatography was more important due to its simplicity and speed. T.l.c. arose from a need to satisfactorily separate lipids which paper techniques could not achieve, but it was soon realized that the technique was also considerably more flexible. Paper chromatography is limited by the cellulose support whereas the thin layer of material on a glass plate can be prepared from a slurry of a wide variety of different chemical types, e.g. silica gel, celite, alumina, cellulose (analogous to paper chromatography) and chemically modified celluloses; and more recently with the advent of reversed phase chromatography, C_2, C_8 and C_{18} silanized and diphenyl silica.

The modern basis of t.l.c. was established by Stahl (1956) and separations were found to be considerably shorter than on paper, spots were more compact, resolution was better, submicrogram samples could be separated and recovered if necessary (by scraping away the spot using a fine spatula). These are now usually re-extracted and injected on to h.p.l.c.

T.l.c. is now generally regarded as a reliable and sensitive qualitative technique for the separation of complex mixtures in stability samples. In a typical analysis, extracted samples are spotted 20 mm from the bottom of a square glass plate, 200 mm × 200 mm coated with a dry slurry of silica (250 μm thick) and placed in a closed tank, containing a 10 mm layer of eluting solvent, which has produced a satured vapour phase. The sample is developed (separated) by the capillary movement of the solvent up the plate and is therefore similar to h.p.l.c. except it is a thin flat column

(stationary phase) with solvent (mobile phase) pumped by capillary flux and much of the theory (see Snyder, 1968; Bristow, 1976) is the same. Consequently t.l.c. and h.p.l.c. are complimentary. T.l.c. will quantify the number of components (since they can be seen) and estimate their concentration by reference to standards run concurrently, when h.p.l.c. can quantify their level, confident that all have been separated. The developing solvent for t.l.c. (particularly h.p.t.l.c. (high performance t.l.c.) and reverse phase) is also a useful guide to identify the mobile phase for h.p.l.c.

For further details of t.l.c. and h.p.l.c. the reader is referred to analytical texts.

High performance liquid chromatography (h.p.l.c.)

High performance (pressure) liquid chromatography is essentially column chromatography performed by elution under pressure. By pumping the eluting solvent (mobile phase) under a pressure of up to 40 MPa (about 6000 p.s.i.) and a flow rate of up to 3 ml min^{-1}, the column can be much smaller and use much smaller particle size packing material (stationary phase). This results in shorter retention times (solute time in column), high sensitivity (typically 1 ng), the need for only a small sample volume (0–50 μl) and yet high selectivity (separation power) for the resolution of complex mixtures is possible.

H.p.l.c. methods can be divided into two distinct modes as follows.

Normal phase h.p.l.c.

Normal phase h.p.l.c. is performed by eluting a silica-packed column, which is hydrophilic, with a non-polar mobile phase. The mobile phase is usually hexane to which is added one or more of the following (in increasing order of polarity), chloroform ($CHCl_3$), tetrahydrofuran (THF), acetonitrile (ACN), isopropyl alcohol (IPA) or methanol (MeOH)). Separation is achieved by a process of partition with differential adsorption and desorption of both the solute and solvents during passage down the column. Polar solutes are retained whereas more lipophilic molecules are not. By increasing the polarity of the mobile phase (e.g. by adding MeOH or IPA), polar solutes are eluted more quickly while non-polar solutes are better retained; their order of retention may also change. Decreasing solvent polarity increases polar solute retention and facilitates the elution of lipophilic molecules.

In general, normal phase h.p.l.c. is used for moderately polar solutes, for example, those freely soluble in methanol. Non-polar hydrocarbon-soluble solutes are difficult to retain and very polar, water-soluble solutes are difficult to elute sufficiently.

Reverse phase h.p.l.c.

When the solute is eluted by a polar (largely aqueous) mobile phase over a hydrophobic stationary phase, the chromatography is known as reverse phase. Solute behaviour is the reverse of that described for normal phase h.p.l.c. and uses a hydrophilic silica stationary phase. Separation between the stationary phase and mobile phase is solvophobic, analogous to partition behaviour (see section 2 of this chapter).

Hydrophobicity of the stationary phase is achieved by bonding a coating on to the silica support. The most common bonded phases are alkyl silanes of C_{18} (octadecylsilane, ODS), C_8 (octylsilane, OS) and C_1 (trimethylsilane). The predominantly aqueous mobile phase usually contains methanol, ACN and/or THF to modify solvent polarity by matching the lipophilicity of the solutes in order to facilitate good chromatography.

Ionization control can be achieved by using pH buffers (phosphate and acetate) in the range pH 2–8. The inclusion of 1–2% acetic acid or diethylamine is used to suppress the ionization of weak acids and bases respectively. This is known as *ion-suppression chromatrography*. This technique is used to increase lipophilicity and improve retention of polar solutes.

In general polar solutes have short retention times on reverse phase h.p.l.c. while non-polar compounds are retained. Increasing the mobile phase polarity (by increasing the water concentration) shortens retention for polar solutes while retaining less polar compounds. Decreasing solvent polarity (by decreasing water concentration) helps retain polar compounds while more lipophilic solutes are eluted more rapidly.

Non-aqueous reverse phase (NARP) h.p.l.c., where THF or methylene chloride replaces water in the mobile phase, is used to separate lipophilic solutes.

The great flexibility of choice in mobile phase (by using solvents ranging from water to hexane), the increasing number of available stationary phases (particularly bonded phases) and the inherent sensitivity of h.p.l.c. produces a powerful analytical technique. Accordingly it is the method of choice in preformulation stability studies.

Further details may be found in the literature of h.p.l.c. equipment manufacturers, in the books of Bristow (1976), Pryde and Gilbert (1979) and Hamilton and Sewell (1977) and in standard analytical chemistry texts.

5 DRUG AND PRODUCT STABILITY

Wherever possible, commercial pharmaceutical products should have a shelf life of 5 years. The potency should not fall below 90% at the recommended storage conditions and the product should still look and perform as it did when first manufactured.

By investigating the intrinsic stability of the drug, it is possible to advise on formulation approaches and indicate types of excipient, specific protective additives and packaging which are likely to improve the integrity of the drug and product. Typical stress conditions are shown in Table 13.11.

Drug degradation occurs by four main processes:

(a) hydrolysis
(b) oxidation
(c) photolysis
(d) trace metal catalysis.

Hydrolysis and oxidation are the most common pathways and in general light (c) and metal ions catalyse a subsequent oxidative process.

Table 13.11 Stress conditions used in preformulation stability assessment

Test	Conditions
Solid	
Heat (°C)	4, 20, 30, 37, 37/75% RH, 50 and 75
Moisture uptake	30, 45, 60, 75 and 90% RH at RT[1, 2]
Physical stress	Ball milling
Aqueous solution	
pH	1, 3, 5, 7, 9 and 11 at RT and 37 °C. Reflux in 1 M HCl and 1 M NaOH
Light[3]	U.v. (254 and 366 nm) and visible (south facing window) at RT
Oxidation[3]	Sparging with oxygen at RT; u.v. may accelerate breakdown

[1] RT is ambient room temperature. Can vary between 15 and 25 °C.
[2] Saturated solutions of $MgBr_2$, KNO_2, NaBr, NaCl and KNO_3 respectively.
[3] At pH of maximum stability in simple aqueous solution.

Temperature

Thermal effects are superimposed on all four chemical processes. Clearly a greater available free energy leads to a more rapid reaction and typically a 10 °C increase in temperature produces a 2–5-fold increase in decay.

Often the increase in reaction rate with temperature follows an Arrhenius-type relationship (see Chapter 7). As long as the Arrhenius relationship holds and a plot of the log of the rate of reaction against the reciprocal of absolute temperature yields a straight line, the reaction rate can be calculated at any temperature. In turn this allows a prediction of shelf life at room temperature by extrapolation. This assumption forms the basis of many accelerated stability tests. However, the mechanism or pathway of the chemical breakdown often changes with temperature. This may be indicated by a discontinuity of 'knee joint' in the Arrhenius plot but often this is not easily detected and this would inevitably lead to erroneous conclusions, based on elevated temperature data, to predict shelf lives at room temperature or under refrigeration.

Order of reaction

The time course of degradation depends on the number of reactants whose concentration influences the rate and the orders of reaction and the mathematical relationships relating decomposition to time are described in Chapter 7.

It is often more convenient to express reaction rates in terms of time. The most common is the *half-life*, the time at which the concentration has halved ($t_{\frac{1}{2}}$ or t_{50}). The shelf life of a product can be likewise expressed as t_{90} (i.e. the time for a 10% loss).

In the absence of a definitive value for the activation energy (E_a), which may normally be obtained from the slope of the Arrhenius plot, it is prudent to assume a low value (e.g. 10 kcal mol^{-1}), since this will lead to higher reaction rates and any prediction of shelf life will be conservative. Values for a wide range of reactions are 10–100 kcal mol^{-1}, but are usually in the range 15–60 kcal mol^{-1} with a mean of 19.8 (Kennon, 1964).

Most breakdowns are first order in nature but some are zero order, e.g. aspirin in aqueous suspension, whilst a few are second order, e.g. chlorbutol hydrolysis.

Hydrolysis

The most likely cause of drug instability is hydrolysis. Obviously water plays a dominant role but in many cases it is implicated passively, particularly in solid dosage forms. Here it acts as a solvent vector between two reacting species in solution. The solution is often saturated so that studies in dilute solution can be completely misleading (see Solid-state stability, below).

Hydrolytic reactions involve nucleophilic attack of labile bonds, e.g. lactam > ester > amide > imide, by water on the drug in solution and are first order. When this attack is by a solvent other than water it is known as *solvolysis*.

A number of conditions catalyse the breakdown:

(a) presence of OH^-
(b) presence of H_3O^+
(c) presence of divalent metal ions
(d) ionic hydrolysis (protolysis) is quicker than molecular
(e) heat
(f) light
(g) solution polarity and ionic strength
(h) high drug concentrations.

The influence of pH

The degradation of most drugs is catalysed by extremes of pH, i.e. high $[H_3O^+]$ and $[OH^-]$, and many drugs are most stable between pH 4 and 8. Where maximum stability dictates wider values, it is important for injections that the buffer has a low capacity to prevent unnecessary challenge to the homoeostatic pH 7.4 of blood.

Weakly acidic and basic drugs are most soluble when ionized and it is then that instability is most likely since the species are charged. This leads to a potential problem since many potent drugs are extremely poorly soluble and pH ionization is the most obvious method to obtain a solution. In some cases, therefore, the inclusion of a water-miscible solvent in the formulation will increase stability by (a) suppressing ionization, (b) reducing the extreme of pH required to achieve solubility, (c) contributing itself to solubility, e.g. 20% propylene glycol in chlordiazepoxide injection and (d) reducing the water activity by reducing the polarity of the solvent.

Reactions in aqueous solution are usually catalysed by pH and this is monitored by measuring degradation rates (usually pseudo first order) against pH, keeping temperature, ionic strength and solvent concentration constant. Suitable buffers include acetate, citrate, lactate, phosphate and ascorbate (the latter having intrinsic antioxidant activity).

Solvolysis

Where the reacting solvent is not water, then breakdown is termed solvolysis. Furthermore the definition can be extended to include any change in solvent polarity (usually measured as dielectric constant) as a result of increased ionic strength, which is equivalent to an increased solvent polarity. For example, phenobarbitone is considerably more stable in preparations containing water-miscible solvents whereas aspirin, which undergoes extensive hydrolysis, is degraded further by aqueous solvents. Both effects are directly related to the dielectric constant (polarity) of the solvent. In general, if a compound produces degradation products which are more polar than itself then the addition of a less polar solvent will stabilize the formulation. If the degradation products are less polar, then the vehicle should be more polar to improve stability. With the hydrolysis of neutral non-polar drugs, e.g. steroids, the transition state will be non-polar and with no net charge. In this case solvents will not affect the rate of decomposition and can be used with impunity to increase solubility.

Finally, although solvolytic breakdown may be significant, the advantages of cosolvent solubility, as in the case of chloramphenicol, may be more attractive provided the intrinsic stability is good.

Oxidation

Whereas in hydrolysis, water (or solvent), pH and temperature are the major factors involved, oxidation is largely controlled by the environment: light, trace metals, oxygen and oxidizing agents. Reduction is a complimentary reaction (Red-Ox) and there is a mutual exchange of electrons. Oxidation is a loss of electrons and an oxidizing agent must be able to take electrons. In organic chemistry, oxidation is synonymous with dehydrogenation (the loss of hydrogen) and this is the mode of action of polyhydroxyphenol antioxidants, e.g. hydroquinone. Most antioxidants function by providing electrons or labile H^+, which will be accepted by any free radical to terminate the chain reaction. A prerequisite for effective antioxidant activity in any particular preparation is that the antioxidant is more readily oxidized than the drug.

Chelating agents

Chelating agents are complexes, which unlike simple ligands, e.g. ferrocyanide $(Fe(CN)_6^{4-})$, which form complex salts by a single bond provided by a lone electron pair, are capable of forming more than one bond. For example, ethylene diamine is bidentate (two links), tripyridyl is tridentate (3) and ethylene diamine tetraacetic acid (EDTA) is hexadentate (6) which means this is particularly effective as a pharmaceutical chelating agent.

Photolysis

Oxidation, and to some extent hydrolysis, is often catalysed by light. The energy associated with the radiation increases as its wavelength decreases, so that the energy of u.v. > visible > i.r., and is independent of temperature (see Table 13.12).

Table 13.12 Relationship between wavelength and associated energy of various forms of light

Type of radiation	Wavelength (nm)	Energy (kcal mol⁻¹)
U.v.	50–400	287–72
Visible	400–750	72–36
I.r.	750–10 000	36– 1

When molecules are exposed to electromagnetic radiation they absorb light (photons) at characteristic wavelengths which causes an increase in the energy state of the compound. This energy can:

(a) cause decomposition
(b) be retained or transferred
(c) be converted to heat
(d) result in emission of light at a new wavelength (fluorescence, phosphorescence).

Natural sunlight lies in the wavelength range 290–780 nm of which only the higher energy (u.v.) range (290–320 nm) causes photodegradation of drugs (and sunburn!). Fluorescent lighting tubes emit visible light and potentially deleterious u.v. radiation in the range 320–380 nm, whilst conventional tungsten filament light bulbs are safe, emitting radiations >390 nm.

Thus photolysis is prevented by suitable packing: low actinic amber glass bottles, cardboard outers and aluminium foil overwraps and blisters. Clear flint glass absorbs around 80% in the 290–320 nm range whereas amber glass absorbs more than 95%. Plastic containers, by comparison, absorb only half this amount of radiation. For further details see Chapter 44.

Solid-state stability

Many of the processes of decomposition mentioned in the preceding paragraphs of this chapter apply generally, particularly when the drug is in solution. However, certain important distinctions arise with the stability of drugs in the solid state, e.g. in tables and capsules. There is limited information in the pharmaceutical literature largely due to the complexities of formulated systems and the difficulties in obtaining quantitative data. This scarcity of data must not be interpreted to mean that this area is unimportant, especially given the popularity of tablets and capsules.

In all solid dosage formulations there will be some free moisture (contributed by various additives or excipients, as well as the drug) and, certainly in tablets, a significant percentage, typically 25% w/w, is required to facilitate good compression. This free water has the ability to act as a vector for chemical reactions between drugs and excipients as saturated solutions.

Because of the differences observed in the behaviour of drugs in the solid state or in contact with limited amounts of water, such as adsorbed moisture films, when compared with their reaction in solution, studies in dilute solution can often be quite meaningless and should not be extrapolated glibly to the solid state.

Hygroscopicity

A substance which absorbs sufficient moisture from the atmosphere to dissolve itself is deliquescent. A substance which loses water to form a lower hydrate or becomes anhydrous is termed efflorescent. These are extreme cases and usually most pharmaceutical compounds either are impassive to the water available in the surrounding atmosphere or either lose or gain water from the atmosphere depending on the relative humidity (RH). Materials unaffected by RH are termed non-hygroscopic while those in dynamic equilibrium with water in the atmosphere are hygroscopic. Ambient RH can vary widely and continually depending on the weather and air temperature and these cyclic changes lead to constant variations in the moisture content of unprotected bulk drug and excipients. For this reason pharmaceutical air conditioning is usually set below 50% RH and very hygroscopic products, which are particularly moisture sensitive, are stored below 40% RH.

Formulated solid products, such as tablets and capsules, must be hydrophilic to facilitate wetting and the process of deaggregation and drug dissolution. As a paradox they must have limited hygroscopicity to ensure good chemical and physical stability under all reasonable climatic conditions. Good packaging will accommodate moisture challenge, e.g. glass bottles, foil blisters and desiccant. However, preformulation studies on the drug and potential excipient combinations should provide the basis for more robust formulations and a wider more flexible choice of pack, while still reducing significantly any hydrolytic instability due to absorbed free moisture.

Stability assessment

The testing protocols used to ascertain the stability of formulated products must be performed both in solution and in the solid state since the same drug may be manufactured both as an injection and a capsule, for example. These protocols have been discussed briefly in Chapter 7 and a suggested scheme is shown in Table 13.11.

6 MICROSCOPY

The microscope has two major applications in pharmaceutical preformulation:

(a) basic crystallography, to determine crystal morphology (structure and habit), polymorphism and solvates and
(b) particle size analysis.

Most pharmaceutical powders have crystals in the range 0.5–300 μm. However, the distributions are often smaller, typically 0.5–50 μm, to ensure good blend homogeneity and rapid dissolution. Accordingly a lamp illuminated mono-objective microscope fitted with polarizing filters above and below the stage is more than adequate to study these materials. For most preformulation work a 10× eyepiece and a 10× objective are ideal, although occasionally, with micronized powders and when following solid–solid and liquid–liquid transitions in polymorphism, 10 × 20 may be required.

Crystal morphology

Crystals are characterized by repetition of the constituent atoms or molecules in a regular three-dimensional structure which is absent in glasses and some polymers. These are six crystal systems (cubic, tetragonal, orthorhombic, monoclinic, triclinic and hexagonal — see a standard chemistry text) which have different internal structures and

spatial arrangement of molecules or atoms. While not changing the internal structure, which occurs with polymorphism, crystals can adopt different external structures. This is known as crystal habit of which five types are recognized:

(a) tabular: moderate expansion of two parallel faces;
(b) platy: excessive plate-like development;
(c) prismatic: columnar form;
(d) acicular: needle-like prism;
(e) bladed: flattened acicular.

These can occur in all six crystal systems.

Conditions during crystallization of the drug will contribute to changes in crystal habit and may well be encountered in early batches of a new drug substance during preformulation until the synthetic route has been optimized. The following examples show ways in which crystal habit can be modified.

(a) Excessive supersaturation tends to transform a prism or isodiametric (granular) crystals to a needle shape.
(b) Cooling rate and agitation is effective in changing habit since it changes the degree of supersaturation. Naphthalene gives thin plates (platy) if rapidly recrystallized in cold ethanol or methanol whereas slow evaporation yields prisms.
(c) The crystallizing solvent affects habit by preferential absorption on to certain faces inhibiting their growth. Resorcinol produces needles from benzene and squat prisms from butyl acetate.
(d) The addition of cosolvents or other solutes and ions may change habit by poisoning crystal growth in one or more directions. Sodium chloride is usually cubic but urea causes an octahedral habit.

Particle size analysis

The particle size of a drug has fundamental effects on two important concerns in solid dosage form formulation:

(a) dose uniformity
(b) dissolution rate.

Small particles are particularly important in low dose, high potency drug candidates since large particle populations are necessary to assure adequate blend homogeneity (coefficient of variation less than 2%), and also for any drug whose aqueous solubility is poor (<1 mg ml^{-1}), since dissolution rate is directly proportional to surface area (i.e. to particle size^{-1}). Cohesion, adhesion and powder flow are also dependent (see Chapter 36).

There are numerous methods of particle sizing. Sieving is usually unsuitable during preformulation due to the lack of bulk material. The simplest, but unfortunately the most tedious, method for small quantities is the microscope. The Coulter counter (a conductivity method based on electrolyte displacement as the sample is drawn through a small hole) and laser light scattering are widely used for routine bulk analysis and research (see Chapter 33 for details).

7 POWDER FLOW PROPERTIES

Of primary importance to the formulator when handling a drug powder is an assessment of its flow properties. Various methods of assessing powder flow are discussed fully in Chapter 36; however, when limited amounts of drug are available these can be evaluated simply by measurements of bulk density and angle of repose of the powder. These are extremely useful derived parameters to assess the impact of changes in drug powder properties as new batches become available. Changes in particle size and shape are generally very apparent; an increase in crystal size or a more uniform shape will lead to a smaller angle of repose and smaller Carr's index (see below and Chapter 36).

Bulk density

Neumann (1967) and Carr (1965) developed a simple test to evaluate flowability of a powder by comparing the poured (fluff) density ($\rho_{B\,min}$) and tapped density ($\rho_{B\,max}$) of a powder and the rate at which it packed down. A useful empirical guide is given by the Carr's compressibility index. Here

'compressibility' is a misnomer since compression is not involved.

Carr's index (%)

$$= \frac{\text{Tapped density} - \text{Poured density}}{\text{Tapped density}} \times 100 \tag{13.12}$$

It is a simple index that can be determined on small quantities of powder and may be interpreted as in Table 13.13.

Table 13.13 Carr's index as an indication of powder flow properties

Carr's Index (%)	Type of flow
5–15	Excellent
12–16	Good
18–21	Fair to passable★
23–35	Poor★
33–38	Very poor
>40	Extremely poor

★ May be improved by the addition of glidant, e.g. 0.2% Aerosil.

A similar index has been defined by Hausner (1967):

$$\text{Hausner ratio} = \frac{\text{Tapped density } (\rho_{B\,max})}{\text{Poured density } (\rho_{B\,min})} \tag{13.13}$$

Values less than 1.25 indicate good flow ($= 20\%$ Carr), while greater than 1.25 indicates poor flow ($= 33\%$ Carr). Between 1.25 and 1.5 added glidant normally improves flow.

Carr's index is a one-point determination and does not always reflect the ease or speed with which consolidation of the powder occurs. Indeed some materials have a high index (suggesting poor flow) but they may consolidate rapidly. Rapid consolidation is essential for uniform filling on tablet machines when the powder flows at $\rho_{B\,min}$ into the die and consolidates, to approach $\rho_{B\,max}$, prior to compression. An empirical linear relationship exists between the per cent change in bulk density and the log number of taps in a jolting volumeter (see Chapter 36). Non-linearity occurs up to two taps and after 30 taps when the bed consolidates more slowly. The slope is a measure of the speed of consolidation and is useful for assessing powders or blends with similar Carr's indices, or the beneficial effects of glidants.

Angle of repose

A static heap of powder, when only gravity acts upon it, will tend to form a conical mound. One limitation exists; the angle to the horizontal cannot exceed a certain value and this is known as the angle of repose (θ). If any particle temporarily lies outside this limiting angle, it will slide down the adjacent surface under the influence of gravity until the gravitational pull is balanced by the friction caused by interparticulate forces. Accordingly, there is an empirical relationship between θ and the ability of the powder to flow. However, the exact value for angle of repose can depend on the method of measurement (see Chapter 36).

The values of angle of repose given in Table 13.14 may be used as a guide to the type of flow

Table 13.14 Angle of repose as an indication of powder flow properties

Angle of repose (degrees)	Type of flow
<25	Excellent
25–30	Good
30–40	Passable★
>40	Very poor

★ May be improved by the addition of glidant, e.g. 0.2% Aerosil.

to expect. A simple graphical relationship between angle of respose, Carr's index and the expected powder flow is shown in Fig. 13.6. When only small quantities of powder are available, an alternative is to determine the 'angle of spatula' by picking up a quantity of powder on the spatula and estimating the angle of the triangular section of the powder heap viewed from the end of the spatula. This is obviously a somewhat crude determination but is useful during preformulation when only small quantities of drug are available.

8 COMPRESSION PROPERTIES

The compression properties of most drug powders are extremely poor and necessitate the addition of compression aids. When the dose is less than 50 mg, tablets can usually be prepared by direct compression with the addition of modern direct compression bases but at higher doses the preferred method would be wet massing (see Chapters 37 and 39).

None the less information on the compression properties of the pure drug is extremely useful. While it is true that the tableted material should

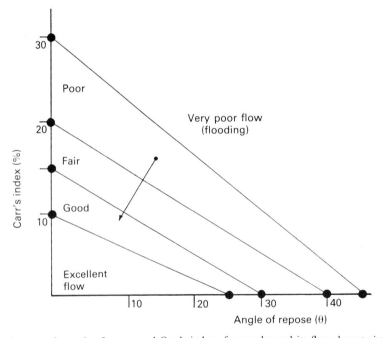

Fig. 13.6 Relationship between the angle of repose and Carr's index of a powder and its flow characteristics

be plastic, i.e. capable of permanent deformation, it should also exhibit a degree of brittleness (fragmentation). Accordingly if the drug dose is high and it behaves plastically, the chosen excipients should fragment, e.g. lactose, calcium phosphate. If the drug is brittle or elastic, the excipients should be plastic, e.g. microcrystalline cellulose, or plastic binders could be used in wet massing. Obviously, as the dose is reduced, this becomes less important as the diluent vehicle dominates compressibility. This is discussed more fully in Chapter 39.

The compression properties (elasticity, plasticity, fragmentability and punch filming propensity) for small quantities of a new drug candidate can be established by the sequence outlined in Table 13.15.

Table 13.15 Scheme for the evaluation of drug compression properties.

	500 mg drug + 1% magnesium stearate		
Sample code	A	B	C
Blend in a tumbler mixer for	5 min	5 min	30 min
Compress 13 mm diameter compacts in a hydraulic press at	75 MPa	75 MPa	75 MPa
for a dwell time of	2 s	30 s	2 s
Store tablets in a sealed container at room temperature to allow equilibration	24 h	24 h	24 h
Perform crushing strength on tablets and record load	A N	B N	C N

Interpretation of the results from the compression scheme

Plastic material When materials are ductile they deform by changing shape (plastic flow). Since there is no fracture, no new surfaces are generated during compression and a more intimate mix of magnesium stearate (as in sample C in Table 13.15) leads to poorer bonding (DeBoer *et al.* 1978). Since these materials bond after viscoelastic deformation, and this is time-dependent, increasing the dwell time at compression (B in Table 13.15) will increase bonding strength. Thus, a material exhibiting tablet crushing strengths in the order B > A > C would probably have plastic tendencies.

Fragmenting material If a material is predominantly fragmenting, neither lubricant mixing time (C in Table 13.15) nor dwell time (B) should affect tablet strength. Thus materials which show tablet crushing strengths which are independent of the scheme of manufacture outlined in Table 13.15 are likely to exhibit fragmenting properties during compression, with a high friability.

Elastic material Some materials, paracetamol is an example, are elastic and there is very little permanent change (either plastic flow or fragmentation) caused by compression; the material rebounds (elastically recovers) when the compression load is released. If bonding is weak, the compact will self-destruct and the top will detach (capping) or the whole cylinder cracks into horizontal layers (lamination). An elastic body will respond as follows to the preparation methods outlined in Table 13.15.

A will cap or laminate.
B will probably maintain integrity but will be very weak.
C will cap or laminate.

Elastic materials require a particularly plastic tableting matrix or wet massing to induce plasticity (see Chapters 37 and 39 for further details).

Punch filming (sticking) Finally, the surface of the top and bottom punches should be examined for adhesion of drug. The punches can be dipped into a suitable extraction solvent and the drug level determined. This will probably be higher for A and B (Table 13.15) since magnesium stearate is an effective anti-adherent and 30 minutes' mixing (C) should produce a monolayer and suppress adhesion more effectively.

Sticky materials can be improved by a change in salt form, by using high excipient ratios, by using abrasive inorganic excipients, by wet massing and/or by the addition of up to 2% magnesium stearate.

9 EXCIPIENT COMPATIBILITY

The successful formulation of a stable and effective solid dosage form depends on the careful selection of the excipients which are added to facilitate administration, promote the consistent release and bioavailability of the drug and protect it from degradation.

Thermal analysis (Section 3) can be used to investigate and predict any physicochemical interactions between components in a formulation and therefore can be applied to the selection of suitable chemically compatible excipients. Primary excipients recommended for initial screening for table and capsule formulations are shown in Table 13.16.

Table 13.16 Suggested primary candidates as excipients for tablet and capsule formulations

Excipient	Function*
Lactose monohydrate	D
Dicalcium phosphate dihydate	D
Dicalcium phosphate anhydrous	D
Calcium sulphate dihydrate	D
Microcrystalline cellulose	D
Maize starch	B, T
Modified starch	B, T
Polyvinylpyrrolidone	B
Hydroxypropyl methylcellulose	B
Sodium starch glycollate	T
Sodium croscarmellose	T
Magnesium stearate	L
Stearic acid	L
Colloidal silica	G

* B, binder; D diluent; G, glidant; L, lubricant; T, disintegrant.

Method

The preformulation screening of drug:excipient interactions only requires 5 mg of drug, in a 50% mixture with the excipient, to maximize the likelihood of observing an interaction. Mixtures should be examined under nitrogen to eliminate oxidative and pyrrolytic effects at a standard heating rate (2, 5 or 10 °C min⁻¹), on the DSC. apparatus, over a temperature range which will encompass any thermal changes due to both the drug and excipient. The melting range and any other transitions of the drug will be known from earlier investigations into purity, polymorphism and solvates. For all potential excipients (Table 13.16) it is sensible to retain in a reference file individual, representative thermograms for later comparison.

Interpretation

A scheme for interpreting the DSC. data from the individual components and their mixtures is shown in Fig. 13.7. Basically, the thermal properties of a physical mixture are the sum of the individual components, and this thermogram can be compared with those of the drug and the excipient alone. An interaction on DSC. will show as changes in melting point, peak shape and

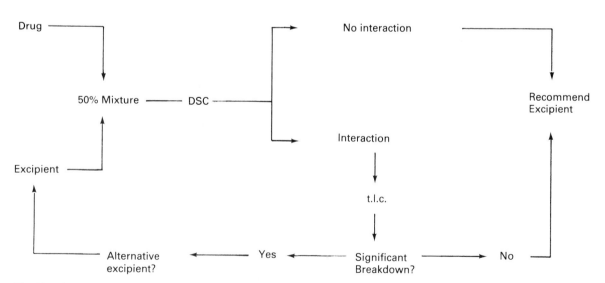

Fig. 13.7 Scheme to identify chemically compatible excipients using DSC with confirmatory t.l.c.

area and/or the appearance of a transition. However, there is invariably some change in transition temperature and peak shape and area by virtue of mixing two components and this is not due to any detrimental interaction. In general, provided that no new thermal events occur or are lost by mixing the two components, no interaction can be assigned. Chemical interactions are indicated by the appearance of new peaks or where there is gross broadening or elongation of an exo- or endothermic change. Second order transitions produce changes in the baseline. Such observations may also be indicative of the production of eutectic or solid solution type melts. The excipient is then probably chemically reactive and incompatible with the drug and should be avoided. Where an interaction is suspected, but the thermal changes are small, the incompatibility can be confirmed by t.l.c.

The advantages of DSC. over more traditional, routine compatibility screens, typically t.l.c., is that no long-term storage of the mixture is required prior to evaluation nor is any inappropriate thermal stress (other than the DSC. itself, which has drug and excipient controls) required to accelerate the interactions. This, in itself, may be misleading if the mode of breakdown changes with temperature and elevated temperatures fail

to reflect the degradative path occurring under normal (room temperature) storage.

Where confirmation is required by t.l.c., samples (50:50 mixtures of drug and excipient) should be sealed in small neutral glass test tubes and stored for either 3 days at 75 °C, 7 days at 50 °C or 14 days at 37 °C depending on whether it is likely, from earlier stability studies (Section 5), that degradation will be atypical at elevated temperatures.

It is important to view the results of such incompatibility testing with caution in cases where the additive is used at low concentration in the product. For example, magnesium stearate is notoriously incompatible with a wide range of compounds when tested as above. Yet, since it is only used at low levels, typically 0.5–1%, such apparent incompatibility rarely produces a problem in practice on long-term storage.

10 CONCLUSIONS

Preformulation studies, properly carried out, have a significant part to play in anticipating formulation problems and identifying logical paths in both liquid and solid dosage form technology (Fig. 13.8). The need for adequate drug solubility

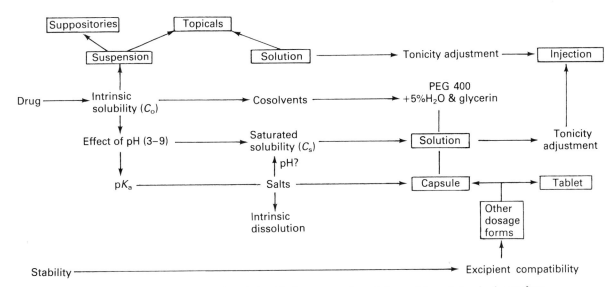

Fig. 13.8 A generic development pathway: the relationship between preformulation and formulation in dosage form development. The formulation stages are shown in boxes and the performulation stages are unboxed

cannot be overemphasized. The availability of sufficient solubility data should allow the selection of the most appropriate salt for development. Stability studies in solution will indicate the feasibility of parenteral, or other liquid, dosage forms and can identify methods of stabilization. In parallel, solid-state stability by DSC., t.l.c. and h.p.l.c. and in the presence of tablet and capsule excipients will indicate the most acceptable vehicles for solid dosage formulations.

Finally, by comparing the physicochemical properties of each drug candidate within a therapeutic group (using C_s, pK_a, melting point, K_w^o) the performulation scientist can assist the synthetic chemist to identify the optimum molecule, provide the biologist with suitable vehicles to elicit pharmacological response and advise the bulk chemist about the selection and production of the best salt with appropriate particle size and morphology for subsequent processing.

REFERENCES

Agharkar, S., Lindenbaum, S. and Higuchi, T. (1976) *J. pharm. Sci.*, **65**, 747–749

Albert, A. A. and Serjeant, E. P. (1984) *Ionization Constants of Acids and Bases*, Wiley, New York.

Bristow, P. A. (1976) *Liquid Chromatography in Practice*, hetp, Macclesfield.

Cadwallader, D. E. (1978) *Br. J. Anaesth.*, **50**, 81.

Carr, R. L. (1965) *Chem. Engng*, **72**(1), 162 and **72**(2), 69.

Collander, R. (1951) *Acta chem. scand.*, **5**, 774.

Cunningham, K. G., Dawson, W. and Spring, F. S. (1951) *J. Chem. Soc. (London)*, 2305.

Davis, S. S. and Higuchi, T. (1970) *J. pharm. Sci.*, **59**, 1376.

DeBoer, A. H., Bolhuis, G. K. and Lerk, C. F. (1978) *Powd. Tech.*, **20**, 75–82.

Dittert, L. W., Higuchi, T. and Reese, D. R. (1964) *J. pharm. Sci.*, **53**, 1325–1328.

Fedors, R. F. (1974) *Polymer Eng. Sci.*, **14**, 147.

Grady, L. T., Hays, S. E., King, R. H., Klein, H. R., Mader, W. J., Wyatt, D. K. and Zimmerci, R. O. (1973) *J. pharm. Sci.*, **62**, 456–464.

Haleblian, J. K. and Biles, J. A. (1967) *Proc. A.Ph.A. Acad. Pharm. Sci.*, Las Vegas.

Hamilton, R. J. and Sewell, P. A. (1977) *Introduction to High Performance Liquid Chromatography*, Chapman and Hall, London.

Hamlin, W. E., Northam, J. I. and Wagner, J. G. (1965) *J. pharm. Sci.*, **54**, 1651–1653.

Hammelt, L. P. (1940) Chapter 7 of *Physical Organic Chemistry*, McGraw-Hill, New York.

Hansch, C. and Dunn, W. J. (1972) *J. pharm. Sci.*, **61**, 1.

Hansch, C. and Fujita, T. (1964) *J. Am. Chem. Soc.*, **86**, 1616–1626.

Hansch, C. and Leo, A. J. (1979) *Substituent Constants for Correlation Analysis in Chemistry and Biology*, Wiley, New York.

Hausner, H. H. (1967) *Int. J. Powd. Metall.*, **3**, 7.

Kaplan, S. A. (1972). *Drug Metab. Revs*, **1**, 15–32.

Kennon, L. (1964). *J. pharm. Sci.*, **53**, 815–818.

Kuhnert-Brandstatter, M. (1965) *Pure appl. Chem.*, **10**, 133.

Leo, A. J., Hansch, C. and Elkins, D. (1971) *Chem. Revs*, **71**, 525.

Levich, V. G. (1962) *Physico-chemical Hydrodynamics*, Prentice Hall, New Jersey.

Long, F. A. and McDevitt, W. F. (1952) *Chem. Revs*, **51**, 119–169.

Meyer, H. (1899) *Arch. Exp. Pathl. Pharmac.*, **42**, 109.

Miller, L. C. and Holland, A. H. (1960) *Mod. Med.*, **28**, 312.

Nelson, E. (1958) *J. pharm. Sci.*, **47**, 297.

Neumann, B. S. (1967) *Adv. Pharm. Sci.*, **2**, 181–220. Academic Press, London.

Overton, E. (1901) *Studien uber die Narkose*, G. Fishcer, Jena.

Paruta, A. N., Sciarrone, B. J. and Lordi, N. G. (1965) *J. pharm. Sci.*, **53**, 1349–1353.

Pearson, J. and Varney, G. (1969) *J. Pharm. Pharmacol.*, **21**, 60S.

Perrin, D. D., Dempsey, B. and Serjeant, E. P. (1981) pK_a *Predictions for Organic Acids and Bases*, Chapman & Hall, London.

Pryde, A. and Gilbert, M. T. (1979) *Applications of High Performance Liquid Chromatography*, Chapman and Hall, London.

Rekker, R. F. (1977) *The Hydrophobic Fragmental Constant*, ed. W. T. Nauta and R. F. Rekker, Elsevier, Amsterdam.

Senior, N. (1973) *J. Soc. Cosmet, Chem.*, **24**, 259–278.

Snyder, L. R. (1968) *Principles of Adsorption Chromatography*, Marcel Dekker, New York.

Spiegel, A. J. and Noseworthy, M. M. (1963) *J. pharm. Sci.*, **52**, 917.

Stahl, E. (1956) *Thin Layer Chromatography, a Laboratory Handbook*, Academic Press, New York.

Tute, M. S. (1971) *Adv. Drug Res.*, **6**, 1 Academic Press, London.

Wagner, J. G. (1961) *J. pharm. Sci.*, **50**, 359.

Yalkowski, S. H., Amidon, G. L., Zografi, G. and Flynn, G. L. (1975). *J. pharm. Sci.*, **64**, 48.

Yalkowski, S. H. and Roseman, T. J. (1981). *Techniques of Solubilization of Drugs*, Chapter 3, ed. S. H. Yalkowski, Marcel Dekker, New York.

BIBLIOGRAPHY (see Table 13.2)

Albert, A. A. and Serjeant, E. P. (1984) *Ionization Constants of Acids and Bases*, Wiley, New York.

Berge S. M, Binghley, L. D. and Monkhouse, D. C. (1977) *J. Pharm. Sci.*, **66**, 1

Bristow, P. A. (1976) *Liquid Chromatography in Practice*, hetp, Macclesfield.

Connors, Amidon and Kennon (1978)

Dalglish, C. (1969) in *Isolation and Identification of Drugs*, ed. E. G. C. Clarke, Pharmaceutical Press, London

DeBoer, A. H., Bolhuis, G. K. and Lerk, C. F. (1978) *Powd. Tech.*, **20**, 75–82.

Haleblian, J. K. (1975) *J. Pharm. Sci.*, **64**, 1269

Haleblian, J. and McCrone, W (1969) *J. Pharm. Sci.*, **58**, 911

Higuchi, T. and Connors, K. A. (1965) *Adv. Anal. Chem. Inst.*, 117

Jaffe, H. H. and Orchin, M. (1962) *Theory and Applications of u.v. Spectroscopy*, John Wiley & Sons, London

Jones, T. M. (1981) *Int. J. Pharm. Tech. Prod. Mfr.*, **2**, 17.

Leo, A. J., Hansch, C. and Elkins, D. (1971) *Chem. Revs*, **71**, 525.

McCrone, W. C., McCrone, L. B. and Delly, J. G. (1978) *Polarized Light Microscopy*, Ann Arbor Science, Michigan

Mader, W. J. (1954) *Organic Analysis*, vol. 2, Interscience, New York.

Mollica, J. A., Ahuja, S. and Cohen, J. (1978) *J. Pharm. Sci.*, **67**, 443

Neumann, B. S. (1967). *Adv. Pharm. Sci.*, **2**, 181–220. Academic Press, London.

Smith, A. (1982) *Anal. Proc.*, **19**, 559.

Swarbrick, J. (1970) *Current Concepts in the Pharmaceutical Sciences: Biopharmaceutics*, Lea & Febiger, Philadelphia.

Wendlandt, W. W. (1974) *Thermal Methods of Analysis*, Interscience, New York.

Yalkowski, S. H. and Roseman, T. J. (1981) *Techniques of Solubilization of Drugs*, Chapter 3, ed. S. H. Yalkowski, Marcel Dekker, New York.

Solutions

An understanding of the properties of solutions, the factors that affect solubility and the process of dissolution is essential because of the importance of solutions in so many areas of pharmaceutical formulation. It is recommended, therefore, that this chapter be read in conjunction with Chapters 3 and 5 for a full understanding of this topic.

A solution is an homogenous one-phase system consisting of two or more components. The solvent is that phase in which the dispersion occurs and the solute is that component which is dispersed as small molecules or ions in the solvent. In general the solvent is present in the greater amount but there are several exceptions. For example, Syrup BP contains 66.7% w/w of sucrose as the solute in 33.3% w/w of water as the solvent.

ADVANTAGES AND DISADVANTAGES OF SOLUTIONS AS AN ORAL DOSAGE FORM

Although tablets and capsules are more widely used than liquid preparations for oral administration the latter do exhibit several advantages.

1 Liquids are easier to swallow than solids and are therefore particularly acceptable for paediatric and geriatric use.

2 A drug must be in solution before it can be absorbed. A drug administered in the form of a solution is immediately available for absorption. Thus the therapeutic response is faster than if using a solid dosage form which must first disintegrate in order to allow the drug to dissolve in the gastrointestinal fluid before absorption can begin. Even if the drug should precipitate from solution in the acid conditions of the stomach it will be in a sufficiently wetted and finely divided state to allow rapid absorption to occur.

3 A solution is a homogenous system and therefore the drug will be uniformly distributed throughout the preparation. In suspension or emulsion formulations uneven dosage can occur due to phase separation on storage.

4 Some drugs, including aspirin and potassium chloride, can irritate and damage the gastric mucosa particularly if localized in one area as often occurs after the ingestion of a solid dosage form. Irritation is reduced by administration of a solution of a drug because of the immediate dilution by the gastric contents.

There are, however, several problems associated with the manufacture, transport, stability and administration of solutions.

1 Liquids are bulky and therefore inconvenient to transport and store. If breakage of the container should occur the whole of the product is immediately and irretrievably lost.

2 The stability of ingredients in aqueous solution is often poorer than if they were formulated as a tablet or capsule, particularly if they are susceptible to hydrolysis. The shelf life of a liquid dosage form is therefore often much shorter than the corresponding solid preparation. Not only is the stability of the drug of importance but also that of other excipients such as surfactants, preservatives, flavours and colours. The chemical stability of some ingredients can, however, be improved by the use of a mixed solvent system. The inclusion of a surfactant above its critical micelle concentration can also help because the hydrolytic degradation of a material may be reduced by its incorporation within the micelles (solubilization).

3 Solutions often provide suitable media for the growth of micro-organisms and may therefore require the incorporation of a preservative.

4 Accurate dosage usually depends on the ability of the patient to use a 5 ml spoon or, more rarely, a volumetric dropper.

5 The taste of a drug, which is usually unpleasant, is always more pronounced when in solution than when in a solid form. Solutions can, however, easily be sweetened and flavoured to make them more palatable.

FORMULATION OF SOLUTIONS

Aqueous solutions

Water is the most widely used solvent for use as a vehicle for pharmaceutical products because of its lack of toxicity, physiological compatibility and its ability to dissolve a wide range of materials.

For most preparations potable water can be used. This is water freshly drawn from the mains system and which is suitable for drinking. If this type is unobtainable then a suitable, though more expensive, alternative is Purified Water BP which has been freshly boiled and cooled before use to destroy any vegetative micro-organisms which may be present. Purified Water BP should be used, however, on all occasions where the presence of salts, often dissolved in potable water, is undesirable. Purified Water BP is normally prepared by the distillation or deionization of potable water.

Water for Injections BP must be used for the formulation of parenteral solutions and is obtained by the sterilization of pyrogen-free distilled water immediately after collection.

For the formulation of aqueous solutions of drugs, such as phenobarbitone sodium or aminophylline, which are sensitive to the presence of carbon dioxide or drugs which are liable to oxidation, such as apomorphine and ergotamine maleate, then Water for Injections BP free from carbon dioxide or free from air must be used. These are both obtained from apyrogenic distilled water in the same way as before, but are then boiled for at least 10 minutes, cooled, sealed in their containers whilst excluding air and then sterilized by autoclaving. For further details on parenteral solutions see Chapter 21.

Approaches to the improvement of aqueous solubility

Although water is very widely used for inclusion in pharmaceutical preparations, it may not be possible to ensure complete solution of all ingredients at all normal storage temperatures. Even if in solution it is important to ensure that the concentration of any material is not close to its limit of solubility as precipitation may occur if the product is cooled or if any evaporation of the vehicle should occur.

In these cases one or more of the following methods may be used in order to improve aqueous solubility.

Cosolvency

The solubility of a weak electrolyte or non-polar compound in water can often be improved by the addition of a water-miscible solvent in which the compound is also soluble. Vehicles used in combination to increase the solubility of a drug are called cosolvents (see Chapter 5) and often the solubility in this mixed system is greater than can be predicted from the material's solubility in each individual solvent.

Because it has been shown (Paruta *et al.*, 1964) that the solubility of a given drug is maximal at a particular dielectric constant of any solvent system, it is possible to eliminate solvent blends possessing other dielectric constants. In some cases, however, the actual solvent system used may be of greater importance (Gorman and Hall, 1964).

The choice of suitable cosolvents is somewhat limited for pharmaceutical use because of possible toxicity and irritancy, particularly if required for oral or parenteral use (Spiegal and Noseworthy, 1963). Ideally, suitable blends should possess values of dielectric constant between 25 and 80, although some oils are available with values of less than unity. The most widely used system which will cover this range is a water/ethanol blend, other suitable solvents including sorbitol, glycerol, propylene glycol and syrup. For example, a blend of propylene glycol and water is used to improve the solubility of co-trimoxazole, and paracetamol is formulated as an elixir by the use of alcohol, propylene glycol and syrup. For external appli-

cation to the scalp betamethasone valerate is available dissolved in a water/isopropyl alcohol mixture.

For further details covering the suitability of different cosolvents see under their individual headings in this chapter.

pH control

If a drug is either a weak acid or a weak base then its solubility in water can be influenced by the pH of the system. A quantitative application of the Henderson–Hasselbalch equation (Chapter 3) will enable the solubility of such a material in water at a given pH to be determined, providing its pK_a and the solubility of its unionized species is known (see Chapter 3). The solubility of a weak base can be increased by lowering the pH of its solution whereas the solubility of a weak acid is improved by a pH increase. Some materials will accept or donate more than one hydrogen ion per molecule and will therefore possess more than one pK_a value and hence will exhibit a more complex solubility profile.

In controlling the solubility of a drug in this way it must be ensured that the chosen pH does not conflict with other product requirements. For example, the chemical stability of a drug may also depend on pH (Norton 1967; Smith, 1967) and in many cases the pH of optimum solubility does not coincide with the pH of optimum stability (Heward *et al.*, 1970). This may also be true for other ingredients especially dyes, preservatives and flavours.

The pH of solutions for parenteral and ophthalmic use, for application to mucous membranes or for use on abraded skin must also be controlled as extremes can cause pain and irritation (Lupton, 1942). This is particularly true for subcutaneous, intramuscular and c.n.s. injections because the solutions will not be rapidly diluted after administration.

In some instances the bioavailability of drugs may be influenced by the pH of their solution (Chapter 9) and changes in pH may also affect preservative activity by altering the degree of its ionization.

Often a compromise must be reached during formulation to ensure that the stability and solubility of all ingredients, physiological compatibility and bioavailability are all adequate for the product's intended purpose.

The values of molar solubilities and dissociation constants of drugs which are reported in the literature or determined during preformulation studies are usually for the drug alone in distilled water. These values may differ in the final formulation due to the presence of other ingredients. For example, the inclusion of cosolvents such as alcohol or propylene glycol will lower the dielectric constant of the vehicle and therefore increase the solubility of the unionized form of the drug (Schumacher, 1969). This lowering of the polarity of the solvent system will also reduce the degree of dissociation of the drug and hence its pK_a will be increased. As this effect will increase the concentration of the unionized (less soluble) species an increase in the pH of the system may be necessary in order to maintain solubility. It must be realized, therefore, that maximum solubility may best be achieved by a judicious balance between pH control and concentration of cosolvent and can be determined as before by the application of the Henderson–Hasselbalch equation by substitution of the new values both for pK_a and for the molar solubilities of the unionized species.

Suitable buffer systems for the control of pH are discussed later in this chapter but care must be taken because the solubilities of sparingly soluble electrolytes can be decreased still further by the addition of a soluble electrolyte should they contain a common ion. The opposite can be true, however, if they do not possess common ions.

As solutions of non-electrolytes are not significantly affected by pH other methods of improving their solubility must be found.

Solubilization

The solubility of a drug which is normally insoluble or poorly soluble in water can often be improved by the addition of a surface-active agent. This phenomenon of micellar solubilization has been widely used for the formulation of solutions.

The amount of surfactant used for this purpose must be carefully controlled. A large excess is undesirable because of cost, possible toxic effects

and its effect on product aeration during manufacture. Excessive amounts may also reduce the bioavailability of a drug due to its strong adsorption within the micelle. An insufficient amount of surfactant, however, may not solubilize all of the drug or may lead to precipitation on storage or on dilution of the product.

Reference to Fig. 6.13 will show that hydrophilic surfactants possessing HLB values above 15 will be of particular value as solubilizing agents. The material chosen must be non-toxic and non-irritant bearing in mind its intended route of administration. It must also be miscible with the solvent system, compatible with the other ingredients, free from disagreeable odour and taste and be non-volatile.

Examples include the solubilization of fat-soluble vitamins such as phytomenadione using polysorbates thus enabling their inclusion with water-soluble vitamins in the same formulation. The solubility of amiodarone hydrochloride can similarly be improved (Ravin et al., 1969) although this drug can exhibit autosolubilization at high concentrations. The solubilization of iodine to produce iodophores is achieved by the use of macrogol ethers. These products exhibit several advantages over simple iodine solutions including an improved chemical stability, reduced loss of active agent due to sublimation, less corrosion of surgical instruments and, in some cases, enhanced activity. Many steroids are also poorly water soluble and alphadolone acetate and alphaxalone are together solubilized with polyoxyethylated castor oil to produce a solution suitable for intravenous administration as an anaesthetic. Other drugs which have been solubilized include antibiotics such as griseofulvin which has been formulated with cetamacrogol (Elworthy and Lipscomb, 1968). Polyoxyethylene/polyoxypropylene copolymers, some of which are also suitable for parenteral administration, are used to maintain the clarity of solutions for oral use. Lanolin derivatives have also been used for the solubilization of volatile and essential oils.

The solubility of phenolic compounds such as cresol and chloroxylenol which are normally soluble in water up to 2% and 0.03% respectively can be improved by solubilization with soaps. Lysol contains 50% cresol in an aqueous system by the use of the potassium soaps of oleic, linoleic and linolenic acids. It may also be possible to combine the beneficial effects of solubilization and cosolvency in one formulation (Boon *et al.*, 1961). A 5% chloroxylenol solution can be formulated by the inclusion of potassium ricinoleate (which is formed *in situ* by the reaction between potassium hydroxide and castor oil), as well as ethanol and terpineol as cosolvents. Glycerol has also been used with polysorbate 80 to improve the solubility of vitamin A (Coles and Thomas, 1952).

For further details see Elworthy *et al.* (1968), Swarbrick (1965), Moore and Bell (1959), Monte-Bovi *et al.* (1954), Applewhite *et al.* (1954), Elworthy and Macfarlane (1965a, b).

To ensure that the optimum concentration of surfactant is chosen, a known weight or volume is added to each of a series of vials containing the solvent. Ensuring adequate temperature control, varying amounts of solubilizate are added to each vial in ascending order of concentration. The maximum concentration of drug which will form a clear solution with a given concentration of surfactant can be determined visually or by optical density measurement and is known as the maximum additive concentration (MAC). This method can be repeated for different amounts of surfactant to enable a graph to be constructed of MAC against surfactant concentration from which the optimum amount of solubilizing agent can be chosen for any required amount of drug (see Fig. 14.1). Alternatively, a ternary phase diagram can be constructed (see Fig. 14.2) which will present a more comprehensive picture of the effects of solubilizate, surfactant and solvent concentrations on the physical characteristics of the system.

The three axes form the three sides of an equilateral triangle each axis representing 0–100% of one of the components. Point A thus represents a formulation consisting of 50% solubilizate, 20% surfactant and 30% water. By plotting at each point a number representing one particular system (e.g. 1 = clear solution, 2 = emulsion etc.) and enclosing each system within a boundary, a phase diagram can be constructed. Suitable formulations which will give clear solutions will be immediately apparent and the best can then be chosen bearing in mind the desirable properties required for this

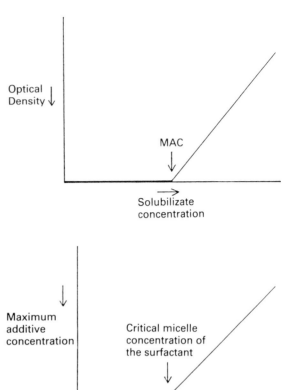

Fig. 14.1(a) Graph of optical density of a solubilizate/surfactant/solvent system versus solubilizate concentration at a fixed surfactant concentration showing the maximum additive concentration (MAC) (b) Determination of the MAC for a range of surfactant concentrations will thus provide this graph enabling the optimum concentration of surfactant to be chosen to solubilize a given amount of active material

type of product. It is also important to ensure that the formulation chosen does not lie too close to a phase boundary as the positions of these can depend on the storage temperature of the product. From this type of phase diagram the physical composition of diluted preparations can also be shown. Point B, for example, represents a product consisting of 40% solubilizate and 60% surfactant. The construction of a straight line from here to point C represents the dilution of the product with increasing concentrations of water. Should the concentration of drug to be included in the product be fixed then the third axis can be used to represent varying concentrations of a third excipient such as a cosolvent. These values must,

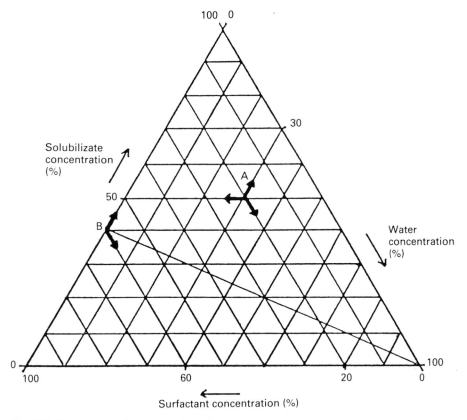

Fig. 14.2 Construction of a ternary phase diagram

however, be plotted as percentage drug plus excipient to ensure a maximum value of 100%.

Complexation

In some cases it may be possible to interact a poorly soluble drug with a soluble material to form a soluble intermolecular complex. As most complexes are macromolecular, however, they tend to be inactive, being unable to cross lipid membranes. It is essential, therefore, that complex formation is easily reversible so that the free drug is released during or before contact with biological fluids.

The term *hydrotropy*, which has been defined as the increase in aqueous solubility of a material by the inclusion of additives (Neuberg *et al.*, 1930), should be considered to be a form of complexation, although this definition also covers the increase in drug solubility which can sometimes be achieved by the inclusion of electrolytes.

It is not easy to predict if a drug will complex with a particular compound to give improved solubility. Many complexes are not water-soluble and may, in fact, be better suited for the prolonged release of the drug. Several well known examples are in general use, however, and include the complexation of iodine with a 10–15% solution of polyvinylpyrrolidone to improve the aqueous solubility of the active agent. Similarly the interaction of salicylates or benzoates with xanthines such as theophylline or caffeine or with carbazochrome is carried out for the same effect.

Chemical modification

As a last resort chemical modification of a drug may be necessary in order to produce a water-soluble derivative. Examples include the synthesis of the sodium phosphate salts of hydrocortisone, prednisolone and betamethasone. The water-soluble chloramphenicol sodium succinate has no antibacterial activity of its own but is suitable for parenteral administration as a solution in order to obtain high blood levels after which it is converted back to the active base. Although many poorly soluble drugs have been modified in this way they are, of course, regarded as new chemical entities and thus full toxicity, pharmacology and preformulation studies may be required for these as well as for their parent compounds.

Particle size control

The size and shape of very small particles, if less than 1 μm diameter, can affect their solubility (May and Kolthoff, 1948). As particle size decreases solubility will increase. In practice, however, this phenomenon has little application in the formulation of solutions, but is of particular relevance in suspension formulation.

Non-aqueous solutions

The use of alternative solvents

If it is not possible to ensure complete solution of the ingredients at all storage temperatures or if the drug is unstable in aqueous systems it may be necessary to use an alternative solvent. The use of non-aqueous systems may also have other advantages. For example, the intramuscular injection of solutions of drugs in oils is often used for depot therapy and some drugs are specifically synthesized to improve their oil solubilities, the propionate and benzoate esters of testosterone and oestradiol, respectively, being good examples. The oily solution remains as a discrete entity within the muscle tissue, releasing the drug slowly into the surrounding tissue whereas a similar aqueous solution would diffuse readily and, being miscible with tissue fluid, would cause the drug to be released quickly.

It must be borne in mind that, in choosing a suitable solvent, its toxicity, irritancy and sensitizing potential must be taken into account as well as its flammability, cost, stability and compatibility with other excipients. It will be obvious that a greater choice of solvent will be available for inclusion into products for external application

than those for internal use, while for parenteral products the choice is even further limited (Spiegal and Noseworthy, 1963).

A far wider range of solvents, however, is available for use during the manufacture of pharmaceutical products when the solvent is removed before packaging and therefore not present in the final product. Examples include acetone, light petroleum and chloroform although the latter is also used as a flavour and preservative in some extemporaneously prepared formulations.

The following is a classification of some of the most widely used non-aqueous solvents in pharmaceutical preparations.

Fixed oils of vegetable origin

These are non-volatile oils which consist mainly of fatty acid esters of glycerol. Almond oil, for example, which consists of glycerides mainly of oleic acid, is used as a solvent for Oily Phenol Injection BP, water being unsuitable because of the caustic nature of aqueous phenol solutions. Of similar chemical composition is arachis oil which is used as the solvent in Dimercaprol Injection BP. Olive oil, sesame oil, maize oil, cottonseed oil, soya oil and castor oil are all suitable for parenteral use, the latter also being used as the solvent in Physostigmine Oily Eye Drops BP and in some formulations of triamcinolone ear drops.

Ethyl oleate, which is a useful solvent for both Calciferol Injection BP and Testosterone Propionate Injections BP, is less viscous than the oils described above, and therefore more easily injected intramuscularly. Of similar viscosity is benzyl benzoate which can be used as an alternative solvent for dimercaprol.

Some fixed oils are sufficiently tasteless and odourless to be suitable for oral use as solvents for such materials as vitamins A and D. Fractionated coconut oil is used as the solvent for phenoxymethylpenicillin which would otherwise hydrolyse rapidly if present in an aqueous system. Veterinary formulations may also contain these solvents, arachis oil, for example, being used for hexachlorophane in the treatment of fascioliasis in ruminants.

Oils tend to be unpleasant to use externally,

however, unless presented as an emulsion. Arachis oil is one of the few examples and is used as the solvent in Methyl Salicylate Liniment BP.

Alcohols

Ethyl alcohol is the most widely used solvent in this class, particularly for external application, where its rapid evaporation after application to the skin imparts a cooling effect to such products as Salicyclic Acid Lotion BP. It is also particularly useful for the extraction of crude drugs being more selective than water. At concentrations greater than 15% it exhibits antimicrobial activity but because of its toxicity it is used orally or parenterally only at low concentrations, usually as a cosolvent with water. If required for external use then industrial methylated spirit (IMS), which is free from excise duty, is usually included rather than the more expensive ethanol. Because IMS contains 5% methyl alcohol as a denaturant it is rendered too toxic for internal use.

An alcohol possessing similar properties is isopropyl alcohol which is used externally as a solvent for dicophane. Its main advantage is that it is less likely to be abused than ethanol and denaturation is not necessary.

Polyhydric alcohols

Alcohols containing two hydroxyl groups per molecule are known as glycols but due to their toxicity are rarely used internally. One important exception to this is propylene glycol

$$CH_3.CH(OH)CH_2OH$$

which is often used in conjunction with water or glycerol as a cosolvent. It is used, for example, in the formulation of Digoxin Injection BP, Phenobarbitone Injection BP and some formulations of Diazepam Injection BP, Co-trimoxazole Intravenous Infusion BP and as the diluent for both Chloramphenicol Ear Drops BP and some brands of hydrocortisone ear drops and in many preparations for oral use.

The lower molecular weight polyethylene glycols (PEG) or macrogols have the general formula

$$OHCH_2(CH_2CH_2O)_nCH_2OH$$

PEG 400, for example, being used as a solvent in Erythromycin Ethylsuccinate Injection USP. They are also widely used as cosolvents with alcohol or water although their main use is in the formulation of water-miscible ointment bases.

There are also other glycols available, which, although rarely included in products for human use, can be used for extraction processes or as solvents in the formulation of veterinary and horticultural solutions. Examples include dipropylene glycol (the diluent in Piperonyl Butoxide Application BP Vet for veterinary use), diethylene glycol, ethylene glycol and their monoethyl ethers.

Glycerol, an alcohol possessing three hydroxyl groups per molecule, is also widely used particularly as a cosolvent with water for oral use. At higher concentrations it is used externally in, for example, Phenol Ear Drops BPC 1973.

Dimethylsulphoxide

This is a highly polar compound and is thought to aid the penetration of drugs through the skin. Although used mainly as a solvent in veterinary formulation, it is used as a carrier for idoxuridine, an antiviral agent, for application to human skin.

Ethyl ether

This material is widely used for the extraction of crude drugs but because of its own therapeutic activity is not used for the preparation of formulations for internal use. It is, however, used as a cosolvent with alcohol in some collodions.

Liquid paraffin

The oily nature of this material makes it unpleasant to use externally, although it is often used as a solvent for the topical application of drugs in emulsion formulations. At one time light liquid paraffin was widely used as the base for oily nasal drops which are now rarely used because of the possibility of causing lipoidal pneumonia if inhaled into the lungs. It has a minor use in veterinary formulation as a solvent in, for example, anthelmintic drenches containing carbon tetrachloride.

Miscellaneous solvents

Isopropyl myristate and isopropyl palmitate are oily materials used as solvents for external use particularly in cosmetics where their low viscosity and lack of greasiness make them pleasant to use.

Dimethylformamide and dimethylacetamide have both been used as solvents in veterinary formulation but their toxicities render them unsuitable for human use. Kerosene too is also limited in its application being used mainly as a solvent for insecticides such as pyrethrum and piperonyl butoxide.

Xylene is present in some ear drops for human use to dissolve ear wax and glycofurol is a constituent of formulations of co-trimoxazole intramuscular injection.

As with aqueous systems it may be possible to improve the solubility of a drug in a particular vehicle by the addition of a cosolvent. For example, nitrocellulose is poorly soluble in both alcohol and ether but adequately soluble in a mixture of both. The formulation of Digoxin Injection BP, too, is best achieved by the inclusion of both ethyl alcohol and propylene glycol.

Formulation additives

Buffers

These are materials which, when dissolved in a solvent, will enable it to resist any change in pH should an acid or an alkali be added. The choice of suitable buffer depends on the pH and buffering capacity required. It must be compatible with other excipients and have a low toxicity.

Most pharmaceutically acceptable buffering systems are based on carbonates, citrates, gluconates, lactates, phosphates or tartrates. Borates can be used for external application but not to mucous membranes or to abraded skin (Windheuser, 1963).

As the pH of most body fluids is 7.4, products such as injections, eye drops and nasal drops should, in theory, be buffered at this value. Many body fluids themselves, however, have a buffering capacity and when formulating low volume intravenous injections or eye drops a wider pH range can be tolerated. This is potentially useful should a compromise be necessary between a pH which is physiologically acceptable and a pH of maximum stability and solubility and optimum bioavaibility. For further details on the use of buffers see Chapter 3.

Colours

Once a suitable flavour has been chosen it is often useful to include a colour which is associated with that flavour to improve the attractiveness of the product. Another reason for the inclusion of colours is to enable easy product identification particularly of poisonous materials including weedkillers or mineralized methylated spirit and, for example, to differentiate between the many types of antiseptic solution used in hospitals for the disinfection of skin, instruments, syringes etc. The development of a strongly coloured degradation product which does not affect the use of the product may occasionally be masked by the presence of a suitable colour.

It is essential to ensure, however, that any colour chosen is acceptable in the country in which the product is to be sold. A colour which is acceptable in one country may not be acceptable in another and as aspects of colour legislation can change quite frequently it is necessary to ensure that only the latest regulations are consulted. The legal departments of most dye manufacturers are usually willing to supply up to date information. The proliferation of nomenclature which exists for most colours can also cause confusion. For example, the water-soluble dye amaranth is also known as Bordeaux S, CI Food Red 9, and CI Acid Red 27. It has been allocated the Colour Index Number 16185 by the Society of Dyers and Colourists and the American Association of Textile Chemists and Colorists. Under the USA Food, Drug and Cosmetics Act it is known as FD and C Red Number 2 and a directive of the Council of European Communities has allocated it the reference number E 123.

As with flavours and perfumes there is available a range of both natural and synthetic colours. The former, which tend to be more widely acceptable, can be classified into carotenoids, chlorophylls, anthocyanins and a miscellaneous group which includes riboflavines, caramel and extracts of red beetroot (Kläui, 1978). They can, however, exhibit the usual problems associated with natural products, namely variations in availability and in chemical composition, both of which may cause formulation difficulties.

Synthetic or 'coal tar' dyes tend to give brighter colours and are generally more stable than natural materials. Most of those which are suitable for pharmaceutical use are the sodium salts of sulphonic acids and therefore they may be incompatible with cationic drugs. Care must also be taken to ensure that any dye used is not adversely affected by pH or by u.v. radiation or by the inclusion of oxidizing or reducing agents (Swartz and Cooper, 1962) or surfactants (Scott et al., 1960).

A useful review on the availability and use of colours can be found in Martindale: The Extra Pharmacopoeia.

Density modifiers

It is rarely necessary to control the density of a solution except when formulating spinal anaesthetics. Solutions of lower density than cerebrospinal fluid will tend to rise after injection and those of higher density will fall. Careful control both of the density of such injections and the position of the patient on the operating table will enable precise control of the area to be anaesthatized to be attained. The terms used to describe the density of injections in relation to that of spinal fluid are isobaric, hypobaric and hyperbaric, meaning of equal, lower and higher density respectively. The most widely used material for this type of density modification is dextrose.

Flavours and perfumes

The simple use of sweetening agents (q.v.) may not be sufficient to render palatable a product containing a drug with a particularly unpleasant taste. In many cases, therefore, a flavouring agent can be included. This is particularly useful in paediatric formulation to ensure patient compliance. The inclusion of flavours has the additional advantage of enabling identification of liquid products to be achieved easily.

Flavouring and perfuming agents can be obtained from either natural or synthetic sources. Natural products include fruit juices, aromatic oils such as peppermint and lemon oils, herbs and spices and distilled fractions of these. They are available as concentrated extracts, alcoholic or aqueous solutions, syrups or spirits and are particularly widely used in the manufacture of products for extemporaneous use. Artificial perfumes and flavours are of purely synthetic origin often having no natural counterpart. They tend to be cheaper, more readily available, less variable in chemical composition and more stable than natural products. They are usually available as alcoholic or aqueous solutions or as powders.

The choice of a suitable flavour can only be made as a result of subjective assessment and, as consumer preferences vary considerably, this task is not easy. Some guidance can, however, be given by reference to Table 14.1 which shows that certain flavours are particularly useful for the masking of one or more of the basic taste sensations of saltiness, bitterness, sweetness and sourness. These tastes are detected by sensory receptors on various areas of the tongue while the more subtle flavours are detected by the olfactory receptors.

Table 14.1

Taste of product	Suitable masking flavour
Salty	Apricot, butterscotch, liquorice, peach, vanilla
Bitter	Anise, chocolate, mint, passion fruit, wild cherry
Sweet	Vanilla, fruits, berries
Sour	Citrus fruits, liquorice, raspberry

In some cases there exists a strong association between the use of a product and its flavour or perfume content. For example, products intended for the relief of indigestion are often mint flavoured. This is because for many years mint has been used in such products for its carminative effect, but even in products containing other active agents, the odour and taste of mint are now firmly associated with antacid activity. Similarly the odour of terpineol is often associated with antiseptic activity and in a competitive market it may therefore be unwise to alter these flavours or perfumes.

The fact that personal preferences for flavours and perfumes often vary with age can also aid the formulator. Children, in general, prefer fruity tastes and smells while adults choose flowery odours and acid flavours.

Other suitable materials for the masking of unpleasant tastes include menthol, peppermint oil and chloroform. In addition to their own particular tastes and odours they also act as desensitizing agents by the exertion of a mild anaesthetic effect on the sensory taste receptors. Flavour-enhancing agents such as citric acid for citrous fruits and glycine or monosodium glutamate for general use are now becoming more widely used.

Isotonicity modifiers

Solutions for injection, for application to mucous membranes and large volume solutions for ophthalmic use must be made iso-osmotic with tissue fluid to avoid pain and irritation. The relevance of osmotic pressure in the formulation of injections is discussed in Chapter 21.

If isotonicity is required it can only be accomplished after the addition of all other ingredients because of their effect on the osmotic pressure of a solution.

Preservatives

When choosing a suitable preservative it must be ensured that adsorption on to the container from the product does not occur or that its efficiency is not impaired by the pH of the solution or by interactions with other ingredients. For example, many of the widely used parahydroxybenzoic acid esters can be adsorbed into the micelles of some non-ionic surfactants (Barr and Tice, 1957) and, although their presence can be detected by chemical analysis, they are, in fact, unable to exert their antimicrobial activity. It is only by full microbiological challenge testing that the efficiency of a preservative system can be properly assessed.

Although most of the information concerning the preservation of emulsions and suspensions is also applicable to the formulation of solutions, a more comprehensive discussion on the preservation of pharmaceuticals can be found in Chapter 27.

Reducing agents and antioxidants

The decomposition of pharmaceutical products by oxidation can be controlled by the addition of reducing agents or antioxidants (see Chapter 13).

Sweetening agents

Low molecular weight carbohydrates and in particular sucrose are traditionally the most widely used sweetening agents. Sucrose has the advantage of being colourless, very soluble in water, stable over a pH range of about 4–8 and by increasing the viscosity of fluid preparations will impart to them a pleasant texture in the mouth. It will mask the tastes of both salty and bitter drugs and has a soothing effect on the membranes of the throat. For this reason sucrose, despite its cariogenic properties, is particularly useful as a vehicle for antitussive preparations. Polyhydric alcohols such as sorbitol, mannitol and to a lesser extent glycerol also possess sweetening power and can be included in preparations for diabetic use where sucrose is undesirable. Other less widely used bulk sweeteners include hydrogenated glucose syrup, isomalt, fructose and xylitol. Treacle, honey and liquorice are now very rarely used having only a minor application in some extemporaneously prepared formulations.

Artificial sweeteners can be used both in conjunction with sugars and alcohols to enhance the degree of sweetness or on their own in formulations for patients who must restrict their sugar intake. They are also termed intense sweeteners because, weight for weight, they are hundreds and even thousands of times sweeter than sucrose and are therefore rarely required at a concentration greater than about 0.2%. At present only four artificial sweeteners are permitted for oral use by the Food Additives and Contaminants Committee, the most widely used being the sodium or calcium salt of saccharin. They exhibit a high water solubility and are chemically and physically stable over a wide pH range. Less widely used are aspartame (a compound of l-aspartic acid and l-phenylala-nine, the use of which is increasing rapidly), acesulfame potassium and thaumatin (Parker, 1978). The main disadvantage of all artificial sweeteners is their tendency to impart a bitter or metallic after-taste and they are, therefore, often formulated with sugars to mask this (Brookes, 1965; Leach, 1970).

TYPES OF PREPARATIONS

Mixtures and draughts

Mixtures are usually aqueous preparations which can be in the form of either a solution or a suspension. Most preparations of this type are manufactured on a small scale as required and are allocated a shelf life of a few weeks before dispensing. Doses are usually given in multiples of 5 ml using a metric medicine spoon.

A draught is a mixture of which only one or two large doses of about 50 ml are given, although smaller doses are often necessary for children.

Elixirs

The terms mixture and elixir are often confused although an elixir refers strictly to a solution of a potent or nauseous drug. If the active agent is sensitive to moisture it may be formulated as a flavoured powder or granulation by the pharmaceutical industry and then simply dissolved in water immediately prior to administration. Dosage is usually given using a 5 ml medicine spoon although smaller volumes can be given using a volumetric dropper.

Linctuses

A linctus is a viscous preparation usually prescribed for the relief of cough. It usually consists of a simple solution of the active agent in a high concentration of sucrose often with other sweetening agents. This type of product, which is also designed to be administered in multiples of 5 ml, should be sipped slowly and not be diluted beforehand. The syrup content has a demulcent action on the mucous membranes of the throat.

For diabetic use the sucrose is usually replaced by sorbitol and/or synthetic sweeteners.

Mouthwashes and gargles

Aqueous solutions for the prevention and treatment of mouth and throat infections can contain antiseptics, analgesics and/or astringents. They are usually diluted with warm water before use.

Nasal products

These are formulated as small volume solutions in an aqueous vehicle, oils being no longer used for nasal administration. Because the buffering capacity of nasal mucous is low, formulation at a pH of 6.8 is necessary. Nasal drops should also be made isotonic with nasal secretions using sodium chloride and viscosity can also be modified using cellulose derivatives if necessary. Active agents for administration by this route are usually for local use and include antibiotics, anti-inflammatories and decongestants.

Ear drops

These are simple solutions of drugs in either water, glycerol, propylene glycol or alcohol/water mixtures for local use and include antibiotics, antiseptics, cleansing solutions and wax softeners.

Enemas

Aqueous or oily solutions, as well as emulsions and suspensions, are available for the rectal administration of medicaments for cleansing, diagnostic or therapeutic reasons.

Preparations for external use

Lotions can be formulated as solutions and are designed to be applied to the skin without friction. They may contain either humectants, so that moisture is retained on the skin after application of the product, or alcohol which evaporates quickly, imparting a cooling effect and leaving the skin dry.

Liniments, however, are intended for massage

into the skin and can contain such ingredients as methyl salicylate or camphor as counter-irritants.

Liquids for application to the skin or mucous membranes in small amounts are often termed paints and are often applied with a small brush. The solvent is usually alcohol, acetone or ether which evaporates quickly leaving a film on the skin containing the active agent and a viscosity modifier such as glycerol to ensure prolonged contact with the skin.

Collodions are similar preparations which, after evaporation of the solvent, leave a tough, flexible film which will seal small cuts or hold a drug in intimate contact with the skin. The film former is usually pyroxylin (nitrocellulose) in an alcohol/ether or alcohol/acetone solvent blend. Often a plasticizer such as castor oil and an adherent like colophony resin are included.

Intermediate products

There are many pharmaceutical solutions which are designed for use during the manufacture of other preparations and which are rarely administered themselves. Aromatic waters, for example are aqueous solutions of volatile materials which are used mainly for their flavouring properties. Examples include peppermint water and anise water which also have carminative properties and chloroform water which also acts as a preservative. They are usually manufactured as concentrated waters and are then diluted, traditionally 1 to 40 in the final preparation.

Infusions, extracts and tinctures are terms used for concentrated solutions of active principles from animal or vegetable sources. Infusions are prepared by extracting the drug using 25% alcohol but without the application of heat. Traditionally these preparations are then diluted 1 to 10 in the final product. Extracts are similar products which are then concentrated by evaporation. Tinctures are alcoholic extracts of drugs but are relatively weak compared with extracts.

Spirits are also alcoholic solutions but of volatile materials which are mainly used as flavouring agents.

Syrups are concentrated solutions of sucrose or other sugars to which medicaments or flavourings are often added. For example Codeine Phosphate

Syrup BPC 1973 is used as a cough suppressant and Orange Syrup BP contains dried bitter orange peel as a flavouring agent. Although syrups are used in the manufacture of other preparations, such as mixtures or elixirs, they can also be administered as products in their own right, the high concentrations of sugars imparting a sweetening effect.

As syrups can contain up to 85% of sugars, they are capable of resisting bacterial growth by virtue of their osmotic effect. Syrups containing lower concentrations of sugars often include sufficient of a polyhydric alcohol such as sorbitol, glycerol or propylene glycol in order to maintain a high osmotic gradient. Wild Cherry Syrup BP, for example, contains 80% sucrose with 5% glycerol. It is possible, however, in a closed container, for surface dilution of a syrup to take place. This occurs as a result of solvent evaporation which condenses on the upper internal surfaces of the container and then flows back on to the surface of the product thus producing a diluted layer which provides an ideal medium for the growth of certain micro-organisms. For this reason syrups often contain additional preservatives.

A further problem with the storage and use of syrups involves the crystallization of the sugar within the screw cap used to seal the containers thus preventing their release. This can be avoided by the addition of the polyhydric alcohols previously mentioned or by the inclusion of invert syrup which is a mixture of glucose and fructose.

STABILITY OF SOLUTIONS

Both the chemical and physical stability of solutions in their intended containers is important. A solution must retain its initial clarity, colour, odour, taste and viscosity over its allocated shelf life.

Clarity can easily be assessed by visual examination or by a measurement of its optical density after agitation. Colour too may be assessed both visually and spectrophotometrically and equipment suitable for the measurement of rheological properties of solutions has been covered earlier. The stability of flavours and perfumes is perhaps more difficult to assess. Although chromatographic methods are used with varying success to quantify these properties, a considerable reliance must be placed on the organoleptic powers of a panel of assessors, who must be screened to ensure that their powers of olfaction and gustation are sufficiently sensitive. If a suitable majority of the panel members are unable to detect a difference between a stored sample and a freshly prepared reference material, it may be assumed that the taste or odour of the sample has not significantly changed.

MANUFACTURE OF SOLUTIONS

For both small and large scale manufacture of solutions the only equipment necessary is suitable mixing vessels, a means of agitation and a filtration system to ensure clarity of the final solution. During manufacture the solute is simply added to the solvent in a mixing vessel and stirring is continued until dissolution is complete. If the solute is more soluble at elevated temperatures it may be advantageous to apply heat to the vessel particularly if the dissolution rate is normally slow. Care must be taken, however, should any volatile or thermolabile materials be present. Size reduction of solid materials to increase their total surface areas should also speed up the process of solution.

Solutes present in low concentrations, particularly dyes, are often predissolved in a small volume of the solvent and then added to the bulk. Volatile materials such as flavours and perfumes are, where possible, added at the end of a process and after cooling if necessary, to reduce loss by evaporation. Finally it must be ensured that significant amounts of any of the materials are not irreversibly adsorbed on to the filtration medium used for final clarification. For discussion on suitable packaging materials and containers for solutions see Chapters 12 and 44.

REFERENCES

Barr, M. and Tice, L. F. (1957) The preservation of aqueous preparations containing nonionic surfactants. *J. Am. Pharm. Ass. (Sci. Edn)*, **46**, 445–451.

Boon, P. F. G., Coles, C. L. J. and Tait, M. (1961) The influence of the variations in solubilising properties of polysorbate 80 on the vitamin A palmitate: polysorbate 80:glycerol:water system. *J. Pharm. Pharmac.*, **13**, 200T–204T.

Brookes, L. G. (1956) The use of synthetic sweetening agents in pharmaceutical preparations and foods. *Chemist and Druggist*, **183**, 421–423.

Coles, C. L. J. and Thomas, D. F. W. (1952) The stability of vitamin A alcohol in aqueous and oily media. *J. Pharm. Pharmac.*, **4**, 898–903.

Elworthy, P. H. and Lipscomb, F. J. (1968) Solubilisation of griseofulvin by nonionic surfactants. *J. Pharm. Pharmac.*, **20**, 817–824.

Gorman, W. G. and Hall, G. D. (1964) Dielectric constant correlations with solubility and solubility parameters. *J.Pharm.Sci.*, **53**, 1017–1020.

Heward, M., Norton, D. A. and Rivers, S. M. (1970) Stability to heat and subsequent storage of chloramphenicol eye drops BPC. *Pharm. J.*, **204**, 386–387.

Kläui, H. (1978) the colouration of liquid galenical forms in fluid oral dosage forms. *Pharm.J.*, **222**, 92.

Leach, R. H. (1970) Factors limiting the use of sugars in paediatric formulations. *Pharm.J.*, **205**, 227–228.

Lupton, A. W. (1942) The pain effects of injections of varying pH. *Pharm.J.*, **148**, 105.

Martindale: The Extra Pharmacopoeia, 28th edn. (1982) Ed. J. E. F. Reynolds, The Pharmaceutical Press, London.

May, D. R. and Kolthoff, I. M. (1948) The aging of precipitates and coprecipitation XL. The solubility of lead chromate as a function of particle size. *J. Phys. Colloid Chem.*, **52**, 836–854.

Neuberg, L. and Weinmann, F. (1930) Theory of hydrotropy. *Biochem. Z.*, **229**, 466–479.

Norton, D. A. (1967) Developments in the formulation and packaging of eye drops. *J. hosp. Pharm.*, **24**, 328–338.

Parker, K. J. (1978) Alternatives to sugar. The search for an ideal non-nutritive sweetener is almost a century old. *Nature*, **271**, 493–495.

Paruta, A. H., Sciarrone, B. J. and Lordi, N. G. (1964) Solubility of salicylic acid as a function of dielectric constant. *J.Pharm.Sci.*, **53**, 1349–1353.

Ravin, L. J., Shami, E. G., Intoccia, A., Rattie, E. and Joseph, G. (1969) Effect of polysorbate 80 on the solubility and 'in vitro' availability of 2-butyl-3-benzofuranyl 4-[2-(diethylamino)ethoxy]-3, 5-diiodophenyl ketone hydrochloride. (SKF 33134A). *J. Pharm. Sci.*, **58**, 1242–1245.

Schumacher, G. E. (1969) Some theoretical aspects of bulk compounding technology I. Ionic equilibria, pH and choice of solvents. *Am. J. hosp. Pharm.*, **26**, 354.

Scott, M. W., Goudie, A. J. and Huetteman, A. J. (1960) Accelerated color loss of certified dyes in the presence of nonionic surfactants. *J. Am. Pharm. Ass. (Sci. Edn)*, **49**, 467–472.

Smith, G. (1967) Eye drops. *Pharm. J.*, **198**, 53–61.

Spiegal, A. J. and Noseworthy, M. M. (1963) The use of nonaqueous solvents in parenteral products. *J. Pharm. Sci.*, **52**, 917–927.

Swartz, C. J. and Cooper, J. (1962) Colorants for

pharmaceuticals *J. Pharm. Sci.*, **51**, 89–95.

Windheuser, J. (1963) The effect of buffers on parenteral solutions. *Bull.Parent.Drug Ass.*, **17**, 1–8.

BIBLIOGRAPHY

Applewhite, R. W., Buckley, A. P. and Lewis Noble, W. (1954) Aqueous solutions of phenobarbital. *J. Am. Pharm. Ass. (Pract. Pharm. Edn.)*, **15**, 164–166.

Elworthy, P. H., Florence, A. T. and Macfarlane, C. B. (1968) *Solubilisation by Surface Active Agents*, Chapman and Hall, London.

Elworthy, P. H. and Macfarlane, C. B. (1965a) The physical chemistry of some nonionic detergents. *J. Pharm. Pharmac.*, **17**, 65–82.

Elworthy, P. H. and Macfarlane, C. B. (1965b) Further aspects of the physical chemistry of some nonionic detergents. *J. Pharm. Pharmac.*, **17**, 129–143.

Foster, A. (1979) Colour legislation and cosmetic and toiletries. *Int. J. cosmet. Sci.*, **1**, 221–245.

Monte-Bovi, A. J., Halpern, A. and Mazzola, P. (1954) Solubilising agents for elixirs. *J. Am. Pharm. Ass. (Pract. Pharm. Edn.)*, **15**, 162–164.

Moore, C. D. and Bell, M. (1959) Solubilisation. *Pharm. J.*, **182**, 171–173.

Swarbrick, J. (1965) Solubilised systems in pharmacy. *J. Pharm. Sci.*, **54**, 1229–1237.

Suspensions

A coarse suspension is a dispersion of finely divided, insoluble solid particles (the disperse phase) in a fluid (the dispersion medium). Most pharmaceutical suspensions consist of an aqueous dispersion medium although in some instances it may be an organic or oily liquid. A disperse phase with a mean particle diameter of up to 1 μm is usually termed a colloidal dispersion and include such examples as aluminium hydroxide and magnesium hydroxide suspensions. A solid in liquid dispersion in which the particles are above colloidal size is termed a coarse suspension. The physical properties of both colloidal and coarse suspensions are discussed in Chapter 6.

Physical properties of a well-formulated suspension

1 The suspension must remain sufficiently homogenous for at least the period between shaking the container and removing the required dose.

2 The sediment produced on storage must be

easily resuspended by the use of moderate agitation.

3 The suspension may be required to be thickened in order to reduce the rate of settling of the particles. The viscosity must not be so high that removal of the product from the container and transfer to the site of application is difficult.

4 The suspended particles should be small and uniformly sized in order to give a smooth, elegant product free from a gritty texture.

PHARMACEUTICAL APPLICATIONS OF SUSPENSIONS

Many people have difficulty in swallowing solid dosage forms and therefore require the drug to be dispersed in a liquid. If the drug is insoluble or poorly soluble in a suitable solvent then formulation as a suspension is usually required. Some eye drops too, notably hydrocortisone and neomycin are available as suspensions because of their poor solubility in a suitable solvent.

The degradation of a drug in the presence of water may also preclude its use as an aqueous solution in which case it may be possible to synthesize an insoluble derivative which can then be formulated as a suspension. For example, oxytetracycline hydrochloride is used in solid dosage forms but in aqueous solution would hydrolyse rapidly. A stable liquid dosage form can, however, be made by suspending the insoluble calcium salt in a suitable aqueous vehicle.

The prolonged contact between the solid drug particles and the dispersion medium can be further reduced by the preparation of the suspension immediately prior to issue to the patient (Ball et al., 1978). Ampicillin, for example, is provided by the manufacturer as either the base or the trihydrate mixed with the other powdered or granulated ingredients. The pharmacist then makes the product up to volume with water immediately before issue to the patient, allocating a suitable shelf life which is usually 7 days at room temperature or 14 days if kept refrigerated.

A drug which degrades in the presence of water may alternatively be suspended in a non-aqueous vehicle. Phenoxymethylpenicillin is available for oral use as a suspension in fractionated coconut oil and in some countries tetracycline hydrochloride

is dispersed in a similar base for ophthalmic use.

Some materials are required to be present in the gastrointestinal tract in a finely divided form and their formulation as suspensions will provide the desired high surface area. Solids such as kaolin, magnesium carbonate and magnesium trisilicate, for example, are used for the adsorption of toxins or to neutralize excess acidity. A dispersion of finely divided silica in dimethicone 1000 is used in veterinary practice for the treatment of 'frothy bloat'.

The adsorptive properties of fine powders are also used in the formulation of some inhalations. The volatile components of menthol and eucalyptus oil would be lost from solution very rapidly during use, whereas a more prolonged release is obtained if the two active agents are adsorbed on to light magnesium carbonate prior to the preparation of a suspension.

The tastes of most drugs are more noticeable if in solution than if in an insoluble form. Paracetamol is available both in solution as Paediatric Paracetamol Elixir BP and also as a suspension. The latter formulation is more palatable and therefore particularly suitable for children. For the same reason chloramphenicol mixtures can be formulated as suspensions containing the insoluble chloramphenicol palmitate.

Suspensions of drugs can also be formulated for topical application (Chapter 22). They can be fluid preparations such as Calamine Lotion BP which is designed to leave a light deposit of the active agent on the skin after evaporation of the dispersion medium. Some suspensions are of semi-solid consistency, for example, pastes which contain high concentrations of powders dispersed, usually, in a paraffin base. It may also be possible to suspend a solid drug in an emulsion base as with Zinc Cream BP.

Suspensions can also be formulated for parenteral administration in order to control the rate of absorption of the drug (Chapter 21). By varying the size of the dispersed particles of active agent, the duration of activity can be controlled. If an aqueous vehicle is used some diffusion of the product will occur along muscle fibres after injection. In order to prolong activity even further, the drug may be suspended in fixed oils such as arachis or sesame oils, in which case the product will remain, after injection in the form of an oil globule thus presenting to the tissue fluid a smaller surface area for release of drug (Woodward, 1952).

Vaccines, for the induction of immunity, are often formulated as suspensions. They may consist of dispersions of killed micro-organisms as in Cholera Vaccine or of the constituent toxoids adsorbed on to a substrate of aluminium hydroxide or phosphate as in Diphtheria and Tetanus Vaccine. Thus a prolonged antigenic stimulus is provided resulting in a high antibody titre.

Some X-ray contrast media are also formulated in this way. Barium sulphate, for the examination of the alimentary tract, is available as a suspension for either oral or rectal administration and propyliodone is dispersed in either water or arachis oil for examination of the bronchial tract.

Chapter 20 describes some aspects of the formulation of aerosols many of which are also available as suspensions of the active agent in a mixture of propellants.

FORMULATION OF SUSPENSIONS

Particle size control

It is first necessary to ensure that the drug to be suspended is suitably subdivided prior to formulation as the rate of sedimentation of a suspended particle can be retarded by a reduction in its size. Large particles, if greater than about 5 μm diameter, will also impart a gritty texture to the product and may cause irritation if injected or instilled into the eyes. The ease of administration of a parenteral suspension may depend upon particle size and shape and it is quite possible to block a hypodermic needle with particles over 25 μm diameter, particularly if they are acicular in shape rather than isodiametric. A particular particle size range may also be chosen in order to control the rate of release of the drug and hence its bioavailability.

Even though the particle size of a drug may be small when the suspension is first manufactured, there is always a degree of crystal growth which occurs on storage (Higuchi, 1958) particularly if temperature fluctuation occurs. This is because the

solubility of the drug may increase as the temperature rises but on cooling the drug will crystallize out. This is a particular problem with slightly soluble drugs such as paracetamol.

If the drug is polydispersed then the very small crystals of less than 1 μm diameter will exhibit a greater solubility then the larger ones. Thus the small crystals will become even smaller while the diameters of the larger particles will increase. It is therefore advantageous to use a suspended drug of narrow size range. The inclusion of surface-active agents or polymeric colloids which adsorb on to the surface of each particle may also help to prevent this.

Different polymorphic forms of a drug may exhibit different solubilities, the metastable state being the most soluble. Conversion of the metastable form in solution to the less soluble stable state and its subsequent precipitation will lead to changes in particle size (Callow and Kennard, 1961; Carless *et al.*, 1968a, b; Pearson and Varney, 1973).

The use of wetting agents

Some insoluble solids may be easily wetted by water and will disperse readily throughout the aqueous phase with minimum agitation. Most, however, will exhibit varying degrees of hydrophobicity and will not be easily wetted. Some particles will form large porous clumps within the liquid while others remain on the surface and become attached to the upper part of the container. The foam produced on shaking will be slow to subside because of the stabilizing effect of the small particles at the liquid/air interface.

To ensure adequate wetting the interfacial tension between the solid and the liquid must be reduced so that the adsorbed air is displaced from the solid surfaces by the liquid. The particles will then disperse readily throughout the liquid particularly if an intense shearing action is used during mixing. If a series of suspensions is prepared each containing one of a range of concentrations of wetting agent, then the concentration to choose will be the lowest which will produce adequate wetting.

The following is a discussion of the most widely used wetting agents in pharmacy.

Surface-active agents

Figure 6.13 shows that surfactants possessing an HLB value of between about 7 and 9 would be suitable for use as wetting agents. The hydrocarbon chains would be adsorbed by the hydrophobic particle surfaces while the polar groups would project into the aqueous medium becoming hydrated. Thus wetting of the solid would occur due to a fall both in interfacial tension between the solid and the liquid and to a lesser extent between the liquid and air.

Most surfactants are used at concentrations of up to about 0.1% as wetting agents and include, for oral use, the polysorbates (Tweens) and sorbitan esters (Spans). For external application sodium lauryl sulphate, sodium dioctylsulphosuccinate and quillaia extract can also be used.

The choice of surfactant for parenteral administration is obviously more limited, the main ones used being the polysorbates, some of the polyoxyethylene/polyoxypropylene copolymers (Pluronics) and lecithin.

Disadvantages in the use of this type of wetting agent include excessive foaming and the possible formation of a deflocculated system which may not be required.

Hydrophilic colloids

These materials include acacia, bentonite, tragacanth, alginates and cellulose derivatives and will behave as protective colloids by coating the solid hydrophobic particles with a multimolecular layer. This will impart a hydrophilic character to the solid and thus promote wetting.

These materials are also used as suspending agents and may, as with surfactants, produce a deflocculated system particularly if used at low concentrations.

Solvents

Materials such as alcohol, glycerol and glycols which are water miscible will reduce the liquid/air interfacial tension. The solvent will penetrate the loose agglomerates of powder displacing the air from the pores of the individual particles thus enabling wetting to occur by the dispersion medium.

Flocculation or deflocculation?

Having incorporated a suitable wetting agent it is then necessary to determine whether the suspension is flocculated or deflocculated and to decide which state is preferable. Whether or not a suspensions flocculated or deflocculated depends on the relative magnitudes of the electrostatic forces of repulsion and the forces of attraction between the particles. The effects of these particle/particle interactions have been adequately covered in Chapter 6 but it must be realized that the incorporation of a wetting agent may result in a suspension exhibiting different physical characteristics from one which contains no additives other than the solid and the dispersion medium.

If a suspension is deflocculated the dispersed particles remain as discrete units and, since the rate of sedimentation depends on the size of each unit, settling will be slow. The repulsive forces between individual particles allow them to slip past each other as they sediment. The slow rate of settling prevents the entrapment of liquid within the sediment which thus becomes compacted and can be very difficult to redisperse. This phenomenon is also called *caking* or *claying* and is the most serious of all the physical stability problems encountered in suspension formulation.

Aggregation of particles in a flocculated system will lead to a much more rapid rate of sedimentation or subsidence because each unit is composed of many individual particles and is therefore larger. The rate of settling will also depend on the porosity of the aggregate since, if porous, the dispersion medium can flow through as well as around each aggregate or floccule as it sediments.

The nature of the sediment of a flocculated system is also quite different from that of a deflocculated one. The structure of each aggregate is retained after sedimentation thus entrapping a large amount of the liquid phase. Although aggregation in the primary minimum will produce compact floccules while a secondary minimum effect will produce loose or 'fluffy' floccules of higher porosity, the volume of the final sediment will still be large and will easily be redispersed by moderate agitation.

The supernatant of a deflocculated system will remain cloudy for an appreciable time after shaking due to the very slow settling rate of the smallest particles in the product. In a flocculated system the supernatant quickly becomes clear as the flocs which settle rapidly are composed of particles of all sizes (Michaels and Bolger, 1964). Figure 15.1 illustrates the appearance of both flocculated and deflocculated suspensions at given times after shaking.

With respect to coarse pharmaceutical suspensions, therefore, deflocculated systems have the advantage of a slow sedimentation rate thus enabling a uniform dose to be taken from the container, but when settling does occur, the sediment is compacted and difficult to redisperse. Flocculated systems form loose sediments which are easily redispersible but the sedimentation rate is fast and there is a danger of an inaccurate dose being administered and the product would look inelegant.

A deflocculated system with a sufficiently high viscosity to prevent sedimentation would be an ideal situation. It cannot be guaranteed, however, that the system would remain homogenous during the shelf life of the product. Usually a compromise is reached in which the suspension is partially flocculated and viscosity is controlled so that the sedimentation rate is at a minimum (Haines and Martin, 1961).

Degree of flocculation

It is important therefore to ensure that the product exhibits the correct *degree* of flocculation. Underflocculation will give those undesirable properties which are associated with deflocculated systems. Overflocculation may be irreversible. The product will look inelegant and its viscosity may be high resulting in difficult redispersion.

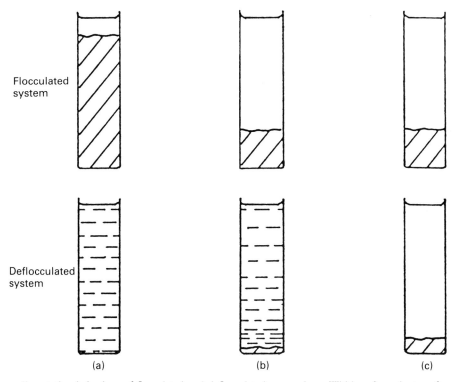

Flocculated system

Deflocculated system

(a)   (b)   (c)

Fig. 15.1 The sedimentation behaviour of flocculated and deflocculated suspensions. Within a few minutes of manufacture (a) there is no apparent change within the deflocculated system compared with its initial appearance. Even after several hours (b), there is still little obvious change except that the concentration of solids in the lower layers has increased at the expense of the upper layers due to slow particle sedimentation. There is a small amount of a compact sediment. After a prolonged storage (c), depending on the physical stability of the system, the supernatant has cleared leaving a compact sediment. In the flocculated system at (a) there is some clear supernatant with a distinct boundary between it and the sediment. At (b) there is a larger volume of clear supernatant with a relatively large volume of a porous sediment which does not change further even after prolonged storage (c)

Controlled flocculation is usually achieved by a combination of particle size control, the use of electrolytes to control zeta potential and the addition of polymers to enable cross-linking to occur between particles. Some polymers have the advantage of becoming ionized in an aqueous solution and can therefore act both electrostatically and sterically. These materials are also termed polyelectrolytes.

Flocculating agents

In many cases, after the incorporation of a non-ionic wetting agent, a suspension will be found to be deflocculated either because of the reduction in solid/liquid interfacial tension or because of the hydrated hydrophilic layer around each particle forming a mechanical barrier to aggregation. The use of an ionic surfactant to wet the solid may produce either type of suspension. If the charge on the particle is neutralized then flocculation will occur. If a high charge density is imparted to the suspended particles then deflocculation will be the result.

If it is necessary for the suspension to be converted from a deflocculated to a flocculated state this may be achieved by the addition of electrolytes, surfactants and/or hydrophilic polymers.

Electrolytes The addition of an inorganic electrolyte to an aqueous suspension will alter the zeta potential of the dispersed particles and if this value is lowered sufficiently then flocculation may occur.

The Schultz–Hardy rule shows that the ability of an electrolyte to flocculate hydrophobic particles depends on the valency of its counter ions. Although more efficient, trivalent ions are less widely used than mono- or divalent electrolytes because they are generally more toxic. If hydrophilic polymers, which are usually negatively charged, are included in the formulation they may be precipitated by the presence of trivalent ions.

The most widely used electrolytes include the sodium salts of acetates, phosphates and citrates and the concentration chosen will be that which produces the desired degree of flocculation (Martin, 1961; Hiestand, 1964). Care must be taken not to add excessive electrolyte or charge reversal may occur on each particle thus forming, once again, a deflocculated system.

Surfactants Ionic surface-active agents may also cause flocculation by neutralization of the charge on each particle thus resulting in a deflocculated system. Non-ionic surfactants will, of course, have little effect on the charge density of a particle but may, because of their linear configurations, adsorb on to more than one particle thus forming a loose flocculated structure.

Polymeric flocculating agents Starch, alginates, cellulose derivatives, tragacanth, carbomers and silicates are examples of polymers which can be used to control the degree of flocculation. Their linear branched chain molecules form a gel-like network within the system and become adsorbed on to the surfaces of the dispersed particles thus holding them in a flocculated state. Although some settling can occur, the sedimentation volume is large and usually remains so for a considerable period.

Care must be taken to ensure that, during manufacture, blending is not excessive as this may inhibit the cross-linking between adjacent particles and result in the adsorption of each molecule of polymer on to one particle only. If this should occur then a deflocculated system may result because the formation of the hydrophilic barrier around each particle will inhibit aggregation. A high concentration of polymer may have a similar effect if the whole surface of each particle is coated. It is essential that areas on each suspended particle remain free from adsorbate so that cross-linking can recur after the product is sheared.

As these polymeric materials will also modify the viscosity of suspensions, further details of their use can be found in the next section.

Rheology of suspensions

An ideal pharmaceutical suspension would exhibit a high apparent viscosity at low rates of shear so that, on storage, the suspended particles would either settle very slowly or, preferably, remain permanently suspended. At higher rates of shear, such as those caused by moderate shaking of the product, the apparent viscosity should fall sufficiently for the product to be poured easily from its container. The product, if for external use, should then spread easily without excessive dragging but should not be so fluid that it runs off the skin surface. If intended for injection, the product should pass easily through a hypodermic needle with only moderate pressure applied to the syringe plunger. It would then be important for the initial high apparent viscosity to be reformed after a short time to maintain adequate physical stability (Hiestand, 1964).

A flocculated system, in part, fulfils these criteria. In such a system pseudoplastic or plastic behaviour (see Chapter 2) is exhibited as the structure progressively breaks down under shear. The product then shows the time-dependent reversibility of this loss of structure which is termed thixotropy.

A deflocculated system, however, would exhibit Newtonian behaviour due to the absence of such structures and may even, if high concentrations of disperse phase are present, exhibit dilatancy.

Although a flocculated system may exhibit a degree of thixotropy and plasticity, unless a high concentration of disperse phase is present, it may not be sufficient to prevent rapid settling, particularly if a surfactant or an electrolyte is present as a flocculating agent. In these cases suspending agent may be used which will enhance the apparent viscosity of the system.

Suitable materials are the hydrophilic polymers which exert their effect by entrapping the solid dispersed particles in their gel-like network thus preventing sedimentation. At low concentrations many suspending agents can be used for controlling flocculation and it must be realized that if high quantities are to be used to enhance viscosity the degree of flocculation may also be altered.

Viscosity modifiers

The following materials are those most widely used for the modification of suspension viscosity.

Polysaccharides

Acacia gum (gum arabic) This natural material is often used as a thickening agent for extemporaneously prepared suspensions. Acacia is not a good thickening agent and its value as a suspending agent is largely due to its action as a protective colloid. It is therefore useful in preparations containing tinctures of resinous materials which precipitate on addition to water. It is essential to ensure that any precipitated resin is well coated by the protective colloid before any electrolyte (which should be well diluted) is added. Acacia is not very satisfactory as a suspending agent for dense powders and it is often, therefore, combined with other thickeners as in Compound Tragacanth Powder BP which contains acacia, tragacanth, starch and sucrose.

Unfortunately, acacia mucilage becomes acidic on storage due to enzyme activity and it also contains an oxidase enzyme which may cause deterioration of active agents which are susceptible to oxidation. This enzyme can, however, be inactivated by heat.

Because of the stickiness of acacia it is rarely used in preparations for external use.

Tragacanth This product will form viscous aqueous solutions. Its thixotropic and pseudoplastic properties make it a better thickening agent than acacia and it can be used both for internal and external products. As with acacia it is mainly, though not exclusively, used for the extemporaneous preparation of suspensions of short shelf life.

Tragacanth is stable over a pH range of 4–7.5 but takes several days to hydrate fully after dispersion in water. The maximum viscosity of its dispersions is not, therefore, achieved until after this time. Its viscosity is also affected by heating of either the powder or the mucilage and care must be taken during its storage. There are several grades of this material available and only the best quality is suitable for use as a pharmaceutical suspending agent.

Alginates Alginic acid, a polymer of d-mannuronic acid, is prepared from kelp and its salts have similar suspending properties to those of tragacanth. Alginate mucilages must not be heated above 60 °C as depolymerization occurs with a consequent loss in viscosity. They are most viscous immediately after preparation after which there is a fall to a fairly constant value after about 24 hours. It exhibits a maximum viscosity over a pH range of 5–9 and at low pH the acid is precipitated. Sodium alginate (Manucol) is the most widely used material in this class but it is, of course, anionic and will be incompatible with cationic materials and with heavy metals. The addition of calcium chloride to a sodium alginate dispersion will cause the calcium salt to be formed with a large increase in viscosity. Several different viscosity grades are commercially available.

Starch Starch is rarely used on its own as a suspending agent but is one of the constituents of Compound Tragacanth Powder BP and it can also be used with sodium carboxymethylcellulose. Sodium starch glycollate (Explotab, Primojel), a derivative of potato starch, has been evaluated for its use in the extemporaneous preparation of suspensions (Farley and Lund, 1976).

Water-soluble celluloses

Several cellulose derivatives are available which will disperse in water to produce viscous colloidal solutions suitable for use as suspending agents (Davies and Rowson, 1957, 1958).

Methylcellulose (Celacol) This is a semisynthetic polysaccharide of the general formula:

$$[C_6H_7O_2(OH_2)OCH_3]_n$$

and is produced by the methylation of cellulose. Several grades are available depending on their degree of methylation and on the chain length. The longer the chain the more viscous is its solution. For example a 2% solution of methylcellulose 20 exhibits a kinematic viscosity of 20 cS $(2 \times 10^{-5} \text{ m}^2\text{s}^{-1})$ and methylcellulose 4500 has a value of 4500 cS $(4.5 \times 10^{-3} \text{ m}^2\text{s}^{-1})$ at 2% concentration. Because these products are more soluble in cold water than in hot, they are often dispersed in warm water and then on cooling with constant stirring a clear or opalescent viscous solution is produced. Methylcelluloses are non-ionic and therefore stable over a wide pH range from 3 to 11 and are compatible with many ionic additives. On heating these dispersions, the methylcellulose molecules become progressively dehydrated and eventually gel at about 50 °C and on cooling the original form is regained.

Hydroxyethylcellulose (Natrosol 250) This compound has hydroxyethyl instead of methyl groups attached to the cellulose chain. It has the advantage of being soluble in both hot and cold water and will not gel on heating. Otherwise it exhibits the same properties as methylcellulose.

Sodium carboxymethylcellulose (Edifas, Cellosize) This material can be represented by:

$$[C_6H_{10-x}O_5(CH_2COONa)_x]_n$$

where x represents the degree of substitution, usually about 0.7, which in turn affects its solubility. The viscosity of its solution depends on the value of n which represents the degree of polymerization. The numerical suffix gives an indication of the viscosity of a 1% solution. For example sodium carboxymethylcellulose 50 at a concentration of 1% will have a viscosity of 50 cP (50 mPa s). This material produces clear solutions in both hot and cold water which are stable over a pH range of about 5–10. Being anionic, this material is incompatible with polyvalent cations and the acid will be precipitated at low pHs. Heat sterilization of either the powder or its mucilage will reduce the viscosity and this must be taken into account during formulation. It is widely used at concentrations of up to 1% in products for oral, parenteral or external use.

Microcrystalline cellulose (Avicel) This material consists of crystals of colloidal dimensions which disperse readily in water (but are not soluble) to produce thixotropic gels. It is a widely used suspending agent often with between 8 and 11% sodium carboxymethylcellulose added to aid its dispersion and to act as a protective colloid (Battista and Smith, 1962; Walkling and Shangraw, 1968). The rheological properties of these dispersions can often be improved by the incorporation of additional hydrocolloid, in particular carboxymethylcellulose, methylcellulose and hydroxypropylmethylcellulose which will also stabilize the dispersion against the flocculating effects of added electrolyte.

Hydrated silicates

There are three important materials within this classification namely bentonite, magnesium aluminium silicate and hectorite and they belong to a group called the montmorillonite clays. They hydrate readily, absorbing up to 12 times their weight of water particularly at elevated temperatures. The gels formed are thixotropic and therefore have useful suspending properties. As with most naturally occurring materials they may be contaminated with spores and this must be borne in mind when considering a sterilization process and when choosing a preservative system (Barr, 1964).

Bentonite This has the general formula:

$$Al_2O_3.4SiO_2.H_2O$$

It is used at concentrations of up to 2 or 3% in preparations for external use such as calamine lotion. As this product may contain pathogenic spores it should be sterilized before use.

Magnesium aluminium silicate (Veegum) This is available as an insoluble flake which disperses and swells readily in water by absorption of the aqueous phase into its crystal lattice. Several grades are available differing in their particle size, acid demand and in the viscosity of their dispersions. They can be used both internally and externally at concentrations of up to about 5% and are stable over a pH range of 3.5–11 (Escabi and DeKay, 1956). Veegum/water dispersions will exhibit thixotropy and plasticity with a high yield value but the presence of salts can alter these rheological properties because of the flocculating effect of their positively charged counter ions. Some grades, however, have a higher resistance to flocculation than others.

This material is often combined with organic thickening agents such as sodium carboxymethylcellulose or xanthan gum to improve yield values, degree of thixotropy and to control flocculation (Huycke, 1950; Wood *et al.*, 1963; Ciullo, 1981).

Hectorite This material is similar to bentonite and can be used at concentrations of 1–2% for external use (Mascardo and Barr, 1955). It is also possible to obtain synthetic hectorites (Laponites) which do not exhibit the batch variability or level of microbial contamination associated with natural products and which can also be used internally. As with other clays it is often advantageous to include an organic gum to modify the rheological properties (Neumann and Sansom, 1970).

Carboxypolymethylene (Carbopol)

This material is a totally synthetic copolymer of acrylic acid and allyl sucrose. It is used at concen-

trations of up to 0.5% mainly for external application although some grades can be taken internally. When dispersed in water it forms acidic, low viscosity solutions which, when adjusted to a pH of between 6 and 11, become highly viscous (Meyer and Cohen, 1959).

Colloidal silicon dioxide (Aerosil, Cab-O-Sil)

When dispersed in water this finely divided product will aggregate forming a three-dimensional network. It can be used at concentrations of up to 4% for external use (Beckerman and Schumacher, 1961) but has also been used for thickening non-aqueous suspensions.

Formulation additives

Buffers

The inclusion of buffers (see Chapters 3 and 21) may be necessary in order to maintain chemical stability, control tonicity or to ensure physiological compatibility. It must be remembered, however, that the addition of electrolytes may have profound effects on the physical stability of suspensions.

Density modifiers

From a qualitative examination of Stokes' law (Chapter 6), it can be seen that if the disperse and continuous phases both have the same densities then sedimentation would not occur. Minor modifications to the aqueous phase of a suspension by incorporating sucrose, glycerol or propylene glycol can be achieved but due to differing coefficients of expansion this can only be possible over a small temperature range.

Flavours, colours and perfumes

The use of these ingredients has been discussed in Chapter 14 and the information there will be directly applicable to suspension formulation.

Because of the high surface area of the dispersed powders in this type of formulation, however, adsorption of these materials may occur thus reducing their effective concentration in solution.

For example, the finer the degree of subdivision of the disperse phase the paler may appear the colour of the product for a given concentration of dye. It must also be realized that the inclusion of these adjuvants may alter the physical characteristics of the system. Either the presence of electrolytes or their effect on pH will influence the degree of flocculation.

Humectants

Glycerol and propylene glycol are examples of suitable humectants which are sometimes incorporated at concentrations of about 5% into aqueous suspensions for external application. They are used to prevent the product from drying out after application to the skin.

Preservatives

The section covering the preservation of emulsions (Chapter 16) is applicable also to suspension formulation. It is essential that a suitable preservative be included particularly if naturally occurring materials are to be used. This is to prevent the growth of micro-organisms which may be present in the raw material and/or introduced into the product during use. Some of the natural products, particularly if they are to be applied to broken skin, should be sterilized before use. Bentonite, for example, may contain *Clostridium tetani* but can be sterilized by heating the dry powder at 160 °C for 1 hour or by autoclaving aqueous dispersions. Care must be taken to ensure that the activity of any of the ingredients is not destroyed by the sterilization process.

As with emulsion formulation, care must be taken to ascertain the extent of inactivation, if any, of the preservative system due to interactions with other excipients. Solubilization by wetting agents, interaction with polymers or adsorption on to suspended solids, particularly kaolin or magnesium trisilicate may reduce the availability of preservatives.

Sweetening agents

Suitable sweeteners have been discussed in Chapter 14. High concentrations of sucrose, sorbitol or glycerol, which will exhibit Newtonian properties, may adversely affect the rheological properties of the suspension. Synthetic sweeteners may be salts and can affect the degree of flocculation.

STABILITY TESTING OF SUSPENSIONS

The physical stability of a suspension is normally assessed by the measurement of its rate of sedimentation, the final volume or height of the sediment and the ease of redispersion of the product.

The first two parameters can be assessed easily by a measurement of the total initial volume or height of the suspension (V_o) and the volume or height of the sediment (V), as shown in Fig. 15.1. By plotting the value of V/V_o against time for a series of trial formulations (all initial values will equal unity) it can be seen by an assessment of the slope of each line which suspension shows the slowest rate of sedimentation. When the value of V/V_o becomes constant this indicates that sedimentation has ceased.

Alternatively the term *flocculation value* can be used which is a ratio of the final volume or height of the sediment and the volume or height of the fully sedimented cake of the same system which has been deflocculated.

Attempts have also been made to equate the zeta potential of the suspended particles with the physical stability, particularly the degree of flocculation, of the system using an electrophoresis apparatus (Stanko and DeKay 1958; Martin, 1961).

The ease of redispersion of the product can be assessed qualitatively by the simple agitation of the product in its container. The use of a mechanical shaker will eliminate variations in shaking ability.

An assessment of these three parameters at elevated temperatures would give a speedier indication of a rank order of degree of instability but it is essential to correlate these results with those taken from suspensions stored at ambient temperatures.

Centrifugation

A qualitative examination of Stokes' law (Chapters 6 and 33) would indicate that centrifugation would also be a suitable method of increasing the rate of sedimentation of a suspension, but again it is not always possible to predict accurately the behaviour of such a system when stored under normal conditions from data obtained after this type of accelerated testing. The process of centrifugation may destroy the structure of a flocculated system which would remain intact under normal storage conditions. The sediment formed would become tightly packed and difficult to redisperse whether or not the initial suspension is flocculated or deflocculated (Jones and Grimshaw, 1963). This method may, however, give a useful indication of the relative stabilities of a series of trial products.

Rheological assessment

Although apparent viscosity measurements are also used as a tool for the assessment of physical stability the high shear rates involved may also destroy the structure of a suspension. Very low rates of shear, using for example the Brookfield viscometer with Helipath stand, can give an indication of the change in the structure of the system after various storage times. It may be possible to combine the results from sedimentation techniques with those from rheological assessments (Foernzler et al., 1960).

A measurement of the residual apparent viscosity, after breaking down the structure of the suspension, can be used as a routine quality control procedure after manufacture.

Temperature cycling

By the exaggeration of the temperature fluctuations that any product is subjected to under normal storage conditions it may be possible to compare the physical stabilities of a series of suspensions. Cycles consisting of storage for several hours at a temperature of about 40 °C followed by freezing have been used successfully. Similarly normal temperature fluctuations can be used but at increased frequencies of only a few

minutes at each extreme. This method of accelerated stability testing is particularly useful for the assessment of crystal growth (Carless and Foster, 1966). Measurement of particle size is usually carried out microscopically, by laser diffraction or by using a Coulter Counter. It is important, of course, to ensure that the suspension is deflocculated to ensure that each individual particle is measured rather than each floccule.

MANUFACTURE OF SUSPENSIONS

It is important to ensure, initially, that the powder to be suspended is in a suitably fine degree of subdivision in order to ensure adequate bioavailability, minimum sedimentation rate and impalpability. Suitable size reduction equipment and the relative merits of wet and dry milling are detailed in Chapter 34.

For the extemporaneous preparation of suspensions on a small scale the powdered drug can be mixed with the suspending agent and some of the vehicle using a pestle and mortar. It may also be necessary, at this stage, to include a wetting agent to aid dispersion. Other soluble ingredients should then be dissolved in another portion of the vehicle, mixed with the concentrated suspension and then made up to volume.

It is often preferable, particularly on a larger scale, to make a concentrated dispersion of the suspending agent first. This is best accomplished by adding the material slowly to the vehicle while mixing. Suitable mixers are described in chapter 16 under 'Manufacture of emulsions' but can include either an impeller type of blender or a turbine mixer. This stage is important as it is necessary to ensure that agglomerates of the suspending agent are fully broken up. If they are not then the surface of each agglomerate may gel and therefore cause the powder inside to remain non-wetted. Very intense shearing, however, can destroy the polymeric structure of the suspending agent, and it may be better to use milder shearing and then allow the dispersion to stand until full hydration has been achieved. This may be instantaneous or may, as with tragacanth, take several hours. If the suspending agent is blended with one of the water-soluble ingredients, such as sucrose, this will also aid dispersion.

The drug to be suspended is then added in the same way along with the wetting agent. For very hydrophobic drugs wetting may be facilitated by mixing under reduced pressure. This has the additional advantage of deaerating the product and thus improving its appearance. Other ingredients should now be added, preferably dissolved in a portion of the vehicle, and the whole made up to volume if necessary. Finally homogenization, as detailed in Chapter 16, would ensure complete dispersion of the drug and the production of a smooth and elegant preparation.

It is also possible, though much less widely used, to suspend an insoluble drug by precipitating it from a solution. This can be accomplished either by double decomposition, or, if a weak acid or a weak base, by altering the pH of its solution or by precipitating the drug from a water-miscible solvent on the addition of water. This method may be of use if the drug is required to be sterile but is degraded by heat or by irradiation. A soluble form of the drug is dissolved in a suitable vehicle, sterilized by filtration and then precipitated to form a suspension.

In normal circumstances aqueous suspensions can be autoclaved as long as the process does not adversely affect either physical or chemical stability.

BIOAVAILABILITY OF SUSPENDED DRUGS

After the oral administration of suspensions, the drug, which is already in a wetted state, is presented to the gastrointestinal fluids in a finely divided form. Thus dissolution occurs immediately from all particles. The rate of absorption of the drug into the blood stream is therefore usually faster than for the same drug in a solid dosage form but not as fast as that from a solution. The rate of release of a drug from a suspension is also dependent upon the viscosity of the product. The more viscous the preparation, the slower is likely to be the release of the drug. Care must therefore be taken to ensure that the physical characteristics of the suspension do not change on addition to an acid medium if this should affect the rate of release of the drug.

Because the rate of release of an active agent from a suspension is usually slower than the release from solution, drugs are often formulated as suspensions for intramuscular, intra-articular or subcutaneous injection in order to prolong the release of the drug (see Chapter 21). This is often termed depot therapy. Penicillin V, for example, which is normally water soluble, can be synthesized as the insoluble procaine salt. After intramuscular injection as a suspension the rate of release is sufficiently slowed to maintain adequate blood levels for up to 24 hours. A further sustained effect can also be achieved by the inclusion of aluminium stearate as a gelling agent in this formulation. If the drug is suspended in an oil, which, after injection, will remain as an oil globule, release of the drug will occur more slowly than from an aqueous suspension when the product may diffuse along muscle fibres thus increasing the area of contact.

Sustained release preparations formulated as suspensions for oral use are not very common but one example is the binding of phentermine on to cationic exchange resins which are then suspended in an aqueous vehicle. After ingestion the drug is slowly released by exchanging with ions present in the gastrointestinal tract. One of the main difficulties in the formulation of this type of product is to ensure that ions are not present in any of its ingredients.

REFERENCES

Ball, D., Lee, T., Ryder, J., Seager, H. and Sharland, D. (1978) Improving the stability of a product containing interactive ingredients. A comparison of different approaches. *J. Pharm. Pharmac.*, **30**, 43P.

Barr, M. (1964) Clays as dispersion stabilisers in pharmaceutical systems. *J. Am. Pharm. Ass. (Pharm Edn)*, **NS4**, 180–183.

Battista, D. A. and Smith, P. A. (1962) Microcrystalline cellulose. *Ind. Engng Chem. (Int. Edn)*, **54** (9), 20–29.

Beckerman, J. H. and Schumacher, G. E. (1961) Experiences with fumed silicon dioxide as a suspending agent. *Am. J. hosp. Pharm.*, **18**, 278–281.

Callow, R. K. and Kennard, O. (1961) Polymorphism of cortisone acetate. *J. Pharm. Pharmac.*, **13**, 723–733.

Carless, J. E. and Foster, A. A. (1966) Accelerated crystal growth of sulphathiazole by temperature cycling. *J. Pharm. Pharmac.*, **18**, 697–708.

Carless, J. E., Moustafa, M. A. and Rapson, H. D. C. (1968a) Dissolution and crystal growth in aqueous suspensions of cortisone acetate. *J. Pharm. Pharmac.*, **20**, 630–638.

Carless, J. E., Moustafa, M. A. and Rapson, H. D. C. (1968b) Effect of crystal form, cortisone alcohol and agitation on the crystal growth of cortisone acetate in aqueous suspensions. *J. Pharm. Pharmac.*, **20**, 639–645.

Ciullo, P. A. (1981) Rheological properties of magnesium aluminium silicate/xanthan gum dispersions. *J. Soc. Cosmet. Chem.*, **32**, Sept/Oct.

Davies, R. E. M. and Rowson, J. M. (1957) Water-soluble cellulose derivatives. Factors affecting the viscosity of aqueous dispersions. Part 1. *J. Pharm. Pharmac.*, **9**, 672–680.

Davies, R. E. M. and Rowson, J. M. (1958) Water-soluble cellulose derivatives. Factors affecting the viscosity of aqueous dispersions. Part 2. *J. Pharm. Pharmac.*, **10**, 30–39.

Escabi, R. S. and DeKay, H. G. (1956) New developments in calamine lotion. *J. Am. Pharm. Ass. (Pract. Pharm. Edn)*, **17**, 30–33, 47–49.

Farley, C. A. and Lund, W. (1976) Suspending agents for extemporaneous dispensing: evaluation of alternatives to tragacanth. *Pharm. J.*, **1**, 562–566.

Foernzler, E. C., Martin, A. N. and Banker, G. S. (1960) The effect of thixotropy on suspension stability. *J. Am. Pharm. Ass. (Sci. Edn)*, **49**, 249–252.

Haines, B. A. and Martin, A. N. (1961) Interfacial properties of powdered material; caking in liquid dispersions Part 2. *J. Pharm. Sci.*, **50**, 753–756, Part 3, 756–759.

Hiestand, E. N. (1964) Theory of coarse suspension formulation. *J. Pharm. Sci.*, **53**, 1.

Higuchi, T. (1958) Some physical chemical aspects of suspension formulation. *J. Am. Pharm. Ass. (Sci. Edn)*, **47**, 657–660.

Huycke, C. L. (1950) Colloidal aluminium magnesium silicate as a suspending agent. *J. Am. Pharm. Ass. Pract. (Pharm. Edn)*, **11**, 170–172.

Jones, W. and Grimshaw, J. T. (1963) Accelerated stability testing of pharmaceutical products. *Pharm. J.*, **191**, 459.

Martin, A. N. (1961) Physico-chemical approach to the formulation of pharmaceutical suspensions. *J. Pharm. Sci.*, **50**, 513.

Mascardo, L. and Barr, M. (1955) A comparison of hectorite and bentonite as suspending agents for pharmaceutical substances. *Drug Stand.*, **23**, 205–208.

Meyer, R. J. and Cohen, L. (1959) *J. Soc. Cosmet. Chem.*, **10**, 143.

Michaels, A. S. and Bolger, J. C. (1964) Particle interactions in aqueous kaolinite dispersions. *Ind. Engng Chem. Fundamentals*, **3**, 14–20.

Neumann, B. S. and Sansom, K. G. (1970) Laponite clay — a synthetic inorganic gelling agent for aqueous solutions of polar organic compounds. *J. Soc. Cosmet. Chem.*, **21**, 237–258.

Pearson, J. T. and Varney, G. (1973) The anomalous behaviour of some oxyclozanide polymorphs. *J. Pharm. Pharmac.*, **25**, 62P–70P.

Stanko, G. L. and DeKay, H. G. (1958) Evaluation of suspensions using electrokinetic measurements. *J. Am. Pharm. Ass. (Sci. Edn)*, **47**, 104–107.

Walkling, W. D. and Shangraw, R. F. (1968) Rheology of microcrystalline cellulose–carboxymethylcellulose gels. *J. Pharm. Sci.*, **57**, 1927–1933.

Wood, J. H., Catacalos, G. and Lieberman, S. V. (1963) A rheological study of the aging of Veegum suspensions. *J. Pharm. Sci.*, **52**, 354–361.

Woodward, W. A. (1952) Recent developments in the pharmacy of antibiotics. *J. Pharm. Pharmac.*, **4**, 1009–1036.

BIBLIOGRAPHY

Hiestand, E. N. (1972) Physical properties of coarse suspensions. *J. Pharm. Sci.*, **61**, 268–272.

Jones, R. D. C., Matthews, B. A. and Rhodes, C. T. (1970) Physical stability of sulfaguanidine suspensions. *J. Pharm. Sci.*, **59**, 518.

Matthews, B. A. and Rhodes, C. T. (1968) Some studies of flocculation phenomena in pharmaceutical suspensions. *J. Pharm. Sci.*, **57**, 569.

Parfitt, G. D. (1973) *Dispersions of Powders in Liquids*, 2nd edn, Applied Science Publications.

Samyn, J. C. (1961) An industrial approach to suspension formulation. *J. Pharm. Sci.*, **50**, (6), 517.

Stortz, G. K. and Kennon, L. (1970) Pharmaceutical suspensions. In: *The Theory and Practice of Industrial Pharmacy* (Ed. L. Lachman), pp. 517–537, Lea and Febiger, Philadelphia, USA.

Emulsions

An emulsion may be defined as two immiscible liquids, one of which is finely subdivided and uniformly distributed as droplets throughout the other. The system is stabilized by the presence of an emulsifying agent. The dispersed liquid or internal phase usually consists of globules of diameters down to $0.1~\mu m$ which are distributed within the external or continuous phase.

Emulsion types

Pharmaceutical emulsions usually consist of mixtures of an aqueous phase with various oils and/or waxes. If the oil droplets are dispersed throughout the aqueous phase the emulsion is termed oil-in-water (o/w). A system in which the water is dispersed throughout the oil is a water-in-oil (w/o) emulsion. It is also possible to form a multiple emulsion. For example, a small water droplet can be enclosed in a larger oil droplet which is itself dispersed in water. This gives a 'water-in-oil-in-water' (w/o/w) emulsion. The alternative o/w/o emulsion is also possible.

If the dispersed globules are of colloidal dimensions (1 nm to 1 μm diameter), the preparation, which is quite often transparent, is called a *microemulsion*. This type of emulsion has similar properties to a micellar system and will therefore exhibit the properties of hydrophobic colloids (see Chapter 6). As the sizes of the dispersed droplets increase, more of the chracteristics of coarse dispersions will be exhibited (see again Chapter 6).

Tests for identification of emulsion type

Several methods are available for distinguishing between o/w and w/o emulsions (see Table 16.1).

Table 16.1 Tests for identification of emulsion type

Oil-in-water emulsions	Water-in-oil emulsions
Miscibility tests	
Are miscible with water but immiscible with oil	Are miscible with oil but not with water
Staining tests by incorporation of an oil-soluble dye	
Macroscopic examination	
Paler colour than a w/o emulsion	More intense coloration than with an o/w emulsion
Microscopic examination	
Coloured globules on a colourless background	Colourless globules against a coloured background
Conductivity tests	
Water, being the continuous phase, will conduct electricity throughout the system. Two metal electrodes, when placed in such a preparation with a battery and suitable light source connected in series will cause the lamp to glow	A preparation in which oil is the continuous phase will not conduct electricity. The lamp will not glow or will only flicker spasmodically

The most common of these involve:

1 miscibility tests with oil or water — the emulsion will only be miscible with liquids that are miscible with its continuous phase,

2 conductivity measurements — systems with aqueous continuous phases will readily conduct electricity whilst systems with oily continuous phases will not, and

3 staining tests — water-soluble and oil-soluble dyes are used one of which will dissolve in and colour the continuous phase.

FORMULATION OF EMULSIONS

Because of the very wide range of emulsifying agents available, considerable experience is required in order to choose the best emulgent system for a particular product. The choice, however, will depend to a large extent on the properties and use of the final product and the other materials required to be present.

Choice of emulsion type

The decision as to whether an o/w or a w/o emulsion is to be formulated will eliminate many unsuitable emulsifying systems.

Fats or oils for oral administration, either as medicaments in their own right, or as vehicles for oil-soluble drugs, are invariably formulated as oil-in-water emulsions. In this form they are pleasant to take and the inclusion of a suitable flavour in the aqueous phase will mask any unpleasant taste.

Emulsions for intravenous administration must also be of the o/w type, although intramuscular injections can also be formulated as w/o products if a water-soluble drug is required for depot therapy.

Emulsions are most widely used, however, for external application. Semisolid emulsions are termed creams and more fluid preparations are either lotions or, if intended for massage into the skin, liniments. Both o/w and w/o types are available. The former are used for the topical application of water-soluble drugs mainly for local effect. They do not have the greasy texture associated with oily bases and are therefore pleasant to use and easily washed from skin surfaces.

Water-in-oil emulsions will have an occlusive effect by hydrating the upper layers of the stratum corneum and inhibiting evaporation of eccrine secretions. This may influence the absorption of drugs from these preparations.

This type of emulsion is also useful for cleansing the skin of oil-soluble dirt, although its greasy texture is not always cosmetically acceptable. Oil-in-water emulsions are less efficient cleansers but are usually more acceptable to the consumer particularly for use on the hands. Similarly, moisturizing creams, designed to prevent moisture loss from the skin and thus inhibit drying of the stratum corneum, are more efficient if formulated as w/o emulsions producing a coherent, water-repellent film on the skin.

Choice of oil phase

In many instances the oil phase of an emulsion is the active agent and therefore its concentration in the product is predetermined. Liquid paraffin, castor oil, cod liver oil and arachis oil are all examples of medicaments which are formulated as emulsions for oral administration. Cottonseed oil, soya bean oil and safflower oil are used for their high calorific value in emulsions for intravenous feeding and examples of externally applied oils which are formulated as emulsions include turpentine oil and benzyl benzoate.

Many emulsions for external use contain an oil which is present solely as a carrier for the active agent. It must be realized, however, that the type of oil used may also have an effect both on the viscosity of the product and on the transport of the drug into the skin (see Chapter 22). One of the most widely used oils for this type of preparation is liquid paraffin. This is one of a series of hydrocarbons which also includes hard paraffin, soft paraffin and light liquid paraffin. They can be used individually or in combination with each other in order to control emulsion consistency. This will ensure that the product can be spread easily but will be sufficiently viscous to form a coherent film over the skin. The film forming capabilities of the emulsion can be further modified by the inclusion of various waxes such as beeswax, carnauba wax or higher fatty alcohols. Thus continuous films can be formed which are sufficiently tough and flexible to prevent contact between the skin and aqueous based irritants. These preparations are called barrier creams and

although many are of the w/o variety, the inclusion of silicone oils, which have exceptional water-repellent properties, may also permit the formulation of o/w products which are equally effective. Dimethicone Cream BPC 1973 is a good example of a silicone based barrier cream.

A variety of fixed oils of vegetable origin are also available, the most widely used being arachis, sesame, cottonseed and maize oils. Those expressed from seeds or fruits are often protein rich and contain useful vitamins and minerals. They are often, therefore, formulated for oral use as emulsions. Because of their lack of toxicity they can be used both internally or externally as vehicles for other materials.

Emulsion consistency

The texture or feel of a product intended for external use must also be considered. A w/o preparation will have a greasy texture and often exhibit a higher apparent viscosity than o/w emulsions. This fact is often used to convey a feeling of richness to many cosmetic formulations. Oil-in-water emulsions will, however, feel less greasy or sticky on application to the skin, will be absorbed more readily due to their lower oil content and can, if necessary, be easily washed from the skin surface.

Ideally emulsions should exhibit the rheological properties of plasticity/pseudoplasticity and thixotropy (see Chapter 2). A high apparent viscosity at the very low rates of shear caused by movement of dispersed phase globules is necessary in order to retard this movement and therefore maintain a physically stable emulsion. It is important, however, that these products should flow freely during agitation, pouring from the container or injecting through a hypodermic needle. Therefore at these high rates of shear a lower apparent viscosity is required. This change in apparent viscosity must be quickly reversible on storage to retard creaming and coalescence.

For an externally applied product a wide range of emulsion consistencies can be tolerated. Low viscosity lotions and liniments can be formulated which can be dispensed from a flexible plastic container via a nozzle on to the skin. Only light shearing is then required in order to spread this type of product over the skin. This is particularly advantages for painful or inflamed skin conditions. The main disadvantage with low viscosity emulsions is their tendency to cream easily especially if formulated with a low oil concentration. It is rarely possible to formulate low viscosity w/o products because of the consistency of the oil phase.

Emulsions of high apparent viscosity for external use are termed creams and are of a semi-solid consistency. They are usually packed into collapsible plastic or aluminium tubes although large volumes or very high viscosity products are often packed into glass or plastic jars.

It is important not to ignore the patient/consumer acceptability of topically applied preparations particularly in a competitive market.

There are several methods by which the rheological properties of an emulsion can be controlled.

Volume concentration of dispersed phase

As discussed in Chapters 2 and 6 Einstein developed an equation relating the viscosity of a suspension to the volume fraction of the particles in that suspension. A qualitative application of this equation to the behaviour of emulsions shows that the vicosity of the product as a whole would be higher than the viscosity of the continuous phase on its own. Thus as the concentration of dispersed phase increases so does the apparent viscosity of the product.

Care must be taken to ensure that the dispersed phase concentration does not increase above about 60% as phase inversion may occur.

Particle size of dispersed phase

It is possible under certain conditions to increase the apparent viscosity of an emulsion by a reduction in mean globule diameter. This can be achieved by homogenization. There are several postulated mechanisms for this occurrence.

A smaller mean globule size may cause increased flocculation. In a flocculated system a significant part of the continuous phase is trapped within aggregates of droplets thus effectively increasing the apparent disperse phase concentration. Emulsions consisting of polydispersed droplets will tend to exhibit a lower viscosity than a monodispersed system due to differences in electrical double layer size and thus in the energy of interaction curves. These variations in interaction between globules during shear may be reflected in their flow behaviour.

If the emulsion is stabilized by a hydrophilic colloid it will act by forming a multimolecular film round the dispersed globules. A reduction in mean globule size will increase the total surface area and therefore more colloid will be adsorbed on to the droplet surface. This will effectively increase the volume concentration of the dispersed phase.

The particle size of the dispersed phase is therefore controlled mainly by the method and conditions of manufacture of the emulsion and by the type of emulgent used and its concentration.

Viscosity of continuous phase

It has been well documented that a direct relationship exists between the viscosity of an emulsion and the viscosity of its continuous phase.

Syrup and glycerol which are used in oral emulsions as sweetening agents will also increase the viscosity of the continuous phase. Their main disadvantage is in increasing the density difference between the two phases and thus possibly accelerating creaming.

Hydrocolloids, when used as emulsifying agents in o/w emulsions, will not only stabilize them by the formation of multimolecular layers around the dispersed globules but also by increasing the continuous phase viscosity. They do not have the disadvantage of changing the density of this phase.

If oil is the continuous phase then the inclusion of soft or hard paraffin or certain waxes will increase its viscosity.

Viscosity of dispersed phase

For most practical applications it is doubtful whether this factor would have any significant effect on total emulsion viscosity. It is possible, however, that a less viscous dispersed phase would be deformed during shear to a greater extent than a more viscous phase and thus the total interfacial area would slightly increase. This may affect double layer interactions and thus the viscosity of the emulsion.

For an excellent review article concerning the flow properties of emulsions see Sherman (1964).

Nature and concentration of emulsifying system

It has already been shown that hydrophilic colloids, as well as forming multimolecular films at the oil/water interface, will also increase the viscosity of the continuous phase of an o/w emulsion. Obviously as the concentration of this type of emulgent increases so will the viscosity of the product.

Surface-active agents forming condensed monomolecular films will, by the nature of their chemical structure, influence the degree of flocculation in a similar way by forming linkages between adjacent globules forming a gel-like structure. A flocculated system will exhibit a greater apparent viscosity than its deflocculated counterpart and will depend on surfactant concentration.

Choice of emulsifying agent

Toxicity and irritancy considerations

The choice of emulgent to be used will depend not only on its emulsifying ability, but also on its route of administration and consequently on its toxicity. Although there is no approved list of emulsifying agents for use in pharmaceutical products there is available the *Emulsifiers and Stabilisers in Food Regulations* (1962) and it can be assumed that emulsifiers contained in this list would be suitable for internally used pharmaceutical emulsions. The regulations mainly include naturally occurring materials and their semisynthetic derivatives such as the polysaccharides, and also include glycerol esters, cellulose ethers, sorbitan esters and polysorbates.

It will be noted that most of these are non-ionic having a tendency to be less irritant and less toxic than their anionic and particularly their cationic counterparts. Ionic emulsifying agents should not be administered orally at the concentrations used for their emulgent properties due mainly to their irritancy on the gastrointestinal tract and consequent laxative effect. Cationic surfactants, in general, are toxic even at lower concentrations and

emulgents such as cetrimide are limited to externally used preparations where its antiseptic properties are of use.

Some emulgents such as the anionic alkali soaps often have a high pH and are thus unsuitable for application to broken skin. Even on normal intact skin with a pH of 5–5.5 the application of such alkaline materials can cause irritancy. Some emulsifiers — wool fat in particular — can cause sensitization reactions in susceptible people.

When choosing an emulgent for parenteral use it must be realised that only certain types of nonionic material are suitable. These include lecithin, polysorbate 80, methylcellulose, gelatin and serum albumin.

Classification of emulsifying agents

The inclusion of an emulsifying agent or agents is necessary to facilitate actual emulsification during manufacture and also to ensure emulsion stability during the shelf life of the product.

The different methods by which emulsifying agents (also called emulsifiers or emulgents) exert their effects have been detailed in Chapter 6, but the one factor common to all of them is their ability to form an adsorbed film around the dispersed droplets between the two phases. There are many types of emulgent available but for convenience of discussion they can be divided into three main classifications — synthetic or semisynthetic surface-active agents, naturally occurring materials and their derivatives and finely divided solids.

These divisions are quite arbitrary and some materials may justifiably be placed in more than one category.

Synthetic and semisynthetic surface-active agents

There are four main categories of these materials depending on their ionization in aqueous solutions: anionic, cationic, non-ionic and amphoteric surfactants.

Anionic surfactants

In aqueous solutions these compounds dissociate to form negatively charged anions which are responsible for their emulsifying ability. They are widely used because of their cheapness but due to their toxicity are only used for externally applied preparations.

Alkali metal and ammonium soaps Emulgents of this group mainly consist of the sodium, potassium or ammonium salts of long chain fatty acids such as:

sodium stearate $C_{17}H_{35}COO^- Na^+$

They produce stable o/w emulsions but may in some instances require the presence of an auxiliary non-ionic emulsifying agent in order to form a complex monomolecular film at the oil/water interface. Because these materials will, in acidic conditions, precipitate out as the free fatty acids, they are most efficient in an alkaline medium.

This type of emulgent can also be formed *in situ* during the manufacture of the product by reacting an alkali such as potassium, sodium or ammonium hydroxide with a fatty acid. The latter may be a constituent of a vegetable oil. Oleic acid and ammonia, for example, are reacted together to form the soap responsible for stabilizing White Liniment BP.

These emulgents are incompatible with polyvalent cations which may cause phase reversal and it is essential, therefore, that deionized water be used for their preparation.

Soaps of divalent and trivalent metals Although many different divalent and trivalent salts of fatty acids exist and would produce satisfactory emulsions, only the calcium salts are commonly used. They are often formed *in situ* during preparation of the product by interacting the appropriate fatty acid with calcium hydroxide. For example oleic acid is reacted with calcium hydroxide to produce calcium oleate which is the emulsifying agent for both Zinc Cream BP and Oily Calamine Lotion BP.

These emulgents will only produce w/o emulsions.

Amine soaps A number of amines form salts with fatty acids. One of the most important types used is based on triethanolamine $N(CH_2CH_2OH)_3$ and is widely used in both pharmaceutical and cosmetic products. For example triethanolamine stearate forms stable o/w emulsions and is usually made *in situ* by a reaction between triethaolamine

and the appropriate fatty acid. Although these emulgents are usually of a neutral pH they are still restricted to externally used preparations. They are also incompatible with acids and high concentrations of electrolytes.

Sulphated and sulphonated compounds The alkyl sulphates have the general formula $ROSO_3^- M^+$ where R represents a hydrocarbon chain and M^+ is usually sodium or triethanolamine. An example is sodium lauryl sulphate which is widely used to produce o/w emulsions but because of its high water solubility and its inability to form condensed films at the oil/water interface, it is always used in conjunction with a non-ionic oil-soluble emulsifying agent in order to produce a complex condensed film. It is used with cetostearyl alcohol to produce Emulsifying Wax BP which stabilizes such preparations as Aqueous Cream BP and Benzyl Benzoate Application BP.

Sulphonated compounds are much less widely used as emulgents. Materials of this class such as sodium dioctylsulphosuccinate are more often used as wetting agents or for their detergency.

Cationic surfactants

In aqueous solutions these materials dissociate to form positively charged cations which provide the emulsifying properties. The most important group of cationic emulgents consists of the quaternary ammonium compounds. Although these materials are widely used for their disinfectant and preservative properties they are also useful o/w emulsifiers. Like many anionic emulgents, if used on their own they will produce only poor emulsions. If used with non-ionic, oil-soluble auxiliary emulgents they will form stable preparations.

Because of the toxicity of cationic surfactants they tend to be used only for the formulation of antiseptic creams where the cationic nature of the emulgent is also responsible for the product's antiseptic properties.

Cationic emulsifying agents are incompatible with anionic surface-active agents and polyvalent anions and are unstable at high pH.

Cetrimide The most useful of these cationic emulgents is cetrimide (cetyl trimethylammonium bromide) $CH_3(CH_2)_{15}N^+(CH_3)_3$ Br^-. Cetrimide Emulsifying Wax BPC 1973, consisting of 90%

cetostearyl alcohol and 10% cetrimide is used in the formulation of Cetrimide Cream BP.

Non-ionic surfactants

These products range from oil-soluble compounds stabilizing w/o emulsions to water-soluble materials giving o/w products. It is usual for a combination of a water-soluble with an oil-soluble emulgent to be used in order to obtain the complex interfacial film necessary for optimum emulsion stability. Non-ionic emulgents are particularly useful due to their low toxicity and irritancy and some, therefore, can be used for orally and parenterally administered preparations. They also have a greater degree of compatibility with other materials than do anionic or cationic emulgents and are less sensitive to changes in pH or to the addition of electrolytes. They do, however, tend to be more expensive.

Being non-ionic the dispersed globules may not possess a significant charge density. In order, therefore, to reduce the tendency for coalescence to occur it is necessary, for an oil-in-water emulsion, that the polar groups be well hydrated and/or be bulky in order physically to prevent close approach of the dispersed droplets.

Most non-ionic surfactants are based on:

1 a fatty acid or alcohol (usually with 12–18 carbon atoms), the hydrocarbon chain of which provides the hydrophobic moiety, and
2 an alcohol (–OH) and/or ethylene oxide grouping ($-OCH_2CH_2-$) which provide the hydrophilic part of the molecule.

By varying the relative proportions of the hydrophilic and hydrophobic groupings many different products can be obtained.

If the hydrophobic part of the molecule predominates then the surfactant will be oil soluble. It will not concentrate at the oil/water interface but tend to migrate into the oil phase. Similarly a water-soluble surfactant will migrate into the aqueous phase and away from the oil/water interface. The best type of non-ionic surfactant to use is one with an equal balance of hydrophobic and hydrophilic groupings. An alternative would be to use two emulgents — one hydrophilic and one hydrophobic. The cohesion between their hydrocarbon chains will then hold both types at the oil/water interface.

Glycol and glycerol esters Glyceryl monostearate (a polyhydric alcohol fatty acid ester) is a strongly hydrophobic material that produces weak w/o emulsions. The addition of small amounts of sodium, potassium or triethanolamine salts of suitable fatty acids will produce a 'self-emulsifying' glycerol monostearate which is a useful o/w emulsifier. Self-emulsifying monostearin is glyceryl monostearate to which anionic soaps (usually oleate or stearate) have been added. This combination is used to stabilize Hydrocortisone Lotion BPC 1973.

Other polyhydric alcohol fatty acid esters are also available either in the pure form or in the 'self-emulsifying' form containing small proportions of a primary emulsifier and include glyceryl mono-oleate, diethylene glycol monostearate and propylene glycol mono-oleate.

Sorbitan esters These are produced by the esterification of one or more of the hydroxyl groups of sorbitan with either lauric, loeic, palmitic or stearic acid. One example is shown below.

This range of surfactants exhibits lipophilic properties and tends to form w/o emulsions. They are, however, much more widely used with polysorbates to produce either o/w or w/o emulsions.

Polysorbates Polyethylene glycol derivatives of the sorbitan esters give us polysorbates. These have the general formula where R represents a fatty acid chain. Variations in the type of fatty acid used and in the number of oxyethylene groups in the polyethylene glycol chains produces a range of products of differing oil and water solubilities. Polyoxyethylene 20 sorbitan mono-oleate, for example, contains 20 oxyethylene groups in the molecule. This number must not be confused with the one given as part of the official name (polysorbate 80) or in the trade name (Tween 80) which is included in order to identify the type of fatty acid in the molecule.

Polysorbates are generally used in conjunction with the corresponding sorbitan ester to form a complex condensed film at the oil/water interface (see Formulation by the HLB method below).

Other non-ionic oil-soluble materials such as glyceryl monostearate, cetyl or stearyl alcohol or propylene glycol monostearate can be incorporated with polysorbates to produce a 'self-emulsifying' preparation. For example Polawax contains cetyl alcohol with a polyoxyethylene sorbitan ester.

Polysorbates are compatible with most anionic, cationic and non-ionic materials. They are of neutral pH and are stable to the effects of heat, pH change and high concentrations of electrolyte. Their low toxicity renders them suitable for oral use and some are also used in parenteral preparations. They have the disadvantage, however, of an unpleasant taste and care must be taken when selecting a suitable preservative as many are inactivated by complexation with polysorbates.

Fatty alcohol polyglycol ethers These are condensation products of polyethylene glycol and fatty alcohols, usually cetyl or cetostearyl, i.e.

$$ROH + (CH_2CH_2O)_n \rightarrow RO(CH_2CH_2O)_nH$$

where R is a fatty alcohol chain.

Perhaps the most widely used is cetomacrogol 1000 which is polyethylene glycol monocetyl ether. This is very useful water-soluble o/w emulgent but due to its high water solubility it is necessary to formulate emulsions including, in addition, an oil-soluble auxiliary emulsifier. Cetomacrogol Emulsifying Wax BP, for example, consists of cetomacrogol 1000 and cetostearyl alcohol and is used to stabilize Cetomacrogol Cream BP.

Also known as macrogol ethers they can be produced with shorter polyoxyethylene groups

and are lipophilic w/o emulsifiers. Combinations of lipophilic and hydrophilic ethers can be used in conjunction to produce stable emulsions.

These materials can be salted out by the addition of high concentrations of electrolyte but are stable over a wide pH range.

Fatty acid polyglycol esters The stearate esters or polyoxyl stearates are the most widely used of this type of emulgent. Polyoxyethylene 40 stearate (in which 40 represents the number of oxyethylene units) is a water-soluble material often used with stearyl alcohol to give o/w emulsions.

Poloxalkols Poloxalkols are polyoxyethylene/polyoxypropylene copolymers with the general formula

$$OH(C_2H_4O)_a(C_3H_6O)_b(C_2H_4O)_a$$

and comprise a very large group of compounds some of which are used as emulsifying agents for intravenous fat emulsions.

Higher fatty alcohols The hexadecyl (cetyl) and octadecyl (stearyl) members of this series of saturated aliphatic monohydeic alcohols are useful auxiliary emulsifying agents. Part of their stabilizing effect comes from their ability to increase the viscosity of the preparation thus retarding creaming. Cetostearyl alcohol will also form complex interfacial films with hydrophilic surface-active agents such as sodium lauryl sulphate, cetrimide or cetomacrogol 1000 and thus stabilize o/w emulsions.

Amphoteric surfactants

This type possesses both positively and negatively charged groups depending on the pH of the system. They are cationic at low pH and anionic at high pH. Although they are not widely used as emulsifying agents, one example, lecithin, is used to stabilize intravenous fat emulsions.

Naturally occurring materials and their derivatives

Naturally occurring materials often suffer from two main disadvantages. They show considerable batch to batch variation in composition and hence in emulsifying properties and also many are susceptible to bacterial or mould growth. For these reasons they are not widely used in manufactured products requiring a long shelf life but rather for extemporaneously prepared emulsions designed for use within a few days of manufacture.

Polysaccharides The most important emulsifying agent in this group is acacia. It stabilizes o/w emulsions by forming a strong multimolecular film round each oil globule and thus coalescence is retarded by the presence of a hydrophilic barrier between the oil and water phases.

Because of its low viscosity creaming will occur readily and therefore a suspending agent such as tragacanth or sodium alginate can also be included. Because of its sticky nature the use of acacia is limited to products for internal use such as Cod-liver Oil Emulsion BPC 1959.

Semisynthetic polysaccharides In order to reduce the problems associated with batch to batch variation, several semisynthetic derivatives are available as o/w emulgents or stabilizers.

Several grades of methylcellulose and sodium carboxymethylcellulose are available and exert their action in a similar way to that of acacia. Methylcellulose 20, for example, is used at a concentration of 2% to stabilize Liquid Paraffin Emulsion BP.

Sterol-containing substances Beeswax, wool fat and wool alcohols are all used in the formulation of emulsions. Beeswax is used mainly in cosmetic creams of both o/w and w/o type in conjunction with borax. Because of the systemic toxicity of boric acid and its salts, however, the use of beeswax/borax preparations is limited although beeswax is used as a stabilizer for w/o creams.

Wool fat (anhydrous lanolin) consists chiefly of normal fatty alcohols with fatty acid esters of cholesterol and other sterols. It will form w/o emulsions of low dispersed phase concentration and it can also be incorporated for its emollient properties. Some individuals exhibit sensitization to this material and because of its characteristic odour and the necessity to incorporate antioxidants it is not widely used. It is, however, to be found in low concentrations in many ointments where its water absorbing properties would be of great value. It can be employed as an emulsion stabilizer with a primary emulsifying agent, for example with

calcium oleate in Oily Calamine Lotion BP, with beeswax in Proflavine Cream BPC 1973 and with cetostearyl alcohol in Zinc Cream BP and ichthammol cream.

Because wool fat has some ideal properties, attempts have been made to improve its other, less desirable, properties by physical and chemical modification. Processes including hydrogenation and fractionation have been carried out with some success. It has also been converted by a reaction with ethylene oxide to give a range of polyoxyethylene lanolin derivatives. These non-ionic products are mainly water soluble and are used as o/w emulgents possessing the properties of emollience.

The principal emulsifying agent in wool fat is wool alcohols which consists mainly of cholesterol together with other alcohols. It is an effective w/o emulgent being more powerful than wool fat and is used in the formulation of Hydrous Ointment BP. It is also incorporated as Wool Alcohols Ointment BP into other ointment bases which, although not emulsions, will readily mix with aqueous skin secretions and easily wash off the skin. Wool alcohols does not have the same strong odour as wool fat but it does require the presence of an antioxidant.

Finely divided solids

Certain finely divided solids can be adsorbed at the oil/water interface forming a coherent film which physically prevents coalescence of the dispersed globules. If the particles are preferentially wetted by the aqueous phase then o/w products will result, while preferential wetting by the oil will produce w/o emulsions.

Montmorillonite clays (such as bentonite and aluminium magnesium silicate) and colloidal silicon dioxide are used mainly for external use. Aluminium and magnesium hydroxides are also used internally. For example, Liquid Paraffin and Magnesium Hydroxide Emulsion BP is stabilized by the incorporation of the magnesium hydroxide.

Formulation by the HLB method

It has already been shown that physically stable emulsions are best achieved by a condensed layer of emulgent at the oil/water interface and that the complex interfacial films formed by a blend of an oil-soluble emulsifying agent with a water-soluble one produces the most satisfactory emulsions (Schulman and Cockbain, 1940 a, b).

Griffin (1949, 1954) devised a useful method for calculating the relative quantities of these emulgents necessary to produce the most physically stable emulsion for a particular oil/water combination. This is called the hydrophile–lipophile balance (HLB) method and was originally applied to non-ionic surface-active agents. Each surfactant is allocated an HLB number representing the relative proportions of the lipophilic and hydrophilic parts of the molecule. High numbers (up to a maximum of 20), therefore, indicate a surfactant exhibiting mainly hydrophilic or polar properties whereas low numbers represent lipophilic or non-polar characteristics. Table 16.2 gives HLB values for some commonly used emulsifying agents. The concept of HLB values is discussed more fully in Chapter 6.

Each type of oil used will require an emulgent of a particular HLB number in order to ensure a stable product. For an o/w emulsion, for example, the more polar the oil phase the more polar must

Table 16.2 HLB values for some pharmaceutical surfactants

Sorbitan trioleate (Span 85)	1.8
Oleic acid	4.3
Sorbitan mono-oleate (Span 80)	4.3
Sorbitan monostearate (Span 60)	4.7
Sorbitan monolaurate (Span 20)	8.6
Polysorbate 60 (polyoxyethylene sorbitan mono stearate	14.9
Polysorbate 80 (polyoxyethylene sorbitan mono-oleate) (Tween 80)	15.0
Polysorbate 20 (polyoxyethylene sorbitan monolaurate) (Tween 20)	16.7
Potassium oleate	20.0
Sodium dodecyl (lauryl) sulphate	40.0

Table 16.3 Required HLB values for a range of oils and waxes

	For a w/o emulsion	*For an o/w emulsion*
Beeswax	5	12
Cetyl alcohol	—	15
Liquid paraffin	4	12
Soft paraffin	4	12
Wool fat	8	10

be the emulgent system. Table 16.3 gives the required emulgent HLB value for particular oil phases for both types of emulsion. If a formulation contains a mixture of oils, fats or waxes the total HLB required can be calculated. The following example of an o/w emulsion will show this.

Liquid paraffin		35%
Wool fat		1%
Cetyl alcohol		1%
Emulsifier system		5%
Water	to	100%

The total percentage of oil phase is 37 and the proportion of each is

Liquid paraffin	$35/37 \times 100 = 94.6\%$
Wool fat	$1/37 \times 100 = 2.7\%$
Cetyl alcohol	$1/37 \times 100 = 2.7\%$

The total required HLB number is obtained as follows.

Liquid paraffin (HLB 12)	$94.6/100 \times 12 =$	11.4
Wool fat (HLB 10)	$2.7/100 \times 10 =$	0.3
Cetyl alcohol (HLB 15)	$2.7/100 \times 15 =$	0.4
Total required HLB		12.1

Thus from theoretical considerations this particular formulations requires an emulgent blend of HLB 12.1 in order to produce the most stable emulsion. It must be realized, however, that the presence of other ingredients, particularly those which may partition into the oil phase, can also affect the required HLB value. It is therefore often necessary to prepare a series of emulsions using blends of a given pair of non-ionic emulsifying agents covering a range of HLB values. This is also important if the required HLB for an oil phase is not available. The HLB value of the emulgent blend giving the most stable emulsion is the required value for that oil phase.

Assuming that a blend of sorbitan mono-oleate (HLB 4.3) and polyoxyethylene sorbitan mono-oleate (HLB 15) is to be used as the emulsifying system, the proportions of each to be used to provide an HLB of for example 12.1, are calculated as follows. Let A be the percentage concentration of the hydrophilic and B the percentage of the hydrophobic surfactants required to give a blend having an HLB value of x. Then

$$A = \frac{100(x - \text{HLB of } B)}{(\text{HLB of } A - \text{HLB of } B)} \text{ and } B = 100 - A$$

In our example therefore

$$A = \frac{100(12.1 - 4.3)}{(15 - 4.3)} = 72.9$$

$$B = 100 - 72.9 = 27.1$$

Since the total percentage of emulgent blend in the formulation is 5 then the percentage of each emulsifier will be

Sorbitan mono-oleate $5 \times 27.1/100 = 1.36$
Polyoxyethylene sorbitan
   mono-oleate $5 - 1.36 = 3.64$

The series of trial emulsions can then be assessed for stability based on the fact that the degree of creaming or separation is at a minimum at the optimal HLB value. Should several of the series show equally poor or equally good stability resulting in an inability to choose a suitable HLB value, then the total emulgent concentration may be increased or reduced respectively and the manufacture of the series repeated.

Having determined the best HLB value for a given pair of emulgents, that value can now be used to assess the suitability of other emulgent blends which may give a better emulsion than that containing the emulgent used for the initial trials.

It must be remembered that in choosing an emulsifier blend the effect of chemical structure on the type of interfacial film must be taken into account. Condensed films are produced by emulgents having long, saturated hydrocarbon groups thus providing maximum cohesion between adjacent molecules. Additionally it has been found in most cases that the most stable emulsions are formed when both emulsifying agents are of the same hydrocarbon chain length.

The use of phase inversion temperature

The use of the HLB system has several disadvantages including the inability to take into account the effects of temperature, the presence of additives and the concentration of the emulsifier. One method proposed by Shinoda (1968) partially overcomes these problems.

An o/w emulsion stabilized by non-ionic emulgents will, on heating, invert to form a w/o product. This is because, as the temperature increases, the HLB value of a non-ionic surfactant will decrease as it becomes more hydrophobic. At the temperature at which the emulgent has equal hydrophilic and hydrophobic tendencies (the phase inversion temperature) the emulsion will invert.

Parkinson and Sherman (1972) have related the stability of an emulsion with the phase inversion temperature (PIT) of its emulsifying agent (see Chapter 6).

Other formulation additives

Antioxidants

Before including an antioxidant in emulsion formulations it is essential to ensure that its use is not restricted in whichever country it is desired to sell the product. In Britain, butylated hydroxyanisole (BHA) is widely used for the protection of fixed oils and fats at concentrations of up to 0.02% and for some essential oils up to 0.1%. A similar antioxidant is butylated hydroxytoluene (BHT) which is recommended as an alternative to tocopherol at a concentration of 10 ppm to stabilize liquid paraffin. Other antioxidants widely used for emulsion formulation include the propyl, octyl and dodecyl esters of gallic acid recommended for use at concentrations up to 0.001% for fixed oils and fats and up to 0.1% for essential oils.

The efficiency of an antioxidant in a product will depend on many factors including its compatibility with other ingredients, its oil/water partition coefficient, the extent of its solubilization within micelles of the emulgent and its sorption on to the container and its closure. It must be realized, therefore, that the choice of antioxidant and the concentration at which it is to be used can only be determined by testing its effectiveness in the final product and in the package in which the product is to be sold.

Humectants

These are added to an emulsion formulation in order to reduce the evaporation of the water either from the packaged product when the closure is removed or from the surface of the skin after application. Propylene glycol, glycerol and sorbitol are all widely used as humectants at a concentration of around 5%. High concentration, if used topically, may actually remove moisture from the skin thus dehydrating it.

Preservatives

Problems associated with the growth of micro-organisms in pharmaceutical products are discussed in Chapter 27. Those microbiological factors of specific importance to the stability of emulsions are discussed later in this chapter. The necessity of including a preservative in an emulsion formulation is discussed below.

Unfortunately there is no theoretical way of choosing a suitable preservatives system, the only reliable methods being based on the results of suitable challenge tests. These methods of testing preservative activity are given in official compendia but essentially involve the addition to the test products of a mixture of Gram-positive and Gram-negative bacteria, yeasts and moulds and comparing their survival with a control sample containing no preservative.

The desirable features of a preservative suitable for use in an emulsion include:

1 a wide spectrum of activity against all bacteria, yeasts and moulds.
2 bactericidal rather than bacteristatic activity. A preservative having a minimal bacteristatic activity may lose it if any physical or chemical changes occur in the system.
3 freedom from toxic, irritant or sensitizing activity.
4 high water solubility. Because the growth of micro-organisms occurs in the aqueous phase it is important that the preservative has a low oil/water partition coefficient. The more polar is the oil phase, the more difficult it is adequately to preserve the product due to the solubility of the preservative in both phases (Bean *et al.* 1969). If the preservative is more soluble in oil than in water, then increasing the proportion of oil will decrease the aqueous phase concentration. Allowance must be made for this when choosing the phase volume ratios.

5 compatibility with the other ingredients and with the container. Certain preservatives are incompatible with particular groups of emulsifying agent. Phenols and the esters of *p*-hydroxybenzoic acid, for example, will complex with certain non-ionic emulgents due either to a reaction with oxyethylene groups or by solubilization within micelles of excess surfactant (Nowak, 1963). In many cases it is possible by chemical assay to detect the correct concentration of preservative in the product even though some of it may not be available for antimicrobial activity. It may be possible in many cases, however, to overcome this problem by increasing the amount of preservative in the product in order to give a satisfactory concentration of free preservative in the aqueous phase (Garrett, 1966). It is important to ensure that during manufacture, the preservative is added after the emulgent has concentrated at the oil/water interface.
6 stability and effectiveness over a wide pH range and temperature.
7 freedom from colour and odour.
8 retention of activity in the presence of large numbers of micro-organisms. Uptake of preservative by bacterial cells may deplete the concentration of preservative in solution thus becoming insufficient to maintain adequate bactericidal activity.

Because of the complex systems involved and the many factors to be taken into consideration, it is necessary to test the efficiency of a new preservative in the finished product and container by suitable challenge testing procedures.

Because of the irritancy and toxicity of certain preservatives, the initial choice will depend on the route of administration of the product. The following is a list of the most widely used preservatives in emulsions.

Organic acids and their salts Benzoic acid is a good antifungal and antibacterial preservative used at a pH of less than 5. A concentration of 0.1% is recommended and an example of its use is with chloroform in liquid paraffin emulsion. Sorbic acid has similar properties to benzoic acid and is also only effective in acidic conditions. Concentrations of 0.1–0.2% are used and both are suitable for oral use.

Parahydroxybenzoic acid esters The methyl, ethyl, propyl and butyl esters and their sodium salts are probably the most widely used group of preservatives. They are active against moulds, yeasts and, to a lesser extent, bacteria and are most effective at a pH of 7–9. Concentrations of 0.1–0.2% are normally used and they are suitable for both external and internal use.

Chlorocresol This is used at concentrations of around 0.1%. Its activity is reduced in alkaline conditions and sometimes in the presence of fixed oils of vegetable or animal origin.

Phenoxyethanol The effective concentration of phenoxyethanol usually lies between 0.5 and 1.0% but due to the relative ineffectiveness against Gram-positive micro-organisms it is usually formulated with other preservatives — particularly the esters of parahydroxybenzoic acid.

Bronopol This is used at a concentration of 0.02% usually in combination with other preservatives and is particularly suitable for oral use.

Quaternary ammonium compounds Because of the toxicity of these materials they are mainly used externally although they are relatively inactive against Gram-negative bacteria and bacterial spores. They are mainly used as antiseptics for topical administration and some, especially cetrimide, can be used as the primary emulsifying agent.

Organic mercurial compounds Phenylmercuric nitrate and acetate are sometimes employed in concentrations up to 0.01% in emulsions stabilized by non-ionic emulgents.

Chloroform This has been used for many years as a preservative for extemporaneously prepared emulsions. Due to its volatility and toxicity, however, its use is now limited.

It must be realized that no single preservative exhibits all of the desirable properties outlined earlier. In many cases a combination is required, the most widely used being a mixture of methyl and propyl *p*-hydroxybenzoates at a ratio usually of 10 to 1.

STABILITY OF EMULSIONS

A stable emulsion is one in which the dispersed globules retain their initial character and remain uniformly distributed throughout the continuous phase. Various types of deviation from this ideal behaviour can occur. Explanations for emulsion stability have been given in Chapter 6. This section will concentrate on methods of improving emulsion stability in practice.

Physical stability

Creaming and its avoidance

This is the separation of an emulsion into two regions one of which is richer in the disperse phase than the other. A simple example is the creaming of milk when fat globules slowly rise to the top of the product. This is not a serious instability problem as a uniform dispersion can be reobtained simply by shaking the emulsion. It is, however, undesirable because of the increased likelihood of coalescence of the droplets due to their close proximity to each other. A creamed emulsion is also inelegant and there is a risk, if the emulsion is not shaken adequately, of the patient obtaining an incorrect dosage.

Consideration of the qualitative application of Stokes' law will show that the rate of creaming can be reduced by the following methods.

Production of an emulsion of small droplet size This factor usually depends on the method of manufacture but an efficient emulsifying agent will not only stabilize the emulsion but also facilitate the actual emulsification process to give a product of fine globule size (Hamill and Petersen, 1966).

Increase in the viscosity of the continuous phase Many auxiliary emulsifying agents, in particular the hydrophilic colloids, have this effect as part of their emulsifying capability. For example, the inclusion of methylcellulose will reduce the mobility of the dispersed droplets in an o/w emulsion. The addition of soft paraffin will have the same effect on water droplets in a w/o emulsion.

Storage of the product at a low temperature (but above freezing point) will increase the viscosity of the continuous phase and also reduce the kinetic energy of the system thus decreasing the rate of migration of the globules of the disperse phase. It is unwise, however, to rely solely on this method of controlling creaming as storage conditions after the product is sold are outside the control of the manufacturer.

Reduction in density difference between the two phases Creaming could be prevented altogether if the densities of the two phases were identical. In practice this method is never used since it could only be achieved over a very narrow temperature range due to differences in the coefficients of expansion between different ingredients.

Control of disperse phase concentration It is not easy to stabilize an emulsion containing less than 20% disperse phase since creaming would occur readily. A higher disperse phase concentration would result in a hindrance of movement of the droplets and hence in a reduction in rate of creaming. Although it is theoretically possible to include as much as 74% of an internal phase, it is usually found that at about 60% concentration phase inversion occurs.

Finally it must be realized that some of the factors above are inter-related. For example homogenization of the emulsion would decrease globule size and, by thus increasing their number, increase the viscosity of the product.

Flocculation prevention

Flocculation involves the aggregation of the dispersed globules into loose clusters within the emulsion. The individual droplets retain their identities but each cluster behaves physically as a single unit. This, as we have already seen, would increase the rate of creaming. As flocculation must precede coalescence, any factor preventing or retarding flocculation would therefore maintain the stability of the emulsion.

Flocculation in the secondary minimum (see Fig. 6.3) occurs readily but redispersion can easily be achieved by shaking. Primary minimum flocculation, however, is more serious and redispersion is not so easy.

The presence of a high charge density on the dispersed droplets will ensure the presence of a high energy barrier and thus reduce the incidence of flocculation in the primary minimum.

Coalescence (synonyms: breaking, cracking)

The coalescence of oil globules in an o/w emulsion is resisted by the presence of a mechanically strong adsorbed layer of emulsifier around each globule. This is achieved either by the presence of a condensed mixed monolayer of lipophilic and hydrophilic emulgents or by a multimolecular film of a hydrophilic material. Hydration of either of these types of film will hinder the drainage of water from between adjacent globules which is necessary prior to coalescence. As two globules approach each other their close proximity causes a flattening of their adjacent surfaces. As a change from a sphere to any other shape results in an increase in surface area and hence in total surface free energy, this globule distortion will be resisted and therefore drainage of the film of continuous phase from between the two globules will be delayed.

The presence of long cohesive hydrocarbon chains projecting into the oil phase will prevent coalescence occurring in a w/o emulsion.

Chemical instability

Although it is not possible to list every incompatibilitiy, the following general points will illustrate the more common chemical problems which can cause the coalescence of an emulsion.

It is necessary to ensure that any emulgent system used is not only physically but also chemically compatible with the active agent and with the other emulsion ingredients. Ionic emulsifying agents, for example, are often incompatible with materials of opposite charge. Anionic and cationic emulgents are thus mutually incompatible.

It has already been demonstrated that the presence of electrolyte can influence the stability of an emulsion either by causing an alteration in the energy of interaction between adjacent globules or by a salting out effect by which high concentrations of electrolytes can strip emulsifying agents of their hydrated layers thus causing their precipitation.

In some cases phase inversion may occur rather than demulsification. If, for example, a sodium soap is used to stabilize an o/w emulsion then the addition of a divalent electrolyte such as calcium chloride may form the calcium soap which will stabilize a w/o emulsion.

Emulgents may also be precipitated by the

addition of materials in which they are insoluble. It may be possible to precipitate hydrophilic colloids by the addition of alcohol. Care must therefore be taken if tinctures are to be included in emulsion formulations.

Changes in pH may also lead to the breaking of emulsions. Sodium soaps may react with acids to produce the free fatty acid and the sodium salt of the acid. Soap stabilized emulsions are therefore usually formulated at an alkaline pH.

Oxidation

Many of the oils and fats used in emulsion formulation are of animal or vegetable origin and can be susceptible to oxidation by atmospheric oxygen or by the action of micro-organisms. The resulting rancidity is manifested by the formation of degradation products of unpleasant odour and taste. These problems can also occur with certain emulsifying agents such as wool fat or wool alcohols. Oxidation of microbiological origin is controlled by the use of antimicrobial preservatives and atmospheric oxidation by the use of reducing agents or, more usually, antioxidants. Some examples are mentioned earlier in this chapter.

Microbiological contamination

The contamination of emulsions by micro-organisms can adversely affect the physicochemical properties of the product causing such problems as gas production, colour and odour changes, hydrolysis of fats and oils, pH changes in the aqueous phase and breaking of the emulsion. Even without visible signs of contamination an emulsion can contain many bacteria and, if these include pathogens, may constitute a serious health hazard. Most fungi and many bacteria will multiply readily in the aqueous phase of an emulsion at room temperature and many moulds will also tolerate a wide pH range. Some of the hydrophilic colloids, which are widely used as emulsifying agents, may provide a suitable nutritive medium for use as an energy source by bacteria and moulds. Species of the genus *Pseudomonas* can utilize polysorbates, aliphatic hydrocarbons and even, in some cases, quaternary ammonium compounds. Some fixed oils including arachis oil

can be used by some *Aspergillus* and *Rhizopus* species and liquid paraffin by some species of *Penicillium*.

A few emulgents, particularly those from natural sources, may introduce heavy contamination into products in which they are used. Because bacteria can reproduce in resin beds, deionized water may be unsatisfactory and even distilled water, if incorrectly stored after collection, can be another source of contamination. Oil-in-water emulsions tend to be more susceptible to microbial spoilage than water-in-oil products as, in the latter case, the continuous oil phase acts as a barrier to the spread of micro-organisms throughout the product and the less water there is present the less growth there is likely to be.

It is necessary, therefore, to include an antimicrobial agent in order to prevent the growth of any micro-organisms which may contaminate the product. Suitable candidates have been discussed earlier in this chapter.

Adverse storage conditions

Adverse storage conditions may also cause emulsion instability. It has already been explained that an increase in temperature will cause an increase in the rate of creaming due to a fall in apparent viscosity of the continuous phase. The temperature increase will also cause an increased kinetic motion both of the dispersed droplets and of the emulsifying agent at the oil/water interface. This effect on the disperse phase will enable the energy barrier to be easily surmounted and thus the number of collisions between globules will increase. Increased motion of the emulgent will result in a more expanded monolayer and thus coalescence is more likely. Certain macromolecular emulsifying agents may also be coagulated by an increase in temperature.

At the other extreme, freezing of the aqueous phase will produce ice crystals that may exert unusual pressures on the dispersed globules and their adsorbed layer of emulgent. In addition, dissolved electrolyte may concentrate in the unfrozen water thus affecting the charge density on the globules. Certain emulgents may also precipitate at low temperatures.

Similarly the effect of the growth of micro-organisms can cause deterioration of emulsions and it is essential, therefore, that these products are protected as far as possible from the ingress of micro-organism, during manufacture, storage and use, and that they contain adequate preservatives.

STABILITY TESTING OF EMULSIONS

Methods of assessing stability

Macroscopic examination

The physical stability of an emulsion can be assessed by an examination of the degree of creaming or coalescence occurring over a period of time. This is carried out by calculating the ratio of the volume of the creamed or separated part of the emulsion and the total volume and comparing these values for different products.

Globule size analysis

If the mean globule size increases with time (coupled with a decrease in globule numbers) it can be assumed that coalescence is the cause. It is therefore possible to compare the rates of coalescence for a variety of emulsion formulations by this method. Microscopic examination or electronic particle counting devices such as the Coulter counter or by laser diffraction sizing are most widely used.

Several other methods have also been reviewed by Sherman (1968).

Viscosity changes

It has already been shown that many factors influence the viscosity of emulsions. Any variation in globule size or number or in the orientation or migration of emulsifier over a period of time may be detected by a change in apparent viscosity. Suitable methods and equipment are detailed in Chapter 2.

In order to compare the relative stabilities of a range of similar products it is often necessary to speed up the processes of creaming and coalescence. This can be achieved by one of the following methods.

Accelerated stability testing

Storage at adverse temperatures

Subjecting an emulsion to extreme variations in temperature is a particularly effective way of assessing its physical stability. Often a temperature cycling method is used where the product is stored at an elevated temperature for up to a week and then refrigerated or even deep frozen for a similar period of time and then repeated until instability is evident.

Centrifugation

The use of a centrifuge at 200–300 rpm will also accelerate the rate of creaming in an emulsion.

MANUFACTURE OF EMULSIONS

It has already been explained that the smaller the globules of the disperse phase the slower will be the rate of creaming in an emulsion. The size of these globules can also affect the viscosity of the product and, in general, it has been found that the best emulsions with respect to physical stability and texture exhibit a mean globule diameter of between 0.5 and 2.5 μm. The choice of suitable equipment for the emulsification process depends mainly on the intensity of shearing required to produce this optimum particle size. Other considerations, however, include the volume and viscosity of the emulsion and the interfacial tension between the oil and water. Thus the presence of surfactants to reduce this will aid the process of emulsification as well as promoting emulsion stability.

In many cases simple blending of the oil and water phases with a suitable emulgent system may be sufficient to produce satisfactory emulsions. Further processing using an homogenizer can also be carried out in order to reduce globule size still further. The initial blending may be accomplished on a small scale by the use of a pestle and mortar or by using a mixer fitted with an impeller type of agitator, the size and type of which will depend primarily on the volume and viscosity of the emulsified product.

A more intense rate of shearing can be achieved using a turbine mixer such as the Silverson mixer–homogenizer. In this type of machine the short, vertical or angled rotor blades are enclosed within a stationary, perforated ring and connected by a central rod to a motor. The liquids are therefore subjected to intense shearing caused initially by the rotating blades and then by the forced discharge through the perforated ring. Different models are available for a variety of batch sizes up to several thousand litres and can include 'in-line' models.

The mixing vessel may also be fitted with baffles in order to modify the circulation of the liquid and may be jacketed so that heating or cooling may be applied.

Homogenizers are often used after initial mixing to enable smaller globule sizes to be produced. They all work on the principle of forced discharge of the emulsion under pressure through fine interstices formed by closely packed metal surfaces in order to provide an intense shearing action.

If two immiscible liquids are subjectd to ultrasonic vibrations alternate regions of compression and rarefaction are produced. Cavities are then formed in the regions of rarefaction which then collapse with considerable force causing emulsification. The required frequency of vibration is usually produced electrically but mechanical methods are also available (Myers and Goodman, 1954; Skauen, 1967). Unfortunately this method of emulsification is limited to small scale production.

Colloid mills are also suitable for preparing emulsions on a continuous basis. The intense shearing of the product between the rotor and stator, which can be variably separated, will produce emulsions of very small globule size.

It is important to ensure that methods of manufacture developed on a laboratory scale can be extended to large scale production easily and without any change in the quality of the product.

During manufacture it is usual to add the disperse phase to the continuous phase during the initial mixing. The other ingredients are dissolved, prior to mixing, in the phase in which they are soluble. This is particularly important when making w/o emulsions. Oil-in-water emulsions, however, are sometimes made by the phase inversion technique. In this method the aqueous phase is added slowly to the oil phase during mixing. Initially a w/o emulsion is formed but as further aqueous phase is added the emulsion inverts to form the intended product. This method often produces emulsions of very low mean droplet size.

Should any of the oily ingredients be of solid or semisolid consistency they must be melted before mixing. It is also essential that the aqueous phase be heated to the same temperature to avoid premature solidification of the oil phase by the colder water before emulsification has taken place. This also has the advantage of reducing the viscosity of the system thus enabling shear forces to be transmitted through the product more easily. Because of the increased kinetic motion of the emulgent molecules at the oil/water interface, however, it is necessary to continue stirring during cooling to avoid demulsification.

Volatile ingredients including flavours and perfumes are usually added after the emulsion has cooled. It must, however, be sufficiently fluid to enable adequate blending to take place.

Ingredients which may influence the physical stability of the emulsion, such as alcoholic solutions or electrolytes, require to be diluted as much as possible before adding slowly and with constant mixing.

RELEASE OF DRUGS FROM EMULSION FORMULATIONS

The main commercial use of emulsions is for the oral, rectal and topical administration of oils and oil-soluble drugs. Lipid emulsions are also widely used for intravenous feeding although the choice of emulgent is very limited and globule size must be kept below 4 μm to avoid the formation of emboli. Quite often, however, the high surface area of dispersed oil globules will enhance the rate of absorption of lipophilic drugs (Lewis et al., 1950; Carrigan and Bates, 1973).

The emulsion can also be used as sustained release dosage form. The intramuscular injection of certain water-soluble vaccines formulated as w/o emulsions can provide a slow release of the antigen and result in a greater antibody response and hence a longer lasting immunity (Lazarus and Lachman, 1967). Other drugs have also been shown to have this effect, the rate of release being mainly dependent upon the oil/water partition coefficient of the drug and its rate of diffusion across the oil phase.

It is also possible to formulate multiple emulsion systems in which an aqueous phase is dispersed in oil droplets which in turn are dispersed throughout another aqueous external phase producing a water-in-oil-in-water (w/o/w) emulsion (Mulley and Marland, 1970). These products can also be used for the prolonged release of a drug which is incorporated into the internal aqueous phase. These products have the advantage of exhibiting a lower viscosity than their w/o counterparts and hence are easier to inject.

Similar o/w/o emulsions can be formulated and are also under investigation as potential sustained release bases.

Multiple emulsions, however, tend to be stable only for a relatively short time although the use of polymers as alternatives to the traditional emulsifying agents (Kumano et al., 1977) may improve their physical stability (Florence and Whitehill, 1982).

REFERENCES

Bean, H. S., Konning, G. K. and Malcolm, S. A. (1969) A model for the influence of emulsion formation on the activity of phenolic preservatives. J. Pharm. Pharmac., 21, 173S.

Carrigan, P. G. and Bates, T. R. (1973) Biopharmaceutics of drugs administered in lipid containing dosage forms.1. G. I. absorption of griseofulvin from an o/w emulsion in the rat. J. pharm. Sci., 62, 1476–1479.

Emulsifiers and Stabilisers in Food Regulations (1962) HMSO, London.

Florence, A. T. and Whitehill, D. (1982) Stabilisation of water/oil/water multiple emulsions by polymerisation of the aqueous phase. J. Pharm. Pharmac., 34, 687–691.

Garrett, E. R. (1966) A basic model for the evaluation and prediction of preservative action. J. Pharm. Pharmac., 18, 589–601.

Griffin, W. C. (1949) Classification of surface active agents by HLB. J. Soc. Cosmet. Chem., 1, 311–326.

Griffin, W. C. (1954). Calculation of HLB values of nonionic surfactants J. Soc. Cosmet. Chem., 5, 249–256.

Hamill, R. D. and Petersen, R. V. (1966) Effects of aging and surfactant concentration on the rheology and droplet size distribution of a non-aqueous emulsion. J. pharm. Sci., 55, 1268–1274.

Kumano, Y., Nakamura, S., Tahara, S., and Ohta, S. (1977) Studies of water in oil (w/o) emulsions stabilised with amino acids or their salts. J. Soc. Cosmet. Chem., 28, 285–314.

Lazarus, J. and Lachman, L. (1967) Parenteral water-in-oil emulsions as adjuvants. Bull. Par. Drug Ass., 22, 184–196.

Lewis, J. M., Cohlar, S. Q. and Messina, A. (1950) Further observations on the absorption of vitamin A. Influence of particle size of vehicle on the absorption of vitamin A. Paediatrics, 5, 425–436.

Mulley, B. A. and Marland, J. S. (1970) Multiple-drop formation in emulsions. J. Pharm. Pharmac., 22, 243–245.

Myers, J. A. and Goodman, J. E. (1954) Pharmaceutical application of ultrasonics. Pharm. J., 173, 422–424.

Nowak,G. A. (1963) The preservation of nonionic emulsions. Soap, Perfumery and Cosmetics, 36, 914.

Parkinson, C. and Sherman, P (1972) Phase inversion temperature as an accelerated method for evaluating emulsion stability. J. Coll. interf. Sci., 41, 327–330.

Schulman, J. H. and Cockbain, E. G. (1940a) Molecular interactions at oil/water interfaces I. Molecular complex formation and the stability of oil-in-water emulsions. Trans. Faraday Soc., 36, 651–660.

Schulman, J. H. and Cockbain, E. G. (1940b) Molecular interactions at oil/water interfaces II. Phase inversion and stability of water-in-oil emulsions. Trans. Faraday Soc., 36, 661.

Sherman, P. (1964) The flow properties of emulsions. J. Pharm. Pharmac., 16, 1–25.

Sherman, P. (1968) Emulsion Science, Academic Press, London.

Shinoda, K. (1968) Using the phase inversion temperature and hydrophile–lipophile balance value for choosing an emulsifier Nippon Kagaku Zasshi, 89(5), 435–442.

Skauen, D. M. (1967) Some pharmaceutical applications of ultrasonics. J. pharm. Sci., 56, 1373–1385.

BIBLIOGRAPHY

Alberman, K. B. (1964) Barrier creams and cleansers. Chemist and Druggist, 182, 200–201.

Alexander, P. (1965) Barrier creams. Manufacturing Chemist, 36(7), 55–58.

Becher, P. (1965) Emulsions: Theory and Practice, 2nd edn, Reinhold, New York.

Blaug, S. M. and Ahsan, S. S. (1961) Interaction of parabens with nonionic molecules. J. pharm. Sci., 50, 441–443.

Davis, S. S. (1976) The emulsion — obsolete dosage form or novel drug delivery system and therapeutic agent. J. clin. Pharm., 1, 11–27.

Fox, C. (1982) The current state of processing technology of emulsions and suspensions. In: Cosmetic Science (Ed. M. M. Breuer), Vol. II, pp. 1–81, Academic Press, London.

Garrett, E. R. (1965) Stability of oil-in-water emulsions. J. pharm. Sci., 54(11), 1557–1570.

Prince, M. (1977) Micro-emulsions. Theory and Practice, Academic Press, London.

Ridout, C. W. (1961) Emulsifying machinery. Manufacturing Chemist, March.

Sherman, P. (1964) The flow properties of emulsions. J. Pharm. Pharmac., 16, 1–25.

Powders and granules

Powders are subdivided solids which are classified in the *British Pharmacopoeia* (BP) according to the size of their constituent particles which can range from less than 1.25 μm to 1.7 mm in diameter. The term powder when used to describe a dosage form, however, describes a formulation in which a drug powder has been mixed with other powdered excipients to produce the final product. The function of the added excipients depends upon the intended use of the product. Colouring, flavouring and sweetening agents for example may be added to powders for oral use.

Conventionally, the title 'powder' should be restricted to powder mixes for internal use and alternative titles are used for other powdered formulations presented in this way, e.g., dusting powders which are for external use. The BP now uses the more descriptive title 'oral powder' to differentiate powders for internal use.

Granules which are used as a dosage form consist of powder particles which have been aggregated to form a larger particle which is usually 2–4 mm diameter. This is much larger than granules prepared as an intermediate for tablet manufacture. The processes involved in forming granules from powders are discussed in Chapter 37.

Powdered and granulated products are often dispensed as:

1 bulk powders or granules for internal use,
2 divided powders or granules (i.e. single dose preparations) for internal use,
3 dusting powders for external use,
4 insufflations for ear, nose or throat use.

Other preparations which may be presented as powders or granules are:

1 antibiotic syrups to be reconstituted before use,
2 powders for injection.

Advantages and disadvantages of powdered and granulated products

The advantages of this type of preparation are as follows.

1 Solid preparations are more stable than liquid preparations. The shelf life of powders for anti-biotic syrups for example is 2–3 years but once reconstituted with water it is 1–2 weeks. The instability observed in liquid preparations is usually the primary reason for presenting some injections as powders to be reconstituted before use.
2 Powders and granules are a convenient form in which to dispense drugs with a large dose. The dose of Compound Magnesium Trisilicate Oral Powder BP is 1–5 g and although it is feasible to manufacture tablets to supply this dose it is often more acceptable to the patient to disperse a powder in water and swallow it as a draught.
3 Orally administered powders and granules of soluble medicaments have a faster dissolution rate than tablets or capsules, as these must first disintegrate before the drug dissolves. Drug absorption from such powdered or granulated preparations will therefore be faster than the corresponding tablet or capsule if the dissolution rate limits the rate of drug absorption.

The disadvantages of powders and granules are as follows.

1 Bulk powders or granules are far less convenient for the patient to carry than a small container of tablets or capsules and are as inconvenient as liquid preparations such as mixtures. Modern packaging methods for divided preparations, however, mean that individual doses can be conveniently carried.
2 The masking of unpleasant tastes may be a problem with this type of preparation. The usual method of attempting this is by formu-lating an effervescent product, but tablets and capsules are a more common alternative for low-dose products.
3 Bulk powders or granules are not a method of

administering potent drugs with a low dose. This is because individual doses are extracted from the bulk using a 5 ml spoon. This method is subject to such variables as variation in spoonfill (e.g. 'level' or 'heaped' spoonfuls) and variation in the bulk density of different batches of a powder, and is therefore not an accurate method of measurement.
Divided preparations can be used for more potent drugs but tablets and capsules have largely replaced them for this purpose.
4 Powders and granules are not a suitable method for the administration of drugs which are inactivated in the stomach; these should be presented as enteric-coated tablets.

Dispensed preparations

Bulk powders

The mixed ingredients are packed into a suitable bulk container such as a wide mouthed glass jar. Because of the disadvantages of this type of prep-aration, the constituents are usually relatively non-toxic medicaments with a large dose, e.g. magnesium trisilicate and chalk which are present in Compound Magnesium Trisilicate Oral Powder BP.

Relatively few proprietary examples exist (examples include Pancrex V, Actonorm) although many dietary/food supplements are packed in this way.

Divided powders

Divided powders are similar formulations to bulk powders but individual doses are separately wrapped. The BP powder quoted above can be dispensed as a bulk or divided powder, illustrating that the only difference between the two prep-arations is one of dose presentation.

Traditionally, single doses were wrapped in paper and if the ingredients were hygroscopic, volatile or deliquescent, a double wrapping of paper lined with waxed or greaseproof paper could be used. Modern packaging materials of foil and plastic laminates have replaced such paper wrap-pings because they can offer superior protective qualities and are amenable to use on high speed packing machines.

Effervescent powders can now be packed in individual dose units because of the protective qualities of laminates. Such powders contain, for example, sodium bicarbonate and citric acid which react and effervesce when the patient adds the powder to water to produce a draught. It is important to protect the powder from the ingress of moisture on storage to prevent the reaction occurring prematurely. The traditional method of preventing this was to pack the acidic and alkaline ingredients in separate wrappings but now this is not necessary.

All powders and granules should be stored in a dry place, however, to prevent deterioration due to ingress of moisture. Even if hydrolytic decomposition of susceptible ingredients does not occur, the particles will adhere and cake, producing an inelegant, often unusable product.

Bulk granules

One disadvantage of bulk powders is that, because of particle size differences, the ingredients may segregate either on storage in the final container or in the hoppers of packaging machines. If this happens the product will be non-uniform and the patient will not receive the same dose of the ingredients on each occasion. This can be prevented by granulating the mixed powders.

Bulk granules therefore contain similar medicaments to powders, i.e. those with a relatively large dose. Methylcellulose Granules BP for example are used as a bulk-forming laxative and have a dose of 1–4 g daily. Many proprietary preparations contain similar bulk-forming laxatives, e.g. Isogel.

Divided granules

These are granulated products in which sufficient for one dose is individually wrapped. Effervescent granules can be formulated and presented in this manner, e.g. Fybogel. The comments on packaging materials discussed under 'Divided powders' above are also equally pertinent to divided granules.

Dusting powders

Dusting powders contain ingredients used for therapeutic, prophylactic or lubricant purposes and are intended for external use.

Only sterile dusting powders should be applied to open wounds, e.g. Chlorhexidine Dusting Powder BP, which is sterilized by the BP method of dry heat sterilization. Dusting powders for lubricant purposes or superficial skin conditions need not be sterile but they should be free from pathogenic organisms. As minerals such as talc and kaolin may be contaminated with spores of organisms causing tetanus and gangrene, these should be sterilized before they are incorporated into the product. In the preparation of Talc Dusting Powder BP, for example, the purified talc used must be sterile and the BP suggests using dry heat sterilization in which the powder is maintained at not less than 160 °C for not less than 1 hour.

Dusting powders are normally dispensed in glass or metal drums fitted with a perforated lid. The powder must flow well from such a container so that it can be dusted over the affected area and therefore the active ingredients are diluted with materials having good flow properties, e.g. purified talc or Sterilisable Maize Starch BP.

Chlorhexidine Dusting Powder BP and Hexachlorophane Dusting Powder BPC 1973 contain antibacterial agents and Talc Dusting Powder BP is used as a lubricant to prevent chafing. Proprietary products are available, usually for the treatment of fungal infections, e.g. Tinaderm and Phytocil which are used for *Tinea* infections such as athlete's foot.

Insufflations

Insufflations are medicated powders which are blown into regions such as the ear, nose and throat using an insufflator. The use of traditional insufflations declined because they were not very acceptable, being more inelegant and less convenient to apply than other topical preparations. A second problem was that if the powder contained a drug which had systemic activity it was difficult, with the conventional insufflator, to ensure that the same dose was delivered on each occasion.

Some potent drugs such as sodium cromoglycate are now presented in this way because they are rapidly absorbed from the lungs when inhaled as a fine powder but poorly absorbed after oral or topical administration. To enhance convenience and ensure a uniform dose is delivered on each occasion, inhalers have been developed to replace the traditional insufflator, e.g. Intal Spinhaler. Sufficient drug for one dose is presented in a hard gelatin capsule diluted with an inert, soluble diluent such as lactose. The capsule is placed in the body of the inhaler and it is broken when the inhaler is assembled. The drug is inhaled by the patient as a fine powder. It is important that the particle size of the drug is controlled to give maximum deposition in the lung (Godfrey *et al.*, 1974; Currey *et al.*, 1975 and see also Sodium Cromoglycate Insufflation BP).

Preparations requiring further treatment at time of dispensing

Oral antibiotic syrups

For patients who have difficulty taking capsules and tablets, e.g. young children, a liquid prep-aration of a drug offers a suitable alternative but many antibiotics are physically or chemically unstable when formulated as a suspension or solution. The method used to overcome this insta-bility problem is to present the dry ingredients of the liquid preparation in a suitable container in the form of a powder or granules. When the phar-macist dispenses the product, a given quantity of water is added to reconstitute the solution or suspension, e.g. Penbritin Syrup, Penicillin V Elixir BP.

Powders for injection

Injections of medicaments unstable in solution must be made immediately prior to use and are presented as sterile powders in ampoules. Suffi-cient diluent, e.g. Water for Injections BP, is added from a second ampoule to produce the required drug concentration and the injection is used immediately. The powder may contain suit-able excipients in addition to the drug, e.g. suffi-cient additive to produce an isotonic solution when the injection is reconstituted.

REFERENCES AND BIBLIOGRAPHY

British Pharmacopoeia (1980) and *Addendum* (1986), HMSO, London.
Currey, S. H., Taylor, A. J., Evans, S., Godfrey, S. and Zeidifard, E. (1975) Disposition of disodium cromoglycate administered in three particle sizes. *Br. J. clin. Pharm.*, **2**, 267.
Godfrey, S., Zeidifard, E., Brown, K. and Bell, J. H. (1974) The possible site of action of sodium cromoglycate assessed by exercise challenge. *Clin. Sci. Mol. Med.*, **46**, 265.

Ryder, J. (1979) The formulation of dry syrup preparations. *Int. J. Phar. Tech. & Prod. Mfr.*, **1**, 14.

Further information on proprietary products can be found in:

The Data Sheet Compendium, Datapharm Publications Ltd. (published annually).
The *Monthly Index of Medical Specialities* (MIMS), Medical Publications Ltd.

Tablets

TABLETS AS A DOSAGE FORM

In December 1843 a patent was granted to the Englishman, William Brockedon, for a machine to compress powders to form compacts. This very simple device consisted essentially of a hole (or die) bored through a piece of metal within which the powder was compressed between two cylindrical punches; one was inserted into the base of the die and at a fixed depth, the other was inserted at the top of the die and struck with a hammer. The invention was first used to produce compacts of potassium bicarbonate and caught the imagination of a number of pharmaceutical companies. Later, Wellcome in Britain was the first company to use the term tablet to describe this compressed dosage form. The *British Pharmacopoeia* defines tablets as being circular in shape with either flat or convex faces and prepared by compressing the medicament or mixture of medicaments, usually with added substances. Tablets are now the most popular dosage form, accounting for some 70% of all ethical pharmaceutical preparations produced. Indeed the importance of tablets as a form of drug administration can be seen from the fact that the *British Pharmacopoeia* (BP) in 1932 included only one tablet monograph (glyceryl trinitrate), which rapidly increased to 82 in the 1953 BP. By 1963 the BP had 183 tablet preparations, and in 1973 this figure had risen to 310 and to 384 in the 1980 edition.

Advantages of compressed tablets

The compressed tablet has a number of advantages as a dosage form. It enables an accurate dosage of medicament to be administered simply. It is easy to transport in bulk and carry by the patient. The tablet is a uniform final product as regards weight and appearance, and is usually more stable than liquid preparations. The release rate of the drug from a tablet can be tailored to meet pharmacological requirements. Finally, the major advantage of the compressed tablet as a dosage form is that tablets can be mass produced simply and quickly and the resultant manufacturing cost is therefore very much lower when compared with other dosage forms.

Types of tablet

Several categories of tablet can be distinguished dependent on the mode of use. The commonest type are those intended to be swallowed whole. A less common type of tablet is that formulated to allow dissolution or dispersion in water prior to administration. Many tablets are formulated to be effervescent and have become increasingly wider used in recent years because of their more rapid release of medicament and reduced chance of causing gastric irritation. Some tablets are designed to be chewed and used where buccal absorption is desired. Alternatively they may be intended to dissolve slowly in the mouth, e.g. lozenges or under the tongue (sublingual). There are now available many types of tablets which provide for the release of the drug to be delayed or allow a controlled, sustained rate of release. Many of these preparations are highly sophisticated and are referred to as 'complete drug delivery systems'. Tablets can also be coated so as to protect the drug against decomposition or to disguise or minimize the unpleasant taste of certain medicaments (see Chapter 40 for further details). Coating also enhances the appearance of tablets and makes them more readily identifiable. In addition, coatings can be applied which are resistant to gastric juices but which readily dissolve in the small intestine. These 'enteric' coatings can protect drugs against decomposition in the acid environment of the stomach. The coating process has traditionally involved the application of surface layers of sucrose so as to build up a thick sugar coat around the tablets. This process can take several days. For this reason the spray application of a film of material is now becoming more popular. This film coating technique can be carried out in a coating pan or alternatively in specialized fluidized bed equipment. Compressed coating around a tablet core has also been developed. These compression machines can produce multilayer tablets with different ingredients in each layer, so that potentially incompatible ingredients can be formulated in the same tablet.

Essential properties of tablets

The major advantage of tablets as a dosage form is that they provide an accurate dosage of medicament. Each tablet must contain a known amount of drug and this must be checked by content uniformity tests. Tablets must also be uniform in weight, appearance and diameter. Another prerequisite of tablets for oral use is that when they are swallowed whole they should readily disintegrate in the stomach. This property represents a great paradox in formulation, since tablets should be produced with sufficient strength to withstand the rigors of processing, coating and packing, yet be capable of rapid breakdown when administered in order to release the drug rapidly. This disintegration involves the bursting apart of the compact by aqueous fluids penetrating the fine residual pore structure of the tablet. These fluids come into contact with tablet components that either swell or release gases and so break apart the intact tablet. Perhaps the most significant property of tablets is that of dissolution rate. The active ingredient must be available pharmacologically and since drugs cannot be absorbed into the blood stream from the solid state, the active ingredient must first dissolve in the gastric or intestinal fluids before absorption can take place (see Chapter 9 for further discussion). Thus dissolution of the drug from tablets into aqueous fluids is a very important property of solid dosage forms (Chapter 5). Tablets should also be stable to air and the temperature of the environment over a reasonable period of time and, in addition, light and moisture should not affect tablet properties. Finally tablets should be reasonably robust and be capable of withstanding normal patient handling and handling during transport. The formulation of a tablet is thus designed so that the final tablet has all these essential properties.

TABLET FORMULATION

Influence of tableting method on formulation

The majority of tablets are not composed solely of the drug. Various materials are usually added that make the powder system more compressible. Indeed powders intended for compression into tablets must possess two essential properties: fluidity and compressibility.

Powder fluidity

Fluidity is required so that the material can be transported through the hopper of a tableting machine. If adequate fluidity does not exist, this gives rise to 'arching', 'bridging' or 'rat-holing' (see Chapter 36). Fluidity is also essential so that adequate filling of the dies occurs in the tableting machine to produce tablets of a consistent weight. If the powder formulation does not flow satisfactorily, variable die filling will result, which will produce tablets that vary in weight and strength and therefore steps must be taken to ensure that fluidity is maintained. Powder flow can be improved mechanically by the use of vibrators. However, the use of these devices can cause powder segregation and stratification and much care needs to be exercised. A better method to enhance powder fluidity is to incorporate a glidant into the formulation (see later). Materials such as fumed silicon dioxide are excellent flow promoters

even in concentrations of less than 0.01%. Another way to improve powder flow is to make the particles as spherical as possible, for example by spray drying or by the use of spheronization machines such as the marumarizor. The most popular method of increasing the flow properties of powders is by granulation. Most powdered materials can be granulated and the improvement in flow can be quite startling. Icing sugar, for example, will not flow, but if it is granulated with water it flows more easily.

Powder compressibility

Compressibility is the property of forming a stable, intact compact mass when pressure is applied. Paracetamol is poorly compressible whereas lactose compresses well. The physics of powder compression and why some materials compact better than others is a subject on its own and is described in Chapter 39. Much research work is in progress to characterize compaction behaviour but suffice to say that little is known about why some materials compress better than others. It is known, however, that in nearly all cases, granulation improves compressibility.

The need for granulation prior to compression

Granulation is the process of particle size enlargement of powdered ingredients (see Chapter 37 for details) and is carried out to confer fluidity and compressibility to powder systems. In addition the ideal properties of a granule include the following:

1 When compacted a tablet granulation should confer physical strength and form to the tablets. The granulation should be capable of being subjected to high compression pressures without defects forming.
2 A good granulation should have a uniform distribution of all the ingredients in the formulation.
3 The particle size range of the granulation should be log normally distributed. There should be a small percentage of both fine and coarse particles.
4 Granules should be as near spherical shape as possible and robust enough to withstand handling, without breaking down.

5 The granulation should be relatively dust free thus minimizing powder spread during tableting.

Tableting methods

The preparation of tablets can be divided into (a) dry methods and (b) wet methods. Dry methods include direct compression, slugging and roller compaction, and wet methods include wet granulation. The reader is referred to Chapter 39 for details.

Direct compression

Dry methods and in particular direct compression are superior to those methods employing liquids, since dry processes do not require the equipment and handling expenses required in wetting and drying procedures and can avoid hydrolysis of water-sensitive drugs. Some drugs, for example aspirin, can be tableted without further treatment, but the vast majority of drugs require the addition of a direct compression vehicle to aid compression. Great interest in direct compression has been evident in recent years and this has resulted in a wide range of direct compression tablet formulations being introduced. A direct compression vehicle is an inert substance which can be compacted with no difficulty and which may do so even when fairly large quantities of drugs are mixed with it. Materials currently available as direct compression diluents may be divided into three groups according to their disintegration properties and their flow characteristics:

1 disintegration agents with poor flow, e.g. microcrystalline cellulose, microfine cellulose and directly compressible starch,
2 free-flowing materials which do not disintegrate, e.g. dibasic calcium phosphate,
3 free-flowing powders which disintegrate by dissolution, e.g. spray-dried lactose, anhydrous lactose, spray-crystallized maltose, dextrose, sucrose, dextrose, mannitol and amylose.

Tablets are produced by mixing the drug with the compression vehicle in a blender. The powder mix is then compressed directly on a tableting machine. The process of direct compression is described in Chapter 39.

Direct compression vehicles should be free flowing, physiologically inert, tasteless, colourless, and have a good mouth feel. Vehicles should also improve the compressibility of poorly compressible drugs, be relatively inexpensive and be capable of being reworked with no loss of flow or compressibility. Finally, direct compression diluents should promote rapid disintegration, be white and able to produce tablets containing a high proportion of non-compressible material (known as *capacity*). In practice, no one single material fulfils all these criteria and it may be necessary to blend two or more compression aids together.

The quantity of medicament which can be mixed with the carrier so that direct compression properties are retained is governed by the capacity of the carrier. The more compressible the active ingredient, the greater the proportion that can be carried successfully by the vehicle. When considering the capacity potential, it is normal to consider the active ingredient as being non-compressible. Generally, unless the drug itself is easily compressible, the amount of drug present is limited to a maximum of about 25% of the tablet weight. Another potential problem with direct compression is static electricity.

The formulation and release of drugs from tablets prepared by direct compression has been extensively investigated. Fox *et al.* (1963) made a detailed study of the tableting properties of microcrystalline cellulose. It was found that extremely hard tablets could be made with ease with no sign of lubrication difficulties. Flowability was very good and tablets exhibited excellent friability and rapid disintegration time. The dissolution of phenobarbitone and prednisone from directly compressed tablets and from tablets prepared by wet granulation was investigated by Kim (1970). It was found that, in general, tablets prepared from soluble direct compression vehicles containing a disintegrant showed faster dissolution times than those prepared by wet granulation. Bolhuis and Lerk (1973) evaluated eleven excipients and found that microcrystalline cellulose and extra fine lactose had the best overall properties.

Microcrystalline cellulose (MCC) is perhaps the most widely used direct compression excipient. It exhibits the highest capacity and compressibility of all known direct compression vehicles (Mendell,

1972), however, its flow properties are relatively poor. MCC is chemically an inert material and is compatible with most drugs. Its high initial moisture content and its hygroscopicity may preclude its use with very moisture-sensitive drugs. However, there is some evidence that MCC may in fact stabilize drugs susceptible to hydrolysis, by perhaps acting as a moisture scavenging agent (Sixsmith, 1976). This has been demonstrated for ascorbic acid and aspirin. It has been reported that MCC has a specific stabilizing effect on nitroglycerine tablets (Richman *et al.*, 1965). It was later found by Goodhart *et al.* (1976), after a very comprehensive study, that nitroglycerine tablets formulated with MCC produced tablets with superior stability and more uniform content than tablets prepared by the popularly used moulded technique.

Another popular direct compression excipient is *dibasic calcium phosphate*, a comparatively cheap insoluble diluent with good flow properties. Khan and Rhodes (1972a, b) and Khan and Rooke (1976) have examined its compressional, disintegration and dissolution properties in the presence of various disintegrants. They have shown that a cationic ion exchange resin and sodium starch glycollate are effective disintegrants for dibasic calcium phosphate system even at low concentration. Dibasic calcium phosphate is slightly alkaline, so must not be used where the active ingredient is sensitive to pH values of 7.3 or above. Shah and Arambulo (1974) have shown from accelerated stability tests that dibasic calcium phosphate (Emcompress) was probably unsuitable for ascorbic acid and thiamine hydrochloride, since deteriorating crushing strength and disintegration properties resulted as well as chemical degradation in the case of ascorbic acid. Calcium salts in general have been shown to adversely effect the absorption properties of several drugs including tetracycline and they should not, therefore, be coformulated. Khan and Rhodes (1976) have shown that for directly compressing griseofulvin, dicalcium phosphate yielded tablets of better weight uniformity than MCC. Direct compression formulations of ampicillin have been successfully produced by Niazi *et al.* (1976) and shown to be better than similar tablets produced by moist granulation.

Dry granulation

Granulation by compression or slugging is one of the dry methods which has been used for many years for moisture- or heat-sensitive ingredients. The blend of powders is forced into dies of a large heavy-duty tableting press and compacted. The compacted masses are called 'slugs'. An alternative technique is to squeeze the powder blend into a solid cake between rollers. This is known as *roller compaction*. The slugs or roller compacts are then milled and screened in order to produce a granular form of tableting material which flows more uniformly than the original powder mix. These processes are described in more detail in Chapters 37 and 39.

Slugging has the advantage over direct compression in that once the slugs are formed, no segregation of drug and excipient can occur. In addition the method is useful for hydrolysable and thermolabile drugs. Although used, slugging is a lengthy process and involves a relatively high capital investment since heavy-duty presses are expensive. Compared with other granulation processes, the throughput is slow.

The effect of various tablet formulations and processing factors on the rate of dissolution of salicylic acid tablets prepared by slugging was investigated by Levy *et al.* (1963). It was found that the dissolution rate increased with decreasing granule size and starch content of the granules. Increasing the slugging pressure of granules caused an increase in dissolution rate due to fracturing of the harder granules into smaller particles with greater specific surface area. Langridge and Wells (1980) have recently shown that precompression or slugging of a mixture of microcrystalline cellulose and dicalcium phosphate dihydrate significantly reduced compressibility of both excipients. Although slugging is one of the oldest and most widely used processes for tableting, it has received very little scientific attention.

Wet granulation

Tableting by the wet granulation process is the most widely used method for pharmaceutical materials. The technique involves a number of stages which are described in detail in Chapter 39. The wet granulation process has a number of advantages over the other granulation methods but it is not readily suitable for hydrolysable and/or thermolabile drugs such as antibiotics. During the development of a tablet formulation, all the physical variables which can affect the resultant granules have to be considered also so as to minimize the effect of process variation on the quality of the final product.

Influence of granulation media In wet granulation, the binder is normally incorporated as a solution or mucilage. The choice of the liquid phase will depend upon the properties of the materials to be granulated. *Water* is the most widely used binder vehicle but non-aqueous granulation using *isopropanol*, *ethanol* or *methanol* may be preferred if the drug is readily hydrolysed. Changes in drug solubility resulting from a change in solvent have been shown by Wells and Walker (1983) to affect granule strength due to solute migration.

In wet granulation, granule growth is initiated by the formation of liquid bridges between primary particles (see Chapter 37). Soluble excipients will dissolve in the binder solution to increase the liquid volume available for wet granulation, consequently granules of large mean size are formed. The soluble components recrystallize on drying to form a greater number of solid bridges. If one of the components absorbs water, this reduces the volume of binder liquid available to form wet granules and so smaller granules will result (Jaiyeoba and Spring, 1980). Thus the choice of binder vehicle can affect the characteristics of the dry granules.

Influence of binder concentration and volume Techniques of binder addition to powders include the incorporation of a concentrated binder solution followed by additional fluid, which maintains a standard binder content. Shubair and Dingwall (1976) studied the rate of release of erythrosine from lactose tablets without disintegrant or lubricant. It was found that release rate was inversely related to starch binder content. Release rates decreased progressively from 2 to 10% w/w mucilage, but an unexpected rapid release followed use of 20% w/w starch mucilage. Further research did not indicate that poor binder distribution gave a complete explanation, since addition of water to dilute the 20% w/w mucilage to 10% w/w did not reduce the dissolution rate. Therefore the method of incorporation of the binder may also have an effect on drug release. The effect of increasing the volume of binder fluid used to granulate blends of lactose and boric acid, has been investigated by Opakunle and Spring (1976). Increasing the volume of binder fluid produced stronger granules, thought to be due to the formation of more binder bonds and the presence of more recrystallized bridges. Thus the amount of binder fluid must be very closely controlled in order to produce granules of a consistent hardness.

Tablet excipients

A tablet does not just contain the active ingredient but also includes other substances, known as excipients, which have specific functions. The various classes of excipients which are normally incorporated into tablet formulations are discussed here.

Diluents

Diluents or 'bulking agents' are 'inert' substances which are added to the active ingredient in sufficient quantity to make a reasonably sized tablet. This agent may not be necessary if the dose of the drug per tablet is high. Generally, a tablet should weigh at least 50 mg and therefore very low dose drugs will invariably require a diluent to bring the overall tablet weight to at least 50 mg. The principal substance employed as a diluent is *lactose*. It has a pleasant taste, rapidly dissolves in water, absorbs very little moisture and is fairly neutral in reaction. Its main disadvantage is that it is somewhat expensive and has poor flow characteristics. Lactose deforms easily under pressure and, as a result of this ductility, good tablets are normally produced. The spray-dried form of lactose flows much more readily and is used as a direct compression vehicle. *Dicalcium phosphate* is another diluent that is used extensively as a tablet diluent. It is insoluble in water and makes good hard, white granules. It absorbs even less moisture than lactose and is therefore used with hygroscopic drugs such as pethidine hydrochloride. The *starches* are used as diluents and as binding agents. They are available as finely divided powders and aid the disintegration process. Starches contain up to 14% moisture and can therefore lead to stability problems for a moisture-sensitive drug. Another very popular diluent is *microcrystalline cellulose*. This substance is supplied as a free-flowing ingredient and is normally used as a direct compression vehicle. It has disintegrating properties and requires less lubricant in the formulation than other diluents. *Dextrose* has been used as a bulking agent, but the granules produced are much softer and not very white. In addition, dextrose absorbs moisture. *Sucrose* is very hygroscopic and goes sticky on exposure to moisture. Its pleasant taste makes it especially useful in lozenges. *Mannitol* is another sugar which, although expensive, is very quick dissolving and is therefore used for tablets that have to be dissolved, e.g. glyceryl trinitrate tablets. Since it has a negative heat of solution, it is used for chewable tablets because it imparts a pleasant taste and a cooling sensation when sucked or chewed. Table 18.1 summarizes the commonly used diluents.

Table 18.1 Tablet diluents used in the wet granulation process

Diluent	Comments
Dextrose	Hygroscopic
Dicalcium phosphate	Inexpensive, insoluble in water
α-Lactose BP	Inexpensive, relatively inert; the most frequently used diluent
Mannitol	Freely soluble; used particularly for chewable tablets
Microcrystalline cellulose	Excellent compression properties; has some disintegrating ability
Sodium chloride	Freely soluble; used for solution tablets
Sucrose	Sweet taste but hygroscopic; may be diluted with lactose

Courtesy of N. A. Armstrong.

Adsorbents

Adsorbents are substances included in a formulation that are capable of holding quantities of fluids in an apparently dry state. Oil-soluble drugs, fluid extracts or oils can be mixed with adsorbents and then granulated and compressed into tablets. *Fumed silica, microcrystalline cellulose, magnesium carbonate, kaolin* and *bentonite* are examples of adsorbents commonly employed.

Moistening agents

In wet granulation, a moistening agent is required which is usually *water*. If the formulated powder contains sucrose, for example, it may only be necessary to add water, since sucrose rapidly dissolves and acts as its own binding agent. In cases where water cannot be used because the drug is hydrolysed, then alcohol is often substituted. Absolute alcohol is expensive and thus *industrial methylated spirits* is used. Care must be taken to remove all traces of the solvent during drying or the tablets will possess an alcoholic odour. *Isopropyl alcohol* is an alternative moistening agent. It is difficult, however, to remove the last traces from granules and it possesses an objectionable odour.

Binding agents (adhesives)

The substances that act as adhesives to bind powders together in the wet granulation process are known as binders. They also help to bind granules together during compression. If too little binding agent is included in a formulation, soft granules result. Conversely, too much binding agent produces large, hard granules.

Binding agents can be added in two ways depending on the method of granulation:

1 as a powder in the formulation as in 'slugging' or in dry granulation methods,
2 as a solution to the mixed powders as in wet granulation.

There are not many examples of (1) since most substances require some moisture present to make them adhesive.

Common binding agents include starch mucilage and gelatin solution. *Starch* is a good and popular binder and needs to be present in an amount equal to 2%. It is incorporated as a mucilage in water. When dry, the starch binder is insoluble in water, unlike gelatin which remains soluble in the dry state. *Gelatin* is often used as a binder in lozenges. Among the other most important binders is *polyvinylpyrrolidone* (PVP). This substance is soluble both in water and in alcohol and has been shown to release drugs faster than with other binders. Rubinstein and Rughani (1978), using four binders in a tablet formulation of frusemide, showed how the choice of binder affects dissolution rate. They observed t_{50} values between 3.65 minutes with PVP to 117 minutes with starch mucilage. Other less common binders include *hydrolysed gelatin*, derivatives of seaweed (such as *alginic acid*, *sodium alginate* and calcium alginate) and cellulose derivatives (in particular *ethyl cellulose* and *hydroxypropylmethylcellulose*).

Common binders used in the wet granulation process are listed in Table 18.2.

Table 18.2 Adhesives (binders) used in the wet granulation process

Adhesive	Concentration in granulating fluid (% w/v)	Comments
Acacia mucilage	up to 20	Yields very hard granules
Gelatin	5–20	Forms gel in cold, therefore warm solution used; strong adhesive, often used in lozenge granules
Glucose	up to 50	Strong adhesive; hygroscopic, so tablet may weaken in humid conditions
Polyvinyl pyrrolidone (PVP)	2–10	Soluble in water and in some organic solvents; therefore can be used for anhydrous granulation
Starch mucilage	5–10	Often used warm; a very commonly used adhesive
Sucrose	up to 70	Hygroscopic; tablets may harden on storage

Courtesy of N. A. Armstrong.

Glidants

Glidants are materials which are added to tablet formulations in order to improve the flow properties of the granulations. They act by reducing interparticulate friction. The most commonly used and effective glidant is *fumed* (or *colloidal*) *silica*. Flow of granules can be dramatically improved by the addition of less than 0.1% w/w of this material to powders and granules. Fumed silica is thought to act by lodging in the surface irregularities of the particles or granules, which effectively smooths the particle surface.

Lubricants

These agents are required to prevent adherence of the granules to the punch faces and dies. They also ensure smooth ejection of the tablet from the die. Many lubricants also enhance the flow properties of the granules. Talc and magnesium stearate appear to be more effective as punch lubricants than stearic acid, which is more effective as a die lubricant.

Magnesium stearate is the most popular lubricant used and is normally effective on its own as both a die and a punch lubricant. It is incorporated by blending with the dry granules prior to compression, up to a concentration of about 1% w/w. A thin layer of magnesium stearate around the granule is just as effective as a thick layer from the lubrication point of view, but increased magnesium stearate quantities reduce the disintegration time, retard drug dissolution and also reduce the bonding forces between granules to produce soft tablets. The reduction in drug release properties is due to the hydrophobic nature of magnesium stearate preventing drug dissolution. It has been shown (Bolhuis et al., 1975) that the extent of mixing time greatly affects the distribution of magnesium stearate around the tablet granules. An increase in mixing time produces a more uniform distribution of lubricant, but adversely affects tablet hardness and dissolution. For many drugs, magnesium stearate is chemically incompatible (e.g. aspirin) and therefore *talc* or *stearic acid* is often used. Microcrystalline cellulose requires less lubricant for effective lubrication of granules, since to some extent it acts as its own lubricant.

Table 18.3 lists the commonly used tablet glidants and lubricants.

Disintegrating agents

Disintegrants are always added to tablets to promote breakup of the tablets when placed in an

Table 18.3 Commonly used tablet glidants and lubricants

Substance	Lubricant or glidant	Concentration in tablet (% w/w)	Comments
Stearates, e.g. magnesium, calcium, stearic acid	Lubricant	0.25–1	Reduce tablet strength; prolong disintegration; insoluble in water; excellent lubricant properties; magnesium stearate is very widely used
Talc	Lubricant and glidant	1–2	Insoluble but not hydrophobic; only a moderate lubricant
Polyethylene glycol	Lubricant	2–5	Molecular weights 4000–6000; soluble in water; moderately effective
Liquid paraffin	Lubricant	up to 5	Dispersion problems; inferior to stearates
Sodium lauryl sulphate	Lubricant	0.5–5	Moderate lubricant with wetting properties; often used in conjunction with stearates
Colloidal silica	Glidant	0.1–0.5	Excellent glidant
Starch	Glidant	2–10	Primary function is that of a disintegrant
Magnesium lauryl sulphate	Lubricant	1–2	Water soluble

Courtesy of N. A. Armstrong.

aqueous environment. The object of a disintegrant is to cause the tablet to disintegrate rapidly so as to increase the surface area of the tablet fragments and so promote rapid release of the drug. Wagner (1969) proposed a scheme which related tablet breakup to drug dissolution and absorption (Fig. 18.1) which had been referred to previously in Chapter 9. Release rate of the drug is greater from disintegrated particles than from the intact tablet or tablet fragments. Thus, a good disintegrant will quickly break up a tablet into primary particles and ensure that the drug is assimilated at a fast rate. The disintegration test, which is included in all pharmacopoeias, measures the time it takes for a tablet to break down and pass through a standard screen.

Disintegrants can act by swelling in the presence of water to burst open the tablet. Starch is the commonest disintegrant in tablet formulation and is believed to act by swelling. However, other effective disintegrants do not swell in contact with water and the mechanisms by which disintegrants act is the subject of some controversy. It is believed that disintegrants that do not swell exert their disintegrating action by capillary action. Liquid is drawn up through capillary pathways within the tablet and ruptures the interparticulate bonds. This action serves to break the tablet apart. Lowenthal (1973) has discussed in detail the various mechanisms of disintegration.

Starch can be incorporated in many ways into a formulation. For example, all the starch can be added to the other ingredients and the homogenous mix wet granulated. Alternatively, about two-thirds of the starch can be added before wet granulation and the remainder added in dry form to the dried granules. Starch can be added in dry form all at once to the dried granules. This last method is not popular because too much starch between the granules inhibits bonding, with the result that a soft tablet is produced. The advantage of incorporating some of the starch outside the dry granules, is that the disintegration time is improved in tablets possessing water repellant drugs, since the surrounding starch acts as a pathway for water penetration into the tablet and for the pushing apart of granules due to the expansion of a localized high concentration of starch.

Other common disintegrants include *cation exchange resins* (Amberlite IRP 88), *cross-linked polyvinylpyrrolidone* (Polyplasdone XL), *modified starches* (sodium starch glycollate) and *cellulose materials* (Avicel) (see Table 18.4).

Specific formulation requirements of other compressed dosage forms

Lozenges

Lozenges are compressed tablets, usually at least 18 mm in diameter, which do not contain a disin-

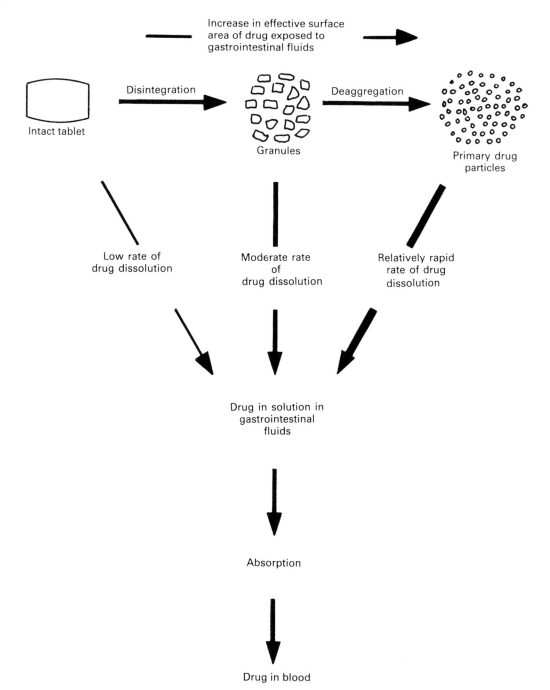

Fig. 18.1 Diagrammatic representation of the disintegration and dissolution steps prior to absorption of a poorly soluble drug from a tablet. (After Wells and Rubinstein, 1976)

tegrant and which are sucked to dissolve in the mouth. Generally there are two types, depending on the required action. The first type produces a local effect in the mouth or throat. Usually this type of lozenge contains an antiseptic (e.g. benzalkonium) or antibiotic. These lozenges must be palatable and slowly soluble. The formulation thus contains some sucrose in fine powder, lactose and

Table 18.4 Tablet disintegrants

Material	Concentration in tablet (% w/w)	Comments
Alginic acid and alginates	2–10	
Carbon dioxide		Created *in situ* in effervescent tablets
Ion exchange resins		Amberlite ®
Magnesium aluminium silicate	up to 10	Veegum ®; often slightly coloured
Microcrystalline cellulose	up to 10	Avicel ®; lubricant properties, directly compressible
Modified corn starch		Starch 1500 ®
Sodium dodecyl sulphate	0.5–5	Primarily a wetting agent but this aids disintegration
Sodium carboxymethylcellulose	1–2	Nymcel ®
Sodium starch glycollate	1–10	Primojel ®; Explotab ®
Starch	2–10	Potato and maize starches are most frequently used
Modified cellulose gum	2	Ac-di-sol ®
Cross-linked polyvinylpyrrolidone		Polyplasdone XL ®

Courtesy of N. A. Armstrong.

gelatin solution to impart a smooth taste. The formulation is compressed between flat-faced punches to allow greater pressures to be applied. Flavours are normally incorporated to assist palatability. The second type of lozenge produces a systemic effect. An example is a lozenge containing vitamin supplements (multivitamin tablets) which is required to be sucked and is a palatable way of administering vitamins. Again flavours are normally included to make the lozenge more acceptable.

Effervescent tablets

Quick dissolution of the active ingredient in water can be very effectively achieved if the tablet is broken apart by the internal liberation of carbon dioxide. This also serves to increase palatability. By combining alkali metal carbonates or bicarbonates with tartaric or citric acid, carbon dioxide can be liberated when the tablet is placed in water. These effervescent mixtures have been known for over 250 years and the famous Rochelle salt (potassium sodium tartrate) dates back to 1731. Effervescent tablets can be produced by wet fusion and heat fusion. With the wet fusion technique, citric acid is moistened and added to sodium bicarbonate and granulated in a suitable mixer, the moist citric acid acting to partially fuse the powders. The granules are then tableted and

the tablets dried in ovens at 70 °C, before being packaged in moisture-proof containers or aluminium foil. The heat fusion technique requires all the powders to be blended dry, with the citric acid being in the form of citric acid monohydrate. The mixed powders are then heated to liberate the water of crystallization in the citric acid, which acts as the granulating agent. The mass is further mixed, whilst being heated, to produce granules which are compressed into tablets.

A water-soluble lubricant is normally used in effervescent tablets to prevent an insoluble 'scum' forming on the water surface. Sweetness is achieved with saccharin, since sucrose is hygroscopic and adds too much bulk to the tablets.

Chewable tablets

For patients who have difficulty in swallowing tablets whole or for children who have not yet learned to wash tablets down with water, chewable tablets present an attractive alternative, with the added advantage that this type of medication can be taken at any time or place when water is not available. Mannitol is normally used as a chewable base diluent, since it has a pleasant, cooling sensation in the mouth and can mask the taste of some objectionable medicaments.

Chewable tablets are prepared by wet granulation. The granules should not be too hard and normally contain a high proportion of flavouring agents to aid palatability, which can include chocolate bases. A disintegrating agent is not required, since the teeth perform this function. Antacid tablets are invariably presented as tablets that should be chewed to obtain quick indigestion relief.

Sublingual and buccal tablets

Tablets placed under the tongue (sublingual) or in the side of the cheek (buccal) can produce an immediate systemic effect by enabling the drug to be directly absorbed through the mucosa. Examples are isoprenaline sulphate (Bronchodilator) and glyceryl trinitrate tablets (vasodilator). These tablets are usually small and flat, do not contain a disintegrant and are compressed lightly to produce a fairly soft tablet. Sucrose is used to impact sweetness.

Implants

Implants are very small pellets composed of drug substance only without excipients. They are normally about 2–3 mm in diameter and are prepared in an aseptic manner to be sterile. Implants are inserted into body tissues by surgical procedures, where they are very slowly absorbed over a period of months. Implant pellets are used largely for the administration of hormones such a stilboestrol, testosterone and dioxycortone acetate. Implants are produced on a single punch machine, normally hand operated. The machine must be appropriately sterilized. The die is filled by hand, since the drug does not normally flow. The particle size of the drug is important and is usually kept large to produce a slow rate of absorption. In addition the implants are made very hard to achieve a gradual release.

Multilayer tablets

A multilayer tablet consists of several different granulations that are compressed, on top of each other, to form a single tablet composed of two or more layers. Each layer is fed from a separate feed frame with individual weight control. Multilayer tablets are mainly used for incompatible substances,

for example, phenylephedrine hydrochloi ascorbic acid in admixture with parac...amol. Paracetamol and phenylephedrine hydrochloride are contained in one layer and paracetamol and ascorbic acid in the other. In spite of the intimate contact at the surface between the two layers, virtually no reaction takes place. Dust extraction is essential during compression to avoid cross-contamination. Each layer, in a multilayer tablet, is individually compressed lightly after each fill. This avoids the granules intermixing if the machine vibrates.

Sustained-release tablets

The advantages, disadvantages and formulation requirements of sustained-release tablets are discussed in the following section. For further details, see the Biopharmaceutics part of this book, particularly Chapters 9 and 11.

Sustained-release tablets

Advantages and disadvantages as a dosage form

In recent years there has been a large increase in the development and use of sustained-release tablets which are designed to release the drug slowly after ingestion. The main factor in the more widespread use of these types of dosage forms is that patient compliance is improved, since only one or two tablets need to be taken daily. Thus the frequency with which the patient has to take these tablets to obtain the desired effect is considerably reduced. In addition, the drug's activity can be extended to take effect throughout the night, so that the patient need not be awakened until morning. A single daily dosage has advantages with psychiatric patients, since this patient group generally forgets to take their medication regularly, and for patients in hospital a decrease in the number of doses administered can result in a time saving for nurses. Another advantage sometimes expressed for sustained-release tablets is that this type of medication reduces the severity or frequency of untoward side effects. Aspirin, for example, has been shown to produce less gastric bleeding when formulated as a sustained-release formulation than conventional aspirin preparations (Treadwell *et al.* 1973). Generally, a sustained-release tablet produces a more constant blood level of drug than repeated doses of a conventional tablet and this may be clinically very significant (see Chapter 11). Aminophylline has a very narrow therapeutic blood level range and many daily dosages must be given in order that the correct therapeutic blood level can be maintained. In practice, this means that conventional tablets must be administered at precise time intervals, which is very inconvenient for the patient. Formulating aminophylline as a sustained-release tablet has resulted in a 12-hourly dosage regimen and the constant blood level that has been achieved has reduced the incidence of toxicity due to blood level peaking. Thus a more efficient utilization of the drug in the body can be effected with some sustained-release formulations.

Although there is no doubt that sustained-release tablets have many advantages to the patient, there are disadvantages with this type of medication. The cost of prolonged action tablets is more per unit dose than conventional dosage forms. Some drugs, such as riboflavin and ferrous sulphate, are more efficiently absorbed in particular regions of the gastrointestinal tract and therefore sustained-release tablets are not very useful, because they release the drug throughout the intestinal tract. Accidental poisoning with sustained-release dosage forms does present special treatment problems not seen with conventional oral tablets. The slow release of the drug into the gastrointestinal tract and its extended absorption, often results in slow clearance of drug from the body. The physical size of the dosage form may present problems. Some patients do experience difficulty in swallowing a 600–650 mg sustained-release tablet and it is often difficult to formulate the tablets so that the overall tablet weight is very much lower than this. In isolated cases, large tablets have been reported lodged in the oesophagus. Sustained-release tablets of potassium chloride have been known to cause ulceration due to delayed gastrointestinal transit time (McCall, 1975). Variability of absorption can be a troublesome problem with sustained-release tablets. After ingestion the tablet should release quantities of drug at much later times to maintain drug absorption over an extended period. This involves a triggering mechanism and the mechanism may exist in the dosage form itself or in the gastrointestinal tract of the patient. Sustained-release tablets can fail because poor formulation can result in all the drug being released at once, or they fail because inconsistent amounts of drug are released. It has been known for sustained-release tablets to be recovered from the faeces of some subjects.

Types of sustained-release tablets

Attempts have been made to classify sustained-release dosage forms according to their mode of release or the blood level–time profiles that they produce. These differences are discussed in Chapter 11. Suffice it to say here that the BNF presently refers to all such preparations as 'sustained release'.

Formulation of sustained-release tablets

Sustained-release tablets can consist of two parts: an immediately available dose and a sustaining part, containing many times the therapeutic dose, for protracted blood drug levels. The immediately available dose is normally directly added to the sustaining part of the tablet or alternatively is incorporated in the tablet coating with the sustaining portion in the core of the tablet. The heart of the system resides with the sustaining portion of the tablet and various methods have been used to retard drug release.

Methods of achieving sustained-release

Diffusion-controlled release Diffusion entails the movement of drug molecules from a region of high concentration in the tablet to one of a lower concentration in the gastrointestinal fluids. The rate at which diffusion occurs will depend upon the surface area, the diffusional pathway, the drug concentration gradient and the diffusion coefficient of the system. In any one dosage form these factors will be kept constant so that a predetermined diffusion rate of drug out of the tablet will be achieved. In practice, diffusion-controlled release can be produced by formulating the drug in an insoluble matrix. The gastrointesinal fluids penetrate the matrix and drug diffuses out of the matrix and is absorbed. Alternatively, the drug particles can be coated with a polymer coat of defined thickness. In this case the portion of the drug which has dissolved in the polymer coat diffuses through an unstirred film of fluid into the surrounding liquid. In both cases a constant concentration of drug and a constant area of diffusion, together with a constant diffusional pathway, are essential to achieve a constant drug release rate.

With matrix tablets the initial dose is normally placed in the coat of the tablet. The coat and the matrix can be tableted together by compression coating or the coat can be applied using a coating pan or air-suspension technique. In non-coated systems the initial dose is normally tableted with the matrix granulation. Matrices can be compoed of polymeric materials such as methylcellulose or insoluble plastic inert substances such as methyl methacrylate. Higuchi (1962) found that for matrix tablets a plot of the square root of time against amount of drug released produced a straight line and this square root plot is often used to record the dissolution rate of matrix tablets.

Dissolution-controlled release Dissolution can be employed as the rate-limiting step in sustained-release tablets. Drugs with poor dissolution rates are inherently prolonged, but with water-soluble drugs it is possible to incorporate a water-insoluble carrier into the tablet formulation to reduce dissolution. Prolonged drug action can also be achieved by leaving out the disintegrating agent in the tablet formulation. Encapsulated drug products also utilize dissolution to control release. With these products, individual drug particles or granules are coated with a slowly soluble coating material such as polyethylene glycol of varying thickness. The time required for dissolution of the coat is proportional to the coating thickness. The coated particles can be compressed directly into tablets. A pulsed dosing effect is obtained by tableting a small number of different thickness coated particles or more usually by utilizing a spectrum of different thickness coatings.

Release controlled by ion exchange Ion exchange materials are water-insoluble resinous materials containing salt-forming groups. Either anionic or cationic groups can be used to produce the desired ion exchange resin. The drug-charged resin is prepared by mixing the resin with drug solution, then washing to remove contaminant ions and then dried to form beads or particles which are tableted. Drug release is achieved in the presence of a high concentration of appropriately charged ions in the gastrointestinal tract; the drug molecule is exchanged and diffused out of the resin to the gastrointestinal fluids. The method is attractive because it relies only on the ionic environment of the resin and not on pH, enzyme content, etc. at the absorption site. The main disadvantage with this type of sustained-release product is that whereas in theory the ionic content of the gastrointestinal tract should remain constant, in practice the ionic content varies with diet and water content, and therefore variable drug release results.

Release controlled by osmotic pressure With this technique, a semipermeable membrane is placed around a tablet or drug particle which allows transport of water into the centre of the tablet by osmosis. As a result of increased internal pressure, drug solution is then pumped out of the tablet through a small hole in the tablet coating. The delivery rate is contant provided that excess drug is present inside the tablet but rapidly declines parabolically to zero once the concentration drops to below saturation. The size of the delivery orifice is very important and this is bored with the use of a laser beam. Since the mechanism is based on osmotic pressure, the system delivers drug at a rate independent of stirring rate and environment pH, factors which make this system an attractive proposition for prolonged drug release from the gastrointestinal tract.

FORMULATION FACTORS AFFECTING THE RELEASE OF A DRUG FROM TABLETS

The effective surface area of the drug

The dissolution rate of a drug is directly related to the surface area exposed to the dissolution media. In order therefore to increase the dissolution rate for a given amount of drug, the effective surface area has to be increased. This can

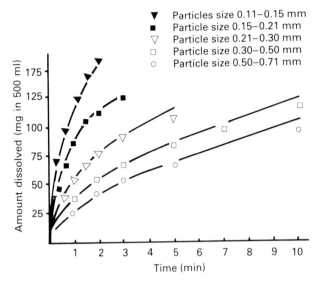

▼   Particles size 0.11–0.15 mm
■   Particle size 0.15–0.21 mm
▽   Particle size 0.21–0.30 mm
□   Particle size 0.30–0.50 mm
○   Particle size 0.50–0.71 mm

Fig. 18.2 Effect of particle size of phenacetin on dissolution rate. (Finholt, P. (1974) Influence of formulation on dissolution rate. In *Dissolution Technology*, L. J. Leeson and J. T. Carstenson, eds, pp. 106–146, Academy of Pharmaceutical Science, American Pharmaceutical Association, Washington, DC).

For the five size ranges examined, the amount of drug dissolving increases as the particle size decreases and surface area increases. However, if the drug is hydrophobic a reduction in particle size may produce a smaller effective surface area and a reduction in dissolution rate. Many *in vivo* studies have also demonstrated the importance of the effective surface area of drug particles. Figure 18.3 shows the effect of administering three different particle sizes of phenacetin on the plasma levels of healthy adult volunteers. Both the rate and extent of phenacetin availability increase as particle size decreases. The effect of particle size reduction on the bioavailability of nitrofurantoin in shown in Fig. 18.4. The microcrystalline form, particle size less than 10 μm, is more rapidly and completely absorbed from tablets than is the macrocrystalline form (74–177 μm) from capsules.

Effect of binding agents

Binding agents are incorporated into tablets during granulation in order to improve the flowability of the drug and to enhance compressibility. These agents coat the drug particles and therefore the rate of solution of the binder in water can determine the release rate from the tableted drug.

simply be accomplished by decreasing the particle size of the drug. See earlier discussion under 'Disintegrating agents' and Fig. 18.1.

Figure 18.2 clearly depicts this phenomenon.

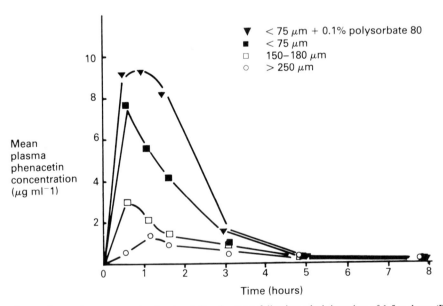

▼   < 75 μm + 0.1% polysorbate 80
■   < 75 μm
□   150–180 μm
○   > 250 μm

Mean plasma phenacetin concentration (μg ml^{-1})

Fig. 18.3 Mean plasma phenacetin concentration in six adult volunteers following administration of 1.5 g doses (Prescott, L. F., Steel, R. F. and Ferrier, W. R. (1970) The effect of particle size on the absorption of phenacetin in man. *Clin. Pharmac. Ther.*, **11**, 496–504)

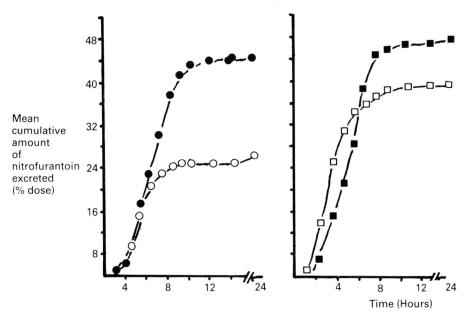

- ● 100 mg macrocrystalline capsule (non-fasting)
- ○ 100 mg macrocrystalline capsule (fasting)
- ■ 100 mg microcrystalline tablet (non-fasting)
- □ 100 mg microcrystalline tablet (fasting)

Fig. 18.4 Mean cumulative urinary excretion of nitrofurantoin after oral administration of a 100 mg capsule or tablet. (Bates, T. R., Sequeria, J. A. and Tembo, A. V. (1974) Effect of food on nitrofurantoin absorption. *Clin. Pharmac. Ther.*, **16**, 63–68

Wells (1980) measured the dissolution rates of chlorpropamide tablets containing starch, hydrolysed gelatin, methylhydroxyethylcellulose (MHEC) and polyvinylpyrrolidone (PVP) as binders. It was found that tablets containing soluble binders (hydrolysed gelatin and PVP) had rapid dissolution rates whereas slow and incomplete disintegration of tablets formulated with starch paste led to protracted release of drug. MHEC produced macrogranular breakdown which gave rise to very slow release rates.

Effect of disintegrants

In order for a drug to be released rapidly from a solid dosage form, the tablet or capsule must disintegrate quickly to liberate a large effective surface area of drug to the dissolving medium. Disintegrants act by either bursting open the tablet and/or by promoting the rapid ingress of water into the centre of the tablet or capsule. In many cases capillarity and therefore the rate of water penetration predominates in causing

disruption. Wells (1980) has found that chlorpropamide tablets containing sodium starch glycollate were superior in dissolution properties from similar tablets containing microcrystalline cellulose and cross-linked polyvinylpyrrolidone. The ion exchange resin Amberlite was found to promote rapid disintegration of chlorpropamide tablets, but dissolution rates were found to be inferior to sodium starch glycollate. Measurement of the swelling capacity and hydration capacity of the disintegrants (Table 18.5) indicated that

Table 18.5 Swelling and hydration characteristics of tablet disintegrants

Disintegrant	Swelling capacity	Hydration capacity
Starch	1.025	1.5620
Microcrystalline cellulose (Elcema)	1.020	4.1778
Cross-linked polyvinylpyrrolidone	1.780	4.8099
Amberlite	2.048	3.7443
Sodium starch glycollate	>3	∞

Amberlite and sodium starch glycollate possesses high swelling capacities and in the case of sodium starch glycollate an exceptionally high hydration capacity.

Effect of lubricants

Most tablets contain a lubricating agent to prevent the dosage form sticking to the processing machinery. Figure 18.5 shows the effect of lubri-

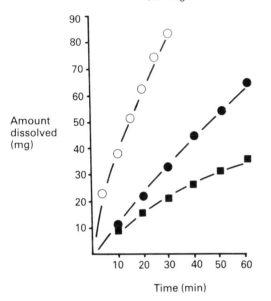

Fig. 18.5 Effect of lubricant on dissolution rate of salicylic acid contained in compressed tablets. (Levy, G. and Gumtow, R. H. (1963) Effect of certain tablet formulation factors on dissolution rate of the active ingredient. III: Tablet lubricants. *J. pharm. Sci.*, **52**, 1139–1141)

cant on the dissolution rate of salicylic acid tablets. The hydrophilic lubricant sodium lauryl sulphate allowed the drug to dissolve more rapidly than the control tablet containing no lubricant. However, incorporation of the popular hydrophobic lubricant magnesium stearate produced a decrease in dissolution rate. The most effective lubricants are very hydrophobic and they must therefore be properly formulated to avoid reducing dissolution rate and bioavailability.

Effect of diluents

Rubinstein and Birch (1977) examined the release rate and bioavailability of 5 mg bendrofluazide tablets containing four different excipients: sorbitol, lactose, calcium orthophospahte and calcium hydrogen orthophosphate. The calcium salts were generally found to be superior to the other diluents. Sorbitol was shown to markedly decrease the release rate of bendrofluazide. This excipient dissolves very slowly and therefore release of the drug occurs by erosion. The calcium salts on the other hand were shown to promote the rapid disintegration of the tablets and therefore to liberate the drug quickly from the dosage form.

Effect of granule size

Rubinstein and Blane (1977) examined the effect of granule size on the *in vitro* and *in vivo* properties of bendrofluazide tablets 5 mg. Extensive investigations showed that in general granule size was not a critical factor affecting the pharmaceutical properties of the tablets.

REFERENCES

Bolhuis, G. K. and Lerk, C. F. (1973) *Pharm. Weekblad*, **108**, 496.
Bolhuis, G. K., Lerk, C. F., Zijlstra, H. T. and De Boer, A. H. (1975) *Pharm. Weekblad*, **110**, 317.
Fox, C. D., Richman, M. D., Reier, G. E. and Shangraw, R. (1963) *Drug Cosmet. Ind.*, **92**, 161.
Goodhart, F. W., Gucluvildiz, H., Daly, R. E., Chapetz, L. and Ninger, F. C. (1976) *J. pharm. Sci.*, **65**, 1466.
Higuchi, T. (1962) *J. pharm. Sci.*, **52**, 1145.
Jaiyeoba, K. T. and Spring, M. S. (1980) *J. Pharm.*

Pharmac., **32**, 386.
Khan, K. A. and Rhodes, C. T. (1972a) *Pharm. Acta Helv.*, **47**, 153.
Khan, K. A. and Rhodes, C. T. (1972b) *Pharm. Acta Helv.*, **47**, 594.
Khan, K. A. and Rooke, D. J. (1976) *J. Pharm, Pharmac.*, **28**, 633.
Khan, K. A. and Rhodes, C. T. (1976) *Drug Dev. Comm.*, **2**, 77.
Kim, Y. (1970) Ph. D. Thesis, University of Maryland, Maryland, USA.

Langridge, L. R. and Wells, J. I. (1980) Paper presented at the British Pharmaceutical Technology Conference, London, April 1980.

Levy, G., Antkowiak, J. M., Procknel, J. A. and White, D. C. (1963) *J. pharm. Sci.*, **52**, 1047.

Lowenthal, W. (1973) *Pharm. Acta Helv.*, **48**, 589.

McCall, A. J. (1975) *Br. med. J.*, **3**, 5.

Mendell, E. J. (1972) *Mfg Chem. Aerosol News*, **43**(3), 47, **43**(4), 40, **43**(5), 43, **43**(6), 31.

Niazi, S., El-Rashidy, R. M. and Eikhwas, F. (1976) *Drug Dev. Comm.*, **2**, 41.

Opakunle, W. O. and Spring, M. S. (1976) *J. Pharm. Pharmac.*, **28**, 806.

Richman, M. D., Fox, C. D. and Shangraw, R. F. (1965) *J. pharm. Sci.*, **54**, 447.

Rubinstein, M. H. and Birch, M. (1977) *Drug Dev. Ind. Pharm.*, **3**(5) 439.

Rubinstein, M. H. and Blane, M. C., *Pharm. Acta Helv.*, **52**, 5.

Rubinstein, M. H. and Rughani, J. M. (1978) *Drug Dev. Ind. Pharm.*, **4**, 541.

Shah, D. H. and Arambulo, A. S. (1974) *Drug Dev. Comm.*, **1**, 495.

Shubair, M. S. and Dingwall, D. (1976) *Mfg Chem. Aerosol News*, **47**, 52.

Sixsmith, M. D. (1976) *Mfg Chem. Aerosol News*, **46**, 27.

Treadwell, B. L. J., Carroll, D. G. and Pomare, E. W. (1973) *N. Z. med. J.*, **78**, 435.

Wagner, J. G. (1969) *J. pharm. Sci.*, **58**, 1253.

Wells, J. I. (1980) Ph.D. Thesis, Liverpool Polytechnic.

Wells, J. I. and Rubinstein, M. H. (1976) *Pharm. J.*, **217**, 629–631.

Wells, J. I. and Walker, C. V. (1983) *Int. J. Pharm.*, **15**, 97.

Capsules

* Introduction and hard gelatin capsules
** Soft gelatin capsules

HISTORICAL DEVELOPMENT OF GELATIN CAPSULES

The word capsule is derived from the latin 'capsula' meaning a small box. In current English usage it is applied to many different articles ranging from flowers to space craft. In pharmacy the word capsule is used to describe an edible package made from gelatin which is filled with medicines to produce a unit dose, mainly for oral use. There are two types of capsule, differentiated by the adjectives 'hard' and 'soft'. The hard gelatin capsule consists of two pieces, a cap and a body, that fit one inside the other. They are produced empty and are filled in a separate operation. The soft gelatin capsule is a capsule which is manufactured and filled in one operation.

The gelatin capsule originated in the first half of the nineteenth century as a means of masking the flavours of the many obnoxious medicines then in vogue. It was devised by a French pharmacy student, F A B Mothes, who made bubbles of gelatin which could be filled with the drug and sealed with a drop of gelatin solution. These one-piece capsules were prepared by dipping small mercury-filled leather sacs into gelatin solutions, emptying out the mercury to collapse the bag, removing the gelatin films and then air drying them. The first patent was filed in Paris in 1834 by Mothes in association with a registered pharmacist, Dublanc. The capsule became immediately popular because it perfectly fulfilled a need. Within 2 years, capsules were being manufactured as far apart as Berlin and New York. Mothes was an astute businessman in that he allowed the market to develop freely and then in 1836 he used his patent and litigation to restrict the manufacture of capsules to himself. Following on from this there were many attempts to get around the patent by using alternative materials or manufacturing methods. Two products emerged from this work: the gelatin-coated pill and the hard two-piece capsule.

In France the one-piece capsule remained the most popular form. Developments were made in the manufacturing process. The moulds were changed to pear-shaped metal ones mounted on disc which simplified the production process. During the 1840s a completely new process was devised; this used a pair of metal plates which had matching sets of cavities on their surface. Two sheets of gelled gelatin mixture were then laid over each of them. The medicine to be filled was placed in the cavities on one sheet, the matching plate was placed on top and the resulting sandwich passed through a pair of pressure rollers which stamped out the capsules. These capsules were much more regular in size than those made previously and were called 'perles'.

The formulation of these shells was a mixture of gelatin, acacia and honey which produced a hard wall. The next significant change in the process occurred in 1873 when another French pharmacist, Taetz, suggested the inclusion of glycerol into the formulation in order to make them soft and elastic and thus easier to swallow. These capsules were now identical to the modern soft gelatin capsule. Finally in 1932, R P Scherer perfected the rotary die process which was the

first continuous method of encapsulation to be implemented and is still the method of choice.

The hard two-piece capsule was invented by a French pharmicist, J-C Lehuby, who took out a patent in 1846 for 'medicinal envelopes'. These were pairs of open-ended cylinders of gelatin which fitted one inside the other. They were produced by dipping silver plated metal moulds into a gelatin solution, drying the resulting films, cutting them to length and joining the two halves together. The performance of these capsules depends upon the accuracy with which the two pieces were made. The development of these capsules was held up until a cheaper accurate mould system could be developed. The problem was solved by an American pharmacist, Mr Hubel of Detroit. He had the idea of using standard gauged iron rod which was widely used in the engineering industry. He cut this into lengths and mounted them into wooden blocks. In 1874, he commenced the first industrial scale manufacture of hard gelatin capsules. From then until after the second World War, this process was confined to the USA.

After Mr Hubel's success, other companies started their manufacture: Eli Lilly & Company of Indianapolis in 1896 and Parke Davis Company of Detroit in 1901. These two companies remain the leading manufacturers in the world. Currently, hard gelatin capsule manufacturing plants are located in all of the major trading blocs.

RAW MATERIALS FOR GELATIN CAPSULES

The raw materials used in manufacture are similar for both hard and soft gelatin capsules. The first stage of the process is to prepare a gelatin solution in demineralized water or a mixture of demineralized water and glycerol. To this are added, colorants, preservatives and process aids depending upon the type of capsule required.

Gelatin

Gelatin is the major component of the capsule and has been the only material from which they have been successfully made. The reason for this is that gelatin possesses four essential basic properties:

1 It is non-toxic. It is widely used in foodstuffs and is acceptable for use in every country in the world.
2 It is readily soluble in biological fluids at body temperature.
3 It is a good film forming material.
4 As a solution in water or a water–glycerol blend it undergoes a reversible phase change from a sol to a gel at temperatures only a few degrees above ambient. This is in contrast to other films which are produced in pharmacy where either volatile organic solvents or large quantities of heat are required to effect this change of state. This property enables films of gelatin to be prepared easily.

Gelatin is a substance of natural origin, but does not occur as such in nature. It is prepared by the hydrolysis of collagen which is the main protein constituent of connective tissues. Thus animal bones and skins are the raw material for the manufacture. There are two main types of gelatin: type A, which is produced by acid hydrolysis, and type B, which is produced by basic hydrolysis. The choice of manufacturing method depends upon the nature of the raw materials, skins are mainly acid processed whereas bones are usually basic processed. Animal bones need additional treatment, in that they first need to be decalcified and to produce ossein, a soft sponge-like material. The properties of the gelatin which are most important for the capsule manufacturer are the bloom strength and the viscosity. The bloom strength is a measure of gel rigidity and is expressed as the load in grams required to push a standard plunger a set distance into a prepared gelatin gel (6.66% solution at 10 °C). The gelatin used in hard capsule manufacture is termed high bloom gelatin whereas for soft capsules, lower bloom material is used (150–200 bloom). The viscosity of the gelatin solution is used by the manufacturers of both types to control the thickness of the films or sheets.

Plasticizers

The walls of hard gelatin capsules are firm and rigid. The walls of soft gelatin capsules on the other hand are more soft and flexible; it is turgid because it is manufactured and filled in one operation which results in the pressure of the contents maintaining the capsule shape. The capsule is soft because it contains a large proportion of a plasticizer. This can be varied to produce capsules for different applications (see Table 19.1). The plasticizer which is most frequently used is glycerol; sorbitol, propylene glycol, sucrose and acacia have been used also.

Table 19.1 Control of the plasticizer content of shells for soft gelatin capsules in conjunction with their intended use. Hard gelatin capsules rarely, if ever, contain added plasticizer

Glycerol:gelatin ratio (parts of dry glycerol to one part of dry gelatin)	Application
0.35	Oral capsules with oil fills where final capsule should be hard
0.46	Oral capsule with oil fills where shell requires to be more elastic
0.55–0.65	Capsules containing oils with added surfactant or products with hydrophilic liquid fills
0.76	Oral capsules where a chewable shell is required

Colorants

The colorants which are used can be of two kinds: soluble dyes or insoluble pigments. The soluble dyes are mainly synthetic in origin and by the use of mixtures of dyes, capsules can be made in all colours of the spectrum. The pigments used are of two types. The one which is used in the largest quantity is titanium dioxide. This is white and is used as an opacifying agent. The other class of pigments is the oxides of iron; three are used, black, red and yellow. The colourants which can be used are governed by legislation which varies from country to country. In the last few years, there has been a move away from the use of soluble dyes over to pigments, particularly the iron oxides. For the manufacture of bicoloured soft gelatin capsules, aluminium lakes are used to prevent colour transfer between the two layers of the capsule.

Preservatives

Preservatives are sometimes added to capsules as an in-process aid in order to prevent micro-biological contamination during manufacture. The manufacturers operate their plants following GMP guidelines to minimize this risk. In the finished capsules, the moisture levels are such that the capsules will not support bacterial growth. Soft gelatin capsules sometimes have antifungal agents added to them to prevent growth on their surfaces when they are stored in non-protective packages.

HARD GELATIN CAPSULES

Sizes of hard gelatin capsule shells

The hard gelatin capsule is made in a range of eight sizes from size 000, the largest, to size 5, the smallest (see Fig. 19.1). These sizes have been standard since the start of industrial manufacture. The most popular sizes in practice are size 0 through to 4. The hard gelatin capsule shape (Fig. 19.1) has basically remained unchanged

since its invention, except for the development of the self-locking capsule. These have a series of indentations on the inside of the capsule cap and sometimes the external surface of the capsule body. When the capsule is closed together after filling, these areas form a frictional or interference lock. This idea was first patented by Eli Lilly & Company in 1963 and since that time the other manufacturers have incorporated similar devices into their capsules.

Determination of capsule fill weight

To determine the size of capsule to be used or the fill weight for a formulation the following practical relationship is used:

Capsule fill weight = tapped bulk density of formulation × capsule volume

For example:

1 A formulation has a theoretical fill weight of

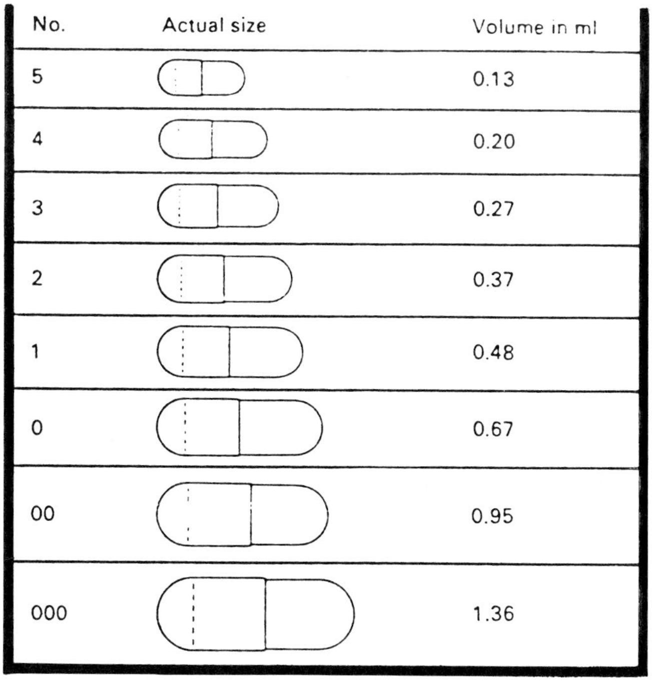

No.	Actual size	Volume in ml
5		0.13
4		0.20
3		0.27
2		0.37
1		0.48
0		0.67
00		0.95
000		1.36

Fig. 19.1 Hard gelatin capsule sizes and fill volumes. The larger, narrower part of the capsules is the body and the smaller, wider part is the cap

350 mg and a tapped bulk density of 0.75 g ml^{-1}. What size capsule is required?

$$\text{Volume occupied by fill weight} = \frac{0.35}{0.75}$$

$$= 0.47 \text{ ml}$$

From Fig. 19.1 it can be seen that a size 1 capsule has a volume of 0.48 ml and is therefore the size required for this particular formulation. This is, of course, fortuitous. What happens when the calculation yields a volume that does not coincide with a standard capsule size?

2 A preliminary mixture has a fill weight of 500 mg and a tapped bulk density of 0.80 g ml^{-1}.

$$\text{Volume occupied by fill weight} = \frac{0.5}{0.8}$$

$$= 0.63 \text{ml}$$

$$\text{Volume of size 0 capsule} = 0.67 \text{ ml}.$$

Thus a size 0 capsule is to be used. How much further diluent could be added to the mixture to improve its performance?

Volume unoccupied = 0.04 ml
Weight additional
diluent 0.04×0.8 = 32 mg

Filling

Hard gelatin capsules are most frequently filled with powders. In the last few years there have been significant developments in formualtion techniques and the filling equipment available which have enabled a range of materials to be handled. The only limitation is that they should not react with the gelatin, e.g. aldehydes, or interfere with the integrity of the shell, e.g. water which will soften the wall. The materials which can be handled are listed in Table 19.2. In addition,

Table 19.2 Types of materials for filling into hard gelatin capsules

Dry solids
    Powders
    Granules
    Pellets
    Tablets
Semisolids
    Thermosoftening mixtures
    Thixotropic mixtures
    Pastes

machines can fill more than one type of substance into the same hard gelatin capsule, e.g. Inderex of ICI Pharmaceuticals which contains a tablet and a quantity of pellets to produce a special release dosage form.

All formulations for filling into capsules must possess two basic requirements. They must:

1 be able to be accurately dosed into the capsule shell,
2 release their active contents in a form which is available to the patient.

To accomplish this the formulation is usually a simple blend of the active ingredients together with adjuvants which aid the process, e.g. diluents, glidants, lubricants and surfactants.

Formulation of powders for filling

The factor which contributes most to a uniformly filled capsule is powder flow. This is because the powder bed from which the dose of mix is measured needs to be homogeneous, packed reproducibly, in order to give uniform fill weights. Good packing is assisted by good powder flow and this is aided by mechanical devices on the filling machine. Low dose drugs can be made to flow well by mixing with free flowing *diluents*, e.g. maize starch. For higher dose drugs the space available within the capsule shell for formulation aids is minimal. Small quantities (up to about 5% w/w) of highly active materials are used: *glidants*, which improve flow by reducing interparticulate friction (e.g. Fumed Silicon Dioxide BP) and *lubricants*, which reduce powder to metal adhesion (e.g. magnesium stearate) thus enabling the dosing devices to function properly.

The literature indicates that the rate-controlling step in disintegration of an encapsulated product is the formulation of the contents. To achieve good drug release the contents should be readily wetted and dispersed by biological fluids. The factors in the formulation which control drug release are the natures of the active ingredient and the adjuvants. Several workers have demonstrated that the smaller particles of drug give higher blood levels than the same dose given as larger particles. This is because the surface area of the drug is greater the smaller the particle size and this influences solution rate. However, this phenomenon cannot be utilized to improve availability in all cases because of particle aggregation. These aggregates may possess large surface areas, but only part of this can be reached by the solution medium. The important measure is the 'available surface area' which is sometimes greater with larger particles.

The adjuvants are often described as the inert components in a formulation. In release terms they can frequently play an active role. The major component of a mixture after the active drug is usually the diluent. This needs to be chosen in relationship to the solubility of the active ingredient. Insoluble drugs are mixed with soluble diluents, e.g. lactose, in order to make the mixture more hydrophilic. Soluble drugs can be mixed with insoluble diluents, e.g. starch, in order to avoid competition for solution.

A formulation has to be designed for both good machine performance and good release properties. Some of the materials used to improve the filling performance, e.g. lubricants, magnesium stearate, are hydrophobic in nature, thus tending to slow down release. This effect can be minimized by using simplex mathematical optimization techniques or by the inclusion of a wetting agent, e.g. sodium lauryl sulphate, into the mix.

Formulation of non-powders for filling

Table 19.2 shows that a variety of materials other than powders can be filled into hard gelatin capsules. The formulation requirements are the same as for powders but are achieved in different ways.

Granules and pellets

Both particles should be as near spherical in shape as possible. Granules are produced by granulation and tend to be more irregular than pellets which are produced by a coating or microencapsulation technique. Both are often formulated to produce modified release patterns.

The machines which fill these materials into capsules use either a gravitational system or more frequently a metering chamber. Uniform filling depends therefore on the granules or pellets being free flowing, regular in shape and size to give uniform packing and non-friable to reduce dust.

Tablets

Tablets are filled into capsules either to produce special release forms or to separate incompatible ingredients. The filling machines use storage hoppers which can release one or more tablets into the open capsule body. A physical sensor then checks for the presence of the tablet before the machine continues.

For ease of filling the tablets need to be smooth, i.e. preferably film coated which also reduces dust, and of a diameter and shape that will easily fit into a capsule body.

Semisolids

This recent innovation in hard gelatin capsule filling is, in fact, a revival of a practice which was common at the beginning of the century. It fell into disrepute because of the problem of capsules coming apart and the product leaking out. This difficulty has been overcome by the use of self-locking capsules and by formulation techniques. Mixtures for filling need only be 'liquid' when filled and should be 'solid' when inside the capsule. This is achieved by using mixtures and materials which are either thermosoftening or thixotropic in nature. They are liquefied for filling by either heat or shearing forces respectively and revert to the solid state within the capsule shell when these are withdrawn. This system can be used for both liquid and solid active ingredients. Filling machines have been developed for handling these formulations which are basically the same as standard powder filling ones except that they have a heated hopper with a stirrer to hold the formulation which is dosed into the capsules through a volumetric pump.

The applications of semisolid filling are only just being investigated. It is a means of safely handling toxic drugs in that it reduces significantly the rate of cross-contamination associated with the filling of powders. For potent drugs it is a way in which uniformity of fill weight and of content can be improved because of the use of solutions and volumetric dosing pumps. Labile materials can be incorporated into a matrix which reduces moisture and oxygen ingress. The release rate of drugs can simply be varied from rapid to prolonged by using excipients with different melting points and HLB values. The more hydrophobic the base, the slower the rate of release. It provides a system for handling liquid mixes which every pharmaceutical manufacturer can perform in-house and not have to go out to a third party contractor.

Bioavailability aspects of hard gelatin capsules

The formulation of a product in a hard gelatin capsule presents the industrial pharmacist with two distinct requirements: first the filling of the powder into the capsule and second, the release of the ingredients into the gastrointestinal tract when the capsule shell disintegrates. These factors are inter-related but for convenience the technology of capsule shell manufacture and filling is discussed in Chapter 41 in the technology section of the book, and the factors in the formulation of products to be filled in hard gelatin capsules which affect drug release are discussed here.

Disintegration and dissolution

The first stage in drug release from a capsule is disintegration of the capsule shell. It has been shown in the literature that whilst products which disintegrate satisfactorily do not necessarily give good results, disintegration must take place for some to occur.

How do capsules disintegrate? When they are placed in a suitable liquid at body temperature the gelatin starts to dissolve, within 1 minute the shell splits, usually at the ends and with a properly formulated product, the contents start to empty before all the gelatin has dissolved.

A formulation for filling into a capsule in the majority of cases is a simple powder mixture of the active ingredients together with diluents, lubricants, glidants or surfactants as required. The powder mass in the capsule should be such that it does not interfere with the dissolution of the gelatin shell and such that it will break up. With this in mind, what factors can be modified in a formulation to ensure that the active ingredients

are released from the capsule and in an optimum form for absorption?

Formulation factors affecting release from hard gelatin capsules

Active ingredient The first consideration is the active ingredient. It is necessary to know its physicochemical properties such as solubility, melting point, crystalline form, etc. Most of the properties of the active ingredient are beyond the control of the formulator but one factor which can be modified is its particle size.

It has been shown for several drugs in capsules that their rate of absorption is governed by their particle size. Fincher et al. (1965) showed that this was true for sulfisoxazole (see Fig. 19.2). They filled three different particle sizes of the drug into capsules and administered them to dogs. The blood levels they obtained demonstrated that the smallest particle size gave the maximum blood level.

This can simply be explained by the fact that solution rate is directly proportional to the surface

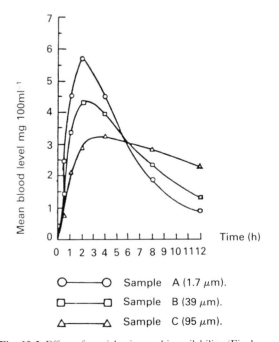

Fig. 19.2 Effect of particle size on bioavailability (Fincher, J. H., Adams, J. G. and Beal, H. M. (1965) *J. pharm. Sci.*, **54**, 704–708)

area of drug. The smaller the particle the greater the relative surface area. Unfortunately, this is not a panacea for all problems because when powders are made smaller they tend to aggregate together and this effect is lost.

The major properties of the active ingredient are out of the control of the formulator. The factors which he can manipulate are the other components in the formulation: diluents, lubricants, glidants and surfactants.

Diluent The material present in the largest quantity is usually the diluent which was always classically described as an inert material added to a formulation to increase the volume of the mixture to a more manageable quantity.

Unfortunately, diluents are not always inert as was demonstrated in the case of the reformulation of diphenylhydantoin which occurred in Australia. The diluent in this case was changed from calcium sulphate to lactose and in the months following the change there was an upsurge in the reported side effects on treatment with this drug.

It was demonstrated that the change of the diluent had a significant effect on the bioavailability of the drug (see Fig. 19.3). The change of diluent to lactose gave higher blood levels, and because this drug is taken by chronic administration the change had a significant effect.

Since this instance the phenomenon has been shown to occur with other drugs. The diluent should be chosen with reference to the solubility and proportion of the active ingredient.

On the other hand for the soluble drug chloramphenicol, it has been shown that an increase in the quantity of lactose in the formulation decreased its dissolution rate. This can be explained by saying that as lactose is readily soluble it passes into solution preferentially and thus the dissolution rate measured is that of chloramphenicol in saturated lactose solution.

Perhaps in the case of a readily soluble drug an insoluble diluent such as starch should be chosen. On disintegration of the capsules the starch grains would help the powder mass to break up without interfering with the solubility of the active ingredient.

Glidants and lubricants Two of the other materials present in a formulation, glidants and lubricants are added to improve the filling properties of the powder mixture. These substances can have an effect on drug release.

The important thing to avoid in the formulation are materials which tend to make the mass hydrophobic. The lubricant which is probably the most commonly used one in the pharmaceutical industry for both tablet and capsule formulations is magnesium stearate which is hydrophobic.

Simmons *et al.* (1972) studied the dissolution rate of chlordiazepoxide formulations with three levels of magnesium stearate, 0, 1 and 5% (see Fig. 19.4). They found that the dissolution was greatly reduced at the highest level of magnesium stearate.

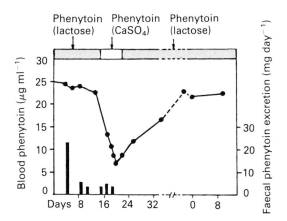

Fig. 19.3 Effect of diluent on bioavailability (Tyrer, J. M., Eadie, M. J., Sutherland, J. M. and Hooper, W. D. (1970) *Br. med. J.*, **4**, 271–273)

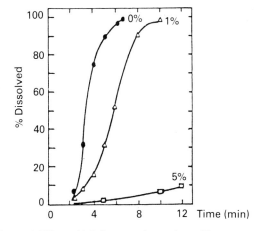

Fig. 19.4 Effect of lubricant on drug release (Simmons, D. L., Frechete, M., Lanz, R. J., Chen, W. S. and Patel, N. K. (1972) *Can. J. pharm. Sci.*, **7**, 62–65)

Wetting; effects of porosity and the addition of surfactants Aguiar *et al.* (1967) with poorly soluble benzoic acid derivatives, measured the dissolution rate of the material presented as a loose powder, and the same quantity of powder filled into a size 00 and a size 1 capsule. The slowest dissolution rate was obtained with the size 1 capsule in which the powder is most tightly packed. They overcame this problem by adding 0.5% of polyol surfactant into the formulation. This greatly improved the dissolution rate which they showed was due to an increase in the deaggregation rate of the material.

If hydrophobic compounds have to be included in formulations because of filling machine requirements, their deleterious effect on drug release can be overcome by the addition of wetting agents, surfactants at levels of 0.1–0.5%. Another solution is by the use of soluble lubricants such as sodium stearyl fumarate which has been recently developed.

The type of filling machine used can affect drug release. The effect of how the powder is packed into the capsule has been shown to be important for some drugs and not for others.

Samyn and Jung (1970) investigated the system, drug, lactose plus magnesium stearate 0% or 5%. This was filled into capsules at a 'normal packing' and a 'dense packing' and measured the dissolution rate. They showed that the denser packing reduced the dissolution rate and also added to the effect of the magnesium stearate (see Fig. 19.5).

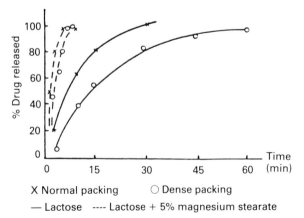

Fig. 19.5 Effect of filling machine on drug release (Samyn, J. C. and Jung, W. Y. (1970) *J. pharm. Sci.*, **59**, 169–175

This effect, however, does not happen with all drugs. In the two cases mentioned above there was an effect but with cephalosporine no difference was found *in vivo*, between 'tight' and 'loose' filled capsules.

The type of filling machine may also have an indirect effect. A capsule formulation is designed for the requirements of both capsule filling and drug release, and these are interdependent.

SOFT GELATIN CAPSULES

Description

Soft gelatin capsules (SGCs, also referred to as soft elastic gelatin (SEG) capsules or softgels) consist of units with a continuous gelatin shell surrounding a liquid fill material. The capsules are formed, filled and sealed in one operation and may be of different sizes and shapes (see Fig. 19.6).

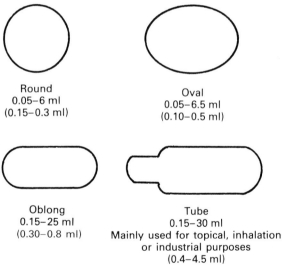

Fig. 19.6 Soft gelatin capsule shapes. The ranges of available fill volumes are indicated. The most common dose volumes suitable for oral administration of drugs are indicated in parentheses

Advantages of soft gelatin capsules as a dosage form

During the development of a new medicinal product, many problems may be experienced by the pharmaceutical scientist. For example:

1 A high dose of a poorly compressible drug may

be difficult to form into tablets and there may be capping problems in production.

2 There may be powder flow or mixing problems and the dose of the drug in each dosage unit may not be uniform.

3 The drug may hydrolyse or oxidize on long term storage.

4 The drug substance may be poorly soluble in water or gastric juice and the bioavailability from some solid dosage forms might be poor.

These difficulties can be resolved in many ways. For example, granulation may facilitate the tableting of compounds. Particle size control or granulation may be used to optimize dose content uniformity. Drugs sensitive to moisture or oxygen can be processed in dry conditions or under nitrogen and packaged in vapour-proof containers. Soluble salts of drugs or pro-drugs may be employed to improve bioavailability. The details of these and other techniques are described elsewhere in this book.

An alternative approach is to consider the use of soft gelatin capsules. The problems mentioned above are overcome for the following reasons.

1 A compression stage is not included in the manufacturing process.

2 The dose content uniformity is optimized because the drug is dissolved or dispersed in a liquid which is then dosed volumetrically into the capsules accurately.

3 Drugs sensitive to oxidation or hydrolysis on long term storage can be protected from the environment by solution or dispersion in oil and encapsulation by gelatin. Such formulations resist gaseous diffusion and contain little labile water.

4 The drug is dissolved or dispersed in a water-miscible or oily liquid and when the capsule is ingested, the capsule breaks and the solution dissolves or is emulsified to give a drug dispersion of high surface area and good bioavailability.

Many compounds which are soluble or dispersible in oil or hydrophilic liquids might benefit from formulation as a soft gelatin capsule and the possibility of using soft gelatin capsules should be explored at an early stage in the development of a new medicinal product.

In this part of the chapter the above problems and the benefits of soft gelatin capsules are discussed in more detail.

Compression

Some drugs are liquids and thus cannot be compressed into tablets. Others melt at the temperature of compaction and cause picking and sticking problems. Many are dusty or cohesive and will not flow. Others compress well at low compaction speeds (pilot plant conditions) but because of a change in the bonding mechanism (i.e. plastic to elastic deformation), they cap and laminate at higher compression speeds (production conditions) or produce weak tablets too friable for further processing (e.g. packaging and film coating). The reader is referred to Chapter 39 for further details.

Compression problems can be minimized by careful choice of excipients and/or by granulation with a plastic binder. However, the cost of granulation can be high and compression can be affected by interbatch variation in material properties. Any compound which is difficult to compress into tablets plus those which are liquids or which melt at the temperature of compaction could be formulated in a soft gelatin capsule.

Mixing and powder flow

Powder flow and mixing problems (see Chapters 36 and 32) may cause dose content variations in both tablets and hard shell capsules. This can result in toxic side effects (e.g. nausea) or poor therapeutic activity in the case of potent compounds with low therapeutic index.

For higher dose drugs, dose content disuniformity may necessitate the use of overages, and therefore the incurring of extra raw material costs. If the dose content varies by ±5% (or ±7.5%, BP limits) of the label claim at the time of manufacture (due to powder flow and mixing problems), the products must contain an overage of 5% (or 7.5%) to avoid 50% of the batch being out of specification (i.e. 90% of label claim) at the end of the shelf life when the product has degraded by 10%. The costs of raw material overages are high and these should be minimized by reducing the dose content variations in all pharmaceutical products.

Fine powders may be cohesive and the formulation may not have uniform flow. Variable weights of material could then be filled into hard shell capsules or fed into the dies of a tableting machine. The fill weight, and therefore the dose content, in these products will vary and in the case of tablets in extreme cases, friable compacts or capped tablets can be produced due to under-compression and overcompaction respectively.

The flow problems of powders can be minimized in many ways, as described in Chapter 36.

The dose content uniformity of soft gelatin capsules is good because the product consists of encapsulated solutions or suspensions which flow readily and are homogeneous. Solutions are produced by mixing and dissolution of all components, and suspensions are manufactured using high speed blenders and homogenizers. The fill liquids are deaerated and then metered into capsules using accurate positive displacement pumps. The fill weight variations due to pump error are negligible and any small differences in the dose content uniformity can be attributed to variations in the suspension uniformity, mechanical setting and machine temperature. A comparison of standard values for dose content uniformity of soft gelatin capsules with published data on dose disuniformities in tablets containing highly potent compounds (Orr, 1981) is shown in Fig. 19.7.

Whereas the dose variations in tablets and hard shell capsules may be up to ±7.5%, the dose disuniformity in soft gelatin capsules is less than ±1% for solutions and between ±1% and ±3% for pastes. Figure 19.8 shows a comparison of riboflavin and vitamin A dose content disuniformity in SEG capsules with the dose content disuniformity in some commercially obtainable tablets.

A comparison of the overages (and therefore extra raw material costs) required for SEG capsules and standard tablets or hard shell capsules shows a potential for reducing costs. For example, if the manufacturing output of a drug substance is 10 000 kg per annum and the cost of the compound is £500 per kg, the annual cost of a 5% overage is £250 000, but the cost of a 1% overage for soft gelatin capsules is £50 000.

Thus improved content uniformity results in improved therapeutic consistency for potent compounds and the potential for reduced costs through the use of smaller overages in the case of high cost products.

Stability

Most drug compounds degrade by oxidation, hydrolysis and by incompatibility reactions during storage after manufacture. Tablets and hard shell capsules contain powders in which moisture may be present as fine films of large surface area

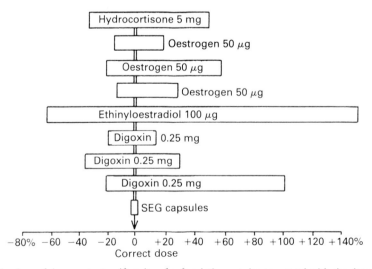

Fig. 19.7 The standard values of dose content uniformity of soft gelatin capsules compared with the dose content variations found in commercially available tablets containing highly potent drugs (Orr, N. (1981) *Progress in the Quality Control of Medicines*, Elsevier Biomedical Press, Amsterdam)

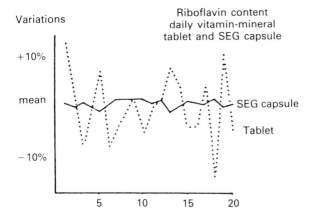

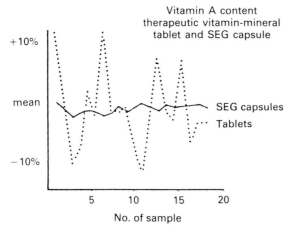

Fig. 19.8 Contrast in the dose content uniformity of riboflavin and vitamin A in commercially available vitamin-mineral tablets and soft gelatin capsules

distributed throughout dosage form. This moisture can arise either because it is left as a residue at the end of the drying stage during manufacture or through the ingress of water vapour from the atmosphere during long term storage.

Water provides a useful medium for chemical interaction. Water-soluble materials within the product, including oxygen, will dissolve to form a saturated solution and decomposition reactions may occur. The problem can be minimized by the correct choice of excipients, by drying the materials prior to encapsulation and tableting (providing the drying process does not cause a compression problem) and by processing or packaging the products at low humidity or under nitrogen in extreme cases and by packaging in vapour-proof containers. Alternatively soft gelatin

capsules in which the drug can be dissolved or dispersed in oil and then encapsulated in a dry shell of gelatin at low relative humidity (RH) (or under nitrogen) can be considered.

The gelatin shell of a soft gelatin capsule provides a good barrier against the diffusion of oxygen from the environment into the liquid contents of the product. The quantity of oxygen (q) that passes through the gelatin is governed by the area (A), thickness (h), partial pressure difference ($p_1 - p_2$), time of diffusion (t) and the permeability coefficient (P) of the shell by the following equation:

$$P = \frac{q\,h}{A\,t\,(p_1 - p_2)} \tag{19.1}$$

The permeability coefficient (P) is related to the diffusion coefficient (D) and the solubility coefficient (S) by the equation $P = DS$. This relationship (i.e. Henry's law) assumes no interaction between the gas and the polymeric film but P is clearly affected by the formulation of the gelatin shell as shown in Fig. 19.9.

Fig. 19.9 shows the relationship between oxygen permeability coefficient and the glycerol concentration in the gelatin shell of SEG capsules at room temperature and relative humidity values from 31 to 80%. The oxygen permeability decreases with the % RH and the glycerol content in the gelatin shell formulation (Hom et al., 1975). For maximum protection against the ingress of

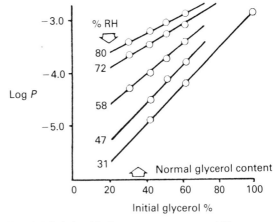

Fig. 19.9 Relationship between oxygen permeability coefficient and the glycerol concentration in the shell of soft gelatin capsules at room temperature and a range of relative humidity values (Hom et al. (1975) J. pharm. Sci., 64, 851)

oxygen, the dry shell of gelatin should be dry and formulated to contain about 30–40% glycerol.

Soft gelatin capsules contain little residual water and compounds which are susceptible to hydrolysis are protected if dissolved or dispersed in an oily liquid fill material and encapsulated as a soft gelatin capsule. Fig. 19.10 shows the relationship between the equilibrium water content and the concentration of glycerol in the gelatin shell of a SEG capsules, stored at room temperature and environmental relative humidities of between 31 and 80%. The data show for example that the minimum water values are found at glycerol levels in the shell of between 30 and 40%. Such a formulation dried at 31% relative humidity has a water content in the shell of about 7% (Hom *et al.*, 1975) and a water content in the fill in equilibrium with the atmosphere. The residual water content of most pharmaceutical compounds stored at 20% relative humidity (the drying condition for SEG capsules) is low and the water levels in the fills of SEG capsules therefore are very small.

The dielectric constant of an oily vehicle is low and the ionization of polar materials is impaired. The tendency for chemical reactions to occur is low and products normally susceptible to oxidation, hydrolysis and chemical incompatibility reactions are relatively stable when formulated as soft gelatin capsules. An example is shown in Fig. 19.11 for comparative long term stability profiles of vitamin A, vitamin C and thiamine,

formulated into soft gelatin capsules and tablets (Tardif, 1965). The stability to oxidation (vitamin C) and hydrolysis (vitamin A and thiamine) is greater when the actives are formulated as soft gelatin capsules.

All pharmaceutical products degrade on storage. To remain within specification, the manufacturer must ensure that the medicine contains 90% of the label claim at the end of its declared shelf life. To achieve this objective, some pharmaceutical products contain an overage. The reduced decomposition within SEG capsules requires lower overages at manufacture and this results in reduced raw material costs.

Thus soft gelatin capsules with oily fills contain little active water and the content of available oxygen is low. Compounds which are susceptible to oxidation or hydrolysis are protected and the possibility of lower initial overages reduces material costs.

Bioavailability

Some drugs, such as neutral compounds or organic acids, are insoluble in water and gastrointestinal fluids and the dissolution rate is slow. When these materials are compounded into tablets or hard shell capsules, the absorption rate is sometimes retarded and the bioavailability may be poor.

The problem can be minimized by presenting the material as a fine suspension using dispersible tablets or powders for reconstitution. Alternatively, the compound can be combined with surfactants or polymers to produce quick dissolving solid solutions. Organic acids can also be given as water-soluble salts or converted chemically into more readily absorbable pro-drugs.

There are a number of problems with the above techniques, however. Liquid products such as fine suspensions may not be the required dosage form for marketing. Solid solutions may be chemically unstable or waxy and difficult to process. Tablets or hard shell capsules containing water-soluble salts of an organic acid may not disintegrate easily due to the precipitation of the free acid and clogging of the dosage form in gastric juice. Pro-drugs must be treated as new chemical entities and examined fully for long term toxicity.

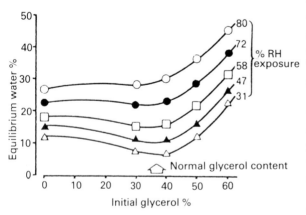

Fig. 19.10 The relationship between equilibrium water content and the concentration of glycerol in the shell of soft gelatin capsules at room temperature and a range of relative humidity values (Hom *et al.* (1975) *J. pharm. Sci.*, **64**, 851)

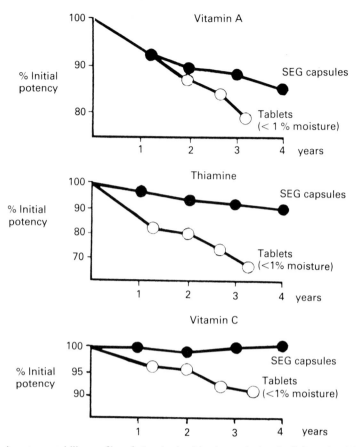

Fig. 19.11 Comparative long term stability profiles of vitamin A, thiamine and vitamin C formulated in soft gelatin capsules (average of 13 multivitamin preparations) and very dry tablets (Tardif (1965) *J. pharm. Sci.*, **54**, 281)

In a soft gelatin capsule formulation the medicament is in solution or is dispersed as a fine suspension in either a hydrophilic vehicle or a hydrophobic base. When a soft gelatin capsule is ingested, the gelatin shell dissolves quickly or breaks open at the heat sealed seam. The liquid medicament is released into the gastric contents where water-miscible vehicles dissolve and oily liquids emulsify.

The drug release and bioavailability of soft gelatin capsules is considered in detail later in this chapter.

Formulation of soft gelatin capsules

There are two main aspects to be considered during the formulation of soft gelatin capsules — the composition of the gelatin shell and the composition of the fill material.

Formulation of the gelatin shell

The composition of the soft capsule shell consists of two main ingredients — gelatin and a plasticizer (e.g. glycerol). Water is used to form the capsule and it may be desirable or even necessary to add other additives such as preservatives, dyes, opacifiers and, rarely, flavours and drugs.

Gelatin

To produce shells with a greater flexibility than hard gelatin capsules it is necessary to control carefully the viscosity and bloom strength of the gelatin used in production. If the viscosity of a standard aqueous gelatin solution is too low, a thin, low strength shell is produced which has the added disadvantage of requiring prolonged drying. If the viscosity of the gelatin solution is too high, a thick film is produced which may be too hard and brittle for this application. High viscosity gelatin formulations also require higher sealing temperatures during manufacture.

The mechanical properties of the gelatin shells are controlled by choice of gelatin grade and by adjusting the concentration of plasticizer in the shell.

Plasticizers

The main plasticizer used for soft gelatin capsules is glycerol. Sorbitol and propylene glycol have also been used but they are normally added in combination with glycerol. Plasticizers are added in relatively large concentrations (particularly when compared with the amounts of plasticizer that may be added to hard gelatin capsules and tablet film coats, for example). The greater the plasticizer content the greater the flexibility of the shell.

Plasticizer concentrations can be expressed as parts of dry plasticizer to 1 part of dry gelatin. In practice these ratios vary widely between 0.3 and 1.0 (see Table 19.1). This wide range encompasses the diversity of plasticizers and fill materials. More specifically, low ratios between 0.3 and 0.5 are used for oily liquid fills, between 0.4 and 0.6 for oily fills with added surfactant and between 0.6 and 1.0 for water-miscible fills and chewable capsules.

Water

The desirable water content of the gelatin solution used to produce a soft gelatin capsule shell depends on the viscosity of gelatin used and ranges between 0.7 and 1.3 parts of water to each part of dry gelatin, with a 1 : 1 ratio being typical. Demineralized water is used.

Preservatives

These have traditionally been added to prevent mould growth in the gelatin shell. Potassium sorbate and methyl, ethyl and propyl hydroxybenzoate (methyl-, ethyl- and propylparaben) are common additives. Current research has shown that the free water content of normal capsule shells is too low to support the growth of micro-organisms and the use of these preservatives is unnecessary.

Colours

A wide range of colours can be incorporated into soft gelatin shells — water-soluble dyes (both synthetic and vegetable, insoluble inorganic and organic pigments and lakes.

Opacifiers

Titanium dioxide is the most common. It is added in concentrations of about 0–0.5%.

Enteric treatment

Enteric properties can be imparted to soft gelatin shells by coating with 4% cellulose acetate phthalate.

Formulation of the capsule contents

It is possible to fill soft gelatin capsules with a very wide range of materials. These range through suspensions and pastes to drugs in solution in oils, self-emulsifying oils and water-miscible liquids. By far the most common situation is to fill them with liquid. Almost any non-aqueous liquid drug or powdered solid made into a suspension can be filled into soft gelatin capsules.

Limitations for fill materials

Drugs or excipients containing high concentrations of water or other gelatin solvents cannot be incorporated. It is not recommended to fill emulsions (whether they be o/w or w/o) since they are unstable and will crack as the water is lost from the shell in the manufacturing process. Surfactants may have a deleterious effect on the capsule seal. Extremes of pH must be avoided. pHs below about 2.5 attack the gelatin leading to hydrolysis and subsequent leakage and pHs above about 7.5 have a tanning effect on the gelatin, affecting the subsequent solubility of the shell. Aldehydes must also be avoided since these have a tanning action on the proteins of the gelatin shell.

Liquid vehicles

These fall into two main categories, water-immiscible oils and water-miscible liquids.

Water-immiscible oils These can be a wide range of volatile and non-volatile oils. They include fixed and aromatic vegetable oils, aliphatic, aromatic and chlorinated hydrocarbons, and liquid ethers and esters.

Water-miscible liquids The following hydrophilic liquids can be used in soft gelatin capsules. Polyethylene glycols — the so-called polyols can be used. Low molecular weight grades (400–600) are used most commonly since they are liquid at ambient temperatures. Alcohols (e.g. isopropyl alcohol), polyglycerols, triacetin, glyceryl esters, sorbitan esters, sugar esters and polyglyceryl esters have also been used.

Propylene glycol and glycerol can be used, but the concentration must be low, e.g. 5–10%, in order to prevent migration into the gelatin and softening of the shell.

Suspensions

Insoluble drugs can be dispersed (with suspending agents and surfactants) in the above vehicles or combinations of vehicles. Suspending agents are added to prevent settling and maintain homogeneity. Examples include beeswax, paraffin wax,

ethylcellulose and hydrogenated vegetable oil for oily bases and solid glycol esters (such as PEG 4000 and PEG 6000) for non-oily bases.

Additives such as surfactants (for example polysorbate 80 (Tween 80)) are often added to promote wetting of the ingredients. The particle size of the solid should be reduced to less than 180 μm in order that they can pass through the filling head. Caking of suspensions in soft gelatin capsules can be avoided by careful rheological control of the vehicle.

Bioavailability aspects of soft gelatin capsules

Acid-soluble drugs, dissolved or dispersed in water-miscible vehicles, are distributed quickly throughout the stomach. Suspended particles dissolve quickly and the bioavailability is good. Soft gelatin capsules have yielded similar blood level curves to those produced by liquids. For example, Fig. 19.12 shows mean serum theophylline levels in 14 subjects after a crossover study using 300 mg of theophylline presented as SEG (polyol liquid fill) capsules and an oral aqueous non-alcoholic solution (Lesko *et al.*, 1979). Similarity between an elixir solution and a soft gelatin capsule (polyol liquid fill) containing 150 mg of papaverine hydrochloride has also been observed (Arnold *et al.*, 1971).

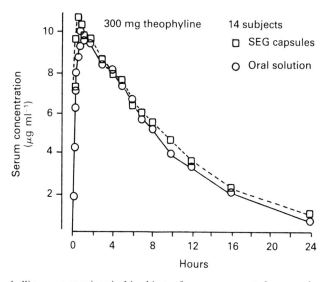

Fig. 19.12 Mean serum theophylline concentrations in 14 subjects after a crossover study comparing soft gelatin capsules (polyol base) with an oral aqueous non-alcoholic solution (Lesko *et al.* (1979) *J. pharm. Sci.*, **68**, 1372)

Acid-insoluble compounds administered as a solution in a soft gelatin capsule precipitate as a fine suspension in the stomach. The surface area is high and the precipitate quickly redissolves to give a solution with optimum bioavailability. Figure 19.13 shows plasma concentrations of digoxin (mean values and standard errors) after oral intake (six subjects in a crossover study) of

0.4 mg digoxin as 2 tablets and 2 SEG capsules (polyol liquid fill) (Binnion, 1976). Figure 19.14 shows the mean serum temazepam levels in five subjects receiving 20 mg of temazepam in a crossover study using tablets (Wyeth) and SEG capsules (polyol fill). The improved bioavailability of temazepam changed the therapeutic effect of a tranquillizer to a hypnotic.

Drugs dissolved in an oil which emulsifies, or drugs which are themselves oils and emulsify, are absorbed directly from the gastrointestinal tract into the lymphatic system through digestion and association with long chain fatty acids as shown schematically in Fig. 19.15 (Palin, 1982). Alternatively, compounds dispersed or dissolved in oil droplets and soluble at low pH, diffuse out into the surrounding aqueous environment or are solubilized in micelles and are absorbed via the hepatic portal vein.

The surface area of emulsified systems is high and the bioavailability is good. Fig. 19.16 shows plasma concentrations (mean values and standard errors) of chlormethiazole after oral intake of 2 tablets (1000 mg solid form, chlormethiazole ethanedisulphonate) and 2 capsules (640 mg as the oil form, chlormethiazole base) in a crossover study using 10 subjects (Frisch and Ortengre, 1966). The oil form gave higher plasma levels.

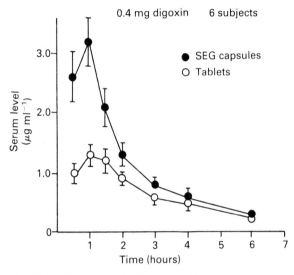

Fig. 19.13 Mean serum levels in six subjects after a crossover study comparing 0.4 mg digoxin as two tablets and two soft gelatin capsules (polyol base). (Binnion (1976) *J. Clin. Pharmacol.*, **16**, 461)

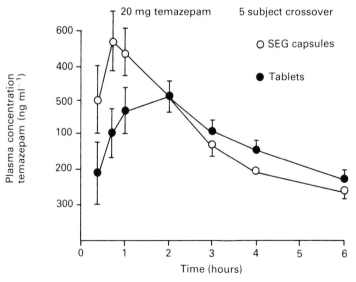

Fig. 19:14 Mean plasma concentrations in five subjects after a crossover study comparing 20 mg temazepam as tablets and soft gelatin capsules (polyol base) (Unpublished data, Wyeth Laboratories)

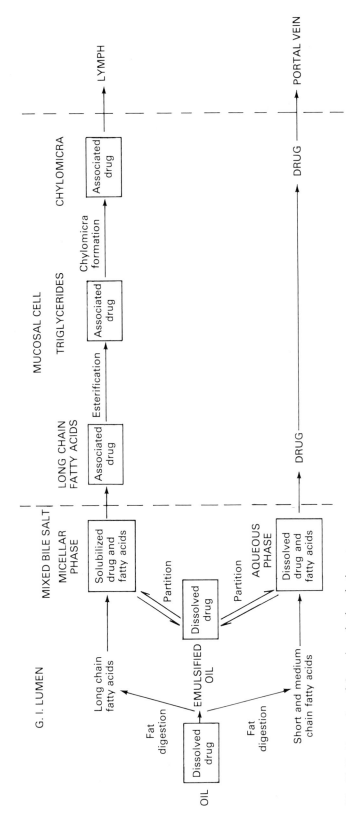

Fig. 19.15 Absorption of drugs into the lymphatic system

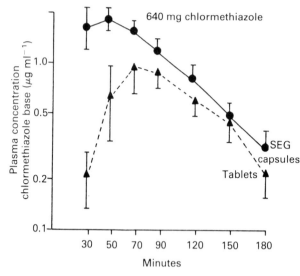

Fig. 19.16 Mean plasma concentrations in 10 subjects after a crossover study comparing 1000 mg chlormethiazole ethanedisulphonate as two tablets with 640 mg chlormethiazole base (an oil) as two soft gelatin capsules. (Frisch *et al.* (1966) *Acta psych. scand.*, **42**, 35)

A number of drugs have been formulated into soft gelatin capsules and found to improve the dissolution rate and enhance bioavailability. An example is phenylbutazone (Hom and Miskel, 1970).

Higher blood levels have been achieved which have enhanced the activity of a drug, e.g. megoestrol, or changed the therapeutic effect of a drug, e.g. temazepam (Fig. 19.14). Alternatively, lower doses have been given in a soft gelatin capsule form to achieve the same steady state blood levels as alternative solid oral dosage forms. This has the benefit of reducing side effects and allowing reductions in raw material costs. It is possible also to administer a lower dose of drug in a SGC than would be necessary in a tablet. The mean digoxin serum levels of eight subjects receiving 0.25 mg digoxin in tablets and 0.2 mg digoxin in SEG capsules (polyol liquid fill) have been compared (Mallis *et al.*, 1975). Repeated dosage showed that the different dosages gave the same steady state blood levels.

REFERENCES AND BIBLIOGRAPHY

Aguiar, A. J., Zelmar, L. E. and Kinkel, A. W. (1967) *J. pharm. Sci.*, **56**, 1243–1252.

Arendano *et al.* (1970) *Am. J. Abstr. Gyrea*, **106**, 122.

Arnold *et al.* (1971) *Int. J. clin. Pharmacol.*, **15**, 230.

Binnion, P. F. (1976) *J. clin. Pharmacol.*, **16**, 161.

Fincher, J. H., Adams, J. G. and Beal, H. M. (1965) *J. pharm. Sci.*, **54**, 704–708.

François, D. and Jones, B. E. (1979) Making the hard capsule with the soft centre. *Manufacturing Chemist and Aerosol News*, **50**(3), 37, 38, 41.

Frisch, E. P. and Ortengre, B. (1966) *Acta psych. scand.*, **42**, 35.

Hom, F. S. and Miskel, J. J. (1970) *J. pharm. Sci.*, **59**(6), 827.

Hom, F. S., Veresh, S. A. and Ebert, W. R. (1975) *J. pharm. Sci.*, **64**(5), 851–857.

Jones, B. E. and Turner, T. D. (1974) Century of commercial hard gelatin capsule manufacture. *Pharm. J.*, **213**, 614–617.

Jones, R. T. (1970) Pharmaceutical gelatin — manufacture.

Proc. Biochem., 5(12), 2–8.

Jones, R. T. (1971) Pharmaceutical gelatin — applications. *Proc. Biochem.*, 6(7), 19–22.

Lesko, L. J., Canada, A. T., Eastwood, G., Walker, D. and Broussea, D. R. (1979) *J. pharm. Sci.*, **68**, 1372.

Mallis *et al.* (1975) *J. Clin. Pharm. Ther.*, **18**, 761.

Newton, J. M. (1972) The release of drugs from hard gelatin capsules. *Pharmaceutische Weekblad*, **107**, 485–498.

Orr, N. (1981) *Progress in the Quality Control of Medicines*, Elsevier Biomedical Press, Amsterdam.

Palin, K., (1982) PhD Thesis, Nottingham University, England.

Samyn, J. C. and Jung, W. Y. (1970) *J. pharm. Sci.*, **59**, 169–175.

Simmons, D. L., Fredhete, M., Lanz, R. J., Chen, W. S. and Patel, N. K. (1972) *Can. J. pharm. Sci.*, **7**, 62–65.

Tardif, J. (1965) *J. pharm. Sci.*, **54**, 281.

Tyrer, J. M., Eadie, M. J., Sutherland, J. M. and Hooper, W. D. (1970) *Br. med. J.*, **4**, 271–273.

Therapeutic aerosols

DEFINITION AND USES OF THERAPEUTIC AEROSOLS

The general public associates the word 'aerosol' with a specific form of presentation of various products in pressurized cannisters which contain the desired materials and the 'propellants' for the expulsion of the contents from the containers. This usage of the word has caused some confusion because the scientific definition of 'aerosol' is rather different:

it is a dispersion of solid or liquid particles (typically smaller than 50 μm) in a gas.

Many types of pharmaceuticals are available in pressurized cannisters. Usually, these preparations are for application to the skin, or into an accessible body cavity (mouth, ear, nose, rectum or vagina). Examples of active ingredients are antiseptics, antibiotics, local anesthetics or dermatological steroids. Spray-on protective films for wound and burn dressings are also used. The pressurized cannisters provide one of the most convenient methods of presenting pharmaceuticals to the user. The active agents can be applied readily to the desired site, with only a minimum mechanical irritation of the affected area. The danger of contamination during or between applications is diminished because the product is dispersed directly from a sealed container. The latter separates the product from the external atmosphere, and therefore improves its chemical and microbiological stability.

Perhaps the most challenging task for a pharmaceutical formulator is the preparation of aerosols for inhalation therapy. This route of drug administration has been known for a long time, and a particularly interesting review of various 'smoke' remedies for asthma appeared towards the end of the last century (Thompson, 1879). Aerosols are unique in that they provide a convenient method of drug delivery directly to the sites of action in the respiratory tract. In order to achieve the same pharmacologically active levels of a drug in the respiratory tract via the gastrointestinal or the parenteral routes, much greater doses of the drug usually have to be administered. One of the chief advantages of inhalation therapy of the diseases of the respiratory tract is therefore the relatively low drug concentration in the systemic circulation. Consequently, the intensity and incidence of side effects of inhaled drugs is in many instances markedly reduced as compared to administration of the same drugs by different routes (Clark, 1972; Neville et al., 1977). The treatment of asthma and bronchitis with aerosol inhalations containing bronchodilators, corticosteroids, anticholinergics or the prophylactic agent sodium cromoglycate (cromolyn sodium) has been particularly successful. Local anesthesia of bronchial airways with lignocaine aerosols has shown promising results. There is less evidence for the safety and efficacy of antimicrobial, antifungal and mucolytic aerosols. Objective evaluations of 'bland' aerosols (i.e. containing only water or saline solutions) have not indicated so far any beneficial effects in clinical studies, although it might be thought that humidification of airways and reduction of the viscosity of sputum would improve the mucociliary clearance in, for example, chronic bronchitis or cystic fibrosis. Aerosol vaccination against certain diseases of the respiratory tract holds some promise; however, this method still requires large scale validation.

There has been a growing interest in the diagnostic application of inhalation aerosols. Thus, aerosolized solutions of bronchospastic agents are administered in provocation tests for the diagnosis and assessment of bronchial asthma. Radio-opaque substances may be inhaled to provide a contrast medium for X-ray examinations of airways. More recently, fine particles labelled with an element emitting gamma radiation (e.g. technetium-99m) have been administered in small quantities as aerosols: upon deposition in the respiratory tract, their location and movement can be followed with suitable external detectors such as scanning scintillation counters and gamma cameras. The observation of the deposition of the particles and their movement with time has been utilized to assess structural and functional abnormalities in the airways.

The human respiratory tract has an extensive blood supply and its total surface area is about 30–100 m^2. Most of the surface area resides in the alveolated regions of the deep lung which contain also a rich capillary network to facilitate rapid gas exchange. Although inhaled drug particles or droplets will typically deposit only on a small fraction of the total available surface area, the possibility of fast drug absorption into the systemic circulation exists. An example of application of the inhalation route for rapid drug absorption and subsequent systemic transport to sites outside the respiratory tract is ergotamine tartrate aerosol for relief of migraine headaches.

Clearly, if inhaled aerosols are to serve their intended purpose, they must first deposit in the respiratory tract. The knowledge of the physicochemical and physiological factors affecting the deposition of aerosols in the airways is therefore a crucial prerequisite for successful design and rational quality control of this dosage form.

IMPORTANT PHYSICOCHEMICAL PROPERTIES OF THERAPEUTIC AEROSOLS

Size distribution

An idealized aerosol, in which the particles or droplets would all have the same size, is said to be 'monodisperse'. In reality, aerosols contain a continuous distribution of liquid or solid components of various sizes. The distribution is usually best described by a logarithmic normal probability function (Chapter 33), characterized by two parameters, the geometric mean diameter and the geometric standard deviation.

Geometric mean diameter

The geometric mean diameter D_g is the nth root of the product of all n diameters. For example, for two particles with $D = 3$ μm, three particles with $D = 4$ μm and one particle with $D = 5$ μm, $D_g = \sqrt[6]{3^2 \times 4^3 \times 5} = 3.77$ μm. The same result is obtained by taking the antilogarithm of the average value of the logarithms of the diameters — hence, this mean is also called 'logarithmic'. *The median diameter* divides the size distribution into two equal halves, i.e. 50% of the particles are below, or above, this size. If the logarithms of diameters conform to the normal probability function, the geometric mean is equal to the median diameter. We shall assume this to be true in the discussion which follows.

If the averaging is done according to the number of particles per given size (as in the example given above), the mean value is called the *count median diameter* (CMD). For most biological applications, however, it is more meaningful to take the average according to the mass of particles in a given size range. This average is called the *mass median diameter* (MMD). The relationship between CMD and MMD is given by a Hatch–Choate equation (Chapter 33).

Geometric standard deviation

The geometric standard deviation σ_g in a logarithmic-normal distribution is the measure of the polydispersity of the aerosol. It is akin to the ordinary standard deviation of the mean in a normally distributed population, σ_N. Thus, a 'monodisperse' population would have $\sigma_N = 1$ and $\ln \sigma_g = 0$ (i.e. $\sigma_g = 1$). Since it is impossible to prepare absolutely monodisperse aerosols, $\sigma_g \sim 1.2$ is conventionally set as the limit at which polydispersity starts.

In analogy with the mean and standard deviation of a normal distribution, the geometric mean and σ_g can be used directly to calculate the fraction of the sample within specified bounds. For example, an aerosol with MMD = 3 μm has 50%

of its mass below this size. Also, for $\sigma_g = 1.7$, approximately 68% of the mass resides in the range antiln $(\ln 3 \pm \ln 1.7) = (1.76 - 5.10)$ μm and 95% of the mass in the range antiln $(\ln 3 \pm 2 \ln 1.7) = (1.04 - 8.67)$ μm.

Aerodynamic diameter

The motion of the disperse phase in a gas stream depends on the size, shape and density of the aerosol particles. The variable which combines these three properties, and is therefore used in the studies of deposition of aerosols in the human respiratory tract, is called the aerodynamic diameter (D_A). It is defined as the diameter of a sphere of unit density (1 kg dm^{-3}) which has the same terminal settling velocity as the particle in question. In principle, it is therefore possible to determine the aerodynamic diameter of any particle by measurement of its free-fall velocity in air and comparing this value with spheres of known dimensions and densities. Alternative techniques for measurement of D_A are described in 'Size analysis' below.

Most particles and droplets in therapeutic aerosols are nearly spherical, with diameters greater than 0.5 μm. For such particles and droplets, the relationship between the diameter D measured microscopically and D_A is described with sufficient accuracy by

$$D_A = D \sqrt{\rho/\rho_o} \tag{20.1}$$

where ρ is the density of the disperse phase and ρ_o is 'unit density' (1 kg dm^{-3}).

More details about sedimentation of particles in fluids and shape factors can be found in Chapter 33.

When the mass median diameter (MMD) and density of a sample are known, the mass median aerodynamic diameter (MMAD) is obtained from Eqn 20.1 as

$$MMAD = MMD \sqrt{\rho/\rho_o} \tag{20.2}$$

MMAD of an inhalation aerosol should refer to the distribution of the drug mass among the particles and droplets of various aerodynamic diameters. The term 'drug mass median aerodynamic diameter' could be used for this purpose (Byron *et al.*, 1977). It gives the aerodynamic size of the disperse phase below or above which 50% of the drug dose resides. The experimental procedures to find this value are described under 'Size analysis' in the 'Testing of aerosols' section of this chapter.

Instability of aerosols

After generation of the aerosol, mass and heat transfer processes between the environment and the disperse phase take place. In particular, the partial vapour pressures of the components of aerosol droplets will be changing as a result of the tendency to equalize with the partial vapour pressures in the environment. Volatile liquids, such as propellants and solvents, evaporate because the surrounding atmosphere effectively acts as an infinite sink for them. The loss of energy in the form of heat of vaporization causes the droplets to cool down but this process may be counteracted by heat transfer from the environment into the droplets.

The atmosphere in human lungs is nearly saturated at 37 °C with water vapour originating from the isotonic fluids covering the surfaces of the respiratory tract. The relative humidity, RH, is defined as

$$RH = 100 \times \frac{p_w}{P_w^o} \qquad (20.3)$$

where p_w is the actual partial vapour pressure and P_w^o is the vapour pressure of pure water at the same temperature at which the measurement is made. Thus, the atmosphere at equilibrium with pure water has RH = 100%. In an aqueous solution, the pressure of solutes depresses the water vapour pressure so that $p_w < P_w^o$. In sufficiently dilute solutions, this depression is described by Raoult's law (Chapter 3). The relative humidity over isotonic solutions at 37 °C is about 99.5%.

The vapour pressure of small droplets of a liquid is greater than the vapour pressure over a large flat surface of the same liquid due to the Kelvin effect (Chapter 4). However, it is permissible to neglect this correction for aqueous droplets of drugs provided that they are greater than about 2 μm (Gonda et al., 1982). Under such circumstances, it may be assumed that droplets

containing isotonic drug solutions at 37 °C have the same partial vapour pressure of water as the fluids covering the lungs.

Suppose now that a dry particle of a water-soluble drug is inhaled. Its initial water vapour pressure is zero, and it will therefore have the tendency to adsorb water, dissolve and accept more water by 'condensation growth' until the drug concentration is isotonic. It can be derived by simple mass balance considerations (Groom et al., 1980) that D_e, the diameter of the droplet containing the isotonic drug solution, is related to the diameter of the original dry particle, D, by

$$D_e = D \sqrt[3]{\frac{\rho}{\rho_e} [1 + \frac{1000}{M \, m_e}]} \qquad (20.4)$$

where ρ and ρ_e are the densities of the dry particle and the isotonic drug solution, respectively, M is the molecular weight of the drug and m_e is its isotonic molality [moles of drug per kg of water]. After correcting for densities (Eqn 20.1), the ratio of the aerodynamic diameter of the equilibrated droplet and the dry particle can be calculated. It has been found that several drugs used in the inhalation treatment of asthma have the capacity to increase their aerodynamic size by a factor of 2–3 as a result of condensation growth (Gonda et al., 1982).

Of course, the particle may deposit in the airways before it has grown to its equilibrium diameter D_e. Several hundred milliseconds are probably necessary for the completion of the growth, and the larger droplets in particular are therefore likely to impact before they reach the isotonic concentration.

Another cause of instability of the particle size distribution of the disperse phase is coagulation. This process depends on the collisions between the aerosol particles. It is therefore important in concentrated systems, especially if there is an appreciable period between the generation of the aerosol and its use.

Corollary

Therapeutic aerosols are usually polydisperse and their particle size distribution may be subject to changes caused by several dynamic processes. Such aerosols are unsuitable for studies aimed at defining the relationship between the size of the dispersed particles and their deposition in the respiratory tract. These investigations necessitate the preparation of 'monodisperse' aerosols ($\sigma_g < 1.2$) which are stable on the time scale of the inhalation experiments. Dilute aerosols made from involatile, non-hygroscopic materials (e.g. polystyrene latex) must be used for this purpose.

DEPOSITION OF AEROSOLS IN THE HUMAN RESPIRATORY TRACT

Aerosols deposit, in general, as a result of the following fundamental mechanisms (Lippmann et al., 1980).

Inertial impaction

A particle carried by a stream of gas has its own momentum which is the product of its mass (inertia) and velocity. When the gas stream encounters an obstacle or a bend, the direction of the gas flow changes. The inertial force of the particle resists this change, causing the particle to fly some distance along the original direction of motion. Therefore, the particle with a high momentum may impact on the surface of the object in front of it, rather than follow the gas streamlines.

In the nasal passages, large particles are captured by impaction on the coarse hair and in the channels serving to adjust the temperature and humidity of the incoming air. The mouth is a less efficient organ for air-conditioning and filtration of coarse particles. The air stream then encounters a sharp bend in the pharynx before it enters the trachea through the laryngeal opening. Only a minute fraction of particles with aerodynamic diameters over 15 μm for mouth breathing, or over 10 μm for nasal breathing, reach as far as this area because the combination of the large particle mass and high air flow velocity in the upper airways make impaction a very efficient mechanism for their capture. The trachea branches (bifurcates) into the left and right pulmonary lobes. The airways then undergo a number of bifurcations, first into 'conductive' branches in the tracheobronchial regions and finally forming the gas exchange spaces of respiratory bronchiole and the alveolar sacs. Due to the successive splitting of the air flow, the gas velocity is gradually decreased from several m s^{-1} to less than 1 mm s^{-1} in the alveolar region. Consequently, impaction ceases to be an important mechanism of deposition in lower airways. Nevertheless, it is still effective at the first few tracheobronchial bifurcations for particles with $D_A > 3$ μm.

Sedimentation (settling)

Particles and droplets suspended in gas are subject to the vertical force of gravitation which acts upon them in all parts of the respiratory tract. The settling velocity increases with the square of the aerodynamic diameter (see Stokes' law, Chapter 6). Sedimentation is therefore an important mechanism of deposition in the lower airways for particles which escape the capture by impaction (0.5 μm $< D_A < 3$ μm).

The sedimentation velocity of particles with $D_A < 0.5$ μm is so low that they would not deposit in the lower airways by settling, unless they were held there over a prolonged period of time.

Diffusion (Brownian motion)

The bombardment of colloidal particles by the molecules and atoms of the surrounding medium causes the colloids to undergo random (Brownian) motion. However, the resultant effect on the colloidal particles is their directional movement (diffusion) from high to low colloid concentration. Consequently, particles or droplets diffuse from the aerosol cloud to the walls of the respiratory tract. The rate of this process is inversely proportional to the particle size and diffusion is therefore the dominant mechanism of deposition in airways for particles smaller than 0.5 μm.

Interception

This mechanism is important for deposition of elongated particles, such as mineral fibres, in lower airways.

Electrostatic precipitation

Electrostatic precipitation of charged aerosol

particles by attraction to a surface of opposite charge is thought to be insignificant for drug aerosols in the respiratory tract.

It should be now apparent that correct instructions for the patient using inhalation aerosols are important (Newman et al., 1980). Slow inspiration of the aerosol reduces impaction in the mouth and pharynx. Breath-holding at the end of inspiration allows the particles which have travelled beyond these regions to deposit by diffusion and sedimentation. Without the breath-holding manoeuvre, most particles with aerodynamic diameter ~0.5 μm are exhaled because they are neither sufficiently large to settle rapidly, nor small enough to deposit by diffusion during normal breathing. The aerosol cloud should enter the patient's mouth during a slow, deep breath so that the bolus of gas containing the medicament travels deeper into the small airways. Of course, the situation may be different if the drug receptors are located in the upper airways, e.g. as in the case of treatment of throat infections with antiseptic sprays.

Marked intersubject variation in the regional distribution of aerosols has been observed in human lungs in carefully controlled studies with normal volunteers. The source of this variation presumably lies in the anatomical and physiological differences between individuals and the effects that these variations have on the mechanisms of deposition. Diseases of the respiratory tract which cause obstruction of airways affect deposition of aerosols. For example, higher tracheobronchial deposition is found in chronic bronchitis, probably due to an excessively thick layer of mucus in the conductive airways.

Our knowledge about the extent to which inhaled substances are retained in various parts of the respiratory tract comes mainly from studies with stable monodisperse aerosols. It is customary to divide the respiratory tract into the head, tracheobronchial and pulmonary regions, and to consider the fraction of a dose depositing in these three locations as a function of the aerodynamic diameter (D_A). An approximation of typical experimental data for normal volunteers at rest inhaling moderately high volumes of aerosols through mouth is shown in Fig. 20.1. The high deposition of very fine aerosols in the pulmonary spaces is the result of rapid diffusion of these small particles. The minimum at $D_A \sim 0.5$ μm has been explained above. The rapid decrease of deposition in the pulmonary region for $D_A > 2$ μm is mainly due to the efficiency of the capture by impaction of large particles in the upper airways.

However, most therapeutic aerosols are neither monodisperse, nor stable. They contain a relatively wide spectrum of particle and droplet sizes. As the aerosol cloud passes from the generator into the airways, the particle size may change by evaporation of the volatile components (solvents and propellants), and by condensation of water vapour from the humid airways upon the particles or droplets containing the drug (see previous section on properties of therapeutic aerosols). The consequences of aerosol instability and polydispersity can be still appreciated from studies such as those represented in Fig. 20.1. For example, we would expect the maximum pulmonary deposition with $D_A = 2–3$ μm. A change of size by a factor of 2 to $D_A \sim 5$ μm would be likely to lead to an increase in the fraction retained in the upper airways and a marked reduction in the dose delivered to the lower airways. A similar effect could be caused by administering an aerosol with a mass median aerodynamic diameter in the optimum range for pulmonary deposition (MMAD ~ 2.5 μm) but having a wide particle size distribution ($\sigma_g > 2$). This is because even a few large particles would be sufficient to carry a substantial part of the dose, and due to their high D_A, they would deposit in the upper airways.

FORMULATION AND GENERATION OF AEROSOLS

The extensive use of several types of portable inhalers, particularly in the treatment of asthma, has been facilitated by the combination of the skills to develop safe and potent drugs and to present them in these rather sophisticated, site-directional delivery systems. Additionally, a selection of aerosol generators is available for use in hospitals. Because the operation of various devices may be based on different principles, the formulation problems must be considered in conjunction with a specific type of aerosol generator.

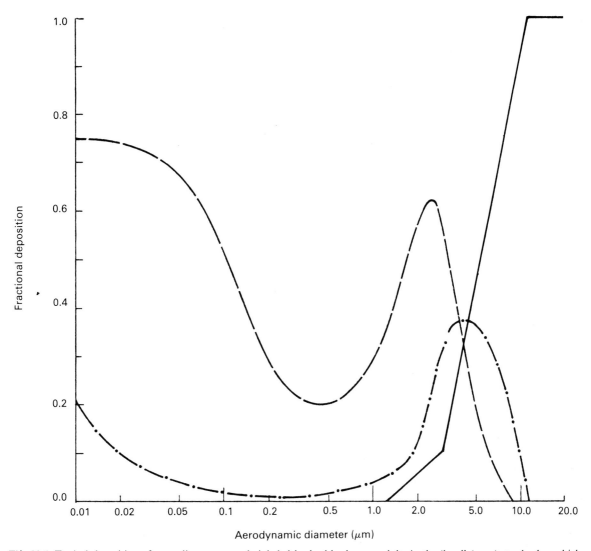

Fig. 20.1 Typical deposition of monodisperse aerosols inhaled by healthy human adults in the 'head' (——), tracheobronchial (—·—) and pulmonary (– – –) regions of the respiratory tract during normal breathing via mouth (Reproduced with copyright permission from Gonda, I. (1981) *J. Pharm. Pharmacol*, **33**, 692)

From a pharmaceutical point of view, there are three important characteristics of an aerosol generator:

1 total output of the drug (e.g. weight of drug per unit time of operation, or weight of drug in a unit spray for metered doses),
2 the drug mass distribution in different aerodynamic size fractions, and
3 reproducibility of operation.

The dose requirements can be satisfied by appropriate scaling of the generator and the number of inhalations provided that the output of the device is stable. The deposition of the aerosol in the respiratory tract depends on the particle and droplet size distribution, and this factor must therefore be carefully controlled.

Generally, aerosols are produced by one of two methods:

1 dispersion of a powder, or liquid, in gas,
2 evaporation of volatile substances which condense to form droplets or fine particles upon cooling to ambient temperature.

Pressurized packages

A large variety of pharmaceutical and cosmetic products is available in this form. Apart from inhalation aerosols, coarse sprays and foams for surface coating are regarded as 'aerosols' in the wider sense of the word. All these products share the convenience of being hermetically sealed in a ready-to-use container. The driving force expelling the formulation out of the package is the pressure P of the propellant which is approximated well by the equation of state for an ideal gas

$$P = \frac{nRT}{V} \qquad (20.5)$$

where n and V are the number of moles and the volume of the propellant gas in the container, respectively, R is the universal gas constant and T is the absolute temperature. If several propellants are used, the total pressure P is calculated from Dalton's law as the sum of the partial vapour pressures p_i ($i = 1, 2. \ldots \ldots n$ for n propellants):

$$P = \sum_{i=1}^{n} p_i \qquad (20.6)$$

Rising temperature causes an elevation of gas pressure inside the container (see Eqn 20.5). It may also increase the pressure of liquefied propellants by increasing their volatility as described by the Clapeyron equation. Storage of pressurized containers in cool places is therefore essential to prevent explosions. Moreover, excessive temperatures lead to chemical and physical deterioration of the product.

Types of propellants

Compressed gases, such as carbon dioxide, nitrogen or nitrous oxide, may be used to expel the product from the package. The disadvantage of this type of generator is that as the volume available to the gas increases as a result of emptying the solid and liquid components, the pressure — and hence the driving force — decreases (see Eqn 20.5). Compressed-gas packages are used mainly for generation of coarse sprays and foams.

Liquefied gases have the advantage that the vapour pressure over the liquid surface stays constant in the cannister at a given temperature since any escaped propellant, or change in the volume available to the gas, is immediately compensated by transfer of more propellant molecules into the gas phase. If a mixture of volatile components, i.e. propellants and solvents, exists in the liquid phase, the partial vapour pressure p_i of a propellant i at a constant temperature may be approximated by Raoult's law for ideal solutions:

$$p_i = x_i \, p_i^{\circ} \qquad (20.7)$$

where x_i and p_i° are the mole fraction and the vapour pressure of the pure propellant i at the given temperature, respectively. The total vapour pressure can be estimated by summing the partial vapour pressures of the major volatile components. Thus, from Eqns 20.6 and 20.7

$$P = \sum_{i=1}^{n} x_i \, p_i^{\circ} \qquad (20.8)$$

The most common propellants are fluorinated and fluorochlorinated hydrocarbons. Non-flammable members of this family which possess low toxicity are used for inhalation aerosols. These propellants are usually gases at, or near, normal ambient conditions. When stored in the aerosol package typically under pressures three to five times the atmospheric value, they form liquids. Alternatively, liquefaction may be forced by reducing the temperature, at normal pressure, below the boiling point of the propellants. This process is employed for the 'cold-fill' manufacture of pressurized packages in large scale production and in the laboratories. The 'pressure-fill' must be used for products which would freeze at reduced temperatures, and for hydrocarbon propellants (e.g. propane and butane) whose vapour concentration could reach explosion limits during the 'cold-fill' process.

Containers

Mechanical strength, chemical inertness and cost are the criteria for selection of the containers. Glass protected with a plastic film against shattering is a suitable material for low pressure packages. Stainless steel containers are expensive but they can withstand high pressures and are virtually non-corrosive. Tin-plated steel is a light material of low cost which can be made chemically non-reactive by suitable plastic coating. The body of the steel container consists usually of three separate pieces, giving it a 'beer can' appearance. Aluminium cannisters may be made by extrusion, thus avoiding the necessity to form seams (cf. tin-plated steel cans). Aluminium, too, can be coated with chemically resistant organic materials.

The plastic films inside metallic containers are particularly important to prevent corrosion by products containing water. Some chlorinated propellants can undergo hydrolysis leading to the formation of the highly corrosive hydrochloric acid. Compatibility of the plastic with the organic materials in the package must also be assured. The presence of air, and oxygen in particular, should be minimized by expelling it with propellants during manufacture. This improves product stability and saves volume in the package.

Formulation aspects

The gas phase containing the propellant gas or vapour is always present in this dosage form. In the simplest system, the second phase, a liquid, is a solution of the active ingredients. Cosolvents, e.g. ethanol, usually have to be added because fluorochlorohydrocarbons are poor solvents. On actuation, the liquid is expelled from the package and the most volatile components evaporate rapidly, leaving behind dry particles or droplets. Fine sprays suitable for inhalation may be obtained with low boiling point propellants (dichlorodifluoromethane and dichlorotetrafluoroethane), provided the concentration of the active ingredients and cosolvents is kept low.

On the other hand, the use of high-boiling point propellants and a large proportion of non-volatile components encourages the formation of coarse droplets suitable for delivery of topical aerosols to the intended areas of the skin only. The absence of fine droplets in such aerosols reduces the potential for accidental inhalation of these products.

An even better localization of substances for topical application to the skin, or for contra-

ception, is achieved by administering them as foam. These can be produced by a 'three-phase' system in which the propellant is in the internal phase of an oil-in-water emulsion. On reaching the atmospheric conditions, expanding bubbles are formed as the propellant evaporates. The bubbles are stabilized by surfactants and the escaping propellant also aids to transform the emulsion into a foam by a 'whipping' action. Depending on the formulation, stable or quick-breaking foams can be produced. The latter, usually containing alcohols and water, are popular for application to the skin. Foams can be produced also with compressed gas propellants which are soluble in the emulsion.

When the propellant is present in the external phase of a water-in-oil system, the released product is a coarse, wet spray rather than a foam, because the internal phase of the emulsion stays largely unchanged by evaporation of the gases.

'Powder aerosols' are prepared by suspending solid dry particles in liquefied propellants containing various additives to prevent agglomeration, caking, crystal growth and clogging of the valves. Sorbitan trioleate and oleic acid are examples of such additives. These systems are used most frequently for therapeutic inhalation aerosols. For this purpose, the drug must be first micronized so that the mass median aerodynamic diameter is in the respirable range. It is particularly crucial for the aerodynamic size distribution to have suitable characteristics at the point of entry into the patient's respiratory tract. This requires good suspension stability and propellants which evaporate rapidly when the product is released. Otherwise, several drug particles may be carried in a relatively large, stable droplet which would deposit in the mouth.

Valves, dip tubes and actuators

The type of valve selected depends on the formulation and the application of the product. Different valves are used for sprays, foams and for delivery of individual unit doses. The latter is achieved by 'metering valves': the first stroke of the valve admits the product into a metering chamber where it stays enclosed. The constant volume of the product is then released from the

(a) Valve at rest

(b) Valve depressed

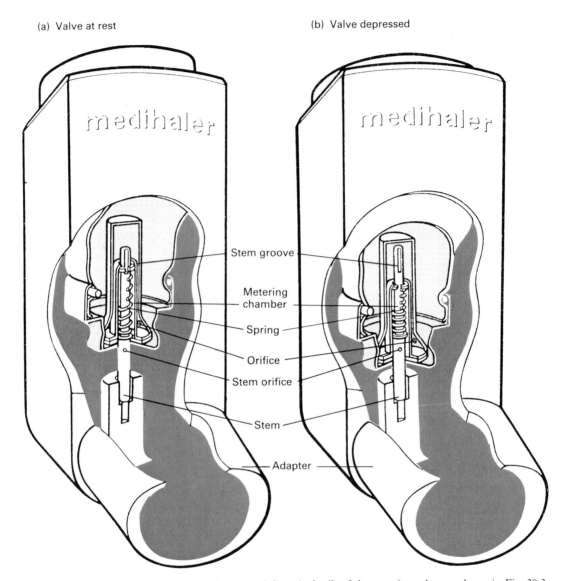

Fig. 20.2 Pressurized cannister placed in an oral actuator (adaptor); details of the metering valve are shown in Fig. 20.3. (a) Valve at rest and (b) valve depressed (Courtesy of Riker Laboratories 3M, Loughborough, UK)

chamber in the reverse stroke of the valve (Figs. 20.2 and 20.3).

In order to assure proper emptying of the package, polyethylene or polypropylene dip tubes reaching the distal end of the container are often connected to the valve. This arrangement also prevents wasteful escape of the propellant.

The valve actuators are shaped in a way which makes the application of the product to the desired part of the body convenient. Thus, different shapes are made for oral, nasal, skin, vaginal or eye administration. Mechanical breakup of the spray can be also assisted by a suitable design of the actuator. The use of 'spacer tubes' for inhalation aerosols is described in the next section.

Performance of pressurized packages as inhalation aerosol generators

The dose output per unit spray ranges from about 50 to several hundred μg. The mass median aero-

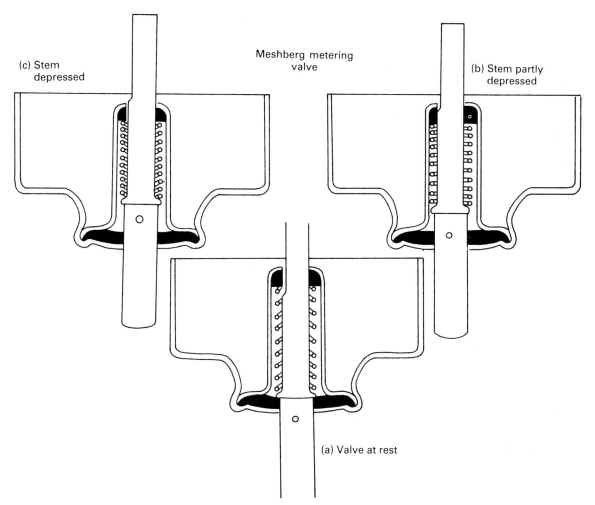

Fig. 20.3 Metering valve: (a) valve at rest: the metering chamber fills with the contents of the cannister by way of the groove; (b) stem of the valve partly depressed: the dose is isolated in the metering chamber; (c) valve depressed: the propellant drives the dose out through the orifice in the stem into the actuator. The spring then returns the stem into the resting position (a) so that the chamber can refill (Courtesy of Riker Laboratories 3M, Loughborough, UK)

dynamic diameters of the particles left after evaporation of the propellant are typically 1.5–4 μm, with geometric standard deviations indicating mild to substantial polydispersity ($\sigma_g \sim 1.7$–3.5). However, much greater aerodynamic diameters exist in the spray before the propellant evaporates. A further problem arises from the high initial velocity of the aerosol components which may cause a large fraction of the medicament to deposit at the back of the mouth by inertial impaction. A simple, but somewhat irreproducible remedy is for the patient to fire the aerosol a little distance away from his mouth. A better solution is to place a

pear-shaped tube up to 250 mm long between the actuator and the patient's mouth (Lindgren et al., 1980). While in the tube, the aerosol has time to slow down and lose most of the propellant. This 'spacer tube' is also advantageous for patients unable to synchronize the valve actuation with the inspiratory manoeuvre.

Air-blast nebulizers

These devices are based on the Venturi tube principle: compressed air enters a narrow tube immersed in a liquid to be aerosolized. As the air exits from the tube it expands, causing a pressure drop which attracts the liquid into the air stream. The former breaks up into droplets whose size distribution depends on the air velocity, and the density, viscosity and surface tension of the liquid (Davis, 1978; Davis *et al.*, 1978). The coarse droplet fraction is removed by one of the many available 'baffle' systems, upon which the particles with the highest momenta deposit (see below under 'Size analysis'); this fraction returns to the liquid reservoir. The remainder of the aerosol leaving the generator is saturated with the vapour of the solvent. Therefore, the temperature of the liquid in the nebulizer falls due to the energy expenditure for vaporization. If the liquid in the reservoir contains dissolved substances, its composition changes during the nebulization. These time-dependent alterations must be borne in mind for long term operation.

It is possible also to nebulize drug suspensions with these generators. However, if it is desired to reproduce the original powder size distribution in the aerosol, the suspension must be sufficiently dilute to prevent formation of aerosols containing more than one drug particle per droplet (Raabe, 1968).

Good quality air-blast nebulizers are capable of producing aqueous aerosols with mass median droplet diameter $MMD_d = 2$–4 μm and geometric standard deviation of about 2. Often, the aerosol is subsequently dried. If the solution contains C (g ml^{-1}) of solute whose density is ρ (g cm^{-3}), the mass median diameter MMD of the dry solid particles is (Mercer, 1973):

$$MMD = MMD_d \, (C/\rho)^{\frac{1}{3}}$$

Ultrasonic nebulizers

The dispersion of liquids in these generators is achieved by mechanical vibrations of a piezoelectric crystal subjected to an alternating electric field. A highly monodisperse aerosol for calibration of instruments may be prepared in a special generator (Berglund and Liu, 1973) in which a constant liquid flow passes through a vibrating orifice which breaks up the flow into uniform cylinders. Large quantities of polydisperse aerosols are prepared in another type of

ultrasonic generator used mainly in hospitals: the piezoelectric vibrations (frequency $\sim$ 1 MHz) are transmitted through a coupling medium to the nebulizer cup. A fountain of liquid is formed which yields droplets. These are transported from the cup by carrier air. The coarse fraction is best removed by baffles.

The mean droplet size decreases with the ultrasonic frequency and the density of the liquid, and it increases with the surface tension of the liquid (Mercer, 1973). Although these generators have typically much higher output than the smaller airblast nebulizers, the character of the particle size distribution is quite similar. In both types of generators, the actual distribution will depend on the operating conditions and the properties of the nebulized formulation.

Dry powder generators

The drug particles to be aerosolized must have the appropriate size distribution for deposition in the desired parts of the respiratory tract because these generators usually do not have the capability to break solid particles. Excipients, such as lactose, may be used in the formulation to dilute the drug and improve its flow properties. The size of these additives should be large enough to prevent their entry into the airways. *Insufflators* are the simplest devices for oral or nasal inhalation of dry solids. The energy for aerosolization is supplied by the patient's breath; in the case of nasal insufflators it may come from air forced out of a rubber balloon. Agglomerates of particles can be broken up by a wire mesh, or a propeller driven by the air flow, placed downstream towards the patient's mouth.

A device which has an electrically operated vertical spinning disc has been tested clinically (Malem *et al.*, 1981). The disc, which is semi-immersed in the powder, rotates rapidly, bringing the solid particles into the gas phase. The carrier air is sucked through the generator when the patient inhales. This device may be used also for dispersion of liquids.

The advantages of dry powder generators are:

1 Their operation is activated by the patient's breath, and therefore the synchronization with the breathing cycle is automatic.

2 In principle, higher drug dose per inspiration may be delivered into the airways because there is no dilution of the medicament with solvents or the dispersion liquid.

However, drug losses occur by adhesion to the walls of the generator and the insufflator capsules in which the formulation is supplied. The simple insufflators tend to produce rather polydisperse aerosols ($\sigma_g \sim 3$). The formation of large compact agglomerates, particularly as a result of storage at high humidity, must be prevented.

Evaporation–condensation generators

These are used very rarely in medicine although some aerosol is invariably formed by this method during the preparation of 'inhalations' from vapour of hot water and menthol or eucalyptus oil.

TESTING OF AEROSOLS

The purpose of this section is to outline the methods which are used specifically in the development and quality control of pharmaceutical aerosols. However, the student should appreciate that this dosage form shares with others the problems of chemical stability (Chapter 13) and microbial contamination (Chapter 27). The theory and practice of control of the properties of suspensions are described in Chapters 6 and 15. Systemic bioavailability tests for all dosage forms are discussed in Part 2 of this book.

Leakage and pressure testing of pressurized cannisters

Since the spray produced by these generators depends on the pressure developed by the propellants, the maintenance of this driving force is essential. In-line leak testing of each container after the filling operation is employed by manufacturers. A detector for halogenated compounds can automatically activate the rejection of a faulty container. In addition there may be compendial requirements (e.g. USP XXI-NF XVI, 1985) to check gravimetrically that the leakage rate from a specified number of containers complies with the official norm.

Non-destructive measurements of the pressure inside the containers can be carried out with gauges which have been prepressurized to the level expected in the cannister. It is necessary to equilibrate the container and its contents beforehand at constant temperature by immersion in a water bath. The method is useful also for a rough identification of liquefied propellants.

In-line pressure testing is important for devices employing compressed gases as the propellants, because it is the only suitable method for checking that an amount of the gas has been put into the pressure pack.

Output, drug concentration and dose delivered

The average total output of the vapour, liquid and solid components can be measured by weighing the aerosol generator, or the part containing the material to be aerosolized, before and after a specified duration of operation (USP XXI-NF XVI, 1985). The drug concentration inside a pressurized cannister may be ascertained by releasing a portion of the contents under the surface of a suitable solvent, assaying for the amount of the drug thus captured (w_1) and noting the weight loss (w_2) from the container (USP XXI-NF XVI, 1985). The density, ρ, of the solution is obtained usually by a pycnometric method. The drug concentration is calculated as $w_1\rho/w_2$.

The tests of inhalation aerosols for the drug content available to the patient's mouth in a unit spray are more directly related to clinical efficacy. The standard method in Britain (BPC 1973) is to release a unit spray under the surface of a specified solvent. From the dose of drug thus captured, the amount retained in the oral actuator when the aerosol is fired into free air, is subtracted to calculate the dose fraction available to the patient. The American standard (USP XX-NF XV, 1980) uses apparatus in which the complete generator is connected to a flow line through which a stream of air is drawn continuously at a rate of 12 dm^3 min^{-1}. After firing a unit spray, the aerosol cloud passes through an intake tube to a sintered-glass bubbler immersed in a suitable absorbing solution. The combined amounts of drug captured in this solution and in the intake tube are then assayed.

None of the above methods can assure that the dose of drug will reach the intended sites in the human respiratory tract because the test results are insensitive to the aerodynamic size distribution of the aerosol.

Size analysis

The reader should refer to Chapter 33 for general information on particle size analysis. Some of the methods described therein (microscopy, Coulter counting) may be used to obtain the size distribution of solid drug particles to be incorporated in suspensions for pressurized cannisters, air-blast nebulizers, or dry powder generators. These preformulation tests, however, do not guarantee that the same drug size distribution will be regenerated in the aerosol. Indeed, some degree of aggregation is likely to occur during the storage and formation of the dispersion in gas phase.

Droplet and particle size can be monitored directly in the aerosol cloud by light scattering and diffraction methods (Chapter 33). The main disadvantage of these techniques is that they do not distinguish between various chemical species in multicomponent aerosols. They are invaluable, however, for the studies of dynamics of droplet growth in simple systems containing, e.g. aqueous solutions of drugs (Bell and Ho, 1981).

The pharmacological effects of a drug depend on the dose fraction reaching the various locations in the human body. The initial fate of the medicament in an aerosol is determined by the aerodynamic diameter of the particle, or droplet, in which it is carried. Therefore, instruments capable of measuring the drug mass distribution among the various aerodynamic size ranges of the aerosol are the most suitable tools for biopharmaceutical assessment of this dosage form *in vitro*. The aerodynamic separation is achieved by utilizing the principles discussed previously in this chapter under 'Deposition of aerosols in the human respiratory tract'.

Cascade impactor (Fig. 20.4) In a typical device, the aerosol passes through a series of stages which have nozzles (jets) of decreasing size.

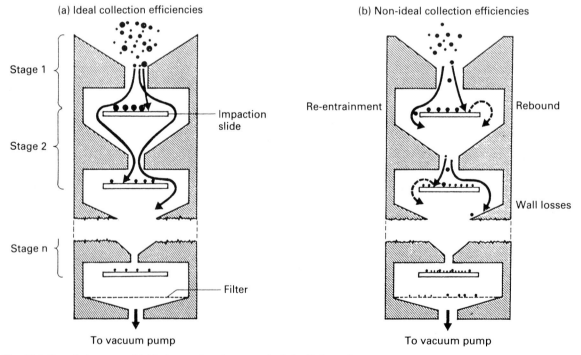

Fig. 20.4 Cascade impactor: (a) ideal operation shown on the left. (b) In reality, some mixing of the particle sizes occurs (see diagram on right), but this can be minimized by suitable coating of the collection surfaces (impaction slides) with viscous fluids. The slides and the filter can be removed for chemical or microscopic analysis.

Perpendicular to each nozzle and some distance downstream from it is located a collection plate. In order to prevent bouncing and blowing off of solid particles, the plates should be coated with a viscous fluid (Groom and Gonda, 1980). The particles with the highest aerodynamic diameters deposit on the first stage because their large momenta will force them to impinge upon the collection plate. The smaller particles follow the air streamlines around the first collection plate and then reach the second, smaller nozzle in which they gain higher velocity and hence higher momenta. Again, some particles will be collected on the second plate whereas the finer fraction continues to the lower stages. The final stage is an 'absolute filter' which should capture the remainder of any droplets or particles contained in the aerosol.

The drug content on every stage is then assayed. The drug mass distribution as a function of the aerodynamic diameter may be calculated from the calibration curves for the individual stages (Gonda *et al.*, 1982). These curves are best obtained by determining the collection efficiency of each stage with monodisperse aerosols (Groom and Gonda, 1980).

The impaction experiments become more realistic when performed at 37 °C in an atmosphere simulating the high relative humidity in the human respiratory tract (Davis and Bubb, 1978). This is important since many therapeutic aerosols have the capacity to grow in size by a factor of two to three because they are hygroscopic under the conditions existing in the respiratory tract. An alternative procedure is to correct the size distribution measured at low relative humidity by a hygroscopic growth factor which can be calculated from the concentration of isotonic drug solutions at 37 °C (see Eqn 20.4 and Gonda *et al.*, 1982).

Multistage liquid impingers are similar to the cascade impactors (Bell *et al.*, 1973). Wet sintered-glass plates serve as the collection surfaces. The penultimate stage, the liquid impinger, consists of a nozzle tangential to the surface of a suitable solvent. An absolute filter is placed at the exit.

Since the aerodynamic diameter is defined in terms of the particle's terminal settling velocity, sedimentation should be the ideal method for assessment of aerosols. In practice, the best results

for particles in the respirable size range are obtained in devices which employ centrifugal, rather than gravitational, force for sedimentation. In the spiral centrifuge aerosol spectrometer (Stöber and Flachsbart, 1969), the sample is introduced into the centre of a spiral channel lined on the outside with a removable foil. The carrier gas flow drives the aerosol from the spiral channel towards the exit at the periphery. However, as the centrifuge rotates, the liquid or solid components deposit along the foil due to the centrifugal force. The distance from the centre at which they deposit is a function of the aerodynamic diameter. This dependence is obtained usually by calibration with monodisperse aerosols. A polydisperse aerosol can be then characterized by microscopic, chemical or radiochemical analysis of the deposits along the length of the foil.

DRUG ABSORPTION AND CLEARANCE FROM THE RESPIRATORY TRACT

Biopharmaceutical considerations of inhalation aerosols differ from other dosage forms in that the problems associated with adequate deposition of drug-containing particles or droplets at the desired sites in the respiratory tract have to be first overcome. Moreover, the drug deposited in the upper airways may be eventually swallowed and follow the gastrointestinal route. This may happen not only to particles deposited in the mouth or the nasopharynx, but also to the material deposited in the other parts of the respiratory tract, with the possible exception of the alveolated regions. Foreign particles, together with cell debris and secretions, are continuously removed from the airways by the mucociliary transport system up to the glottis where they are swallowed. Whether a drug particle will follow this fate depends on the relative rates of this transport route and the processes of drug dissolution, absorption and metabolism in the airways.

Experimental studies (Chowhan and Amaro, 1976) indicate that the rate of drug absorption from the airways into the blood circulation may be limited by the slower dissolution rate of compounds with relatively low aqueous solubility. However, most drugs currently employed in therapeutic inhalation aerosols have good aqueous solubility, and therefore they may be expected to exist as aqueous solutions prior to, or soon after, landing on the surface of airways. The depth of aerosol penetration into the lung is likely to affect the rate of absorption because the nature of the pulmonary surface changes along the tract. Both lipophilic and hydrophilic drugs appear to permeate through the pulmonary epithelium at appreciable rates (Schanker, 1978). Animal studies with many common drugs, e.g. sulphonamides and antitubercular agents, have shown that these compounds are absorbed by a passive non-saturable process. The rate of absorption is dictated by the apparent oil/water partition coefficient of the drugs at the pulmonary pH ($\sim$7.4) except for highly lipid-insoluble compounds. These observations are analogous to the results obtained in the gastrointestinal tract. They indicate that the predominant mechanism of absorption of lipid-soluble compounds from the pulmonary spaces is diffusion through the lipid-like membrane of the pulmonary epithelium. Compounds with low lipid solubility probably diffuse through water-filled pores. Interestingly, disodium cromoglycate — the prophylactic agent used in asthma — is absorbed both by passive diffusion and by a saturable, specific transport system from the respiratory tract, although it is practically unabsorbable from the gastrointestinal tract. Nevertheless, it is believed that when this drug is inhaled, the pharmacological effect is due to its local activity in airways.

It is now recognized that the lung is an important metabolic organ in human and animal bodies. Whether the inhaled drug is intended for local treatment, or for systemic absorption, the possiblity of metabolic conversion must be considered. The spectrum of enzymatic activity in the lung is somewhat different from the liver. Such differences may be advantageous in delivery of drugs which are inactivated by the 'first pass' through the intestine and the liver when administered orally (Davies, 1979).

None of the aforementioned mechanisms is particularly effective in removing solid, insoluble particles lodged deep in the lung. The 'muco-ciliary escalator' is not operating in the unciliated alveolar regions. There, the foreign particles may become engulfed in pulmonary macrophages before they are transported upwards to be removed by the mucociliary system, or translocated into the lymph. However, a large fraction of these particles can disappear from alveoli only by a slow process of dissolution which may take several months or even years. This has important implications for environmental and occupational exposure to fine dusts, as well as for the testing of inhalation aerosols for solid residues.

In summary, the respiratory tract possesses a number of systems for the clearance of inhaled substances. The mechanisms of disposition of drugs deposited in the airways are frequently unique, or quantitatively different from other parts of the body. These findings are helpful in identifying the drugs whose administration in the form of inhalation aerosols may have advantages over other routes of drug delivery.

FURTHER IMPORTANT FACTORS TO BE CONSIDERED IN DESIGN OF THERAPEUTIC AEROSOLS

In contrast to almost any other dosage form, aerosols pose unique toxicological problems associated with their ability to penetrate into the airways. The propellants, formulatory agents and chemical and microbiological contaminants may also accompany the drug into the respiratory tract. The presence of particles or droplets in the respirable range (aerodynamic diameters <15 μm) containing substances not intended for inhalation should be avoided as much as possible. The gaseous propellants can reach all parts of the respiratory tract and be absorbed into the systemic circulation. There is evidence that unless inhaled in excessive quantities, these gases have no serious adverse effects. It has been suggested that release of large amounts of fluorocarbons into the environment by domestic and industrial users of aerosols might deplete the atmospheric ozone level which is important in the control of ultraviolet radiation reaching the earth (Molina and Rowland, 1974). This theory and its implications have not been fully evaluated yet; nevertheless other propellants or alternative presentation of non-essential aerosol products may be desirable in future.

The respiratory tract has anatomical and physiological features which make the entry and retention of foreign particles in the airways difficult. The design of therapeutic inhalation aerosols attempts to overcome these barriers. In a single inspiration, only minute quantities of the drug, typically less than 100 μg, deposit in the airways. Thus, it is not feasible to administer drugs with low potency by this route without prolonged, repeated inhalations. For such administration, usually in hospitals, ultrasonic and air-blast nebulizers are employed. This equipment must be kept scrupulously clean in order to avoid introduction of unwanted material into the patient's lungs. Particular attention has to be paid to prevention of microbial contamination because the size of the aerosol droplets would facilitate the transport of micro-organisms deep into the patient's airways.

One of the primary reasons for the use of inhalation aerosols is that drugs which cause serious systemic side effects may be applied in safe and adequate quantities locally in the airways. Although these drugs can still be absorbed into the systemic circulation from the respiratory tract, the potential for systemic adverse reactions is usually minimized since the total dose of the drug thus applied is very small. For example, amphotericin B is tolerated well by patients when administered as an aerosol for the treatment of fungal infections of the respiratory tract (Eisenberg and Oatway, 1971). This drug is not absorbed from the gastrointestinal tract; its administration by the parenteral route is reserved for life-threatening infections only because it may induce very serious side reactions. In general, however, any advantages that may be gained by local application of drugs by inhalation must be weighed against the potential for adverse reactions in the airways of a patient whose respiratory tract is usually already under stress from the pathological process.

Some vehicles and drugs in aerosols, e.g. certain antibiotics, can provoke bronchospasm. This adverse reaction may necessitate the coadministration of bronchodilators. However, the need to introduce one therapeutic agent in order to combat the toxicity of another drug can be justified only in situations where alternative modes of therapy are dangerous, or less effective.

Fungal colonization of the upper airways can take place during treatment with steroid aerosols. This adverse phenomenon may be controlled by inhalation of antifungal drugs. A potentially more serious hazard is the emergence of antibiotic-resistant bacterial strains during the treatment of Gram-negative respiratory tract infections with antibiotic aerosols. Careful clinical judgment must therefore be made to decide whether inhalation therapy of the patient's infection should be initiated in addition to, or instead of, systemic administration of antibiotics (Hodson et al., 1981).

There are considerable quantitative interindividual differences in the regional deposition of aerosols in the respiratory tract even in well trained subjects. To some extent this variability is reduced in groups containing subjects with similar pathophysiological features. None the less, drugs with a sufficiently wide safety margin between efficacious and toxic doses must be at present employed in therapeutic inhalation aerosols. This applies particularly to the personal inhalers which are often used by patients unable to comply with the manufacturers' instructions for correct application. Although techniques to overcome some of the dependence on the patient's skills have been introduced (e.g., breath-actuated devices and spacer tubes for pressurized cannisters), these problems require further attention.

REFERENCES

Bell, J. H., Brown, K. and Glasby, J. (1973) Variation in delivery of isoprenaline from various pressurised inhalers. *J. pharm, Pharmacol.*, **25** (Suppl.), 32P–36P.

Bell, K. A. and Ho, A. T. (1981) Growth rate measurements of hygroscopic aerosols under conditions simulating the respiratory tract. *J. Aerosol Sci.*, **12**, 247–254.

Berglund, R. N. and Liu, B. H. Y. (1973) Generation of monodisperse aerosol standards. *Env. Sci. Tech.*, **7**, 147–152.

British Pharmaceutical Codex (B.P.C) (1973) pp. 643–646.

Byron, P. R., Davis, S. S., Bubb, M. D. and Cooper, P.

(1977) Pharmaceutical implications of particle growth at high relative humidities. *Pest. Sci.*, **8**, 521–526.

Chowhan, Z. T. and Amaro, A. A. (1976) Pulmonary absorption studies utilizing *in situ* rat lung model: designing dosage regimen for bronchial delivery of new drug entities. *J. pharm. Sci*, **65**, 1669–1672.

Clark, T. J. H. (1972) Effect of beclomethasone dipropionate delivered by aerosol in patients with asthma, *The Lancet*, **i**, 1361–1364.

Davies, D. S. (1979) Pharmacokinetics of inhaled substances. *Scand. J. Resp. Dis.*, **Suppl. 103**, 44–49.

Davis, S. S. (1978) Physico-chemical studies on aerosol solutions for drug delivery I. Water–propylene glycol systems. *Int. J. Pharm.*, **1**, 71–83.

Davis, S. S. and Bubb, M. D. (1978) Physico-chemical studies on aerosol solutions for drug delivery III. The effect of relative humidity on the particle size of inhalation aerosols. *Int. J. Pharm.*, **1**, 303–314.

Davis, S.S., Elson, G. and Whitmore, J. (1978) Physico-chemical studies on aerosol solutions for drug delivery II. Water–propylene glycol–ethanol systems. *Int. J. Pharm.*, **1**, 85–93.

Eisenberg, R. S. and Oatway, W. H. (1971) Nebulization of amphotericin B. *Am. Rev. resp. Dis.*, **103**, 289–292.

Gonda, I., Kayes, J. B., Groom, C. V. and Fildes, F. J. T. (1982) Characterisation of hygroscopic inhalation aerosols. In: *Particle Size Analysis 1981* (Eds. N. G. Stanley-Wood, and T. Allen), pp. 31–43, Wiley Heyden Ltd, New York.

Groom, C. V. and Gonda, I. (1980) Cascade impaction: the performance of different collection surfaces. *J. Pharm. Pharmacol.* **32** (Suppl.), 93P.

Groom, C. V., Gonda, I. and Fildes, F. J. T. (1980) Prediction of equilibrium aerodynamic diameters for inhalation aerosols. *2nd Int. Conf. Pharm. Technol.*, *APGI*, *Paris*, Vol. 5, pp. 124–131.

Hodson, M. E., Penketh, A. R. L. and Batten, J. C. (1981) Aerosol carbenicillin and gentamicin treatment of *Pseudomonas aeruginosa* infection in patients with cystic fibrosis. *The Lancet*, **ii**, 1137–1139.

Lindgren, S. B., Formgren, H. and Morén, F. (1980) Improved aerosol therapy in asthma: Effect of actuator tube size on drug availability. *Eur. J. resp. Dis.*, **61**, 56–61.

Lippmann, M., Yeates, D. B. and Albert, R. E. (1980) Deposition, retention and clearance of inhaled particles. *Br. J. ind. Med.*, **37**, 337–362.

Malem, H., Henery, D., Ward, M., Roderick-Smith, W. H. and Gonda, I. (1981) Early experience with a vertical spinning-disc nebuliser. *The Lancet*, **ii**, 664–666.

Mercer, T. M. (1973) *Aerosol Technology in Hazard Evaluation*, Academic Press, New York.

Molina, M. J. and Rowland, F. S. (1974) Stratospheric sink for chlorofluoromethanes: chlorine atom-catalysed destruction of ozone. *Nature*, **249**, 810–812.

Neville, A., Palmer. J. B. D., Gaddie, J., May, C. S.,

Palmer, K. N. V. and Murchison, L. E. (1977) Metabolic effects of salbutamol: comparison of aerosol and intravenous administration. *Br. med. J.*, **1**, 413–414.

Newman, S. P., Pavia, D. and Clarke, S. W. (1980) Simple instructions for using pressurized aerosol bronchodilators. *J. Roy. Soc. Med.*, **73**, 776–779.

Raabe, O. G. (1968) The dilution of monodisperse suspensions for aerosolization. *Am. Ind. Hyg. Assoc. J.*, **29**, 439–443.

Schanker, L. S. (1978) Drug absorption from the lung. *Biochem. Pharmacol.*, **27**, 381–385.

Stöber, W. and Flachsbart, H. (1969) Size-separating precipitation of aerosols in a spinning spiral duct. *Env. Sci. Tech.*, **3**, 1280–1296.

Thompson, R. E. (1879) Drug smoking. *Pharmaceut. J.*, **10**, 386 (extract in *Pharmaceut. J.*, 1979, **223**, 535).

United States Pharmacopoeia XXI-National Formulary XVI (USP XXI-NF XVI) (1985) pp. 573–574 and pp. 1219–1220.

BIBLIOGRAPHY

Brandenburger Brown, E. A. (1974) The localization, metabolism and effects of drugs and toxicants in lung. In: *Drug Metabolism Reviews* (Ed. F. J. DiCarlo), Vol. 3, pp. 33–87, Marcel Dekker, New York.

Gonda, I. and Byron, P. R. (1978) Perspectives on the biopharmacy of inhalation aerosols. *Drug Dev. ind. Pharm.*, **4**, 243–259.

Hinds, W. C. (1982) *Aerosol Technology*, John Wiley & Sons, Chichester.

Junod, A. (1976) Uptake, release and metabolism of drugs in the lungs. *Pharmac. Ther. B.*, **2**, 511–521.

Lippmann, M. (1977) Regional deposition of particles in the human respiratory tract. In: *Handbook of physiology — Section 9: Reactions to Environmental Agents*. (Eds D. H. K. Lee, H. L. Falk and S. D. Murphy), Ch. 14, pp. 213–232. Am. Physiol. Soc. and The Williams & Wilkins Co., Washington and Baltimore.

Lourenco, R. V. and Cotromanes, E. (1982) Clinical aerosols, I. Characterization of aerosols and their diagnostic uses. *Archs intern. Med.*, **142**, 2163–2172. II. Therapeutic Aerosols, *ibid.*, 2299–2308.

Morén, F. (1981). Pressurized aerosols for oral inhalation. *Int. J. Pharm.*, **8**, 1–10.

Sciarra, J. J. (1980) Aerosols. In: *Remington's Pharmaceutical Sciences* (Ed. A. Osol, *et al.*), 16th Edn, Ch. 92, pp. 1614–1628, Mack Publishing Co., Easton, Pennsylvania.

Sciarra, J. J. and Stoller, L. (1974) *The Science and Technology of Aerosol Packaging*, John Wiley & Sons, Chichester.

Swift, D. L. (1980) Aerosols and humidity therapy: generation and respiratory deposition of therapeutic aerosols. *Am. Rev. resp. Dis.*, **122** (Part 2, Suppl.), 71–77.

Parenteral products

STERILIZATION OF INJECTIONS

Injections are sterile products intended for administration into the bodily tissues. Their formulation involves careful consideration of all the following inter-relating factors:

1 the proposed route of administration,
2 the volume of the injection,
3 the vehicle in which the medicament is to be dissolved or suspended,
4 the osmotic pressure of the solution,
5 the use of preservative,
6 the pH of the solution,
7 the stability of the medicament and methods of sterilization,
8 the specific gravity of the injection,
9 the properties of suspensions for injection,
10 the properties of emulsions for injection,
11 containers or closures for injections,
12 particulate contamination,
13 biopharmacy of injections.

THE BIOPHARMACY OF INJECTIONS

Injections are administered into the body by many routes. The route of administration affects the formulation and biopharmaceutics of the preparation. There now follows a description of routes of administration to clarify nomenclature used throughout the rest of the chapter. Fig. 21.1 shows the sites of injection.

Routes of administration

The most important routes are as follows.

Intracutaneous or intradermal route

Injections are made into the skin between the inner layer (dermis) and the outer layer (epidermis). The volume that can be injected intradermally is small, usually 0.1–0.2 ml, due to the poor vascularity of the site which gives poor dispersion of the drug, and leaves blisters or weals at the site of the injection. The route is used mainly for diagnostic tests.

Subcutaneous or hypodermic route

Injections are made under the skin into the subcutaneous tissue. The volume injected is usually 1 ml or less. This route is not used for aqueous suspensions or oily suspensions and fluids since these would cause pain and irritation at the injection site.

Intramuscular route

Injections are made by passing the needle into the muscle tissue via the skin, subcutaneous tissue and membrane enclosing the muscle. The volume is usually no greater than 2 ml and should not exceed 4 ml. This route is used for aqueous and oily suspensions and oily solutions, since if they were injected intravenously blockage of small blood vessels might occur leading to poor vascular supply of local tissues possibly resulting in gangrene.

Intravascular routes

These are either intra-arterial (into arteries) or intravenous (into veins). The intra-arterial route is used for an immediate effect in a peripheral organ, e.g. to improve circulation to the extremities when arterial flow is restricted by arterial spasm or early gangrene. Tolazoline hydrochloride, a peripheral vasodilator, is sometimes administered by this route.

Substances are introduced directly into the blood stream by the intravenous route. The most common site is the median basilic vein at the anterior surface of the elbow. The volume can vary from less than 1 ml to in excess of 500 ml. Small volumes may be administered for a rapid effect (e.g. anaesthetics) and large volumes (perfusion or infusion fluids) to replace body fluid loss in shock, severe burns, vomiting and diar-

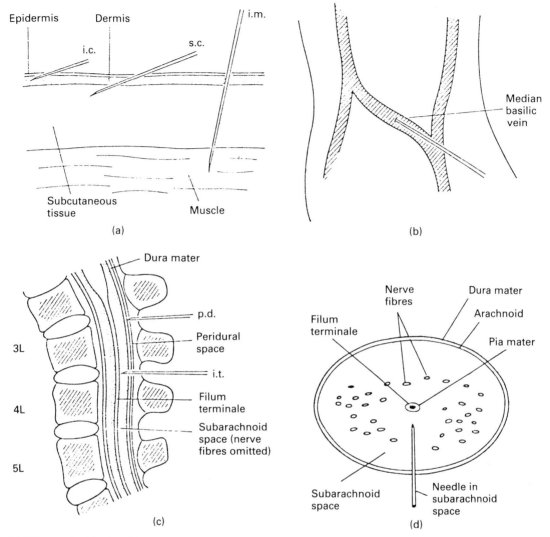

Fig. 21.1 Routes for injection. Key: (a) i.c., intracutaneous route; s.c., subcutaneous route; i.m., intramuscular route: (b) i.v., intravenous route into the median basilic vein at the anterior surface of the elbow: (c) p.d., peridural route; i.t., intrathecal route: (d) subarachnoid route.

rhoea. The route ensures rapid body dispersion and generally administration of volumes in excess of 10 ml is termed intravenous infusion. Oil-in-water emulsions may be administered by this route if the globule size is controlled but the route cannot be used for w/o emulsions.

Intracardiac route

This is used for emergencies only when stimulants, e.g. adrenaline or isoprenaline sulphate, are given directly into the heart muscles or ventricles.

Intraspinal routes

These routes involve access into or around the spinal cord. Single dose injections, no greater than 20 ml, are used. Intrathecal or subarachnoid injections are made into the subarachnoid space that surrounds the spinal cord which is enclosed in three coats. The outer one is known as the dura mater, the middle one as the arachnoid and the inner one as the pia mater. The subarachnoid space lies between the arachnoid and pia mater and contains the cerebrospinal fluid (c.s.f.). The route is used for spinal anaesthetics (e.g. bupivacaine) and antibiotics (e.g. streptomycin in the treatment of tubercular meningitis).

Intracisternal injections are made into the cisterna magna which lies directly below the medulla. Although the route is primarily used to remove c.s.f., it is occasionally used for antibiotic treatment or for the investigation of the c.s.f. circulation by dye injection.

Peridural injections are made into the peridural space which is located between the dura mater and the inner aspect of the vertebrae. This space extends throughout the full length of the spinal column and injections may be made at different regions, e.g. thoracic, lumbar or sacral. The route is used for spinal anaesthesia although careful consideration of the specific gravity of the injection has to be made to allow exact positioning of the injection.

Great care should be taken to ensure that any chosen buffering agent does not damage the delicate nervous tissue or its coats.

Intra-articular and intrabursal routes

Intra-articular injections are made into the synovial fluid which lubricates the articulating ends of bones in a joint. Intrabursal injections are similar, being given into the bursae which are small sacs of fluids between movable parts such as tendons and bones. The common sites are the subacromial bursa in the shoulder and the olecranon bursa in the elbow. Both solutions and suspensions may be administered by these routes.

Ophthalmic routes

Because of the restricted target areas the dose-volume is never greater than 1 ml. Four routes are used; the subconjunctival route (beneath Tenon's capsule, close to the eye but not into it), the intravitreous route (into the vitreous chamber), the intracameral route (into the anterior chamber) and the intraocular route (into the posterior segment of the globe). Great care should be given to the choice of any prospective buffering agent.

Other routes which may be used include the intra-ossicular route, the intracerebral route, the intraperitoneal route (for dialysis solutions), the intrapleural route and, in cattle, the intra-mammary route.

Bioavailability of drugs from injections

Injections are often used for either rapid or localized activity. An injection directly into the blood stream ensures that the drug is spread rapidly throughout the body before other factors, like plasma bonding, binding to selective sites and metabolism will reduce the achieved concentration. Intrathecal, instracisternal, intracardiac and the intravenous routes can be used for rapid onset of drug action. Unlike tablets, where there are disintegration and dissolution stages prior to absorption, injections achieve a rapid high blood level. However, formulation, coupled with variation in the site of administration may affect markedly the biopharmacy of drugs. The pH of an injection may effect the degree of ionization of a drug, rendering it more or less likely to pass through biological membranes. Increasing the viscosity of an injection will slow the absorption, especially from intramuscular injections, and drug solubility, dependent on polymorphism, will affect the activity of drugs. Thus the polymorphism of novobiocin and chloramphenicol can alter their biological properties. For suspensions, the particle size of the drug influences absorption rate and increasing the particle size of a drug, e.g. insulin, will decrease the available surface area and decrease its absorption from an injection site, giving a sustained release effect. Similarly, the blood levels of procaine penicillin G increase as the particle size of the suspension decreases.

The routes of administration markedly affect the disposition and biopharmacy of drugs. The intravenous route gives immediate and total access of the drug molecules to the body. Maximum plasma concentrations may be achieved after 4 minutes. The duration of action may be affected by dose, distribution, metabolism and excretion of the drug but the elimination usually follows first order kinetics. Constant blood levels may be obtained by intravenous drips. Intramuscular and subcutaneous routes can act as sustained release routes but this depends on the dosage form. Aqueous solutions are most rapidly absorbed into the blood stream and aqueous suspensions show retarded release due to the dissolution step introduced into the absorption process. The use of oleaginous vehicles may further delay absorption due to a partitioning of the drug from the oil to the aqueous body fluids and oleaginous suspensions provide a retarding dissolution process prior to partitioning. For these routes, viscosity, drug concentration and the patient's movement may further alter absorption rates. Even differences in the choice of muscle may influence absorption. Generally the subcutaneous route provides slower absorption due to the low vascular supply to the skin (for further information see Gibaldi, 1977).

FORMULATION OF INJECTIONS

Throughout this section, reference is made to injections of the *British Pharmacopoeia*. These are included as illustrative examples for which the full formula can be obtained. The reader can extrapolate the principles discussed to other, non-official or novel formulations.

Volume of the injection

The volume of an injection primarily depends on the solubility of the medicament, but may be influenced by preference for a particular route. Intracutaneous injections have to be small to prevent the formation of blisters. Only the intravenous route is suitable for large volumes which must be made isotonic. Intravenous injections with doses greater than 15 ml must not contain a bactericide and therefore cannot be sterilized by heating with a bactericide. When the volume is in excess of 15 ml the injection should be free from pyrogens.

The volume should be convenient to administer. Volumes greater than 20 ml are unsuitable for injections by a syringe and infusions are not worth setting up for less than 250 ml. The volume can often be reduced by dispensing a hypertonic solution and administering by slow intravenous infusion.

The vehicle

Any vehicle used should be pharmacologically inert, non-toxic (i.e. compatible with blood, non-sensitizing, non-irritating), maintain the solubility of the drug, be chemically and physically stable and be unaffected by pH changes. Vehicles should not interfere with the therapeutic activity of the injection. They must be exhaustively tested for freedom from toxicity, they must be pure and have no pharmacological activity of their own.

Water is the ideal vehicle for most injections since aqueous preparations are well tolerated by the body and are the safest and easiest to administer. However, a change from water may be required for a variety of reasons. Hydrolysis of certain drugs may result in the formation of inert or toxic byproducts. Some poorly water-soluble drugs may be so insoluble that they cannot be administered in water. Consequently, the use of cosolvents, e.g. propylene glycol for Dimenhydrinate Injection BP or oily vehicles such as benzylbenzoate and arachis oil for Dimercaprol Injection BP, is permitted. Oily vehicles often give a depot effect over their aqueous counterparts and steroid drugs, e.g. progesterone, which are poorly water soluble are formulated in ethyl oleate or fixed oils to enable depot release to continuously replace deficient secretions. Oily media may indeed be preferable to aqueous vehicles. Propyliodone, although present in the *British Pharmacopoeia* as both an aqueous suspension and an oily suspension in arachis oil, is often preferred in oily suspension as a contrast medium of X-ray examination of the respiratory tract because this is less irritating than the aqueous suspension.

Oily injections suffer from many disadvantages including the following.

1 They may be too viscous in cold weather to administer without warming.
2 They often cause pain at the site of the injection.
3 They will contaminate the syringe and needle making them difficult to clean.
4 They must be used only by the intramuscular route, since their accidental intravenous injection may lead to thrombosis.

However, contrast media, e.g. Iodised Oil Fluid Injection BP or Propyliodone Oily Injection BP, may be given by other routes because they are not injected into tissues but into the internal cavities that are under investigation, e.g. the lungs. Very occasionally alcohol is used to dissolve the medicament but the solution must be diluted with an aqueous vehicle shortly before administration to avoid pain and tissue damage.

Water and pyrogens

Before potable water can be rendered suitable for use in injections it has to be specially purified. The injection of distilled water may cause a rise of body temperature; water producing this reaction is said to be pyrogenic (fever producing) and water free from this effect is described as apyrogenic. Substances which are pyrogenic may be produced by many micro-organisms including moulds, yeasts and bacteria. The most potent are those associated with Gram-negative bacteria and are endotoxins originating from the cell wall. The main causative substance is lipid in nature but its potency is enhanced by protein and especially polysaccharide fractions which appear to increase the solubility of the lipid fraction. Pyrogenic molecules have a high molecular weight often in excess of 1 000 000.

The sources of pyrogens may be the solvent, the medicament, any added buffering or stabilizing substance, the apparatus used in manufacture, the final containers and the method of storage between preparation and sterilization. Undoubtedly, the major source is the solvent and especially Water for Injections BP.

Injection of pyrogens into the body produces various physiological responses including erythema at the injection site, pain in the legs and trunk with general discomfort and high temperature. It is this last response that the *British Pharmacopoeia* uses as the basis to estimate pyrogens by studying temperatures in specially treated rabbits, although other methods especially the limulus amoebocyte lysate test have been developed (Thomas *et al.*, 1980).

Pyrogen tests are applied to all injections claimed to be apyrogenic, i.e. to Water for Injections BP, to single dose injections of volume greater than 15 ml and powders which require making up to a solution with vehicle prior to administration, when the reconstituted injection is tested. However, it is vital that intravenous infusions should be free from pyrogens since a large volume injection will contain a correspondingly large amount of pyrogen. As large volume injections (perfusion fluids) are usually given intravenously the pyrogen will have a more rapid effect. Patients receiving infusion fluids are often dangerously ill and the effect of rise of temperature could be fatal.

Water for Injections BP is sterilized distilled water free from pyrogens and is prepared from potable water. Since tap water may be pyrogenic, the first aim in the preparation of Water for Injections BP must be to remove or destroy pyrogens. This is complicated as pyrogens are thermostable, water soluble and are unaffected by common bactericides and, therefore, none of the methods used to sterilize injections can be relied upon to eliminate pyrogens.

However, pyrogens are also non-volatile and they can be removed from water by distillation. Ordinary distillation is not satisfactory since pyrogens may be carried over in the receiver, dissolved in the spray which is entrailed in the steam. Therefore, a trap is fitted to the distilling flask to stop this entrainment. Certain bacteria are able to multiply in distilled water. Inadequate protection from air and storage at a temperature that favours bacterial growth may cause a rapid increase in the bacterial count. Ideally distilled water for parenteral solutions should be sterilized immediately after collection from the still. The exception is when the water is used at once for making an injection that requires sterilization. Then, provided the injection is sterilized immediately after preparation (i.e. within 4 hours), freshly distilled non-sterilized water may be used. Distilled water may be used after a much longer storage provided it is maintained at a high temperature, e.g. 80 °C, when bacterial growth and hence pyrogen production will be prevented. Because of the great danger from pyrogens in large volume infusion fluids, the *British Pharmacopoeia* gives a special warning of the need for their immediate sterilization, e.g., Laevulose Intravenous Infusion BP.

For further information on the preparation of Water for Injections BP see Perkins, 1969; Ridgway, 1973; or Groves, 1973a. Another method of preparing water for injections is reverse osmosis which is accepted by the USP (see Frith *et al.*, 1976).

Water for Injections BP is suitable as a vehicle for many official preparations. However, it may sometimes be necessary to further improve its quality by removing dissolved gases. Some medicaments, e.g. the barbiturates and sulphonamides, are weakly acidic and only slightly soluble in water and they are therefore administered as the more soluble sodium salts. For instance, amylobarbitone sodium (solubility 1 in less than 1) when dissolved in water containing carbon dioxide will rapidly precipitate the free base amylobarbitone (solubility 1 in 1500) rendering it dangerous and unsuitable for injection. Examples of other injections requiring water free from carbon dioxide are Aminophylline Injection BP, Methohexitone Injection BP and Sodium Bicarbonate Intravenous Infusion BP. However, Water for Injections BP free from carbon dioxide is unnecessary for thiopentone injection BP because the official substance is a mixture of thiopentone and sodium carbonate and the latter will keep the salt in solution. Carbon dioxide may be removed from water for injections by boiling the water for 10 minutes.

Water for injections free from dissolved air is produced in a similar manner and the residual air space at the top of the ampoules is replaced by nitrogen or another inert gas after packing, before sealing. This product replaces normal water for injections in products containing medicaments which are sensitive to low levels of oxygen and hence can be protected from oxidation. Examples include Chlorpheniramine Injection BP, Chlorpromazine Injection BP, Phenylephrine Injection BP, Sulphadimidine Injection BP and Promazine Injection BP.

Water-miscible vehicles

It is often not possible to dissolve the medicament in water for injections. To increase the solubility, non-toxic solvents can be used and these include ethyl alcohol, glycerol, propylene glycol, liquid macrogols and benzyl alcohol.

Ethyl alcohol is used only when other methods of presentation are impracticable. Its own physio-

logical activity and the pain and tissue damage it causes unless administered with special care, are serious disadvantages. It is not the main solvent in any official injection but a few (e.g. Digoxin Injection BP, Ergotamine Injection BP and Phenytoin Injection BP) contain a low concentration to facilitate solution of the active ingredient. Melphalan Injection BP is a solution in a vehicle containing 95% ethyl alcohol but is diluted before use.

Propylene glycol is included in several preparations including Cotrimoxazole, Digoxin, Dimenhydrinate, Melarsoprol, Phenobarbitone and Phenytoin injections BP. In the *British Pharmacopoeia* (1958), Digoxin Injection BP contained 70% ethyl alcohol which had to be diluted with Sodium Chloride Injection BP 1958 and given intravenously by slow injection to ensure rapid dilution with blood. The official preparation is now a stable solution in a solvent containing 40% propylene glycol, 10% ethyl alcohol and water buffered to about pH 7 and does not require dilution before use.

Until 1968, Phenobarbitone Injection BP was prepared by aseptically dissolving sterile phenobarbitone sodium in Water for Injections BP free from carbon dioxide immediately before use. The current injection is a solution in 90% propylene glycol which is stable enough to be sterilized at 98–100 °C and has a satisfactory storage life.

Although propylene glycol is relatively non-toxic (possibly because it is rapidly metabolized and excreted), it causes severe irritation on subcutaneous and intramuscular injection and preferably should not be given by these routes, unless an anaesthetic such as benzyl alcohol is included, e.g. Dimenhydrinate Injection BP. Although the liquid macrogols have been recommended as prospective vehicles (Carpenter and Shaffer, 1952) care must be taken during their sterilization as formaldehyde can be generated.

Water-immiscible vehicles

Eight of the oily injections of the *British Pharmacopoeia* are simple solutions (e.g., deoxycortone Acetate Injection BP, Hydroxyprogesterone Injection BP and Oestradiol Benzoate Injection BP).

Their prescribed solvents are a suitable fixed oil, a suitable ester (e.g. ethyl oleate) or a mixture of both. Suitable alcohols may be included in the solvents for Deoxycortone Acetate, Oestradiol Benzoate and Progesterone Injections BP.

Fixed oils must not contain mineral oils or solid paraffins as these cannot be metabolized by the body and might eventually cause tissue reaction and even tumours. They must be free from rancidity (since rancid oils contain free fatty acids) and from any material that might cause irritation.

Arachis oil is specified for Dimercaprol Injection BP and Propyliodone Oily Injection BP but has the disadvantages of thickening slowly on exposure to air and becoming rancid. Alternatives include sesame oil (probably the most stable because it contains natural substances that prevent rancidification), cotton seed and maize oils. Sensitivity to these oils may cause problems.

Esters give less viscous preparations that are easier to inject, particularly in cold weather. However, a reduction in the length of action of depot preparations has been found when ethyl oleate has been used instead of oil. The maximum prolongation effect is obtained from the depot if it is spherical and, therefore, absorption is probably more rapid from the less viscous ester preparations because of their greater tendency to spread and offer a larger surface to the tissue fluid.

Peroxide-free ethyl oleate is the solvent for Calciferol Injection BP. Peroxides are the intermediates in the auto-oxidative rancidification of oils and fatty acids, and they are undesirable in injections, particularly when the medicament is susceptible to oxidation. Calciferol injection also requires storage in ampoules from which the air has been displaced by an inert gas.

Alcohols may be used in three official preparations because occasionally the medicament concentration may be greater than its solubility in fixed oils, ethyl oleate or a mixture of both. Either benzyl alcohol or ethyl alcohol can improve the solvent properties of these vehicles in concentrations that are harmless and non-irritant by the intramuscular route.

Table 21.1 indicates the advantage of using a

Table 21.1 Solubility of steroids in different vehicles

	Water	Arachis oil	Ethyl oleate	Alcohol 95%
Deoxycortone acetate	Almost insoluble	1 in 140	1 in 150	1 in 50
Oestradiol benzoate	Insoluble	1 in 500	1 in 200	1 in 150
Progesterone	Insoluble	1 in 60	1 in 60	1 in 8
Testosterone	Insoluble	1 in 35	1 in 20	1 in 6

solvent containing an alcohol for deoxycortone acetate, progesterone and to a less extent oestradiol benzoate. Conversely the high solubility of testosterone propionate in arachis oil and ethyl oleate makes the use of alcohols unnecessary.

Other oily bases include almond oil (for Oily Phenol Injection BP), poppyseed oil, isopropyl myristate and polyoxyethylene oleic triglycerides (Labrafils). Another solvent, benzyl benzoate is used for Dimercaprol Injection BP. Dimercaprol is a liquid formulated in oil because aqueous solutions are unstable. For strong preparations, the required amount of dimercaprol would not completely dissolve in arachis oil but was miscible with benzyl benzoate. The resulting mixture can be diluted with arachis oil to give an injection that is stable, even to dry heat sterilization, if protected from air. Although the official strength is below that which gives solubility problems, the *British Pharmacopoeia* uses benzyl benzoate because of its stabilizing effect.

Osmotic pressure

Great care has to be taken to make certain injections isotonic with plasma. Husa and his colleagues (Husa and Adams, 1944; Hartman and Husa, 1957; Thomasson and Husa, 1958) have reported that certain medicaments in solutions iso-osmotic with plasma can pass through the red blood cell membrane, i.e. these solutions are not isotonic and may be harmful in use. Although normal practice is to adjust solutions to iso-osmoticity with plasma, iso-osmotic solutions of new drugs should be checked for isotonicity and haemolytic activity on red cells before using them by the intravenous route.

Intravascular injections

Solutions with a lower osmotic pressure than blood are said to be hypotonic and those with higher pressure are hypertonic. Both may be termed paratonic, i.e. not isotonic. Blood cells swell rapidly and burst (haemolysis) in hypotonic solutions. This damage is irreversible and dangerous if a large number of cells is involved. A very hypotonic solution or a large volume of less hypotonicity can cause this damage on intravascular injection. When placed in hypertonic solutions, water passes outwards from blood cells and they shrink, becoming crenate in outline. When the osmotic pressure returns to normal the blood cells assume their normal shape. Therefore, grossly hypertonic solutions may be administered without damage to blood cells. Consequently, although isotonicity is preferred, hypertonic solutions are normally used since to produce isotonic solutions of many medicaments would require large volumes of water which would be difficult to administer. Thus injections which are hypertonic are slowly injected intravenously to ensure rapid dilution in the blood stream and minimal crenulation of red blood cells.

Certain injections may irritate and damage the walls of veins. This may be used intentionally, e.g. in the treatment of varicose veins where the circulation is sluggish and an injection may remain undiluted for a considerable time. Hypertonic solutions are used for sclerosing varicose veins, e.g. Morrhuate Sodium Injection USP and Ethanolamine Oleate Injection BP which is preferred as it is more stable and less toxic. For Quinine Dihydrochloride Injection BP a 30% solution is standard strength but is very hypertonic (5% is isotonic) and has an acid pH (1.5–3.0). Sclerosis may occur if this injection is used undiluted, so it must be diluted at least 10 times with Water for Injections BP before use and injected slowly.

Intrathecal injections

These must be isotonic. The c.s.f. has a slow circulation and even the injection of a small volume of paratonic solution would cause a local disturbance of osmotic pressure. Also the volume of the c.s.f. is low (100–160 ml) and a comparatively small injection will affect the osmotic pressure throughout, causing headache and vomiting.

Intramuscular injections

The osmotic pressure will vary according to the type of injection and its desired therapeutic use. Aqueous solutions of medicaments intended to be absorbed quickly should be slightly hypertonic. This encourages a mild local effusion (exosmosis) of tissue fluids which will promote rapid absorption. Medicaments intended to be absorbed slowly and produce a depot effect are formulated as either an aqueous suspension (containing an insoluble form of the drug) or as a solution or suspension in a hydrophobic vehicle.

Intracutaneous injections

The intracutaneous route is used for diagnostic preparations. As the diagnosis is dependent on the subsequent development of an immune response involving inflammation, it is essential that the active principle should be the only cause of this reaction. Since paratonic solutions can irritate the skin, diagnostic intradermal injections are usually made isotonic.

Subcutaneous injections

The injection volume is very small, and since injection is made directly into fatty tissue, a wide range of paratonicity is possible without untoward effects. Isotonic solutions are preferable to reduce pain.

Comparison of the official injections shows that these principles have been followed. Thus the intracutaneously administered diagnostic preparation Schick test toxin is made isotonic. Small volume injections given subcutaneously, intramuscularly or intravenously are not adjusted, e.g. Atropine Sulphate and Methadone Injections BP. In other cases where small volumes are injected, particularly by the intramuscular or intravenous routes, the solutions are hypertonic. However, large volume infusion fluids are usually formulated to be isotonic, or nearly isotonic with blood plasma, e.g. Sodium Chloride Injection USP, Compound Sodium Lactate Injection BP and Dextrose Injection USP.

Hydrogen ion concentration (pH)

The pH of many official preparations is adjusted to a definite pH or to within a pH range. The use of buffers to stabilize the pH is often permitted. Some of the reasons for pH adjustment are as follows.

To increase the stability of the injection

An unfavourable pH is one of the major causes of instability in pharmaceuticals. It is imperative that unstable medicaments have their pH adjusted to the optimum for maximum stability. This is especially important for injections which have to withstand a heat sterilization process or have a long shelf life. The utilization of an optimum pH is used to stabilize injections of antibiotics (e.g. benzylpenicillin, tetracycline), alkaloids (e.g. ergometrine injection to a pH of 2.7–3.5), vitamins (e.g. cyanocobalamin to a pH of 4.0–5.5) and polypeptides (e.g., oxytoxin to a pH of 3.0–4.5).

To minimize pain, irritation and necrosis on injection

The optimum for stability may not, however, prove a suitable formulation. Very acid or alkaline solutions are painful on injection and may cause irritation or even necrosis of the tissues, especially with the subcutaneous or intramuscular routes. Intravenous injections, if given slowly, are rapidly diluted and the pH is further neutralized by the buffering power of the blood plasma. Consequently, injections should not be more acid or alkaline than stability dictates. Intrathecal, peridural and intracisternal injections should be adjusted to between pH 7.0 and 7.6 and ideally pH 7.4, since non-neutral solutions can cause aseptic meningitis.

When acidic or basic substance are used in the preparation of injections e.g., ethylenediamine (Aminophylline Injection BP) or sodium hydroxide

(Compound Sodium Lactate Injection BP), the pharmacopoeia ensures that no significant excess of these substances is present.

To provide unsatisfactory conditions for growth of micro-organisms

Use can be made of low and high pHs to prevent the growth of micro-organisms. Solutions of pH below 4 are bactericidal to many micro-organisms and may not require additional protection against bacteria. However, this effect is less marked with moulds because these can tolerate acid pHs. The antibacterial activities of Ethanolamine Injection BP, which does not require a bactericide in multiple-dose containers, is partly due to its high pH of 8–9.

To enhance physiological activity

For some preparations the free bases are more active than the salts themselves. However, as these substances are generally more stable at acid pHs it is often difficult to produce satisfactory preparations without using the salts. For instance, solutions of procaine and adrenaline produce the greatest anaesthetic effect when buffered to slight alkalinity yet are only stable for a few hours. Solutions of pH less than 4, although less potent, can be autoclaved with little loss of activity and the injection therefore has a pH of 3.0–4.5.

Therefore, where maximum physiological activity is shown by neutral or alkaline solutions while maximum stability is found in acid media, the pH should be kept as high as physiologically possible with an acceptance level of stability.

Buffers

Buffer systems suitable for injections should have no toxicity, be compatible with the medicament and other added substances and should have a high buffer capacity. The pH of a completed injection can be altered by the decomposition of the medicament but leaching of alkali from the glass of the container or extraction of acid or alkaline impurities from the rubber closure can be avoided by careful selection and preparation of containers and closures.

Suitable buffers include citric acid/sodium phosphate (Digoxin Injection BP), sodium acetate (Insulin Zinc Suspension Injection BP), sodium phosphate (Isophane Insulin Injection BP) and dipotassium hydrogen phosphate (Melphalan Injection BP). Borates are too toxic for use in injections.

Examples illustrating the use of buffers include Benzylpenicillin Injection BP and depot injections of insulin. The optimum pH range for the stability of penicillin solutions is 6.0–7.0. Hydrolysis readily occurs in aqueous solutions with the formation of inactive benzylpenicilloic acid. This is accompanied by a fall in pH which further catalyses hydrolysis leading to progressively greater acidity and more rapid hydrolysis until the antibiotic has been destroyed. Decomposition can be retarded by buffering the pH of the solution to 6.0–7.0 with 4.5% w/v sodium citrate. The life of the injection is, therefore, increased from 7 days (without buffer) to 14 days, if stored at 2–10 °C.

The used of insoluble forms of medicaments to prolong drug action has been mentioned earlier. The effect of protamine zinc insulin lasts longer (24–36 hours) than that of plain insulin (6–8 hours) because in the former insulin is in a very insoluble complex from which it is only slowly made available to the body. Because this complex is most insoluble over the very narrow pH range 6.9–7.4, a phosphate buffer is used to prevent variations.

Specific gravity of injections

This is of importance in spinal anaesthesia. If the upper part of the patient's body is raised by sloping the operating table, solutions of lower specific gravity than the spinal fluid will tend to rise on injection and those of higher specific gravity will tend to sink. On the other hand, the opposite effects will occur if, as is sometimes necessary for operations on the lower part of the body, the patient is tilted head downwards. Careful choice must be made of the specific gravity of the solution and the position of the patient so that the movement of the injection will be in the right direction. Although the specific gravity of the c.s.f. is not constant an average figure is 1.0059 at 37 °C. The terms used to describe the specific gravity of solutions in relation to that of the c.s.f. are isobaric, hypobaric and hyperbaric, i.e. of equal, lower and higher specific gravity respectively.

For example, cinchocaine hydrochloride, 1 in 1500 in 0.5% saline is hypobaric and has a weight per ml of 1.0036 at 37 °C. Alternatively cinchocaine hydrochloride, 1 in 200 in 6% dextrose, is a hyperbaric solution and has a weight per ml of 1.02.

Suspensions for injection

It is sometimes necessary to formulate the drug to be injected as a suspension. For example, formulation of a drug of low solubility in an aqueous vehicle requires a suspension, increased stability of a drug can be attained by formulation as a suspension and suspensions provide an effective depot release (Nash, 1972).

However, the use of suspensions as injections leads to further problems. The drug must remain suspended for a time sufficient to enable withdrawal of a uniform dose, especially if packed in a multiple-dose container. Therefore, the following processes must be understood.

Wettability

Some substances, e.g. cortisone acetate and procaine penicillin, are not only poorly soluble in water but are also poorly wetted by it. This problem may also be linked to particle size since very fine particles are difficult to wet. It would be difficult, therefore, to break up the clumps in any simple aqueous suspensions prepared from them and the foam produced by shaking would take a long time to disperse because it is stabilized by the film of unwettable powder at the liquid/air interfaces. To ensure satisfactory wetting of the solid it is necessary to reduce the interfacial energy between it and the liquid. This may be achieved by adding a suitable wetting agent and non-ionic types are widely employed, e.g. the polysorbates and sorbitan trioleate.

Sedimentation rate

Despite the presence of wetting agents, a suspension will be difficult to use if the particles sediment quickly. To counteract this a hypophilic colloid may be added to increase the viscosity of the vehicle, which then holds the particles in suspension long enough for an accurate dose to be removed and at the same time helps to prevent the reformation of clumps. A desirable property of a suitable colloid is rapid solution because suspensions have to be reconstituted just before use. Choices of colloids include sodium carboxymethylcellulose, polyvinylpyrrolidone, gelatin and methylcellulose.

Claying

A deflocculated suspension is often unsatisfactory because when small particles settle they produce a very tightly packed sediment that is hard to disperse and is said to have clayed. This can be avoided by reducing the amount of wetting agent; sufficient is added to take the powder into suspension but the quantity added is not enough to break down the smaller aggregates. Such a suspension (partially deflocculated) will settle more quickly but the sediment is loose and easy to disperse.

Macek (1963) illustrated these problems with procaine penicillin suspensions. Very small quantities of aluminium trichloride produced flocculated suspensions which were unsightly. Partial flocculation was achieved using monosodium citrate, together with a small quantity of a protective colloid or sorbitol.

Size and shape of particles

The depot effect of a suspension is influenced by both the size and shape of the suspended particles. Larger particles produce a greater depot effect because they take longer to be absorbed, e.g. larger crystals in crystalline insulin-zinc suspensions cause a protracted hypoglycaemic effect. However, large crystals sediment quickly, cause more pain on injection and tend to block syringe needles. Similarly, crystals which are approximately isodiametric (cubic, e.g. insulin or platelet, e.g. procaine penicillin) are better than long acicular crystals since the latter are more likely to cause needle blockage. In certain cases, e.g. cortisone acetate, care must be taken to

prepare crystals by a method that will produce a stable structure. Some are unstable and on storage in suspension may either change into a more stable polymorphic form or show crystal growth, becoming too large and leading to the difficulties mentioned above.

Thioxotropy

Although claying can be prevented by flocculation, it is possible to overdo this and produce a preparation in which the particles are so highly flocculated that the preparation becomes an unpourable paste. By careful choice of the particle size and percentage of powder, these pastes can become thixotropic, i.e. they are solid in the absence of a shearing force but become fluid if tapped or shaken, the original structure being resumed after a few minutes at rest. Thixotropic preparations have the advantage that the particles remain in more or less permanent suspension during storage and yet when required for use, the pastes are readily made fluid by tapping or shaking. The shearing force on the injection as it is pushed through the needle ensures that it is fluid when injected but the rapid resumption of the gel structure prevents excessive spreading in the tissues and, consequently, a more compact depot is produced than with non-thixotropic suspensions.

Preparation of aqueous suspension injections

Nash (1972) summarized the preparation of aqueous suspensions for injection. The sequence of manufacturing processes is:

1 recrystallization of the drug followed by particle size reduction,
2 sterilization of the drug,
3 sterilization of the vehicle,
4 aseptic wetting of the powdered drug by the vehicle,
5 aseptic dispersion and milling of the bulk suspensions, followed by
6 aseptic filling into the final sterile containers which can be sealed.

Suspensions in oily vehicles

As depot preparations, oily suspensions have the

potential advantage of combining the retarding effect of a hydrophobic vehicle and an insoluble medicament. However, because of the disadvantages of oily vehicles, aqueous formulations are preferred even though they do not have as powerful a depot effect.

Addition of a gelling agent   In Sterile Penicillin G Procaine with Aluminium Stearate Suspension USP (an oily procaine penicillin injection) the medicament is suspended in peanut or sesame oil that has been gelled with 2% of aluminium stearate. The latter produces a molecular lattice structure that gives rigidity to the preparation and renders it thixotropic. Procaine penicillin tends to clay if allowed to sediment; the rigid gel prevents this.

Particle size   Crystalline zinc insulin has been used to illustrate that in an aqueous suspension large particles give a greater depot effect. However, for preparations of procaine penicillin in oil containing aluminium stearate reduction of particle size gives increased prolongation. Particles of procaine penicillin are coated with the water-repellent aluminium stearate and are, therefore, less easily reached by aqueous tissue fluids and absorption will be further delayed. The greater the subdivision of the powder, the greater its surface area and consequently the greater the area of protective coating. Fine particles, majority under 5 μm, are required for this type of suspension.

Emulsions for injection

Emulsions are thermodynamically unstable systems which require stabilizers in the form of either surface-active agents or finely divided particles, the latter are unsuitable for parenteral use. Ideally, emulsions should be formulated so that the dispersed droplets are 0.5–1.0 μm in diameter. This corresponds to the size of the chylomicra, which are the natural transport systems for fat through the blood stream. Few of the globules should be greater than 3 μm in diameter. Unstable emulsions are dangerous since their storage may result in increased globule size due to coalescence which would result in thrombosis if injected.

Sterile emulsions are used to make feasible the safe injection of oily substances by the intravenous route. The emulsifiers and stabilizers used should be non-toxic e.g. lecithin, polysorbate 80, gelatin, methylcellulose and serum albumin. An example is Phytomenadione Injection BP (vitamin K) where lecithin is used as an emulsifying agent.

Intravenous therapy and emulsions

Intravenous therapy is used to correct deficiencies in the electrolyte and fluid balance of the body but may also be used to provide parenteral hyperalimentation when the patient is unable to use his gastrointestinal tract, e.g. following abdominal surgery. Solutions for intravenous infusions are clear and may contain ethanol, amino acids, carbohydrates, electrolytes and vitamins. However, glucose metabolism will provide only 14.3 kJ g^{-1} of energy whereas fat metabolism can provide up to 37.7 kJ g^{-1}.

Consequently for parenteral nutrition it is desirable to use intravenous fat emulsions as a concentrated source of energy. The aqueous phase of such emulsions will by necessity contain surface-active agents and since these can cause haemolysis of erythrocytes, the aqueous phase is made isotonic to plasma by the addition of, for example, glucose, sorbitol or glycerol. The oily phase can consist of sesame, cod-liver, linseed, peanut, olive or more commonly cotton seed or soya bean oils. Gelatin and/or cellulose derivatives may be included to increase the viscosity of the emulsion thereby preventing coalescence. Emulsifiers, like synthetic lecithins or fractionated egg yolk phospholipids together with surface-active agents like Pluronic F68 or the polysorbates are used to stabilize the emulsion. Sterilization of the emulsion is a problem since heat would coalesce the emulsion and filtration is impossible. Rapid growth of micro-organisms is possible in such emulsions since there is no preservative present.

A typical simple composition is 15% cotton seed oil, 4% dextrose, the oil being emulsified by 1.2% lecithin or soya bean phosphatide, 1% of a polyoxalkol, e.g. Poloxamer 188, and water to 100%. To further illustrate this KabiVitrum Ltd produce an oil-in-water emulsion (Intralipid 20%) to the following formula (see KabiVitrum Ltd,

1984/85):

Fractionated soya bean oil	100 g
Fractionated egg phospholipids	6 g
Glycerol	11 g
Water for injections	to 500 ml

The emulsion is formulated to pH 7 and the estimated energy provided by one litre of this preparation is 8.4 MJ compared with 4.7 MJ for one litre of Sorbitol Intravenous Infusion BP For further details of parenteral products and their formulation see Irvine (1978).

Colloidal dispersions and solubilized products

Colloids can be prepared and used for injections. Albumin, proteins, dextrans and carbohydrate polymers dissolve in water to form hydrophilic solutions. Certain injections are colloidal solutions, e.g. Iron Dextran Injection BP and Iron Sorbitol Injection BP, the latter being a complex of ferric ions, sorbitol and citric acid stabilized with dextran and sorbitol. Solubilized products also can potentially be used as injections. Above their critical micelle concentration, surfactants in solution form micelles whose centre will act as a solvent for lipid-soluble materials. By selective use of 1 or 2 surfactants and a cosolvent it is possible to solubilize many drugs.

QUALITY ASSURANCE OF INJECTIONS

Microbiological preservation

The use of bactericides in aqueous single-dose injections

Bactericides may be found in injections which are prepared either by heating with a bactericide or by aseptic techniques. They are allowable in aseptically produced products to supress the growth of micro-organisms inadvertantly added during preparation. Thus chlorocresol (0.2% w/v), phenylmercuric nitrate (0.002% w/v) and phenylmercuric acetate (0.002% w/v) are recommended by the *British Pharmacopoeia* as being suitable for heating with a bactericide. The bactericide is included in the preparation at the concentration recommended and the contents are maintained at 98–100 °C for 30 minutes to effect sterilization.

Aseptic preparation of injections involving sterilization by membrane filtration (i.e. they are not sterilized in their final containers) requires a high degree of manipulative skill to prevent accidental contamination. The *British Pharmacopoeia*, therefore, allows (it is *not* obligatory) the addition of a suitable bactericide to the solution before filtration. If the injection solution contains a bactericide it is important to remember that single-dose injections will also contain the bactericide and cannot be used for the intra-ocular or intracardiac routes or others giving access to the cerebrospinal fluid.

The use of bactericides in multiple-dose injections

Injections are frequently dispensed in containers holding several doses. These are known as multiple-dose injections and are supplied in bottles usually closed with a rubber cap which should allow the withdrawal of single doses of the injections with minimal risk of contaminating the remainder.

Contamination may arise from many causes including failure to sterilize the cap before withdrawing a dose, failure in sterilization of the needle or syringe, injection of unsterile air or inrush of unsterile air as the needle is withdrawn. The danger in introducing bacteria into an injection is the rapidity with which they can multiply. The last dose from a bottle may contain millions of organisms. Consequently, the *British Pharmacopoeia* states:

'Aqueous preparations supplied in containers for use on more than one occasion contain a suitable antimicrobial preservative in appropriate concentration except when the preparation has adequate antimicrobial properties.'

A multiple-dose injection sterilized by the process of heating with a bactericide should not require additional bactericide.

The bactericides used in multiple-dose containers destroy vegetative bacteria in a few hours at room temperature but they are not usually capable of killing bacterial spores (i.e. sporicidal). However, spores are unlikely to germinate in their presence and, therefore, the number of contaminations will remain small. Some bacteria and moulds have a destructive action on medicaments.

Bactericides suitable for aqueous injections

The desirable features of a suitable preservative for multiple-dose injections were summarized by Sykes (1958):

1 ability to prevent the growth of, and preferably to kill, contaminating organisms,
2 compatibility with the medicament, even on long storage and should not interfere with the therapeutic efficacy of the product,
3 low absorption rate into rubber,
4 absence of toxicity to the patient.

In addition Allwood (1978) considered further properties to be desirable including:

5 a broad spectrum of activity to include fungi as well as vegetative bacteria,
6 activity over a wide pH range,
7 the preservative should be uninfluenced by the container, and
8 stability in aqueous solution at high temperatures if the injection is to be sterilized by moist heat processes.

The *British Pharmacopoeia* suggests *o*-cresol (0.3%), chlorocresol (0.1%), benzyl alcohol (1%) and phenylmercuric salts (0.002%). In addition the *Pharmaceutical Codex* includes phenol (0.5%), chlorbutol (0.5%), and phenylmercuric acetate or nitrate (but at 0.001%). This list provides a choice that allows for incompatibilities with medicaments but only phenol is not appreciably absorbed by rubber and may not always prove suitable. However, pH may affect activity (Allwood, 1978). Phenol, *o*-cresol and chlorocresol are active up to a pH of about 9, but chlorbutol is less active above a pH of 5.0 and unstable above pH 6.0. Phenylmercuric acetate is active only above pH 6.0. Care has to be taken with solubility, for instance at room temperature the saturated solubility of phenylmercuric nitrate and phenylmercuric borate are respectively 0.08% and 0.33%. Interactions of preservatives with containers may include the leaching of hydroxyl ions, reducing the activity of phenol by increasing the pH. Toxicity may envolve hypersensitivity.

However, the substances listed are only suggestions and others may be substituted if they are more satisfactory in particular cases. The *Pharmaceutical Codex* requires that such alternatives should have a bactericidal activity at least equivalent to that of 0.5% phenol. The *British Pharmacopoeia* recommends that the number of bacteria recovered per ml is reduced by a factor of not less than 10^3 within 6 hours of challenge and no organism is recovered from 1 ml at 24 hours and thereafter. In addition the number of moulds or yeasts recovered per ml is reduced by a factor of not less than 10^2 within 7 days of challenge and there is no increase thereafter. Thiomersal 0.01–0.02% is used in certain immunological preparations while Procainamide Injection BP and some commercial cortisone injections contain 0.9% benzyl alcohol.

An additional preservative is unnecessary in multiple-dose injections prepared by heating with a bactericide since they already contain one; nor is one necessary when the medicament has bactericidal activity, e.g. Ethanolamine Oleate Injection BP. This contains 2.0% benzyl alcohol as a local anaesthetic and, therefore, even if the active ingredient had no antibacterial activity there would be no need for an additional bactericide.

Bactericides suitable for oily injections

The bactericides mentioned previously are more soluble in fats and oils than in water and, therefore, when present in an aqueous liquid containing bacteria, will tend to leave the water and concentrate in the lipoid constituents of the bacteria. Oily solutions of these substances have lower antibacterial activity because the bactericides will not leave the oil as readily as they will leave an aqueous solution, i.e. the partition coefficient is not in favour of the bactericide concentrating in the bacteria.

The *Pharmaceutical Codex* recommends as bactericides for oily preparations in multiple-dose containers phenol (0.5%), cresol (0.3%) and chlorocresol (0.1%). These are exactly the same concentrations as for the aqueous products. It is not a failure to take their reduced activity into account but a reflection of the difficulty of investigating the efficiency of bactericides in oily media. The *Codex* acknowledges their probable poor effectiveness since it includes the statement:

'these bactericides *may* afford *some* protection from contamination with *vegetative* micro-organisms but are *ineffective* against *sporing* organisms.'

Evidence suggests that micro-organisms are

unlikely to multiply in an anhydrous environment. Eisman *et al.* (1953) studied the sporicidal activities in sesame oil of a number of substances including commonly used preservatives. Since a phenylmercuric salt, even at 0.01%, was one of the least active compounds tested it is understandable that phenylmercuric nitrate is not in the list recommended in the *Codex*.

Limitations in the use of bactericides

If bactericides were included in large volume intravenous injections, there would be a risk of adminstering a toxic dose. They must not be included if the dose exceeds 15 ml. Bactericidal agents cannot be used in infusion fluids which cannot be packed in multiple-dose containers nor sterilized by heating with a bactericide. There is no objection to the inclusion of a bactericide when the dose of an intravenous injection is less than 15 ml.

Bactericides should not be used in intracardiac and intra-arterial injections in case they further damage the affected tissues or organs. Similarly bactericides should never be used in intrathecal, intracisternal and peridural injections. The meninges are very easily irritated and serious inflammation (aseptic meningitis) may be set up by bactericides. As the c.s.f. is a favourable medium for bacterial growth it would be dangerous to inject even a few organisms from a contaminated multiple-dose injection. Therefore, injections for intrathecal, intracisternal and peridural use should be packed in single-dose containers, sealed by fusion of glass. Injections for ophthalamic routes should also not contain bactericides.

Parenteral solutions of radionucleides are often supplied in multiple-dose containers because decay constantly changes the dose volume and opened, partly used ampoules are less easy to store safely until the contents have decayed sufficiently for disposal. The choice of bactericide is limited by the instability of many under the influence of radiation.

Incompatibilities of common bactericides

A bactericide must be compatible with the medicaments and with the auxiliary substances present in a solution that it is required to preserve. Incompatibility with the four common bactericides is not uncommon. Phenol is incompatible with procaine penicillin, quinine hydrochloride and thiamine hydrochloride, cresol with carbachol, ergometrine and quinine hydrochloride and phenylmercuric acetate with ascorbic acid, ergometrine, hyoscine hydrobromide, pethidine hydrochloride and thiamine hydrochloride. Chlorocresol is less satisfactory and incompatible with many substances, including benzylpenicillin, calcium chloride, carbachol, chlorpheniramine maleate, diamorphine hydrochloride, ergometrine, heparin, mersalyl, methadone, papaveretum and quinine hydrochloride. Some of these incompatibilities are due to salting out of the bactericide by strong solutions of the medicaments, others may have been caused by the use of chlorocresol of insufficient purity. Phenol and cresol do not have many incompatibilities and are particularly valuable for the majority of protein preparations, e.g. immunological products.

Chemical stability of the medicament

Adjustment of pH

Adjustment of the pH is a major method of stabilizing injections since decomposition is often catalysed by hydrogen or hydroxyl ions. Often a pH can be found at which the loss of activity is negligible, provided the preparation is packed and stored correctly, but in some cases breakdown still occurs, although at a reduced rate. Four methods can be used to increase the stability of injections.

Addition of a reducing agent or antioxidant

The most popular reducing agents for injections are sulphurous acid salts (Smith and Stevens, 1972) which include sodium sulphite, sodium metabisulphite and sodium bisulphate. They are used principally to retard the oxidation of drugs that are readily oxidized in aqueous solution to form coloured decomposition products. Sodium metabisulphite is used to prevent the decomposition of adrenaline injections and prevent the green colour due to the oxidation of apomorphine and the darkening of morphine sulphate in morphine sulphate injection (Yeh and Lach,

1961). However, the same researchers (1971) have shown that morphine reacts with sodium metabisulphite to form a product which is insoluble in water and dilute hydrochloric acid. Sodium metabisulphite is most suitable for injections of low pH but when the stability range of the medicament extends to the alkaline side of neutral (e.g. Gallamine Injection BP) sodium sulphate is more appropriate. Sodium thiosulphate is included in Sodium Iodide (^{131}I) Injection BP and Sulphadiazine Injection BP.

The reducing action of dextrose may be used, e.g. Carbachol Injection BP and Phentolamine Injection BP. Ascorbic acid has been examined but it is not as effective as sodium metabisulphite. Thiourea has been recommended as an antioxidant for ascorbic acid injections and an antioxidant, e.g. propylgallate, is usually included in injectable oils and ethyl oleate to prevent rancidification. Lachman (1968) comprehensively reviewed antioxidants and their uses.

Intrathecal injections must not contain antioxidants and, therefore, careful consideration of the formulation must be made. For instance, morphine injection may be formulated for intrathecal use without an antioxidant but will degrade to pseudomorphine and morphine IV oxide (Deeks et al., 1983). Their presence must be balanced off against the risk which the presence of an antioxidant would cause.

Replacement of air by an inert gas

In injections where oxygen is a serious cause of decomposition, improved stability may be obtained by replacement of the air in the final containers with an inert gas. Nitrogen satisfactory fulfils the requirement of inertness and availability. The method may be used alone as in injections containing ergot alkaloids (e.g. ergotamine) and in Tubocurarine Injection BP, or together with one or more reducing agents, as in Apomorphine Injection BP (sodium metabisulphite) and Chlorpromazine Injection BP (sodium metabisulphite and ascorbic acid).

Use of sequestering agents

Trace quantities of many heavy metal ions often catalyse destructive changes in medicaments, e.g.

the breakdown of the sulphur-containing ring of benzylpenicillin (copper, lead, mercury and zinc), the oxidation of adrenaline (copper, iron and chromium), the degradation of thiomersal (copper) and the decomposition of oxytetracycline (copper). These effects can often be prevented by adding a substance, termed a sequestering agent, that will form a soluble coordination compound with the metal in which the latter is held in a non-ionizable form. Then the catalytic property of the ion is often, but not always, suppressed.

The agent that has been most widely used for this purpose is ethylenediamine tetra-acetic acid (EDTA), usually as its di- or tri- sodium or calcium disodium salts. Sodium polymetaphophate and dimercaprol have been investigated as sequestering agents. Other examples include the use of disodium edetate in Sodium Bicarbonate Injection BP and citric acid in Digoxin Injection BP, Propranolol Injection BP and Urea Injection BP. When sequestering agents are used to prevent metal-catalysed oxidation, they are usually more effective if a reducing agent is present.

Inclusion of specific stabilizers

Calcium Gluconate Injection BP Calcium gluconate is sparingly soluble in cold water (1 in 30) but readily forms a supersaturated solution. A 10% injection (BP strength) can be prepared by dissolving the salt in hot water. This solution tends to deposit crystals, particularly if it has not been carefully filtered to remove foreign particles that can act as nuclei for crystal formation. To reduce this tendency to crystallize, not more than 5% of the gluconate may be replaced by calcium d-saccharate or another suitable harmless calcium salt (e.g. the lactobionate, glucoheptonate or laevulinate salts).

Sodium Bicarbonate Injection BP Solutions of sodium bicarbonate, when heated, form sodium carbonate and liberate carbon dioxide. Unfortunately, the carbonate may cause harmful effects, e.g. haemolysis and calcium precipitation. Therefore, to prevent decomposition, the container should be thoroughly sealed to prevent gas loss during sterilization and the injection should be saturated with carbon dioxide before sterilization. Precipitation of calcium or magnesium carbonate may occur due to impurities in the bicarbonate or to the extraction of calcium or magnesium ions from the glass container. To minimize this problem it is permissible to add 0.01% disodium edetate to sequester the troublesome ions.

Mersalyl Injection BP   Mersalyl, the sodium salt of a complex organic acid containing mercury, decomposes in solution liberating toxic mercuric ions. Sodium chloride, in plasma, would induce this breakdown if mersalyl alone was injected. However mersalyl combines with compounds containing an acidic nitrogen atom, e.g. theophylline, and makes its liberation more difficult. The acid and the stabilizer, theophylline, are suspended in water and sodium hydroxide is added until solution has been effected. The pH is adjusted to 7.6–8.2 which is the optimum for stability.

Limitations in the use of additives

No matter what the formulation or type of injection, any added substance(s) should not interfere with the activity of the drug. They should be safe, effective at low concentrations and be stable to both heat and storage. Additives should not be used unless their value is unquestionable. Ideally a patient should receive only the drug prescribed.

Particulate contamination

The origins, nature and hazards of particulate contamination have been covered extensively elsewhere (Chapter 27 and Groves *et al.*, 1973b) but need mention.

Particulate contamination may arise from four main sources:

1 materials arising from the drug, vehicle or added substances not filtered out at clarification prior to filling the final container,
2 materials present in the final container which were not removed by rinsing prior to filling,
3 materials falling by chance into the final container during the filling process.

Such materials from 1, 2, and 3 above may include cellulose fibres, dust, cotton fibres, hair, dandruff and loose skin from human origin as well as microbial contamination. Some filters may shed particles during use.

4 The container or closures may be sources of particles either during storage or removal of doses prior to administration. Thus constituents of closures may deposit into the injection during sterilization, e.g. carbon black, whiting, zinc oxide and clay. To prevent this problem the closure may be coated with a lacquer but this may also subsequently flake into the medicament. On withdrawal of a dose the penetration of the needle through the closure may result in coring or forcing rubber particles into the injection. Even glass containers are sources of contamination since the injection may react with the glass causing flaking and the physical force required to open ampoules may cause glass spicules to be deposited into the injection.

The physical damage caused by particles following injection has been discussed (Dempsey and Webber, 1983). It has been suggested that such particles can cause inflammatory responses, tissue growths possibly leading to neoplasms, antigenic reactions and occlusion of blood vessels leading to damage especially to the brain, kidney, liver and eyes.

PACKAGING OF INJECTIONS

Containers for injections

Ideal properties

The ideal properties for containers of injections are as follows.

1 The container should not affect its contents.
2 There should be no surface changes of the container at the temperatures and pressures associated with sterilization.
3 They should protect from light when the contents are photosensitive.
4 The containers should either be cheap enough to dispose of after one use or be easy to clean and reuse.
5 The contents should be easy to examine through the container to detect particles, contamination and decomposition.

Types of container

Several types of container have been developed for injections. *Ampoules* are single-dose glass containers with capacity of 0.5–50 ml. They are usually made from neutral or soda (lime-soda) glass and tend to liberate glass particles on opening into the product. Ampoules are sealed by heat fusion to exclude micro-organisms and may be used either for solutions or for powders. *Cartridges* are cylindrical glass tubes sealed by rubber at each end, holding slightly more than 1 ml. For use they are inserted into a metal syringe barrel and are used for one occasion only. *Prepacked syringes* were first introduced in the 1960s and contain one dose of medicament; there is no danger of particulate contamination due to the glass. *Antibiotic vials* and *multiple-dose containers* are rubber capped and allow withdrawal of a dose via a needle once it has penetrated the rubber cap. Antibiotic vials allow easy addition of a vehicle through the rubber closure (via a needle) and facilitate dissolving of the powder immediately prior to administration. Multiple-dose containers provide flexibility in the dose to be withdrawn. However, there is a greater risk of contamination (and hence the inclusion of a bactericide in multiple-dose injections) than in ampoules.

Containers for large volume fluids (greater than 50 ml) may be constructed from either glass or plastics. Glass bottles tend to be thick walled and are sealed with materials other than glass, e.g. plastic or rubber discs with an aluminium screw cap. Plastic containers are unbreakable, light and disposable. They are less transparent than glass containers, are easily punctured and there is difficulty in estimating unused volumes.

Single-dose versus multiple-dose containers

Single-dose ampoules are difficult to manipulate during use. However, their closures are completely airtight and their use is essential for drugs which need to be packed in an atmosphere of nitrogen. There is no possibility of solvent loss. In comparison, multiple-dose containers allow variation in the dose that can be withdrawn. The presence of the rubber seal may cause problems like preservative loss and particulate contamination from rubber coring during removal of the dose. Indrawing of air may lead to contamination of unused product.

Materials for injection containers

Glass

Glass produced by fusion of silica alone is resistant to chemical attack, thermal shock and the risks of handling but is expensive and difficult to manufacture. Other substances are added to give glasses of lower melting points, e.g., alkaline oxides, oxides of divalent elements and boric or aluminium oxides.

Types of glass Soda glass is unsuitable as a container material for injections because it yields appreciable quantities of alkali to aqueous solutions, flakes comparatively easily, loses brilliance on repeated use and is liable to fracture with sudden changes of temperature. Soda glass is, however, specified for thiopentone sodium since alkali stabilizes this medicament. Borosilicate glass was developed to avoid alkali extraction but is expensive and difficult to mould. It has been superseded by neutral glass which is soft and easier to manipulate, having good resistance to autoclaving and to solutions of pH up to 8. Neutral glass is used for alkali-sensitive injections and to produce ampoules, small vials and large transfusion bottles. Lead-free glass is required for ampoules intended for Sodium Calciumedetate Injection BP and Trisodium Edetate Injection BP. These medicines are sequestering agents which would take up lead ions from the glass.

Leaching of alkali can be further reduced by pretreatment of the glass surface. Sulphuring is used to give lime-soda glass a neutral surface through which the extraction of alkali ions is small. However, none of the glasses used for pharmaceutical containers is completely free from extractable alkali and, therefore, limit tests are given in the pharmacopoeias for extractable alkali. (For further information on glass composition, see Chapter 44 and Sanga, 1979.)

Associated problems for parenterals Glass may cause the following pharmaceutical problems.

Alkalinity Glass containers easily yield alkali ions to aqueous preparations. Alkaloidal salts in injection (e.g. apomorphine hydrochloride, ergotamine tartrate) may precipitate the free alkaloid if the pH rises. Similarly insulin injections (pH 3.0–3.5) may precipitate the free insulin if the pH rises to the isoelectric point of insulin (pH 5.5–5.6). Rises in pH can also increase the chemical instability of formulated drugs. Although methods of stabilization may be used, e.g. pH adjustment, replacement of air by nitrogen and the inclusion of antioxidants, trace quantities of alkali will decompose apomorphine hydrochloride, atropine (hydrolysis) and morphine sulphate. Vitamins are similarly sensitive. All these injections need low-alkali content glasses. Injections prepared as the powder and dissolved immediately prior to use need not be packed in low alkalinity glasses.

Loss of brilliance and flaking
Extraction of weakly bonded alkali ions from the glass under damp conditions may result in dissolution of some of the surface silica due to the high alkalinity of the deposit resulting in a loss of surface brilliance. This makes visualization of contents difficult and may be the first stage of cracking of the glass surface leading to flaking into the contents of the injection. Flakes rapidly form by alkaline solutions etching away into the silica structure, e.g. injections containing sodium citrate or phosphate. They develop more slowly in solutions of chlorides of sodium, potassium or calcium. The *British Pharmacopoeia* warns that in certain injections (e.g. Sodium Chloride, Sodium Lactate and Compound Sodium Lactate) small particles may separate from a glass container.

Plastics

Types of plastics
The plastics used to pack injections are thermoplastic in nature. These soften on heating to a viscous fluid and harden on cooling. Those used include high density polyethylene, polyvinylchloride (PVC) and polypropylene. PVC is poorly flexible and, therefore, plasticizers are added to produce the flexible material required for bags for infusion fluids. Polypropylene is similar to high density polyethylene but with a higher heat resistance. All three types may be sterilized by autoclaving.

Associated problems for parenterals
The *British Pharmacopoeia* stresses the importance of knowledge of the plastic composition. Injections packed in plastic should be examined under 'in use' simulations for sensory, chemical and physical changes, changes in quantity of the contents due to permeability of the plastic, change in pH, the effects of light and changes in assay results. Attention should be given to extractable substances (which, if released, should be innocuous and compatible with contents), to permeability of gases and solvent vapours and to absorption of active ingredients, bactericides and other adjuncts.

Examples of these problems include the liberation of cyclohexanone (a solvent for PVC) from PVC bags into intravenous solutions (Ulsaker and Korsnes, 1977) and the presence of liquid particles of di-2-ethylhexylphthalate (a plasticizer) in intravenous fluids (Horioka *et al.*, 1977). Many drugs, e.g. diazepam, hydralazine hydrochloride and thiopentone sodium, are adsorbed on to PVC. Such problems vary to factors including pH, concentration, octanol–water partition coefficients, lipid solubility and the extent of ionization of molecules in solution. Plastic containers should not yield more than a minimum of soluble matter. In addition plastic containers must comply with texts for toxicity, ether-soluble extractives and metal additives (heavy metals, tin and barium).

Closures

Types and properties of closure materials
Closures are made from rubbers and the ideal rubber should show good ageing properties with no deterioration with age or oxidation. The hardness and elasticity should be sufficient to allow a needle to pass through without blunting yet on withdrawal of the needle the puncture should close immediately. The properties of the rubber should not be altered by the selected sterilization process and the rubber should not be permeable to air and moisture, the latter of which might degrade water-sensitive drugs, e.g. penicillin. However, injections which are sensitive to oxygen should be packed in glass-fused containers (ampoules).

Two types of rubber may be used for closures, natural or synthetic. Natural or raw rubber is unsuitable for use before additives are used to give it better physical and chemical properties. Added substances include vulcanizing agents (e.g. sulphur), accelerators to reduce this amount of sulphur (e.g. thiazoles and thiurans) and activators (e.g. stearic acid or stearates) to increase the activity of accelerators. Fillers (e.g. carbon black or magnesium carbonate) reinforce the physical properties and extending agents (e.g. talc) reduce the cost. Antioxidants are added (e.g. phenols) to reduce oxidation of rubber which is catalysed by light, copper and manganese. Rubbers may be coloured by pigments (e.g. iron oxides, sulphides and coal tar dyes) and softening agents and lubricants may be added.

In comparison with natural rubber, synthetic rubbers are more resistant to high temperature, more resistant to ageing and more expensive. However, as they are harder than natural rubbers a substantially higher level of softening agents, e.g. dibutylphthalate, is used to improve resilience. Often carbon black or fine clay is used as filler. Four types are used for closures. Butyl rubbers are resistant to chemical attack and ageing but their oil and solvent resistance is low. Nitrile rubbers are oil and heat resistant but absorption of bactericides and leaching of extractive are considerable. Chloroprene rubbers are resistant to oxygen and oils and zinc oxide rather than sulphur is used for vulcanization. Water permeability is low. Silicone rubbers are heat resistant and show low permeability to water. The advantages and disadvantages of rubbers have been reviewed by Stafford (1981).

Associated problems for parenterals The various added substances used in the preparation of the rubber should not be released into the medicament, and care should be taken that no toxic materials are released nor should inactivation of the medicament by pH changes occur. Similarly there should be no extraction of injection ingredients by the rubber. This is the biggest problem with rubber closures. Loss of bactericides from injections may occur by two processes which may similarly effect the medicament or other substances present in the injection.

Absorption by the rubber The bactericide is partitioned between the injection and the rubber according to its partition coefficient. Phenol and benzyl alcohol are attracted to the water and are not absorbed. However, others like chlorocresol and phenylmercuric nitrate are strongly attracted to the rubber and are strongly absorbed. To minimize these problems the *British Pharmacopoeia* prescribes a method of treating the rubber where closures are treated with solutions containing bactericides in concentrations twice that found in the injection. The solution should contain other ingredients that may similarly be absorbed from the injection.

Loss through volatilization from the outer surface of the rubber cap Once equilibrium has been reached the bactericide volatilizes into the atmosphere from the surface of the closure. Loss can be limited by sealing the closure with a less permeable material (e.g. paraffin wax). The choice of such a material is limited because it should not fragment. Loss can be reduced by reduction in the upper surface area of the closure exposed and by increasing its thickness.

Some rubber caps have been reported to reduce the antioxidant activity of sodium metabisulphite or sulphur dioxide by adsorption from solution.

Care should also be taken that the closure intended for oily injections should be constructed from oil-resistant materials.

STERILIZATION OF INJECTIONS

Wherever possible, injections should be sterilized in their final container to reduce to a minimum the possibility of contamination. The principles of sterilization are discussed in Chapter 26 and industrial sterilization procedures are described in Chapter 43.

Dry heat sterilization is used for oily injections, e.g. Progesterone Injection BP. However propyliodone is thermolabile and hence, to prepare the injection, the sterile powder is added by aseptic technique to arachis oil, previously sterilized by dry heat.

Moist heat sterilization, i.e. autoclaving, is used for most thermostable aqueous preparations.

Closures may be sterilized by autoclaving them in solutions containing preservatives (and medicaments) at concentrations twice those found in the injection.

Heating with a bactericide may be used for injections that are thermolabile to autoclaving. However, the use of this method of sterilization is forbidden when the injections are intended for certain routes, e.g. intrathecal.

Sterilization by filtration may be used as an alternative to dry heat for oils and may avoid slight changes in heat sterilized products. No heat is used and therefore the method is suitable for aqueous preparations which are thermolabile and stable in solution. Examples include Betamethasone Sodium Phosphate Injection BP, Diazepam Injection BP and Ergotamine Injection BP. Care

should be taken, however, as certain drugs may adsorb to the filter.

Certain injections may not, however, be sufficiently stable to enable sterilization by filtration. Therefore, the powders are packed, sterile in ampoules, to be reconstituted at the time of injection by *aseptic processes*. Examples include Amylobarbitone Sodium Injection BP, Pentamidine Injection BP, Tetracyline Injection BP and Thiopentone Injection BP. The powders may be sterilized by dry heat (if thermostable in dry state) or by bacterial filtration prior to aseptic precipitation or crystallization. Terminal sterilization with gaseous disinfectants (e.g. ethylene oxide) may be used provided no chemical changes occur in the drug. Erythromycin, tetracycline and penicillins are unharmed by this process.

REFERENCES

Allwood, M. C. (1978) Antimicrobial agents in single and multi-dose injections. *J. appl. Bact.*, **44**, SVII–SXVII.

Carpenter, C. P. and Shaffer, C. B. (1952) Polyethylene glycols as injection vehicles. *J. Am. Pharm. Ass. (Sci. Ed.)*, **41**, 27–29.

Deeks, T., Davis, S. and Nash, S. (1983) Stability of an intrathecal morphine injection formulation. *Pharm. J.*, **230**, 495–497.

Dempsey, G. and Webber, G. S. (1983) Hazards of particle injection. *Pharm. J.*, **231**, 63–64.

Eisman, P. C., Jaconia, D. and Mayer, R. L. (1953) The preservation of parenteral vegetable oils by chemical agents. *J. Am. Pharm. Ass. (Sci. Ed.)*, **42**, 659–662.

Frith, C. F., Dawson, F. W., Sampson, R. L. (1976) Water for Injection U.S.P. XIX by reverse osmosis. *Bull. Parent Drug Assoc.*, **30**, 118–127.

Gibaldi, M. (1977) *Biopharmaceutics and Clinical Pharmacokinetics*, 2nd edn, Lea and Febiger, Philadelphia.

Groves, M. J. (1973a) *Parenteral Products*, William Heinemann, London.

Groves, M. J. (1973b). Particulate contamination in intravenous fluids. 1. Nature, origin and hazard. *Pharm. J.*, **210**, 185–187; 2. The detection of particulate contamination. *Pharm. J.*, **211**, 163–166; 3. Standards for control of cleanliness. *Pharm. J.*, **211**, 166–168.

Hartman, C. W. and Husa, W. J. (1957) Isotonic solutions, V. The permeability of red corpuscles to various salts. *J. Am. Pharm. Ass. (Sci. Ed.)*, **46**, 430–433.

Horioka, M., Aoyama, T. and Karasawa, H. (1977) Particles of di-2-ethylhexyl phthalate in intravenous infusion fluids migrating from polyvinyl chloride bags. *Chem. Pharm. Bull.*, **25**, 1791–1796.

Husa, W. J. and Adams, J. R. (1944) Isotonic Solutions, II. The permeability of red corpuscles to various substances *J. Am. Parm. Ass. (Sci. Ed.)*, **33**, 329.

KabiVitrum Ltd. (1984/85) Data in A.B.P.I. *Data sheet Compendium (1984/85)*, DataPharm. Publications Ltd, London.

Irvine, M. K. A. (1978) Products for parenteral nutrition. *Pharm. J.*, **221**, 216–219.

Lachman, L. (1968) Antioxidants and chelating agents as stabilisers in liquid dosage forms. *Drug. Cosmet. Ind.*, **102**(1), 36–40, 146–148; **102**(2), 43–45, 146–149.

Macek, T. J. (1963) Preparation of parenteral despersions. *J. pharm. Sci.*, **52**, 694–699.

Nash, R. A. (1972) Parenteral Suspensions. *Bull. Parent Drug Assoc.*, **26**, 91–95.

Perkins, J. J. (1969) *Principles and Methods of Sterilisation*, 2nd edn, Charles C Thomas, Springfield, Illinois.

Ridgway, K. (1973) Pyrogens and pyrogen free water. *Proc. Biochem.*, **8**(7), 9–12.

Sanga, S. V. (1979) Review of glass types available for packaging parenteral solutions. *J. Parent Drug. Assoc.*, **33**, 61–67.

Smith, G. and Stevens, M. F. G. (1972) Sulphur dioxide — preservative and potential mutagen. *Pharm. J.*, **209**, 570–572.

Stafford, P. (1981) Rubber and its pharmaceutical applications. *Manufacturing Chemist and Aerosol News*, **52**(6), 25, 27.

Sykes, G. (1958) The basis for sufficient of a suitable bacteriostatic in injections. *J. Pharm. Pharmac.*, **10**, 40T–46T.

Thomas, W. H., Thomson, R. and Hui, L. K. (1980) Evaluation of non-official methods of pyrogen testing of injectables. *Pharm. J.*, **224**, 259–261, 270.

Thomasson, C. L. and Husa, W. J. (1958) Isotonic solutions, VII. The permeability of red corpuscles to various alkaloidal salts. *J. Am. Pharm. Ass. (Sci. Ed.)*, **47**, 711–714.

Ulsaker, G. A. and Korsnes, R. M. (1977) Determination of cyclohexanone in intravenous solutions stored in PVC bags by gas chromatography. *Analyst*, **102**, 882–883.

Yeh, S. Y. and Lach, J. L. (1961) Stability of morphine in aqueous solutions, III. *J. pharm. Sci.*, **50**, 35–42.

Yeh, S. Y. and Lach, J. L. (1971), Stability of morphine in aqueous solution IV. *J. pharm. Sci.*, **60**, 793–794.

Topical preparations

The main purpose of this chapter is to show how the physicochemical properties of a drug in a topical dosage form affect the drug's percutaneous absorption. This process, and the drug's topical bioavailability, depend on the medicament leaving a formulation (cream, ointment, etc.) and penetrating through the stratum corneum into the viable epidermis and dermis. Within the living tissues the molecule usually produces its characteristic pharmacological response before the systemic circulation removes it. The ultimate aim in dermatological biopharmaceutics is to design active drugs, or pro-drugs, and incorporate them into vehicles or devices which deliver the medicament to the active site in the biophase at a controlled rate.

The plan of the chapter is to introduce the reader to the structure, function and topical treatment of human skin; to deal with the principles of membrane diffusion, skin transport, the properties influencing percutaneous absorption and the methods for studying the process; and to close with a brief discussion of dermatological vehicles and a protocol for producing a dermatological formulation. The reader may then see that skin therapy is a paradox; at first sight it appears to be a simple form of treatment yet closer examination reveals that sound dermatological design represents one of the most difficult aspects of the science of formulation.

STRUCTURE, FUNCTION AND TOPICAL TREATMENT OF HUMAN SKIN

The skin combines with the mucosal linings of the urogenital, digestive and respiratory tracts to protect the internal body structure from a hostile external environment of varying pollution, temperature, humidity and radiation. The skin safeguards the internal organs, limits the passage of chemicals into and out of the body, stabilizes blood pressure and temperature, and mediates the sensations of heat, cold, touch and pain. It expresses emotions (such as the pallor of fear, the redness of embarrassment and anger, and the sweating of anxiety). The integument identifies individuals through the characteristics particular to man, e.g. colour, hair, odour and texture.

Skin damages easily, mechanically, chemically, biologically, and by radiation. Thus the tissue suffers cuts, bruises, burns, bites and stings; detergents, chemical residues, organic solvents and pollutants attack and penetrate the surface, and micro-organisms and plants deliver contact allergens. Topical and systemic drugs, toiletries and cosmetics, and many diseases may all harm the skin.

Anatomy and physiology

The human skin comprises three tissue layers: the stratified, avascular, cellular epidermis, the underlying dermis of connective tissue, and the subcutaneous fat layer (Fig. 22.1). Hairy skin contains hair follicles and sebaceous glands; glabrous skin of the soles and palms produces a thick epidermis with a compact stratum corneum but there are no hair follicles or sebaceous glands.

The epidermis

The multilayered epidermis varies in thickness, ranging from about 0.8 mm on the palms and soles to 0.006 mm on the eyelids. The cells of the basal layer (stratum germinativum) divide and migrate upwards to produce the stratum corneum or horny layer. Man survives in a non-aqueous environment because of the almost impermeable

nature of this dead, dense layer, which is crucially important in controlling the percutaneous absorption of drugs and other chemicals. The stratum corneum may be only 10 μm thick when dry but swells several fold in water. There are two main types of horny layer, the pads of the palms and soles adapted for weight bearing and friction and the remaining flexible, impermeable membranous layer. The basal cell layer also includes melanocytes which produce and distribute melanin granules to the keratinocytes.

The dermis

The dermis (or corium), at 3–5 mm thick, consists of a matrix of connective tissue woven from fibrous proteins (collagen, elastin, and reticulin) which are embedded in an amorphous ground substance of mucopolysaccharide. Nerves, blood vessels and lymphatics traverse the matrix and skin appendages (eccrine sweat glands, apocrine glands, and pilosebaceous units) pierce it. The dermis needs an efficient blood supply to convey nutrients, remove waste products, regulate pressure and temperature, mobilize defence forces and to contribute to skin colour. Branches from the arterial plexus deliver blood to sweat glands, hair follicles, subcutaneous fat, and the dermis itself. This supply reaches to within 0.2 mm of the skin surface, so that it quickly absorbs and

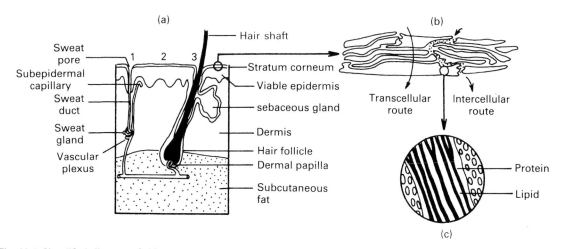

Fig. 22.1 Simplified diagram of skin structure and routes of drug penetration. (a) Route (1) Via the sweat ducts; route (2) across the continuous stratum corneum; or route (3) through the hair follicles with their associated sebaceous glands. (b) Representation of the stratum corneum membrane, illustrating two possible subroutes for diffusion. (c) Idealized representation of protein filaments in lipid matrix within stratum corneum cell

systemically dilutes most compounds passing the epidermis. The generous blood volume in the skin usually acts as a 'sink' for diffusing molecules reaching the capillaries, keeping penetrant concentrations in the dermis very low, maximizing epidermal concentration gradients, and thus promoting percutaneous absorption.

The subcutaneous tissue

The subcutaneous fat (subcutis, hypoderm) provides a mechanical cushion and a thermal barrier; it synthesizes and stores readily available high-energy chemicals.

The skin appendages

The *eccrine sweat glands* (2–5 million) produce sweat (pH 4.0–6.8) and may also secrete drugs, proteins, antibodies and antigens. Their principal function is to aid heat control, but emotional stress can also provoke sweating (the clammy palm syndrome).

The *apocrine sweat glands* develop at the pilosebaceous follicle to provide the characteristic adult distribution in the armpit (axilla), the breast areola, and the perianal region. The milky or oily secretion may be coloured and contains proteins, lipids, lipoproteins and saccharides. Surface bacteria metabolize this odourless liquid to produce the characteristic body smell.

Hair follicles develop over all skin except the red part of the lips, the palms and soles, and parts of the sex organs. One or more sebaceous glands, and in some body regions an apocrine gland, open into the follicle above the muscle which attaches the follicle to the dermoepidermal junction.

Sebaceous glands are most numerous and largest on the face, forehead, in the ear, on the midline of the back and on anogenital surfaces; the palms and soles usually lack them. These holocrine glands produce sebum from cell disintegration; its principal components are glycerides, free fatty acids, cholesterol, cholesterol esters, wax esters and squalene. Abnormal sebaceous activity may lead to seborrhoea (excess sebum), gland hyperplasia without clinical seborrhoea, obstruction of the pilosebaceous canal (acne and comedones — whiteheads or blackheads), and other types of dysfunction — the dyssebacias.

The *nails*, like hair, consist of 'hard' keratin with a relatively high sulphur content, mainly as cysteine. Unlike the stratum corneum, the nail behaves as a hydrophilic matrix with respect to its permeability.

Functions of the skin

The skin performs many varied functions but we need only consider some aspects of its containment and protective roles.

The mechanical function

The dermis provides the mechanical properties of skin, with the epidermis playing a minor part. Our skin is elastic but once it has taken up its initial slack, it extends further only with difficulty. With age, the skin wrinkles and becomes more rigid. The thin horny layer is quite strong and depends for its pliability on a correct balance of lipids, water-soluble hygroscopic substances and particularly water. The tissue requires some 10–20% of moisture to act as a plasticizer and so maintain its suppleness.

The protective function

Microbiological barrier The stratum corneum provides a microbiological barrier and the sloughing of squames with their adhering microorganisms aids the protective mechanism. However, microbes penetrate superficial cracks and damaged stratum corneum may allow access to the lower tissues, where infection may develop. The so-called acid mantle (produced by sebaceous and eccrine secretions at pH 4.2–5.6) probably does not defend the skin against bacteria via its acidity, as was once thought. However, skin glands also secrete short chain fatty acids which inhibit bacterial and fungal growth. Bacteria are unlikely to enter the tiny opening of the inner duct of the eccrine gland; the entrances to the apocrine gland and the hair follicle are much wider and these appendages may become infected.

Chemical barrier An important function of human skin is to bar the entry of unwanted molecules from outside while controlling the loss of water, electrolytes and other endogenous constituents. The horny layer is very impermeable to chemicals and usually contributes the rate-limiting step in percutaneous absorption. The intact skin is a very effective barricade because the diffusional resistance of the horny layer is large and the appendageal shunt route provides only a small fractional area (about 0.1%).

Radiation barrier   For skin exposed to sunlight, ultraviolet light of 290–400 nm is the most damaging. Three main acute reactions follow irradiation: erythema, pigmentation, and epidermal thickening. Ultraviolet light stimulates melanocytes to produce melanin which partially protects the skin. In a severe photosensitive disease such as xeroderma pigmentosum, sunlight may induce changes even in negroes, whose intense racial pigmentation makes them less susceptible to sunburn. Chronic reactions to sunlight include skin 'ageing', premalignancy and malignancy. Sun-damaged skin may produce solar keratoses, progressing to a squamous cell carcinoma. Bowen's disease, malignant melanomata, and basal cell carcinoma may evolve.

Heat barrier and temperature regulation   The stratum corneum is so thin over most body areas that it does not effectively protect the underlying living tissues from extremes of cold and heat; it is not an efficient heat insulator. The skin, however, is the organ primarily responsible for maintaining the body at 37 °C. To conserve heat, the peripheral circulation shuts down to minimize surface heat loss; shivering generates energy when chilling is severe. To lose heat, blood vessels dilate, eccrine sweat glands pour out their dilute saline secretion, water evaporates and removal of the heat of vaporization cools the body.

Electrical barrier   In dry skin, resistance and impedance are much higher than in other biological tissues.

Mechanical shock   An acute violent blow bruises and blisters the skin; friction may blister or thicken the epidermis, producing callosities and corns. Accidental minor trauma to patients on corticosteroids may severely damage their skin.

Rational approach to topical formulation

Three main methods attack the problem of formulating a successful topical dosage form. We can manipulate the barrier function of the skin: for example, topical antibiotics and antibacterials help a damaged barrier to ward off infection; sunscreening agents and the horny layer protect the viable tissues from u.v. radiation; and emollient preparations restore pliability to a desiccated horny layer. Or we can direct drugs to the viable skin tissues without using oral, systemic, or other routes of therapy. The third approach uses skin delivery for systemic treatment, for example, transdermal therapeutic systems provide systemic therapy for motion sickness, angina and hypertension.

In dermatology, we aim at five main target regions — skin surface, horny layer, viable epidermis and upper dermis, skin glands, and systemic circulation (Figs. 22.1 and 22.2).

Surface treatment

We care for the skin surface mainly by using a simple camouflage or cosmetic application, by forming a protective layer, or by attacking bacteria and fungi. Some examples include protective films, sunscreens, and barriers which hinder moisture loss and so avert chapping. For topical antibiotics, antiseptics and deodorants, the surface micro-organisms are the target and effective surface bioavailability requires that the formulation should release the antimicrobial so it can penetrate the surface skin fissures and reach the organisms. Developmental studies should at least confirm that the formulation releases and does not bind the medicament.

Stratum corneum treatment

The main therapies aimed at the horny layer improve emolliency by raising water content or stimulating sloughing (keratosis) with, for example, salicylic acid. The insertion of moisturizing agents or keratolytics into stratum corneum involves release from the vehicle and penetration into the tissue. Ideally, the medicament should not enter viable skin; this may be difficult to prevent.

Skin appendage treatment

We may reduce hyperhydrosis of the sweat glands with antiperspirants such as aluminium or other

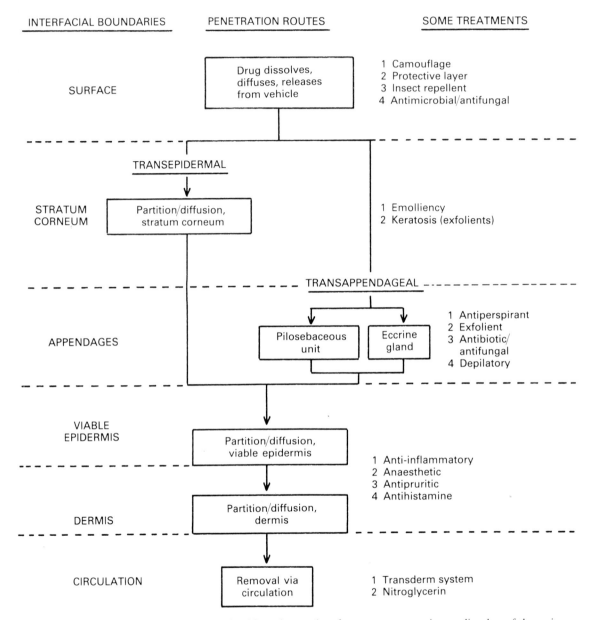

Fig. 22.2 The routes by which drugs penetrate the skin and examples of treatments appropriate to disorders of the various strata (Source: Barry 1983. Reproduced with permission of the copyright owner)

metal salts. In acne, we use topical exfolients such as salicylic acid, tretinoin (retinoic acid) and benzoyl peroxide; topical antibiotics include tetracycline, erythromycin and clindamycin. Depilatories usually contain strontium or barium sulphides, or thioglycolates. Topical clotrimazole, miconazole and thiobendazole treat fungal diseases of the nails, stratum corneum and hair.

Getting the medicament to the diseased site is a problem with appendage treatment. For example, it is difficult to achieve a high antibiotic concentration in a sebaceous gland when, as in acne, a horny plug blocks the follicle. The drug may not be sufficiently hydrophobic to partition from the water-rich viable epidermis and dermis into the sebum-filled gland.

Viable epidermis and dermis treatment

We can treat many diseases provided that the preparation efficiently delivers drug to the receptor. However, many potentially valuable drugs cannot be used topically as they do not readily cross the stratum corneum. Hence, investigators use penetration enhancers to diminish this layer's barrier function (see later). Another approach develops pro-drugs which reach the receptor and release the pharmacologically active fragment. The efficacy of many topical steroids depends partly on molecular groups which promote percutaneous absorption but which may not enhance drug–receptor binding.

Drug examples include topical steroidal and non-steroidal anti-inflammatory agents; corticosteroids may also be used in psoriasis. Anaesthetic drugs like benzocaine reduce pain, and anti-pruritics and antihistamines alleviate itch but they may cause sensitization. Topical 5-fluorouracil and methotrexate eradicate premalignant and some malignant skin tumours and treat psoriasis.

Systemic treatment via percutaneous absorption

Generally, healthy skin is not used as a drug route during systemic attacks on disease. The body absorbs drugs slowly and incompletely through the stratum corneum and much of the preparation is lost by washing, by adherence to clothes and by shedding with stratum corneum scales. Other problems include marked variations in skin permeability with subject, site, age and condition, which make control difficult. However, the route has been used to treat motion sickness (hyoscine), angina (nitroglycerin) and hypertension (clonidine).

Figure 22.2 illustrates drug penetration routes and examples of treatments appropriate to various skin strata.

BASIC PRINCIPLES OF DIFFUSION THROUGH MEMBRANES

A useful way to study percutaneous absorption is to consider first how molecules penetrate membranes and then move on to the special case of skin transport.

The diffusion process

In passive diffusion, matter moves from one region of a system to another following random molecular motions. The basic hypothesis underlying the mathematical theory for isotropic materials (which have identical structural and diffusional properties in all directions) is that the rate of transfer of diffusing substance per unit area of a section is proportional to the concentration gradient measured normal to the section. This is expressed as Fick's first law of diffusion, Eqn 22.1:

$$\mathcal{J} = -D\frac{\partial C}{\partial x} \qquad (22.1)$$

where $\mathcal{J}$ is the rate of transfer per unit area of surface (the flux), C is the concentration of diffusing substance, x is the space coordinate measured normal to the section, and D is the diffusion coefficient. The negative sign indicates that the flux is in the direction of decreasing concentration, i.e. down the concentration gradient. In many situations D is constant but in more complex materials D depends markedly on concentration; its dimensions are (length)^2 (time)$^{-1}$, often specified as cm^2 s^{-1}.

Fick's first law contains three variables, $\mathcal{J}$, C and x, of which $\mathcal{J}$ is additionally a multiple variable, dm/dt, where m is amount and t is time. We therefore usually employ Fick's second law which reduces the number of variables by one. For the common experimental situation in which diffusion is unidirectional, i.e. the concentration gradient is only along the x-axis, Eqn 22.2 expresses Fick's second law as:

$$\frac{\partial C}{\partial t} = D\frac{\partial^2 C}{\partial x^2} \qquad (22.2)$$

Many experimental designs employ a membrane separating two compartments, with a concentration gradient operating during a run and 'sink' conditions (essentially zero concentration) prevailing in the receptor compartment. If we measure the cumulative mass of diffusant, m, which passes per unit area through the membrane as a function of time, we obtain the plot shown in Fig. 22.3. At long times the plot approaches a straight line and

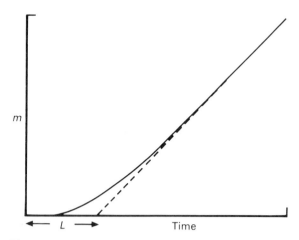

Fig. 22.3 The time course for absorption for the simple zero order flux case obtained by plotting m, the cumulative amount of diffusant crossing unit area of membrane, as a function of time. Steady state is achieved when the plot becomes linear; extrapolation of the linear portion to the time axis yields the lag time L

we obtain the steady state flux, dm/dt, from Eqn 22.3:

$$\frac{dm}{dt} = \frac{DC_0 K}{h} \qquad (22.3)$$

Here C_0 is the constant concentration of drug in the donor solution, K is the partition coefficient of the solute between the membrane and the bathing solution, and h is the thickness of the membrane.

If a steady state plot is extrapolated to the time axis, the intercept so obtained at $m = 0$ is the lag time, L:

$$L = \frac{h^2}{6D} \qquad (22.4)$$

From Eqn 22.4, D is easily estimated provided that the membrane thickness, h, is known. Knowing these and C_0, and measuring dm/dt, Eqn 22.3 provides one way of assessing K. Eqn 22.3 shows why this permeation procedure may be referred to as a zero order process. By analogy with chemical kinetic operations, Eqn 22.3 represents a zero order process with a rate constant of DK/h.

Sometimes with biological membranes we cannot separate the value of D from that of K. We then often employ a composite parameter, the

permeability coefficient, P, where $P = KD$ or $P = KD/h$. The latter definition is used when h is uncertain, e.g. diffusion through skin.

Complex diffusional barriers

Barriers in series

The treatment above deals only with the simple situation in which diffusion occurs in a single isotropic medium. However, skin is a heterogeneous multilayer tissue and in percutaneous absorption the concentration gradient develops over several strata. In terms of a laminate, each layer contributes a diffusional resistance, R, which is directly proportional to the layer thickness, h, and is indirectly proportional to the product of the layer diffusivity, D, and the partition coefficient, K, with respect to the external phase. The total diffusional resistance of all the layers in a three-ply membrane such as skin (stratum corneum, viable epidermis and dermis) is given by the expression

$$R_T = \frac{1}{P_T} = \frac{h_1}{D_1 K_1} + \frac{h_2}{D_2 K_2} + \frac{h_3}{D_3 K_3} \qquad (22.5)$$

Here R_T is the total diffusional resistance, P_T is the thickness-weighted permeability coefficient, and the numerals refer to the separate skin layers.

If one segment has a much greater resistance than the other layers (e.g. that of the stratum corneum compared with that of the viable epidermis or dermis) then the single high resistance phase determines the composite barrier properties. Then $P_T = K_1 D_1 / h_1$ where 1 refers to the resistant phase.

Barriers in parallel

Shunts and pores, such as hair follicles and sweat glands, pierce human skin (Fig. 22.1). Investigators often idealize this complex structure and consider the simple situation in which the diffusional medium consists of two or more diffusional pathways linked in parallel. Then the total diffusional flux per unit area of composite, $\mathcal{J}_T$, is the sum of the individual fluxes through the separate routes. Thus

$$\mathcal{J}_T = f_1 \mathcal{J}_1 + f_2 \mathcal{J}_2 \ldots \qquad (22.6)$$

where f_1, f_2 etc. denote the fractional areas for

each diffusional route. In general, for independent linear parallel pathways during steady state diffusion

$$\mathcal{J}_{\mathrm{T}} = C_{\mathrm{o}} \, (f_1 P_1 + f_2 P_2 + \ldots \ldots) \quad (22.7)$$

where P_1, P_2, ... represent the thickness-weighted permeability coefficients.

If only one route allows diffusant to pass, i.e. the other routes are impervious, then the solution reduces to the simple membrane model with the steady state flux determined by the fractional area and the permeation rate through the open channel.

Influence of material properties on diffusion

This section briefly reviews the physicochemical properties of solute and barrier phase which affect diffusion.

Diffusant solubility

We saw previously that the flux of solute is proportional to the concentration gradient across the entire barrier phase. Thus, one requirement for maximal flux is that the donor solution should be saturated. A formulator can optimize the solubility of a drug such as a corticosteroid by controlling the solvent composition of the vehicle. Then a saturated solution may be obtained at a selected concentration of the drug by experimenting with a series of solvents or, more usually, by blending two liquids to form a miscible binary mixture with suitable solvent properties.

Partition coefficient

The partition coefficient is important in establishing the flux of a drug through a membrane. When the membrane provides the sole or major source of diffusional resistance, then the magnitude of the partition coefficient is very important. This often occurs in percutaneous absorption when the impermeability of the stratum corneum usually provides the rate-limiting step in absorption. The stratum corneum-to-vehicle partition coefficient is then crucially important in establishing a high initial concentration of diffusant in the first layer of the membrane.

Effective concentrations

Although the concentration differential is usually considered to be the driving force for diffusion, the chemical potential gradient or activity gradient is the fundamental parameter. Often the distinction is unimportant but sometimes we must consider it. Thus, the thermodynamic activity of a penetrant in the donor phase or the membrane may be radically altered by, e.g. pH change, complex formation, or the presence of surfactants, micelles or cosolvents. Such factors also modify the effective partition coefficient.

pH variation According to the simple form of the pH-partition hypothesis, only unionized molecules pass readily across lipid membranes. Now weak acids and bases dissociate to different degrees depending on the pH and their pK_a or pK_b. Thus, the proportion of unionized drug in the applied phase determines the effective membrane gradient, and this fraction depends on pH.

Cosolvents Polar cosolvent mixtures such as propylene glycol with water may produce saturated drug solutions and so maximize the concentration gradient across the stratum corneum (see above under Diffusant solubility). However, the partition coefficient of a drug between the membrane and the solvent mixture generally falls as the solubility in the solvent system rises. Thus, these two factors — increase in solubility and magnitude of the partition coefficient — may oppose each other in promoting flux through the membrane. Hence it is important not to over-solubilize a drug if the aim is to promote penetration; the formulation should be at or near saturation.

Surface activity and micellization Here there are two main complicating situations in membrane transport — one where the drug is surface active and forms micelles and the other where additional surfactant is present. When the drug micellizes its total apparent solubility increases dramatically but the apparent partition coefficient decreases. However, the free monomer concentration remains constant as does the true (monomer) partition coefficient. Then, if the micelle cannot cross the membrane, this aggregate has little effect on the permeation process other than by serving as a reservoir to replace monomers and maintaining constant donor concentration.

When drug and surfactant are present the effect of surfactant on drug transport is complicated. The drug in the surfactant solution partitions between the micellar and non-micellar pseudophases. The absorption of micellar drug may be negligible and the effective concentration of the unassociated diffusing species may be so lowered that its flux falls drastically. However, all these effects are more important for membranes such as gastrointestinal or buccal tissue.

Surfactants have effects on skin which relate to lowering of interfacial tension in hair follicles and changes in protein conformation in the stratum corneum. These features will be dealt with later.

Complexation Complex formation is analogous in many ways to micellar solubilization in the manner in which it affects drug permeation. Thus, when complexes form, the apparent solubility and the apparent partition coefficient of the drug change. An increase in the apparent partition coefficient may promote drug absorption, e.g. some caffeine–drug complexes.

Diffusivity

Diffusional speed depends mainly on the state of matter of the medium. In gases and air, diffusion coefficients are large because the void space available to the molecules is great compared to their size, and the mean free path between molecular collisions is big. In liquids, the free volume is much smaller, mean free paths are decreased, and diffusivities are much reduced. In skin, the diffusivities drop progressively and reach their lowest values within the compacted stratum corneum matrix. The diffusion coefficient of a drug in a topical vehicle or in skin depends on the properties of the drugs and the diffusion medium and on the interaction between them.

SKIN TRANSPORT

The skin is very effective as a selective penetration barrier. The epidermis provides the major control element — most small water-soluble non-electrolytes diffuse into the capillary system a thousand times more rapidly when the epidermis is absent, damaged, or diseased. Furthermore, in the intact skin, substances penetrate at rates which may differ by a factor of 10^5. It is important that formulation pharmacists predict and control this selective permeability by relating the physiological and physicochemical attributes of the skin to the properties of the penetrant in a vehicle. We need to correlate the intrinsic properties of the skin barrier with the molecular requirements for breaching it as modified by interactions with the components of topical vehicles. The eventual aim in dermatological biopharmaceutics is to design drugs with selective penetrability for incorporation into vehicles or devices which deliver the medicament to the active site at a controlled rate and concentration for the necessary time.

Routes of penetration

When a molecule reaches intact skin it contacts cellular debris, micro-organisms, sebum, and other materials. The diffusant then has three potential entry routes to the viable tissue — through the hair follicles with their associated sebaceous glands, via the sweat ducts, or across the continuous stratum corneum between these appendages (Fig. 22.1). We can summarize relevant features before arriving at a general conclusion.

Sebum and surface material

The layer of sebum mixed with sweat, bacteria, and dead cells is thin (0.4–10 μm), irregular, and discontinuous; it hardly affects percutaneous absorption.

Skin appendages

Their fractional area available for absorption is small (about 0.1%) and this route usually cannot contribute appreciably to the *steady state* flux. However, the route may be important for ions and large polar molecules which cross intact stratum corneum with difficulty. Diseases which disrupt the horny layer, such as eczema and exfoliative dermatitis, allow easy access.

Skin appendages may act as shunts, important

at short times prior to steady state diffusion, e.g. in bioassays which use pharmacological reactions. Thus minute concentrations of nicotinates or corticosteroids penetrating rapidly down the shunt route may trigger erythema or blanching.

Epidermal route

The epidermal barrier function resides mainly in the horny layer, but what about other skin tissues? The viable layers (particularly the epidermis) may metabolize and inactivate a drug, or activate a pro-drug. The dermal papillary layer contains so many capillaries that the average residence time of a drug in the dermis may only be about a minute. Usually, the deeper dermal layers do not influence percutaneous absorption. However, the dermis may bind a hormone such as testosterone, decreasing its systemic removal. If the penetrant is very lipophilic, it crosses the horny layer to meet an aqueous phase in which it is poorly soluble. The chemical potential immediately below the barrier may then become high, approaching that in the barrier. The potential gradient (stratum corneum to viable tissue) falls, together with the flux. The rate-determining step in percutaneous absorption then becomes barrier clearance not barrier penetration.

Because stratum corneum is dead, it is assumed that there are no active transport processes and no fundamental differences between *in vivo* and *in vitro* permeation processes. However, there may be discrepancies in how some substances permeate excised skin and skin *in vivo*. These differences arise because we manipulate the skin to insert it into the diffusion apparatus.

Within the stratum corneum, molecules penetrate either intercellularly or transcellularly. Electron micrographs of intercellular material suggest a segregation of lipid between protein filaments. In hydrated tissue, these lipid and polar regions would provide parallel pathways for diffusion. Molecules would partition into, and diffuse through, either network according to their polarities. The intercellular route is rich in neutral lipid and this pathway may be more important in percutaneous absorption than previously thought.

Topically applied agents such as steroids, hexachlorophane, griseofulvin, sodium fusidate and fusidic acid may form a depot or reservoir by binding within the stratum corneum.

General conclusions

The stratum corneum develops as a thin, tough, relatively impermeable membrane, which usually provides the rate-limiting step in percutaneous absorption. The entire horny layer, not just some specialized region, provides the diffusional resistance. The membrane allows no drug to pass readily, but nearly all penetrate to some extent. The intracellular keratin presents a mosaic of polar and non-polar regions in which substances dissolve and diffuse according to their chemical affinities; the neutral lipid of the intercellular route provides an alternative pathway. Diffusion is passive, governed by physicochemical laws in which active transport plays no part.

For electrolytes and large molecules with low diffusion coefficients, such as polar steroids and antibiotics, the appendages may provide the main entry route.

Once past the horny layer, molecules permeate rapidly through the living tissues and sweep into the systemic circulation.

The fraction of a drug which penetrates the skin via any particular route depends on the physicochemical nature of the drug, the time scale of observation, the site and condition of the skin, the fomulation and how vehicle components change the skin.

PROPERTIES THAT INFLUENCE PERCUTANEOUS ABSORPTION

When we apply a preparation to diseased skin, the clinical result arises from a sequence of processes:

1 release of the medicament from the vehicle, followed by
2 penetration through the skin barriers, and
3 activation of the pharmacological response.

Effective therapy optimizes these steps as they are affected by three components — the drug, the vehicle and the skin.

Figure 22.4, which represents the flux arising from an ointment suspension, illustrates the

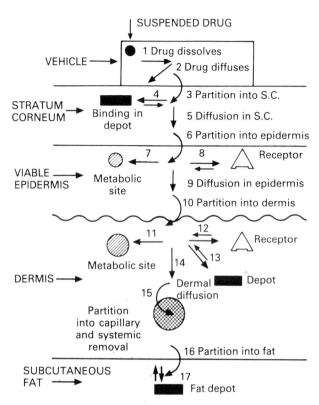

Fig. 22.4 Some stages in percutaneous absorption from a suspension ointment. Emulsion vehicles may also include dissolution and partitioning processes in the internal phase. (Source: Barry 1983. Reproduced with permission of the copyright owner)

complexity of percutaneous absorption. The drug particles must first dissolve so that molecules may diffuse towards the vehicle/stratum corneum interface. They then partition into the stratum corneum and diffuse through it. Some drug may bind at a depot site; the remainder permeates further, meets a second interface, and partitions into the viable epidermis. For a lipophilic species, this partition coefficient may be unfavourable, i.e. less than one. Within the epidermis enzymes may metabolize the drug or it may interact at a receptor site. After passing into the dermis, additional depot regions and metabolic sites may intervene as the drug moves to a capillary, partitions into its wall and out into the blood for systemic removal. A fraction of the diffusant may partition into the subcutaneous fat to form a further depot.

However, there are further complications. The following factors may be important — the non-homogeneity of the tissues, the presence of lymphatics, interstitial fluid, hair follicles and sweat glands, cell division, cell transport to and through the stratum corneum, and cell surface loss. The disease, the healing process, the drug, and vehicle components may progressively modify the skin barrier. As vehicle ingredients diffuse into the skin, cellular debris, sweat and sebum pass into the dermatological, changing its physico-chemical characteristics. Emulsions may invert or crack when rubbed in and volatile solvents may evaporate.

To discuss this complicated process we review the material under headings of biological factors and physicochemical factors. However, because percutaneous absorption is a dynamic process, if one variable changes, it usually causes several effects on drug flux.

Biological factors

Skin age

It is usually assumed that the skins of the fetus, the young and the elderly are more permeable than adult tissue. Children are more susceptible to the toxic effects of drugs and chemicals, partly because of their greater surface area per unit body weight; potent topical steroids, boric acid and hexachlorophane have produced severe side effects and death.

Skin condition

The intact skin is a tough barrier but many agents damage it. Vesicants such as acids and alkalis injure barrier cells and thereby promote penetration, as do cuts, abrasions and dermatitis. In heavy industry, workers' skins may lose their reactivity or 'harden' because of frequent contact with irritant chemicals.

Many solvents open up the complex dense structure of the horny layer. Mixtures of non-polar and polar solvents such as chloroform and methanol remove the lipid fraction, forming artificial shunts through which molecules pass more easily. Solvents such as dimethylsulphoxide (DMSO), dimethylacetamide (DMA) and dimethylformamide (DMF) may be employed clinically to potentiate drug absorption.

Disease commonly alters skin condition; fortunately, for biopharmaceutical purposes, we need only an elementary understanding of the gross changes in deranged skin. We are mainly interested in visible damage. Is the skin inflamed, with loss of stratum corneum and altered keratinization? Then permeability increases. Is the organ thickened with corns and calluses or as in ichthyosis? Drug permeation should now decrease. In diseases characterized by a defective stratum corneum, percutaneous absorption usually increases.

After injury or removal of the stratum corneum, within 3 days the skin builds a temporary barrier which persists until the regenerating epidermis can form normal keratinizing cells. Even the first complete layer of new stratum corneum cells formed over a healing layer can markedly reduce permeation.

Regional skin sites

Variations in cutaneous permeability depend on the thickness and nature of the stratum corneum and the density of skin appendages. However, the absorption rate varies widely for a specific substance passing through identical skin sites in different healthy volunteers; the most permeable regions in some individuals compare with the least permeable sites in others. Investigators produce different rank orders for the permeabilities of skin sites; for simple small molecules, the *diffusivity* decreases in the order: plantar, palmar and dorsum of hand, scrotal and postauricular, axillary and scalp, arm, leg, and trunk. (Note that this grading takes no account of different horny layer thicknesses at these sites.)

Because of the relatively high permeability and ease of access, the hyoscine Transderm system employs the postauricular skin to insert drugs percutaneously into the blood stream. Here, the layers of stratum corneum are thinner and less dense, there are more sweat and sebaceous glands per unit area and many capillaries reach closer to

the surface, increasing its temperature by 4–6 °C relative to the thigh.

Skin metabolism

The skin metabolizes steroid hormones, chemical carcinogens and drugs. Such metabolism may determine the therapeutic efficacy of topically applied compounds (particularly pro-drugs) and the carcinogenic responses in the skin.

Circulatory effects

Theoretically, changes in the peripheral circulation could affect percutaneous absorption; an increased blood flow could reduce the time a penetrant remains in the dermis and also raise the concentration gradient across the skin. Usually, the effect is negligible. In clinically hyperaemic skin, any increase in absorption almost always arises because the disease damages the skin barrier. Potent rubefacients such as nicotinic acid esters would also only have a significant effect after damaging the skin. Potent vasoconstricting agents such as topical steroids could reduce their own clearance rate or that of another drug.

Species differences

Mammalian skins differ widely in characteristics such as horny layer thickness, sweat gland and hair follicle densities and pelt condition. The capillary blood supply and the sweating ability differ between humans and common laboratory animals. Such factors affect the routes of penetration and the resistance to permeation. Frequently, mice, rats and rabbits are used to assess percutaneous absorption, but their skins have more hair follicles than human skin and they lack sweat glands. Subtle biochemical differences between human and animal skin may alter reactions between penetrants and skin.

Comparative studies on skin penetration indicate that, in general, monkey and pig skins are most like that of man; hairless mouse skin has some similar characteristics. Rabbit, rat, and guinea pig skins are highly permeable and the skin of a Mexican hairless dog has different characteristics to those of man.

Physicochemical factors

Factor interactions

The factors controlling the passive diffusion of a solute from a vehicle into the skin arise from the molecular properties of the diffusant, the vehicle, and the skin. We can identify three interactions composed of two factors, i.e. drug/skin, vehicle/skin, drug/vehicle, and one three-factor interaction, i.e. drug/vehicle/skin.

Drug/skin interactions

Skin hydration When water saturates the skin, the tissue swells, softens, and wrinkles and its permeability increases markedly. A compound which efficiently hydrates the skin could improve the treatment of dry, scaly dermatoses. The search for a *natural moisturizing factor* (NMF) has been an important project in the cosmetic industry. There are many candidates for the title of NMF, including free fatty acids, pyrrolidone carboxylic acid, urea, sodium, calcium, potassium, lactate, a sugar/protein complex, or mixtures of these.

Urea moisturizes the skin and is a mild keratolytic. Both effects promote skin penetration and therefore some topical anti-inflammatory steroid preparations include urea (e.g. Alphaderm and Calmurid HC).

Drug/skin binding This may be important, particularly for surface-active agents, sunscreens (where skin substantivity may be important), for drugs such as the topical steroids which form reservoirs in the stratum corneum, and for the priming dose of drugs released from the Transderm system and other controlled release devices.

Vehicle/skin interactions

A pharmaceutical vehicle may change the physical state and permeability of the skin. The mechanism will probably be a solvent action on the stratum corneum, a hydration effect, or an alteration of skin temperature. Often more than one process operates but we shall consider each effect separately.

Vehicle effects on skin hydration Occlusive vehicles such as fats and oils reduce water loss, increase the moisture content of the skin, and thus promote drug penetration. A dramatic example is the use of occlusive plastic films in topical steroid treatment, when the penetration of the steroid often increases tenfold.

Water-in-oil emulsions are less occlusive than lipid material but more occlusive than oil-in-water emulsions.

Powders, either as dusting powders or in lotions, provide a large surface area for evaporation and dry the skin.

Commercial products are often promoted as skin softeners with the presumption that they increase the skin's moisture content. However, they often contain humectants such as glycerol, propylene glycol or polyethylene glycol and emulsifiers which actually withdraw moisture from the skin.

Table 22.1 summarizes the effects which dermatological bases may exert on skin hydration and permeability.

Effect of temperature The penetration rate of material through human skin can change tenfold for a large temperature variation. Adequate clothing on most of the body would prevent wide fluctuations in temperature and penetration rates. Occlusive vehicles increase skin temperature by a few degrees, but any consequent increase permeability is small compared to the effect of hydration.

Penetration enhancers Substances exist which temporarily diminish the impermeability of the skin. Such materials, if they are safe and non-toxic, can be used clinically to enhance the penetration rate of drugs and possibly even to treat patients systemically by the dermal route. The attributes of the ideal penetration enhancer are:

1 The material should be pharmacologically inert.
2 It should be non-toxic, non-irritating, and non-allergenic.
3 The action should be immediate and the effect should be suitable and predictable.
4 Upon removal of the material, the skin should immediately and fully recover its normal barrier property.
5 The enhancer should not cause loss of body fluids, electrolytes or other endogeneous materials.

Table 22.1 Expected effects of common vehicles on skin hydration and skin permeability — in approximate order of decreasing hydration

Vehicle	Examples/constituents	Effect on skin hydration	Effect on skin permeability
Occlusive dressing	Plastic film, unperforated waterproof plaster	Prevents water loss; full hydration	Marked increase
Lipophilic	Paraffins, oils, fats, waxes, fatty acids, alcohols, esters, silicones	Prevents water loss; may produce full hydration	Marked increase
Absorption base	Anhydrous lipid material plus water/oil emulsifiers	Prevents water loss; marked hydration	Marked increase
Emulsifying base	Anhydrous lipid material plus oil/water emulsifiers	Prevents water loss; marked hydration	Marked increase
Water/oil emulsion	Oily creams	Retards water loss; raised hydration	Increase
Oil/water emulsion	Aqueous creams	May donate water; slight hydration increase	Slight increase?
Humectant	Water-soluble bases, glycerol, glycols	May withdraw water; decreased hydration	Can decrease or act as penetration enhancer
Powder	Clays, organics, inorganics, 'shake' lotions	Aid water evaporation; decreased *excess* hydration	Little effect on stratum corneum

Source: Barry (1983). Reproduced with permission of the copyright owner.

6 It should be compatible with all drugs and excipients.

7 The substance should be a good solvent for drugs.

8 The material should be cosmetically acceptable (good spreadability and skin 'feel').

9 The chemical should formulate into all the variety of preparations used topically.

10 It should be odourless, tasteless, colourless and inexpensive.

No single material possesses all these desirable properties. However, some substances exhibit several of these attributes and they have been investigated clinically or in the laboratory.

Probably the most effective penetration enhancers are aprotic solvents such as dimethylsulphoxide (DMSO), dimethylformamide (DMF) and dimethylacetamide (DMA) (see Fig. 22.5). They accelerate the skin penetration of many compounds including water, dyes, barbiturates, steroids, griseofulvin, phenylbutazone, local anaesthetics, antibiotics and quaternary ammonium compounds. The solvents may also enhance reservoirs in the stratum corneum, e.g. topical corticosteroids and griseofulvin. Although the discovery of the rapid skin penetration of DMSO suggested a major advance in dermatological therapy, the initial enthusiasm has been tempered because of irritant action, odour and toxicity. However, it appears that toxicity dangers were over-rated and DMSO is again being used in topical products, although its metabolite, dimethylsulphide, produces a foul breath.

The pyrrolidones can be used with a variety of compounds to promote penetration and to establish drug reservoirs in the stratum corneum and in the nails. A newcomer to the market is Azone (an azacycloalkane-2-one) which has been used with antibacterials, antifungals, steroids, iododeoxyuridine and 5-fluorouracil.

Surface-active agents may promote absorption down the appendages by reducing interfacial tensions. Surfactants (particularly anionics) alter stratum corneum penetration by changing the protein helices. The surfactant attaches to the protein and forces polar groups into the interior of the helices. In this configuration fewer charged groups are available on the helix surface to interact with, and slow down, the permeation of water, ions and hydrogen bonding solutes. Long chain derivatives of sulphoxides, such as decylmethylsulphoxide, probably exert their penetration enhancing effect at low concentrations via their surface-active properties.

Combinations of oleic acid or oleyl alcohol with

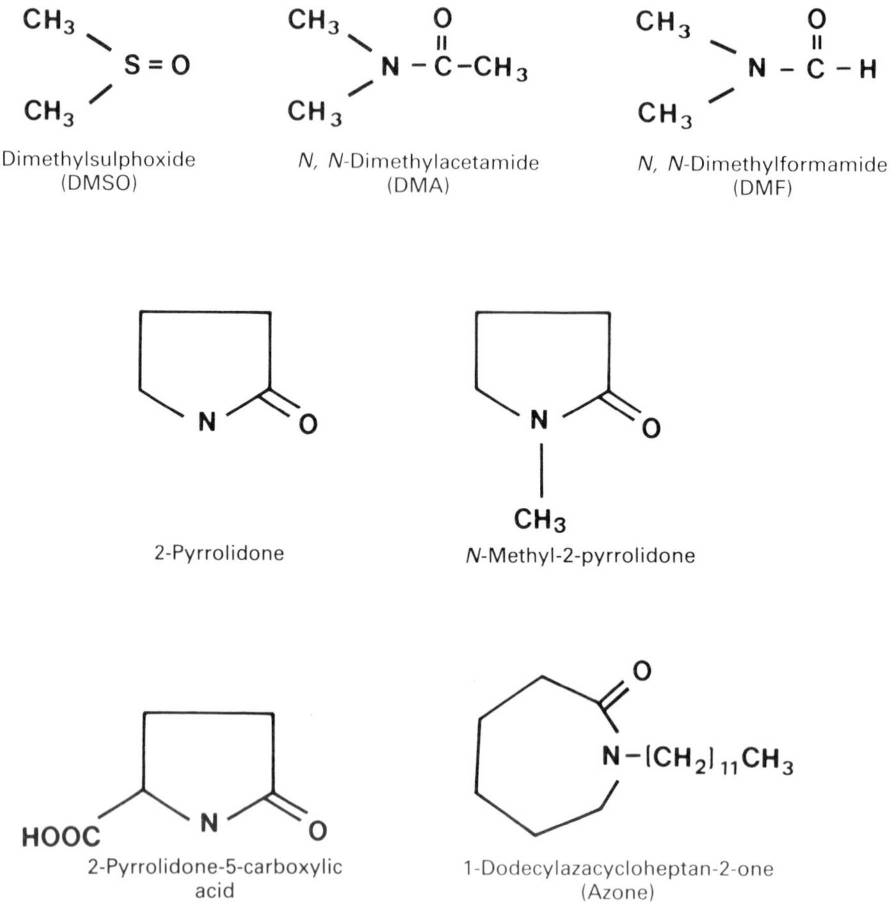

Dimethylsulphoxide
(DMSO)

N, N-Dimethylacetamide
(DMA)

N, N-Dimethylformamide
(DMF)

2-Pyrrolidone

N-Methyl-2-pyrrolidone

2-Pyrrolidone-5-carboxylic
acid

1-Dodecylazacycloheptan-2-one
(Azone)

Fig. 22.5 Formulae of some penetration enhancers

propylene glycol are efficient enhancers for some molecules. Low concentrations of propylene glycol or ethanol are not potent enhancers.

For safety and effectiveness, the best penetration enhancer of all is water. Nearly all substances penetrate better through hydrated stratum corneum than through the dry tissue. Thus, any chemical which is pharmacologically inactive, non-damaging and which promotes horny layer hydration, can be considered as a penetration enhancer. Examples include the natural moisturizing factor and urea.

Drug/vehicle interactions

Here we consider situations in which the impermeability of the stratum corneum is not important. Then the release of the drug from the vehicle provides the rate-limiting step and the skin functions as a sink. This could happen to a patient with a disrupted or absent horny layer or when drug diffusion in the vehicle is exceptionally slow. The vehicle also provides the rate-controlling mechanism in many release studies which use either no membrane or an artificial permeable membrane. Such experiments may correlate with clinical treatment only for patients with severely damaged skin. We can also consider here the Transdermal Therapeutic System (TTS) and similar delivery systems, in which the appliance provides the rate-limiting step for percutaneous absorption leading to systemic therapy.

When diffusion within the vehicle provides the rate-controlling step, our mathematical treatment assumes that the skin is a sink and maintains essentially zero concentration of the penetrating material by rapidly passing it to the circulation. Then the concentration gradient develops solely in the applied material. Two important cases are absorption from solution and from suspension.

Absorption from solution: skin a perfect sink
We can deduce an equation applying to the release of penetrant from one side of a layer of vehicle on the skin under the following conditions.

1 Only a single drug species is important, in true solution, initially uniformly distributed through the vehicle.
2 Only the drug diffuses out of the vehicle. Other components do not diffuse or evaporate and skin secretions do not pass into the vehicle.
3 The diffusion coefficient does not alter with time or position within a vehicle.
4 When the penetrant reaches the skin it absorbs instantaneously.

Under these limitations Eqn 22.8 represents the relationship between m, the quantity of drug released to the sink per unit area of application, with C_o, the initial concentration of solute in the vehicle, D_v, the diffusion coefficient of the drug in the vehicle and t, the time after application.

$$m \simeq 2C_o \left(\frac{D_v t}{\pi}\right)^{\frac{1}{2}} \qquad (22.8)$$

Differentiating this equation provides the release rate, dm/dt, from

$$\frac{dm}{dt} \simeq C_o \left(\frac{D_v}{\pi t}\right)^{\frac{1}{2}} \qquad (22.9)$$

Figure 22.6 illustrates plots of a typical release experiment for betamethasone 17-benzoate dissolved at various concentrations in a polar gel and diffusing into a chloroform sink. According to Eqn 22.8 a plot of m versus $t^{\frac{1}{2}}$ should provide a straight line, as Fig. 22.7 illustrates. A relationship such as Eqn 22.8 or a modification in which m is still proportional to $t^{\frac{1}{2}}$ often fits data outside the limits used originally to define the equation, i.e. up to 65% release instead of only about 30%.

According to these equations we may alter the release rate of a drug from solution and hence its bioavailability by changing drug concentration or the diffusion coefficient.

Absorption from suspensions: skin a perfect sink The amount released and the rate of release

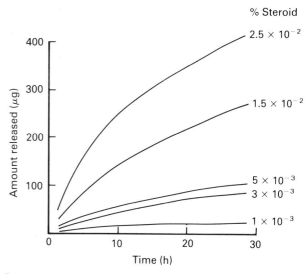

% Steroid

Fig. 22.6 *In vitro* release of betamethasone-17-benzoate from gel formulations as a function of time: steroid strength indicated on plots. (Source: Barry 1983. Reproduced with permission of the copyright owner)

of a drug suspended in a vehicle such as an ointment may be related to time and to the variables of the system. The relevant equations are derived for a simple model system under the following conditions:

1 The suspended drug is micronized so that particle diameters are much smaller than the vehicle layer thickness.
2 The particles are uniformly distributed and do not sediment in the vehicle.
3 The total amount of drug, soluble and suspended, per unit volume (A) is much greater than C_s, the solubility of the drug in the vehicle.
4 The surface to which the vehicle is applied is immiscible with the vehicle, i.e. skin secretions do not enter the vehicle.
5 Only the drug diffuses out of the vehicle; vehicle components neither diffuse nor evaporate.
6 The receptor, which is the skin, operates as a perfect sink.

We can then obtain an equation which relates m to t in the form

$$m = [D_v t(2A - C_s)C_s]^{\frac{1}{2}} \qquad (22.10)$$

This equation holds essentially for all times less than that corresponding to complete depletion of

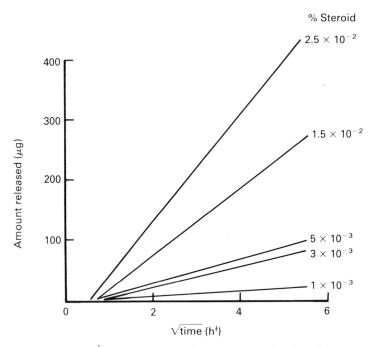

Fig. 22.7 *In vitro* release of betamethasone-17-benzoate from gel formulations as a function of the square root of time: steroid strength indicated on the plots. (Source: Barry 1983. Reproduced with permission of the copyright owner)

the suspended phase. If we differentiate Eqn 22.10 with respect to time, we obtain the instantaneous rate of release dm/dt given by

$$\frac{dm}{dt} = \frac{1}{2}\left(\frac{D_v(2A - C_s)C_s}{t}\right)^{\frac{1}{2}} \quad (22.11)$$

For a common condition in which the solubility of the drug in the vehicle is very small and A is appreciable (i.e. $A >> C_s$), Eqn. 22.10 simplifies to

$$m \simeq (2AD_vC_st)^{\frac{1}{2}} \quad (22.12)$$

Then Eqn 22.11 becomes

$$\frac{dm}{dt} \simeq \left(\frac{AD_vC_s}{2t}\right)^{\frac{1}{2}} \quad (22.13)$$

These equations indicate that the formulator can manipulate drug bioavailability from ointment suspensions by altering the diffusion coefficient, the total concentration, or the solubility. However, Eqn 22.13 predicts that $dm/dt \propto A^{\frac{1}{2}}$; doubling A only increases dm/dt by about 40%.

For obvious reasons Eqns 22.8–22.13 are often referred to as 'square root of time' equations.

Transdermal Therapeutic Systems   A Transdermal Therapeutic System (TTS, Transiderm or Transderm) is a device which releases drug to the skin at a controlled rate well below the maximum that the tissue can accept. Thus, the device, not the stratum corneum, controls the rate at which a drug diffuses through the skin.

A TTS tries to provide systemic therapy in a more convenient and effective way than a parenteral or oral therapy. The claimed advantages for the percutaneous over the oral route include:

1 Drug administration through skin eliminates variables which influence gut absorption, such as changes in pH along the gastrointestinal tract, food and fluid intake, stomach emptying time and intestinal motility and transit time (see Chapter 9).
2 Drug enters the systemic circulation directly, eliminating the 'first pass' effect of the liver, the body's main metabolizing organ. (But note that skin produces enzymes.)

3 Transdermal input may provide controlled, constant drug administration, displaying a single pharmacological effect. The continuity of input may permit the use of drugs with short half-lives and improve patient compliance.

4 Percutaneous administration could eliminate pulse entry into the circulation. Peaks in plasma concentrations often produce undesirable effects and troughs may be subtherapeutic.

5 The transdermal route can use drugs with a low therapeutic index.

Transdermal systems only contain potent drugs, e.g. with dosage not exceeding about 2 mg per day. The compounds must not irritate or sensitize the skin and they must be stable and have the correct physicochemical properties to partition into the stratum corneum and permeate to the vasculature.

A TTS has been considered for, e.g. ephedrine, chlorpheniramine, hyoscine, clonidine, oestradiol and nitroglycerin, together with some experimental drugs. Figure 22.8 is a diagram of the hyoscine device; the multilayer laminate contains a reservoir of drug in a polymeric gel sandwiched between an impermeable backing sheet and a rate-controlling microporous membrane. A contact adhesive (containing additional hyoscine) secures the system to the skin behind the ear and liberates priming drug to saturate skin binding sites. The controlled input of hyoscine acts as an antiemetic during motion sickness, prevents the nausea and vomiting which are side effects of anticancer agents, and treats vertigo.

Drug/vehicle/skin interactions

Usually we cannot disregard the impermeability of the stratum corneum as this layer provides the rate-limiting step in percutaneous absorption. The assumptions made in analysing relevant data include:

1 Stratum corneum provides the rate-limiting step.

2 Skin is a homogeneous intact membrane; appendages are unimportant.

3 Only a single non-ionic drug species is important, dissolving to an ideal solution unaffected by pH, and dissolution is not rate-limiting.

4 Only drug diffuses from the vehicle. Formulation components neither diffuse nor evaporate and skin secretions do not dilute the vehicle.

5 Diffusion coefficient is constant with time or position in the vehicle or horny layer.

6 Penetrant reaching viable tissue sweeps into the circulation, maintaining sink conditions below the stratum corneum.

7 Donor phase depletes negligibly, i.e. constant drug concentration in the vehicle.

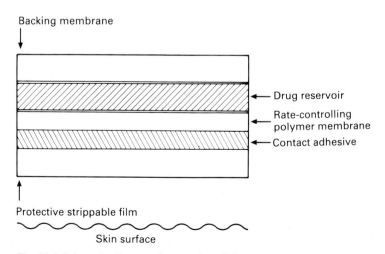

Fig. 22.8 Schematic diagram of a transdermal therapeutic system

8 Vehicle does not alter skin permeability during an experiment by, for example, changing stratum corneum hydration or by acting as a penetration enhancer.

9 Drug remains intact and unaltered.

10 Flux estimates are steady state values.

Most analyses use Eqn 22.3, assume that h, the stratum corneum thickness, is constant and relate changes in the penetration rate to variations in the other three parameters.

An alternative form of Eqn 22.3 uses thermodynamic activities. Thus

$$\frac{\mathrm{d}m}{\mathrm{d}t} = \frac{aD}{\gamma h} \qquad (22.14)$$

where a is the thermodynamic activity of the drug in its vehicle and γ is the effective activity coefficient in the skin barrier. To obtain the maximum rate of penetration we should use the drug at its highest thermodynamic activity, i.e. the pure form. The conclusion, therefore, is that all vehicles which contain the drug as a finely ground suspension (in which the solution activity is maximal and equal to that of the solid) should produce the same penetration rate, *provided that assumptions 1–10 remain valid*.

A few additional comments on diffusion parameters in skin permeation are relevant here. The diffusion coefficient, D, measures how easily a molecule diffuses through the stratum corneum; the measured value may reflect influences other than intrinsic mobility. For example, some drug may bind and become immobilized within the stratum corneum and this affects the magnitude of D. However, regardless of such complications, the value of D measures the penetration rate of a molecule under specified conditions and is therefore useful to know.

The drug flux is related to the partition coefficient K. Once it was incorrectly thought that good skin penetration required a K close to unity. However, many congeneric series of molecules display an *optimal* K, well below which they are too water soluble to partition well into the horny layer. At higher values, the compounds are so lipid soluble they do not readily pass from the stratum corneum into the water-rich viable tissue.

For a drug series, this behaviour produces a parabolic or bilinear relation between pharmacological activity and partition coefficient.

Topical steroids provide a good example of the importance of the partition coefficient. Thus, triamcinolone is five times more active systemically than hydrocortisone but it exhibits only about one-tenth the topical activity. Triamcinolone acetonide, with a more favourable K value, shows a 1000-fold increase in cutaneous activity. Betamethasone possesses only 10 times the topical potency of hydrocortisone although it is some 30 times stronger systemically. Of the 23 esters of betamethasone tested, the 17-valerate has the highest topical activity and this coincides with the most balanced lipid/water partition coefficient. The anti-inflammatory responses to hydrocortisone and its C-21 esters behave similarly. As the side chain lengthens from 0 to 6 carbon atoms, the partition coefficient increases as does the anti-inflammatory index. Thereafter the activity declines as the homologous series extends and the partition coefficient further increases.

METHODS FOR STUDYING PERCUTANEOUS ABSORPTION

Experiments in percutaneous absorption may be designed to answer many questions, such as

1 What is the drug flux through the skin and how do the apparent diffusion coefficient, partition coefficient, and structure activity relationships control it?

2 What is the main penetration route — across the stratum corneum or via the appendages?

3 Which is more important clinically or toxicologically — transient diffusion (possibly down the appendages) or steady state permeation (usually across the intact stratum corneum)?

4 Does the drug bind to the stratum corneum, the viable epidermis or the dermis; does it form a depot in the subcutaneous fat?

5 What is the rate-limiting step — drug dissolution or diffusion within the vehicle, partitioning into, or diffusion through, the skin layers, or removal by the blood, lymph, or tissue fluids?

6 How do skin condition, age, site, blood flow and metabolism affect topical bioavailability? Are differences between animal species important?

7 How do vehicles modify the release and absorption of the medicament? What is the optimal formulation for a specific drug — an aerosol spray, a solution, suspension, gel, powder, ointment, cream, paste, tape, or delivery device?

8 Are vehicle components inert, or do they modify the permeability of the stratum corneum if only by changing its hydration?

9 To increase drug flux, should we use penetration enhancers; alternatively, does a potent drug need retarding?

10 Is the formulation designed correctly to treat intact stratum corneum, thickened epidermis or damaged skin?

11 Should the experimental design produce a pharmacokinetic profile, measuring absorption, distribution, metabolism and excretion?

No single method can answer all questions and provide a full picture of the complex process of percutaneous absorption. We will deal with the important general techniques, dividing them into in vivo and in vitro procedures. The former class uses the skins of living humans or experimental animals in situ, whereas the latter employs isolated membranes and includes simple release studies.

In vitro methods

Because the investigator closely controls laboratory conditions, these are valuable techniques for screening and for measuring fluxes, partition coefficients and diffusion coefficients.

Release methods without a rate-limiting membrane

These procedures record drug release to a simple immiscible phase. They measure only those drug/vehicle interactions which affect release characteristics and they do not determine skin absorption. Typical arrangements are shown in Fig. 22.9; Eqns 22.8–22.13 may be used to analyse results.

Diffusion methods with a rate-controlling membrane

Simulated skin membrane Because human skin is variable and difficult to obtain, workers use other materials, e.g. cellulose acetate, silicone

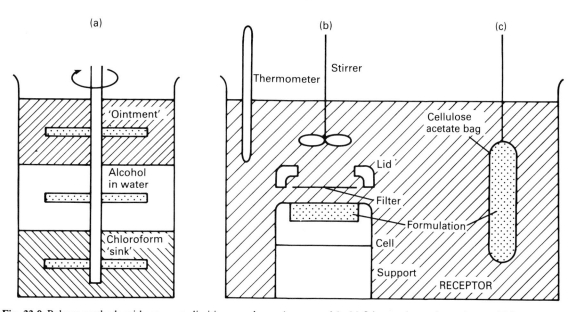

Fig. 22.9 Release methods without a rate-limiting membrane (not to scale). (a) Stirrer agitates three phases which represent the formulation, the skin and the blood supply. (b) Release from an open container to a stirred immiscible receptor phase. (c) Release through a simple dialysis membrane. (Source: Barry 1983. Reproduced with permission of the copyright owner)

rubber, isopropyl myristate, or egg shell membrane. However, these membranes are not as complex as human skin.

Natural skin membrane Excised skins from rats, mice (normal and hairless), rabbits, guinea pigs, hamsters, pigs, hairless dogs, monkeys etc. have been mounted in diffusion cells. However, mammalian skin varies widely in stratum corneum properties and the number density of appendages. Thus, it is best to obtain human skin from autopsies, amputations or cosmetic surgery. Investigators use either stratum corneum or whole skin clamped in a diffusion cell and measure the compound passing from the stratum corneum side through to a fluid bath.

Diffusion cells: steady state flux A well-stirred donor solution at constant concentration releases penetrant through a membrane into an agitated 'sink' receptor liquid simulating the blood supply (Fig. 22.10). Figure 22.11 shows how three important quantities vary with time — that entering the membrane, that passing through (see also Fig. 22.3 and Eqns 22.3 and 22.4) and that remaining in the membrane.

Diffusion cells: simulation of in vivo conditions Cells for imitating topical therapy use an

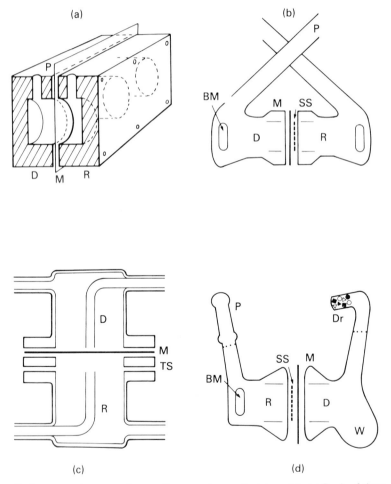

Fig. 22.10 Diffusion cells for zero order or steady state flux experiments (not to scale). (a) Bank of three cells drilled from a Perspex block. (b) Simple glass diffusion cell suitable for human skin. (c) Glass cell with continuously circulating donor and receptor solutions. (d) Glass cell used for determining vapour diffusion through the skin. *Key:* D, donor compartment; R, receptor compartment; M, membrane; P, sampling port; BM, bar magnet; SS, stainless steel support; TS, Teflon support; W, well; Dr, drierite. (Source: Barry 1983. Reproduced with permission of the copyright owner)

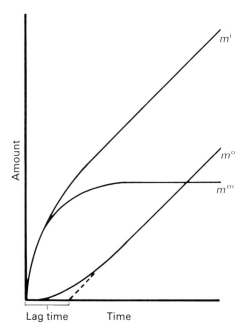

Fig. 22.11 Amount of penetrant entering the membrane (m^i), diffusing through (m^o) and being sorbed (m^m) under zero order flux conditions. (Source: Barry 1983. Reproduced with permission of the copyright owner)

agitated receptor solution to correspond to the blood and an unmixed donor phase to represent the formulation (Fig. 22.12). The donor compartment may be closed or open to ambient conditions or to controlled temperature and humidity; the skin may be washed or materials added during an experiment. The test formulation may be a solid deposited from a volatile solvent, a liquid, a semisolid, a film or a drug device.

In vivo methods

Animal models

Most animals differ significantly from man in features which affect percutaneous absorption: the thickness and nature of the stratum corneum, the density of hair follicles and sweat glands, the nature of the pelt, the papillary blood supply and biochemical aspects. Few techniques produce animal diseases similar to human afflictions. Thus animal models are valuable for studying the anatomy, physiology and biochemistry of skin, for screening topical agents, for detecting possible hazards, and for biopharmaceutical investigations.

However, experience with animals cannot substitute for studies in man.

Techniques

Observation of a pharmacological or physiological response If the drug stimulates a reaction in the viable tissues we may use it to determine penetration kinetics. Local allergic, toxic or physiological reactions include sweat gland secretion, pigmentation, sebaceous gland activity, vasodilatation, vasoconstriction, vascular permeability, epidermal proliferation and keratinization. The most productive biopharmaceutical technique has been the vasoconstrictor or blanching response to topical steroids. For example, Fig. 22.13 illustrates the blanching profiles of betamethasone benzoate in a quick-break aerosol foam, in the foam concentrate and in semisolids, compared with Betnovate Cream. The superiority of the aerosol foam and the inferiority of the benzoate cream are apparent. We use the vasoconstrictor test to screen novel synthetic steroids and develop topical formulations, to test marketed products for bioavailability and clinical efficacy, to perform fundamental studies in percutaneous absorption, and to develop dosage regimens.

Other response methods include changes in blood pressure (e.g. topical application of nitroglycerin), reduction in pain threshold, and production of convulsions.

Physical properties of the skin Relevant methods include measurement of transepidermal water loss, thermal determinations, mechanical analysis, use of ultrasound, classification of function and dimension, spectral analysis, and the use of photoacoustic and electrical properties.

Analysis of body tissues or fluids When urinary analysis is used, all drug penetrating the skin should be accounted for by 'calibrating' the subject with a slow intravenous injection and a simultaneous determination of blood levels, to allow for all pharmacokinetic factors inherent in drug absorption, distribution, storage, metabolism and excretion. Analysis of circulating blood can present difficulties with dilution, extraction and detection, although nanogram drug quantities may

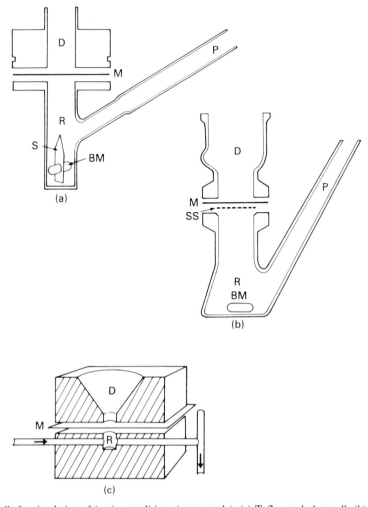

Fig. 22.12 Diffusion cells for simulation of *in vivo* conditions (not to scale). (a) Teflon and glass cell. (b) Glass cell with stainless steel support for the membrane. (c) Stainless stell cell with flow through receptor solution.
Key: D, donor compartment; R, receptor compartment; M, membrane; P, sampling port; BM, bar magnet; S, polyethylene sail; SS, stainless steel support. (Source: Barry 1983. Reproduced with permission of the copyright owner)

now be detected. Faeces analysis alone has limited use. Sometimes the drug has an affinity for an animal organ which can be removed and analysed, e.g. for iodine, iodides and mercury. Tissue biopsies may be analysed and even individual sections measured.

Surface loss We should be able to determine the flux of material into skin from the loss rate from the vehicle (see Fig. 22.11). However, because of skin impermeability, the concentration decrease would generally be small and analytical techniques would have to be sensitive and accu-

rate. Also those differences detectable would probably arise because the vehicle changed by evaporation or by dilution with sweat or transepidermal water. Alternatively, any drug decrease may only reflect deposition on the skin surface or combination with the stratum corneum rather than penetration to the systemic circulation. Loss techniques have mainly been used to monitor radioactive species.

Histology Experimenters may try to locate skin penetration routes from microscopic sections; however, the cutting, handling and development

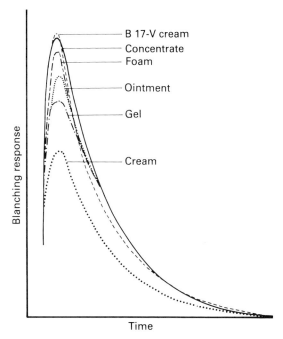

Fig. 22.13 Blanching response to betamethasone benzoate formulations containing 0.025% steroid and 0.1% betamethasone 17-valerate (B 17-V) cream. (Source: Barry 1983. Reproduced with permission of the copyright owner)

of skin sections encourages leaching and translocation of materials away from their original sites, a problem with histological methods in general.

Histochemical techniques have been used for those few compounds which produce coloured end products after chemical reaction. A common mistake is to colour a penetrant with a dye and examine skin sections to locate the penetrant. However, each species partitions and diffuses separately and so the dyed complex dissociates and results are valid only for the dye. Added dye or other different tracer molecule should not be used.

A few compounds fluoresce, revealing their behaviour by microscopy, e.g. vitamin A, tetracycline and benzpyrene.

Microscopic autoradiography cannot be applied to diffusable substances without modification. Substances emit alpha and beta rays and there may be considerable scattering on the autoradiogram; reducing substances reacting with the photographic emulsion — or an incorrect technique — can produce shadowing. Tritium-labelled isotopes are useful because of their weak emissions; strong beta emitters darken areas up to 2 or 3 mm away, a great distance at the cellular scale.

Bioassays

Many specialized bioassays screen topical formulations prior to clinical trial, including those for antibacterials, antifungals, antiyeast preparations, antimitotics, antiperspirants, sunscreen agents, antidandruff, anaesthetic–analgesic formulations, antipruritics, antiwart, poison oak/ivy dermatitis, antiacne and psoriasis. Topical corticosteroid bioassays are the most sophisticated and refined of all such bioassays (see previously); other steroid bioassays include antigranuloma, thymus involution, inflammation, cytological techniques and psoriasis bioassays.

FORMULATION OF DERMATOLOGICAL VEHICLES

People apply many skin preparations ranging from powders, through semisolids, to liquids. Formulators have often developed such preparations for stability, compatibility, and patient acceptability rather than considering the influences that the components may have on drug bioavailability.

The best method of approach in designing a vehicle for optimum bioavailability is to use fundamental permeation theories, while remembering that the treatment regimen and the diseased skin usually violate the constraints of simple diffusion theory. However, with our present knowledge, such a formal approach may limit the investigator to a single-phase system such as a polar gel; multiphase systems usually provide intractable theoretical problems. But physicians usually want a topical application to provide several therapeutic effects as well as good absorption. These aims include anti-inflammatory efficacy in acute inflammation, symptomatic relief of pain and itch, protection from irritation, cleansing, and lubricant and emollient actions. A single-phase vehicle cannot readily achieve so much; we need complex multicomponent bases.

This section considers the formulation of bases

mainly in terms of *unmedicated* preparations. A good base must foster the remarkable recuperative capability of skin. It is often as important to select a vehicle which promotes healing and does no further damage as it is to apply a therapeutic agent. A general rule is that for wet lesions the patient should use an aqueous dressing, and for dry skin a lipophilic base is best. Most vehicles are blended from one or more of three main components — aqueous, powder and oil — together with thickening and emulsifying agents, buffers, antioxidants, preservatives, colours, propellants etc. We shall consider typical examples of the main types of skin preparation.

Dermatological formulations

Liquid preparations

Liquid preparations for external application include simple soaks or baths, applications, liniments, lotions, paints, varnishes, tinctures, and ear drops. A simple soak provides an active ingredient in aqueous solution or suspension, sometimes with water-miscible solvents. Gums and gelling agents may vary the consistency from mobile liquids to stiff ringing gels. Bath additives such as Oilatum Emollient deposit a layer of liquid paraffin on the stratum corneum in an attempt to maintain its moisture content. Applications may be liquid or viscous preparations and often incorporate parasiticides, e.g. dicophane, benzyl benzoate, gamma benzene hexachloride, and malathion. Liniments may be alcoholic or oily solutions or emulsions which should not be applied to broken skin. Lotions are aqueous solutions or suspensions from which water evaporates to leave a thin uniform coating of powder. Evaporation cools and soothes the skin, making lotions valuable for treating acutely inflamed areas. Alcohol enhances the cooling effect and glycerol sticks the powder to the skin. Lotions may also be dilute emulsions, usually of the oil-in-water type. Paints, varnishes and tinctures present solutions of active ingredients in volatile solvents such as water, industrial methylated spirits, acetone, or ether. Ear drops are often aqueous solutions although glycerol and alcohol may also be used.

Gels (jellies)

Gels are two-component semisolid systems rich in liquid. Their one characteristic feature is the presence of a continuous structure providing solid-like properties. In a typical polar gel, a natural or synthetic polymer builds a three-dimensional matrix throughout a hydrophilic liquid. Typical polymers used include the natural gums tragacanth, carrageenan, pectin, agar and alginic acid; semisynthetic materials such as methylcellulose, hydroxyethylcellulose, hydroxypropylmethylcellulose, and carboxymethylcellulose; and the synthetic polymer Carbopol. We may also use certain clays such as bentonite, Veegum and Laponite. Provided that the drug does not bind to the polymer or clay, such gels release medicaments well; the pores allow relatively free diffusion of molecules which are not too large.

Powders

Dusting powders for application to skin folds have finely divided (impalpable) insoluble powders which dry, protect and lubricate, e.g. talc, zinc oxide, starch and kaolin. Dusting powders should not contain boric acid since abraded skin may absorb it in toxic amounts.

Ointments

Ointments are greasy, semisolid preparations, often anhydrous and containing dissolved or dispersed medicaments.

Hydrocarbon bases These usually consist of soft paraffin or mixtures with hard paraffin. Paraffins form a greasy film on the skin, inhibiting moisture loss and improving hydration of the horny layer in dry scaly conditions. This hydration is also a main reason why ointments are so effective in encouraging percutaneous absorption.

The Plastibases are a series of hydrocarbons containing polyethylene which forms a structural matrix in systems which are fluid at the molecular scale but are typical dermatological semisolids. They are soft, smooth, homogeneous, neutral, colourless, odourless, non-irritating, non-sensitizing, extremely stable vehicles. Plastibases are compatible with most medicaments and they maintain their consistency even at high concentrations of solids and under extremes of temperature. The bases apply easily and spread readily, adhere to the skin, imparting a velvety, non-greasy feel, and can readily be removed.

Soap-base greases may be produced by, for example, incorporating aluminium stearate in a heavy mineral oil. A random arrangement of metallic soap fibres weave throughout the oil, producing a product which changes its consistency only slightly when heated; the base readily incorporates drugs and the addition of lanolin permits the absorption of a little water.

Fats and fixed oil bases Dermatological vehicles have frequently contained fixed oils of vegetable origin, consisting essentially of the mono-, di-, and triglycerides of mixtures of saturated and unsaturated fatty acids. The most common oils include peanut, sesame, olive, cotton seed, almond, arachis, maize and persic. Such oils can decompose on exposure to air, light and high temperatures and may turn rancid. Trace metal contaminants catalyse oxidative reactions which the formulator combats with antioxidants such as butylated hydroxytoluene, butylated hydroxyanisole or propyl gallate or with chelating agents such as the salts of ethylenediaminetetra-acetic acid (EDTA). However, antioxidants may be incompatible with the drug or they may sensitize some patients.

Silicones Dimethicones or dimethyl polysiloxanes have properties similar to hydrocarbon bases. They are water repellent with a low surface tension and are incorporated into barrier creams to protect the skin against water-soluble irritants.

Absorption bases Absorption bases soak up water to form water-in-oil emulsions while retaining their semisolid consistencies. Generally, they are anhydrous vehicles composed of a hydrocarbon base and a miscible substance with polar groups which functions as a water-in-oil emulsifier, e.g. lanolin, lanolin isolates, cholesterol, lanosterol and other sterols, acetylated sterols or the partial esters of polyhydric alcohols such as sorbitan monostearate or mono-oleate. Bases such as Wool Alcohols Ointment BP and Simple Ointment BP deposit a greasy film on the skin similar to a hydrocarbon base but they suppress less the transepidermal water loss. However, they may hydrate the stratum corneum by applying a water-in-oil emulsion, thus prolonging the time during which the horny layer can absorb moisture. Some individuals are sensitive to lanolin and this may be important because the sensitization occurs unexpectedly and physicians frequently overlook it, especially in atopic patients who may apply large quantities of lanolin-containing emollients for protracted periods.

Emulsifying bases These essentially anhydrous bases contain oil-in-water emulsifying agents which make them miscible with water and so washable or 'self-emulsifying'. There are three types, depending on the ionic nature of the water-soluble emulsifying agents — anionic (e.g. Emulsifying Ointment BP), cationic (e.g. Cetrimide Emulsifying Ointment BP), or non-ionic (e.g. Cetomacrogol Emulsifying Ointment BPC 1973). Because they contain surfactants, emulsifying bases may help to bring the medicament into more intimate contact with the skin. The bases mix with aqueous secretions and readily wash off the skin; thus they are useful for scalp treatment.

Water-soluble bases Formulators prepare water-soluble bases from mixtures of high and low molecular weight polyethylene glycols (macrogols, Carbowaxes). Suitable combinations provide products with an a ointment-like consistency which soften or melt on skin application. They are non-occlusive, mix readily with skin exudates and do not stain sheets or clothing; washing quickly removes any residue. The macrogols do not hydrolyse, deteriorate, support mould growth or irritate the skin. Examples include Macrogol Ointment BP and Polyethylene Glycol Ointment USNF; because they are water soluble they will not take up more than 8% of an aqueous solution before losing their desirable physicochemical characteristics. To enable a base to incorporate more water we can substitute stearyl alcohol for some of the macrogol component. Macrogol bases are used with local anaesthetics such as lignocaine, but they are incompatible with many chemicals including phenols, iodine, potassium iodide, sorbitol, tannic acid and the salts of silver, mercury and bismuth. The bases diminish the antimicrobial activity of quaternary ammonium compounds and methyl and propyl parahydroxybenzoates and rapidly inactivate bacitracin and penicillin.

Creams

Creams are semisolid emulsions for external application. Oil-in-water emulsions are most useful as water-washable bases whereas water-in-oil emulsions are emollient and cleansing. Patients often prefer a w/o cream to an ointment because the cream spreads more readily, is less greasy and the evaporating water soothes the inflamed tissue. O/w creams ('vanishing' creams) rub into the skin; the continuous phase evaporates and increases the concentration of a water-soluble drug in the adhering film. The concentration gradient for drug across the stratum corneum therefore increases, promoting percutaneous absorption. To minimize drug precipitation a formulator may include a non-volatile, water-miscible cosolvent such as propylene glycol. An o/w cream is non-occlusive because it does not deposit a continuous film of water-impervious liquid. However, such a cream can deposit lipids and other moisturizers on and in the stratum corneum and so restore the tissue's hydration ability, i.e. the preparation has emollient properties.

It is difficult to predict the role which an emulsion plays in percutaneous absorption. This is because, added to all the physiological and physicochemical considerations already discussed in this chapter, must be: the partitioning of the medicament between the emulsion phases; the addition of preservatives; the determination of a true viscosity for the diffusing molecules in the vehicle; and the possibility of phase inversion or cracking of the emulsion when applied to the skin. Drug may also be trapped in micelles present in the continuous phase. Emulsions are complex systems and thus all medicaments must be considered individually with respect to emulsion design, and there are no worthwhile formulation guidelines additional to the principles already discussed.

Pastes

Pastes are ointments containing as much as 50% powder dispersed in a fatty base. They may be useful for absorbing noxious chemicals such as the ammonia which bacteria release from urine. Because of their consistency, pastes localize the action of an irritant or staining material, such as dithranol or coal tar. They are less greasy than ointments because the powder absorbs some of the fluid hydrocarbons. Pastes lay down a thick, unbroken, relatively impermeable film that can be opaque and act as an efficient sun filter. Skiers use such formulations on the face to minimize wind burn (excessive dehydration) and to block out the sun's rays.

Aerosols

Aerosols may function as drug delivery systems for solutions, suspensions, powders, semisolids and emulsions.

Solution aerosols are simple products, with the drug dissolved in a propellant or a propellant/solvent mixture. Typical agents incorporated are steroids, antibiotics, and astringents. The powder aerosol methodology is useful for difficult soluble compounds such as steroids and antibiotics. Semisolid preparations, such as ointments and creams, may be prepared in a flexible bag with compressed nitrogen used for expulsion instead of a volatile propellant. Emulsion systems produce foams which may be aqueous or non-aqueous and stable or quick-breaking. Medicinal stable foams are aqueous formulations used for preoperative shaving, for contraception, and for the treatment of ulcerative colitis. The stable foam, which is similar to a medicated shaving cream, varies in stability depending on the selection of surfactant, solvent and propellant.

Cosmetic or aesthetic criteria for dermatological formulations

However well we design a topical vehicle for maximum drug bioavailability we must still make the preparation acceptable to the patient; a poor product may lead to non-compliance. Patients generally prefer a formulation which is easy to transfer from the container, spreads readily and smoothly, leaves no detectable residue and adheres to the treated area without being tacky or difficult to remove.

Stiff pastes may be hard to rub into the skin or to apply evenly; application to damaged areas may be painful. However, a thick layer of material can occlude the tissue or protect it from mechanical, chemical, or light damage. Ointments and pastes do this and the viscous drag imposed on application may dislodge scales, dead tissue and the remnants of previous doses so that the medicament makes intimate contact with the diseased site. A stiff preparation also helps to delineate the area of treatment.

The sensations of greasiness and tackiness arise from those constituents which form the skin film. For creams, stearic acid and cetyl alcohol produce non-tacky films. Formulations which include synthetic or natural gums should use the minimum amount as the polymers tend to leave a tacky coating on the skin.

Insoluble solids leave an opaque layer, often appearing powdery or crusty. However, as therapy requires such solids in lotions and pastes, the formulator can do little to vary the film's nature and patients accept the residue as part of the treatment.

Physicochemical criteria for dermatological formulations

The developer of dosage forms must note the physical and chemical behaviour of the drug and the dosage form during preformulation studies, throughout bench-scale work, pilot studies and batch processing, at the manufacturing level and during storage and use of a product. Table 22.2 lists general factors which a pharmacist evaluates for a new semisolid during developmental studies and storage.

The first difficulty arises in assessing the chemical stabilities of the drug (in its complex vehicle) and the adjuvants. A general method establishes a shelf-life by using an accelerated stability test at elevated temperatures and the Arrhenius relationship. However, for a multiphase system such as a cream, heat may change the phase distribution and may even crack the emulsion. Thus, the investigator may have to assess the preparation for a long time at the storage temperature. Because of vehicle complexity it may be difficult to separate the labile components for analysis.

Many dermatologicals contain volatile solvents and batches may lose some solvent through the walls of plastic containers or through faulty seams or ill-fitting caps.

Heterogeneous systems may suffer phase changes when stored incorrectly. Emulsions may crack and cream, suspensions can agglomerate and cake, and ointments and gels may 'bleed' as their matrices contract and squeeze out constituents. High temperatures can produce or accelerate such adjustments. Multipoint rheological assessments can readily quantify structural changes in colloidal systems.

For suspensions and emulsions, a particle size analysis may often detect a potentially unstable formulation long before any other parameter changes markedly. Emulsion globules may grow through coalescence as gel networks break down on storage; crystals may enlarge or change their habit or revert to a more stable, less active polymorphic form. Such alterations in crystal form may affect the therapeutic activity of the formulation.

The apparent pH of a topical product may change on storage. Although pH measurements of complex vehicles have no fundamental meaning, investigators sometimes use a pH electrode to monitor formulations as they age.

It can be difficult to manufacture creams and ointments completely free from foreign particles. Aluminium and tin tubes may contaminate a topical with 'flashings' — metal slivers and shavings formed during container fabrication. Their presence is particularly undesirable in ophthalmic ointments and various pharmacopoeial tests limit the extent of such contamination.

In addition to instrumental tests the pharmacist should note any qualitative changes during

Table 22.2 Some physicochemical criteria for pharmaceutical semisolids

Stability of the active ingredients

Stability of the adjuvants

Rheological properties — consistency, extrudability

Loss of water and other volatile components

Phase changes — homogeneity/phase separation, bleeding

Particle size and particle size distribution of dispersed phase

Apparent pH

Particulate contamination

Source: From Flynn (1979).

product storage. The colour may vary, e.g. natural fats, oils and lanolin brown as they oxidize, becoming rancid with a disagreeable odour. The texture may alter as phase relationships vary.

Microbial contamination and preservation; rancidity and antioxidants

Topical bases often contain aqueous and oily phases together with carbohydrates and even proteins and thus bacteria and fungi readily attack them. Microbial growth spoils the formulation and is a potential toxic hazard and a source of infection. Conditions which lower immunity such as injury, debilitating diseases or drug therapy, may encourage organisms that are usually not highly infectious to infect the host, i.e. to become opportunistic pathogens. In 1969, 33 samples of 169 cosmetics and topical drugs surveyed were microbially contaminated, half with Gram-negative organisms which were a health hazard. In the mid-1960s, an outbreak of serious eye infection was traced to an antibiotic ophthalmic ointment contaminated with *Pseudomonas*.

There are many potential sources of microbial contamination. It can occur in raw material and in the manufacturing water, in processing and filling equipment, in packing material, if there is poor plant hygiene or an unclean environment and if plant operatives fail to comply with good manufacturing procedures.

Because of the complexity of dermatological vehicles and their manufacturing processes, there exists no universal preservative, although we can summarize the essential requirements for selecting a material to preserve a specific formulation. The additive must be compatible with all ingredients; it should be stable to heat, prolonged storage and product use conditions; and it must be non-irritant, non-toxic and non-sensitizing to human tissue.

Many prototype pharmaceutical preparations could deteriorate on storage because some components oxidize when oxygen is present. This decomposition can be particularly troublesome in emulsions because emulsification may introduce air into the product and because of the high interfacial contact area between the phases.

The ideal antioxidant would possess the following properties: effective at low concentrations; it and its decomposition products should be non-toxic, non-irritant, non-sensitizing, odourless and colourless; stable and effective over a wide pH range; neutral — should not react chemically with other ingredients; non-volatile.

PROTOCOL FOR DESIGNING, DEVELOPING AND TESTING A DERMATOLOGICAL FORMULATION

Below are listed steps which may help a pharmacist to design a satisfactory formulation. The treatment, although condensed, is valuable for providing a check list to control the development programme.

1 Identify the disease or condition to be treated.
2 Determine the site for drug action — skin surface, stratum corneum, viable epidermis, dermis, appendages or systemic circulation. Consider the body region, e.g. scalp, trunk, feet, nails etc.
3 Note the receptor site within the target area (this may be unknown).
4 Estimate the condition of the average patient's skin — thickened (e.g. ichthyosis), broken and inflamed (e.g. acute eczema), pilosebaceous unit blocked (acne), etc. Remember that successful treatment may rapidly change the condition of the skin. For example, a weeping, wet skin without an intact horny layer may heal quickly to produce a few cell layers with a dry surface.
5 Choose the best drug or pro-drug for the disorder; consider its pharmacological and pharmacokinetic profiles, toxicity, sensitizing potential, stability, susceptibility to skin enzyme metabolism and physicochemical properties (particularly the diffusion coefficient and partition coefficient relevant to the horny layer).
6 Evaluate the optimum kinetics for drug delivery to the target site. Consider pulsed or steady state treatment, amount and strength of dosage form and frequency of application.
7 In the light of points 1–6, select the type of

formulation needed, e.g. cream, ointment, aerosol, delivery device.

8   Decide if and where there is a rate-limiting step in the treatment, e.g. solely within the vehicle, permeation across the stratum corneum or clearance from the viable tissues. Concentrate on maximizing this rate.

9   Choose vehicle ingredients which are stable, compatible, and cosmetically and therapeutically acceptable. Be aware that these adjuvants may have their own therapeutic effects, e.g. occlusive vehicles moisturize the skin.

10   If the intention is to promote drug penetration, optimize the formulation to the maximum chemical potential of the drug. Remember that vehicles often change after application to skin as components evaporate or penetrate the skin and secretions mix with the formulation.

11   If the drug is a poor penetrant, consider using a penetration enhancer but remember that a new enhancer will need a full toxicological screen.

12   Perform *in vitro* tests with trial formulations using a simple synthetic membrane (or no membrane) and a suitable sink; ensure that the drug releases readily from the vehicle.

13   Repeat 12 with human skin to monitor permeation. Such experiments may include a steady state design and a scheme which mimics clinical use.

14   Conduct *in vivo* studies in animals and human volunteers to check for efficacy, safety and acceptability; determine the pharmacokinetic profile and the topical bioavailability.

15   Do clinical trials.

16   Throughout the programme, review the physicochemical behaviour and stability of the dosage form and package during preformulation studies, scale-up procedures, manufacture, storage and use.

REFERENCES AND BIBLIOGRAPHY

Barry, B. W. (1983) *Dermatological Formulations: Percutaneous Absorption*. Dekker, New York and Basel.

Chien, Y. W. (1982) *Novel Drug Delivery Systems*, Chapter 5. Dekker, New York and Basel.

Flynn, G. L. (1979) *Modern Pharmaceutics* (Eds G. S. Banker and C. T. Rhodes), Chapter 8. Dekker, New York and Basel.

Idson, B. (1975) Percutaneous absorption. *J. pharm. Sci.*, **64**, 901–924.

Katz, M. (1973) *Drug Design — Medicinal Chemistry*, Vol. 4 (Ed. E. J. Ariens), Chapter 4, Academic Press, London.

Katz, M. and Poulsen, B. J. (1971) *Handbook of Experimental Pharmacology*, Vol. 28, Pt 1 (Eds B. B. Brodie and J. Gillette, Chapter 7, Springer-Verlag, Berlin.

Poulsen, B. J. (1973) *Drug Design — Medicinal Chemistry*, Vol. 4 (Ed. E. J. Ariens), Chapter 5, Academic Press, London.

Scheuplein, R. J. (1978) *The Physiology and Pathophysiology of the Skin*, Vol. 5 (Ed A. Jarrett), Chapters 54, 55 and 56, Academic Press, London.

Scheuplein, R. J. and Blank, I. H. (1971) Permeability of the skin. *Physiol. Rev.*, **51**, 702–747.

Suppositories and pessaries

SUPPOSITORIES

Introduction

The administration of drugs by routes other than the oral one has to be considered in several circumstances and for a great many varying reasons. Arguments for choosing the rectal route for drug administration include:

1 The patient is not able to make use of the oral route. This may be the case when the patient has an infliction of the gastrointestinal tract, is nauseous, or is postoperative (when the patient may be unconscious or not able to ingest a drug orally). Furthermore several categories of patients, i.e. the very young, the very old or the mentally disturbed, may more easily use the rectal than the oral route.
2 The drug under consideration is less suited for oral administration. This may be so in cases where oral intake results in gastrointestinal side effects, also the drug may be insufficiently stable at the pH of the g.i. tract, or susceptible to enzymatic attack in the g.i. tract or during the first passage of the liver after absorption. Also drugs with an inacceptable taste can be administered rectally without this inconvenience to the patient. The formulation into suppositories of certain drugs that are candidates for abuse, as in suicide, has also been considered.

Besides these apparent advantages, the rectal route also has several drawbacks. Depending on tradition, there are strong feelings of aversion in certain countries, such as the UK and the USA, to rectal administration of drugs, whereas there is complete acceptance on the continent and in Eastern Europe. More rational points in this respect are slow and sometimes incomplete absorption that has been reported and the considerable inter- and intrasubject variation. Also the development of proctitis has been reported. There are also problems with the large scale production of suppositories and of achievement of a suitable shelf life (the latter demanding stringent storage conditions).

It can thus be concluded that rectal administration should certainly not be the route of first choice, but can in certain circumstances be of great advantage to the patient.

The rectal route is used in many different therapies, intended either for local or for systemic effect. *Local effect* is desired in the case of pain and itching mostly due to the occurrence of haemorrhoids. Locally active drugs which are used include astringents, antiseptics, local anaesthetics, vasoconstrictors, anti-inflammatory compounds and soothing and protective agents. Also some laxatives fall into this category. For the attainment of a *systemic effect* all orally given drugs can be used and many are, bearing in mind the limitations discussed above. Antiasthmatic, antirheumatic and analgesic drugs are very much used for this purpose.

Anatomy and physiology of the rectum

Rectal dosage forms are introduced in the body through the anus and are thus brought in the most caudal part of the g.i. tract, i.e. the rectum, Anatomically the rectum is part of the colon, forming the last 150–200 mm of the g.i. tract.

The rectum can be subdivided into the anal canal and the ampulla, the latter forming approximately 80% of the organ. It is separated from the outside world through a circular muscle, the anus. The rectum can be considered as a hollow organ with a relatively flat wall surface, without villi and with only three major folds, the rectal valves. The rectal wall is formed by an epithelium which is one cell layer thick, and is composed of cylindrical cells and of goblet cells which secrete mucus. A diagram of part of the rectal wall and the rectum's veinous drainage is shown in Fig. 23.1.

The total volume of mucus is estimated as approximately 3 ml, spreaded over a total surface area of approximately 300 cm². The pH of the

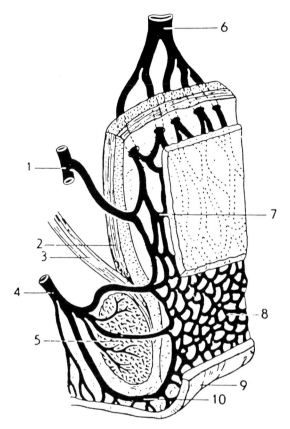

Fig. 23.1 Veinous drainage of the human rectum (after Töndury, 1981): 1 middle rectal vein; 2 tunica muscularis: stratum longitudinale; 3 m. levator ani; 4 inferior rectal vein; 5 m. sphincter ani externus; 6 superior rectal vein; 7 and 8 plexus venosus rectalis (submucosus); 9 skin; 10 v. marginalis. (Source: Töndury G. (1981) *Angewandte und Topographische Anatomie*, 5th edn. Georg Thieme Verlag, Stuttgart. Reproduced by permission of the publishers)

mucous layer is reported as approximately 7.5. Furthermore there seems to be little buffer capacity. This point will be discussed in relation to absorption later on.

Under normal circumstances the rectum is empty and filling provokes a defaecation reflex which is under voluntary control. Data comparing absorption from freshly prepared and aged, more viscous suppositories suggest that there is enough motility to provoke spreading even of rather viscous suppositories.

Absorption of drugs from the rectum

Blood supply, especially veinous drainage, is important for the understanding of drug absorption. As can be seen from Fig. 23.1 there are three separate veins. The lower and middle haemorrhoidal veins drain directly into the general circulation, while the upper one drains into the portal vein which flows to the liver. This means that drug molecules can enter the general circulation directly or by passing through the strongly metabolizing liver. In the latter case only a proportion of the drug molecules (if they are of the high clearance type) will enter the general circulation intact. Thus the bioavailability may be less than 100%. Compared to the small intestine this situation is still more favourable. Recent investigations have shown that avoiding the first passage through the liver is possible; the extent of this effect cannot be generalized since it will depend on the actual part of the rectum through which the drug is absorbed. Thus keeping the drug in the lower part of the rectum would be advisable.

Insertion of a suppository into the rectum results in a chain of effects leading to the bioavailability of the drug. This is represented in a simplified scheme in Fig. 23.2.

Depending on the character of its vehicle (see later) a suppository will either dissolve in the rectal fluid or melt on the mucous layer. Since the volume of rectal fluid is so small dissolution of the complete vehicle will be difficult and require extra

water. Due to osmotic effects (of the dissolving vehicle) water is attracted, with the unpleasant consequence of a painful sensation for the patient. Independent of the vehicle type, drugs that are dissolved in the suppository will diffuse out towards the rectal membranes. Suspended drugs will first have to leave the vehicle (if it is water immiscible) under the influence of either gravity or motility movements and then can start dissolving in the rectal fluid. The dissolved drug molecules will have to diffuse through the mucous layer and then into and through the epithelium forming the rectal wall. The process of absorption will be a passive diffusion process as it is throughout the whole g.i. tract for almost all drugs.

For a generalized discussion on drug absorption the reader is referred to Part 2 of this book. However, some specific points concerning rectal absorption will be discussed here. Table 23.1 gives

Table 23.1 Physiological factors affecting absorption from the rectum

Quantity of fluid available

Properties of rectal mucus

Contents of the rectum

Motility of the rectal wall

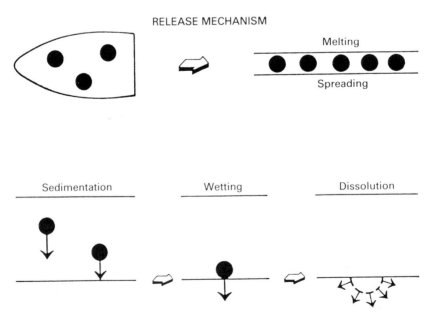

Fig. 23.2 Release process of a drug from a suspension suppository

a survey of the physiological factors in rectal absorption.

The quantity of fluid available for drug dissolution is very small (approximately 3 ml, spread in a layer of approximately 100 μm thick over the organ). Only under non-physiological circumstances is this volume enlarged, e.g. by osmotic attraction by water-soluble vehicles or diarrhoea. Thus the dissolution of slightly soluble substances, as e.g. for phenytoin, can easily be the slowest step in the absorptive process.

Properties of the rectal fluid, such as composition, viscosity and surface tension, are essentially unknown and have to be estimated from data available for other parts of the g.i. tract. The pH and the buffer capacity of the rectum have been mentioned earlier in this chapter. The rectum is usually empty except temporarily when faecal matter arrives from higher parts of the colon. This material is either expelled or transported back into the colon, depending on the voluntary control exhibited on the sphincter of the anus. The rectal wall may exert a pressure on a suppository present in the lumen by two distinct mechanisms. First the abdominal organs may simply press on to the rectum, especially when the body is in upright position. This may stimulate spreading and thus promote absorption. The second source of pressure is the motility of the muscles of the rectal wall, which may originate from the normally occurring colonic motor complexes. These are waves of contractions running over the wall of the colon in caudal direction and are associated with the presence of food residues in the colon.

Formulation of suppositories

Suppositories are mainly used for the administration of drugs via the rectal route, but not exclusively. Application via other routes, such as the vagina, is less common but of distinct use in the treatment of locally occurring infections. Administration of other suppository-type products (bougies) through other body orifices, e.g. ear, nose and urethra, is used very seldomly and is not discussed here. Alternatively dosage forms for the rectal and/or vaginal route are tablets, capsules, ointments and enemas. These will be discussed later on. We will concentrate first on rectal suppositories. Suppositories are formulated in different shapes and sizes (usually 1–4 g). Their drug content varies widely from less than 0.1% up to almost 40%. A more detailed description, together with the methods of preparation can be found in *Dispensing for Pharmaceutical Students* (Carter, 1975). Generally the suppositories consist of a vehicle in which the drug is incorporated and in some cases additives are coformulated.

The vehicle (suppository base)

There are two main classes of vehicles in use, i.e. the glyceride-type fatty bases and the water-soluble ones. Although the ideal vehicle has not been found, the large variety of bases which are available enables a well considered choice for every drug that has to be formulated as a suppository.

Choosing the optimum base requires a lot of practical experience and can at present only partly be guided by scientifically sound data. Much remains to be learned here. However, some general guidelines can be given.

Requirements of the vehicle There is no doubt that a suppository should either melt after insertion in the body or dissolve in (and mix with) the available volume of rectal fluid. For fatty bases this means a melting range lower than appproximately 37 °C (one has to be aware of the fact that the body temperature might be as low as 36 °C at night). The melting range should be small enough to give rapid solidification after preparation, thus preventing separations of suspended, especially high density, drug particles and agglomeration. When the solidification rate is high this may result in fissures, especially when rapid cooling is applied. The melting range, on the other hand, should be large enough to permit easy preparation, which may take a considerable length of time on an industrial scale.

During solidification a suppository should exhibit enough volume contraction to permit removal from the mould or plastic former. The viscosity of the molten base plays an important role both from a technological and from a biopharmaceutical point of view. During preparation the viscosity determines the flow into the moulds but also the separation of drug particles. Clearly a compromise has to be found here. During and after melting in the rectal cavity the suppository mass is forced to spread over the absorbing surface, the rate of which may be determined partly by its viscosity. Drug particles that have to be transported through the base to the interface with the rectal fluid and have to pass this interface to be released will evidently also see viscosity as a determining factor in their journey.

A good suppository base should further be chemically and physically stable during storage as a bulk product and after preparation into a suppository. It should have no incompatibility with drug molecules and should permit an optimal release of the drug it contains.

Clearly this list of requirements cannot always be completely fulfilled and often an acceptable compromise is the best that one can expect.

Fatty vehicles The fatty vehicles in use nowadays are almost exclusively semi- or fully synthetic ones. Cocoa butter is no longer used because of its many disadvantages, such as its well known polymorphic behaviour, insufficient contraction at cooling, low softening point, chemical instability, poor water absorptive power and its price. These points have been discussed extensively in older texts and will be omitted here.

The semisynthetic type of fatty vehicles (sometimes termed *adeps solidus*) have few or none of the problems mentioned above. A comparison is made in Table 23.2. The general composition of both types is mixed triglycerides with C_{12}–C_{18} acids. In the semisynthetic vehicles these acids are saturated, while cocoa butter contains a considerable amount of the unsaturated oleic acid (see iodine number in the table, which for reducing drugs should be <0.5). The presence of oleic acid is almost solely responsible for the special properties of this vehicle. The melting range of the (semi)synthetic bases is usually approximately 3 °C and higher than that of cocoa butter; the acid

content is lower (mostly <0.5) which is one of the reasons that the ageing of aminophylline suppositories is slower when (semi)synthetic vehicles are used. The hydroxyl number in the table refers directly to the amount of mono- and diglycerides present in the fatty base. A high number means that the power to absorb water is high. This may lead to an increased rate of decomposition for drugs that are easily hydrolysed, as acetylsalicylic acid. It should be realized that this capacity could lead to the formation of a w/o emulsion in the rectum which is generally to be avoided because of its very low drug release rate. An advantage of high hydroxyl number is the larger melting and solidifying range which permits easier manufacture.

Water-soluble vehicles Water-soluble (or miscible) vehicles are much less in use for reasons to be discussed below. They comprise the classical glycerol–gelatin or soap bases which are used exclusively for laxative purposes or in vaginal therapy and are further discussed here.

The macrogols are also used. They consist of mixtures of polyethylene glycols of different molecular weight. The melting point is well over body temperature, which means that they mix with the rectal fluid. For true dissolution the available volume of rectal fluid (1–3 ml) is too small. Because of their high melting point they are especially suited for application in tropical climates, but several disadvantages have to be considered. They are hygroscopic and therefore attract water, resulting in a painful sensation for the patient. Incorporation of at least 20% water and moistening before insertion can help to reduce this problem. A considerable number of incompatibilities with various drugs (e.g. phenols, sulphonamides) has been reported. Due to the solubilizing character of this base (low dielectric constant) drugs may tend to remain in the base and release may be slow.

Choice of vehicle A summary of the points which are important for the choice of a suppository base is given in Table 23.3. The parameters

Table 23.2 Some properties of fatty suppository bases

	Melting range	Acid content	Hydroxyl number	Iodine number
Cocoa butter	31–34 °C	<5	0	34–38
Adeps solidus	33–37.5 °C	<2	<5–30	<3

Table 23.3 Formulation parameters of suppository bases

Composition

Melting behaviour

Rheological properties

mentioned in Table 23.3 are evidently not independent of each other. One interesting parameter can be added to this list, i.e. the volume of the suppository. Usually suppositories for adults are 2 ml and for children 1 ml. It has been suggested that the larger volume may provoke a reaction of the rectal wall, thus helping to spread the melt over a larger area. Indeed the increase of volume of, for example, paracetamol suppositories, resulted in faster and more complete absorption of the drug.

The drug

In Table 23.4 the factors related to the drug substance are listed which are of possible consequence for the quality of suppositories.

Table 23.4 Drug-substance related factors

Solubility in water and vehicle

Surface properties

Particle size

Amount

pK_a

Drug solubility in vehicle The drug solubility in the vehicle is of especial interest from the biopharmaceutical point of view. It determines directly the type of product, i.e. solution suppository or suspension suppository. The drug solubility in the rectal fluid determines the maximum attainable concentration and thus the driving force for absorption. When a drug has a high vehicle to water partition coefficient it is likely to be in solution to an appreciable extent (or completely) in the vehicle. This generally means that the tendency to leave the vehicle will be small and thus the release rate into the rectal fluid will be low. This is obviously unfavourable for rapid absorption. On the other hand a certain lipid solubility is required for penetration through the rectal membranes (see above under Absorption of drugs from the rectum). The optimal balance between these two requirements is usually found using the rules listed in Table 23.5.

This table assumes that the release from the dosage form is considered as the rate-limiting step. Thus the tendency to remain in the base should

Table 23.5 Drug solubility and suppository formulation

Solubility in		
fat	water	Choice of base
Low	High	Fatty base (rule 1)
High	Low	Aqueous base (rule 2)
Low	Low	Indeterminate

be lowered as much as possible (rules 1 and 2). When the solubility in fat and water are both low no definite rule can be given. It may well be that the dissolution rate will become the controlling step and thus it seems advisable to use micronized drug particles.

It should be stated as a general rule that emulsion-type suppositories (w/o) are strongly discouraged. The transfer of drug molecules present in dissolved state in the inner phase will be very slow and thus the absorption will be very much retarded.

It seems logical therefore that the first choice of a formulation would be a readily water-soluble form of the drug dispersed in a fatty base. This lays special emphasis on the water solubility of drugs and the methods to improve this. The role of pK_a in this respect should also be considered. For a detailed discussion of these points, see Chapters 3, 5, 9 and 13.

Surface properties The surface properties of drug particles are also important as these particles will be transferred from one phase to another (see Fig. 23.2). This happens first when the drug is brought into contact with the vehicle and air has to be displaced from its surface. When this is not achieved particles may form agglomerates. This adversely affects final content uniformity by an increased tendency to separate. If wetting by the vehicle has taken place displacement by rectal fluid will be required to let the drug go into solution, which is the prerequisite for absorption. This is the underlying reason why people have tried the addition of surfactants to their formulation (see later).

Particle size The particle size of the drug is an important parameter, both technologically and biopharmaceutically. To prevent undue sedimentation during or after preparation the particle size should be limited. The available literature data do not allow us to define an exact limit; however, the use of particles smaller than approximately 150 μm is an indication rather than a rule.

It is, of course, assumed that no agglomeration is taking place. The smaller the particles the less the possible mechanical irritation to the patient (esp. < 50 μm) and the higher the dissolution rate and therefore drugs with a low water solubility will be dispensed in small, preferably micronized, particles. One should be aware of the increased tendency of these particles to agglomerate due to strongly increased van der Waals forces in that case, however. Also an unnecessary size reduction operation should be avoided when possible.

There are good indications that size reduction is not a good decision for all drugs. It has been shown, especially for readily water-soluble drugs, that large particles give blood levels which are higher than or at least equivalent to small particles. This would lead to the suggestion to use particles in the size range 50–100 μm in that case. The lower limit of 50 μm to increase transport through the molten vehicle (see Fig. 23.2) and the upper limit of 100 μm is a safe protection against undue sedimentation during preparation. No clear-cut picture stands, however, for which solubility class this would be the rule to follow. For example paracetamol (solubility in water approximately 15 mg ml^{-1}) gave the best blood levels when the particle size was smaller than 45 μm.

It should also be kept in mind that the spreading suppository mass should drag the suspended particles along to maximize the absorption surface. For heavy compounds it has become clear that this is a problem, but so far little or no proof is available that organic drugs (density usually 1.2–1.4 g cm^{-3}) suffer from this disadvantage when dispersed in, for example, 150 μm size particles. Principally this may be expected, but care is needed to prevent too rapid formulation decisions in this respect.

Amount of drug A complicating factor is the amount of drug present in a suppository. If the number of particles increases, this would also increase the rate to form agglomerates. This will very much depend on the particle size and on the presence of additives. The theory describing the agglomeration behaviour of dispersed systems (DLVO theory, see Chapter 6) can be applied in the non-aqueous systems we are dealing with, but

certain refinements are necessary. Another consequence of the presence of suspended particles is the increased viscosity of the molten base. Also in this case we have to rely largely on empirical data rather than on theory. It seems therefore advisable to include a decision on particle size in the development plan of an actual suppository formulation.

Other additives

For several widely varying reasons formulators of suppositories make use of additives to improve their product. Most of these additions are based on empirical data and will be dealt with in the accompanying, dispensing volume (in preparation). The dispensing aspects include formulations for specific drugs which affect the melting point of the suppository; it may become depressed (by a soluble liquid compound) or increased (by a high amount of soluble high melting active compound). The important point to consider in these situations is the possible influence of formulation changes on the release characteristics. We will further limit the discussion to fatty suppository where this plays a role especially.

The addition of viscosity increasing additives (e.g. colloidal silicon oxide or aluminium monostearate, both approximately 1–2%) will create a gel-like system with a slower release rate of the drug. Data from the literature are not consistent on this point. *In vitro* this can be easily established, but whether the actual release *in vivo* will also be depressed cannot be easily predicted, since the rectal motility will in certain cases be able to overcome this problem. The addition of lecithin is a worthy possibility when high amounts of solid drug are used. The reason why, clearly has to be found in a decreased attraction between the drug particles, altering the flow properties of the dispersion in the positive sense.

The addition of surface-active agents has been practised extensively but still remains a source of great uncertainty. When these compounds are used to create an emulsion system (thus w/o) this has certainly to be discouraged since the release will be unacceptably slow. It may well be, however, that surfactants act as wetting agents. This can influence the release in a positive sense, but so far very little convincing information is available showing that wetting (i.e. displacement of base by rectal fluid) exists as a real problem. Surfactants may also act as deglomerators, which may prevent the formation of cake in the melting suppository, which in turn would certainly slow down the release. Also here no firm conclusions can be drawn since only very scarce research work has been performed on the agglomeration in non-aqueous media. The role of surfactants as spreading enhancers has never been clarified either and this factor is strongly inter-related with the occurrence of rectal motility. There are good indications that the presence of surfactants in a concentration higher than the critical micelle concentration can retard the release from the suppositories.

The finished product

Manufacture

Suppositories are manufactured both on a small scale in batches of 10–20 and on a (semi) automatic scale in batches up to 20 000 per hour. Essentially the mode of manufacture is similar in both cases and involves melting of the vehicle, mixing the drug and the molten vehicle, dispensing in a former, cooling to solidify and, if necessary, packing in the final container. This includes a number of technological processes for which the relevant theory should be considered (see, for example, Chapter 32 for the mixing of semi-solids). Most suppositories nowadays are packed individually in a plastic (PVC) or aluminium foil pack. Requirements leading to a good protection against moisture and oxygen can be deduced from the individual needs of the drug and the properties of the packaging material.

Quality control

A list of properties that should be controlled is given in Table 23.6.

The *appearance* of a suppository includes odour, colour, surface condition and shape. These are organoleptically controlled and will be discussed in the accompanying volume (in preparation).

The requirements for *weight* and *disintegration*

Table 23.6 Control parameters of suppositories

Appearance
Weight
Disintegration
Melting (dissolution) behaviour
Mechanical strength
Content of active ingredient
Release

are given in the *European* and national *pharmacopoeias*. *The melting* and *dissolution behaviour* is in fact reflected in the disintegration test. Many other methods are available, but none of them has been shown to provide more relevant information. The present *European Pharmacopoeia* method proves to be rather insensitive and not too much value should be attributed to the passing of this test.

The *mechanical strength* can be valuable to avoid problems with formulations in which the melting range has been depressed. It can be tested by several methods including a tablet crushing strength tester.

No official requirements are published as yet with regard to the *content uniformity*. This, however, has been shown recently to be a potential problem in semiautomatic manufacture of batches of a few kg. Especially due to sometimes insufficient mixing, the uniformity of content was insufficient. Giving careful attention to the design and control of the filling apparatus could solve most of the problems. However, the beginning and the end of the production process still gives poor results necessitating some degree of rejection.

Drug release from suppositories

Perhaps the most important thing to realize is that for the patient the release characteristics are the determining step towards the success of his therapy. What we really want is an optimal bioavailability (for details see Part 2) which for the formulator means ensuring optimal and reproducible release *in vivo*.

Since there are very little means of obtaining *in vivo* release information this will usually have to be interpreted from *in vitro* release, which introduces the problem of *in vitro/in vivo* correlation.

The present knowledge does not permit the choice of an *in vitro* method with a high predictive power for *in vivo* performance. Some aspects can be discussed, however, to give helpful pointers in this respect. Table 23.7 lists the parameters to be examined in testing suppository release *in vitro*.

Table 23.7 *In vitro* release parameters

Temperature
Contact area
Release medium
Movements
Membranes

The *temperature* to be chosen for testing rectal dosage forms is easily defined as the body temperature. Although for most practical purposes this temperature can be set at 37 °C, this is not so for, especially, fatty suppository testing. Most available vehicles have melting ranges below 37 °C, but this does not necessarily mean that their viscosity at 37 °C is the same. Since the body temperature may be as low as 36 °C at night, this implies that the release rate at 37 °C may be an overestimate. Also comparing bases at 37 °C may lead to erroneous conclusions. The temperature at which testing is performed might be crucial, especially when ageing has occurred. Special attention should therefore be given to the actual testing temperature.

In the set-up shown in Fig. 23.3 the temperature at the surface of the water layer inside the tube, where molten suppository material is gathered may be a few degrees lower than the bulk temperature. By choosing the right dimension and closing the tube at the upperside this problem is eliminated here.

The *contact area* in the rectum over which spreading occurs cannot be standardized without introducing either an overestimate or an under-estimate. In Fig. 23.3 the area is relatively small (i.e. approximately 10 cm²) compared to the total surface area of the rectum (approximately 300 cm²). This type of apparatus therefore is clearly intended to be used for comparative studies only and not for a complete *in vivo* simulation. At present no method is available which closely mimics the *in vivo* situation.

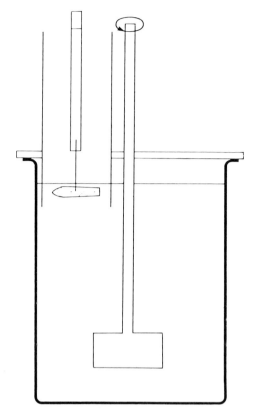

Fig. 23.3 Tube apparatus for sedimentation-controlled release testing from suppositories

Another parameter to be considered is the *release medium*. Whereas not enough information is available on the actual composition and structure of the rectal fluid, a choice is usually made for a relatively large volume of water or buffer solution. Since the rate-limiting step in the bioavailability from fatty suppositories is very often the release from the suppository it seems reasonable enough not to include mucins which control the viscosity *in vivo*. The large volume in most *in vitro* methods would then not be so important either. More difficult is the choice of buffer and especially its strength, since little is known about this factor in the *in vivo* situation (see • above). For water-soluble vehicles the problem is even larger, and essentially no ideal solution has yet been found to the problem of choosing the volume and composition of the release medium. Only recently has interest been created towards the inclusion of one or another way of incorporating a *pressure* feature in release testing. It is clear that rectal motility exists and that it may influence the bioavailability. Not yet clear, however, is how to incorporate this knowledge in the design of a release tester. Attempts have been made, but no conclusive answer is possible as yet.

Very often *membranes* have been used in release testers, usually to envelop the suppository in a small volume of release medium. As has been shown recently this has the enormous drawback that the release as measured in the outer compartment is not equal to the actual release taking place in the inner compartment. Most results published do not take into account that the membrane may form a resistance to passing drug molecules and that the actual release may be underestimated. By a calculation procedure it is possible to obtain the actual release if certain conditions can be met. It seems advisable therefore to avoid membranes in a release tester, whenever possible.

The actual true validation of *in vitro* release testing remains the *in vivo* performance. Several possibilities exist to obtain such data. Bioavailability determination should consider both rate and extent of absorption. Whenever possible these data should be obtained in man, since at present no animal model is available which is sufficiently reliable. For a more detailed discussion on the general aspects of bioavailability testing and *in vitro/in vivo* correlations Chapter 10 can be consulted.

Rectal formulations other than suppositories

Apart from suppositories, many formulations can be used for rectal administration of drugs. For the treatment of *local* disturbances, like haemorrhoids, fatty ointments are used widely. In the treatment of rectocolitis enemas are used with a rather large volume, e.g. 100 ml. This enables the drug to reach the upper part of the rectum and the sigmoid colon.

For the *systemic* administration of drugs, delivery forms such as tablets, capsules and microenemas are in use. Tablets are not very attractive because they cannot disintegrate rapidly, due to the low amount of water present in the rectum. Tablets releasing CO_2 after insertion can be applied, thus stimulating defaecation.

Capsules used to achieve a systemic effect are usually filled with a solution or suspension of the drug in vegetable oil or paraffin. These capsules are mostly of the soft-shell type. With this dosage form limited experience has been obtained, but it seems that no striking differences exist between the bioavailability from rectal capsules and fatty suppositories.

Microenemas are solutions or dispersions of the drug in a small volume (approximately 3 ml) of water or vegetable oil. This form is supplied in a small plastic container, equipped with an application tube. After insertion of the tube, the container is emptied by compression of the bulb. The advantage of this delivery system is obvious, since no melting and dissolution process is necessary before drug release can start, if water is used as a vehicle. Many good results have been obtained with drugs delivered in microenemas, but this form is still of limited applicability, because of its relatively high cost compared to, for example, suppositories. Moreover, administration can not be performed easily by patients themselves, and it is rather difficult to deliver the total content of the plastic container.

PESSARIES

Vaginal administration of drugs

The vaginal route is mainly used for the achievement of local effects, e.g. in the case of *Trichomonas* and *Candida* infections. Some drugs are, however, vaginally administered to achieve systemic effects. In some cases the drugs given by intravaginal route had a higher bioavailability compared to the oral route, because the drug enters immediately into the systemic circulation without passing the metabolizing liver (as is the case with drugs absorbed from the lower part of the rectum).

The vaginal wall is very well suited for the absorption of drugs for systemic use, since it contains a vast network of blood vessels. Only few drugs are administered by this route at present, however. Among these are oestrogens and prostaglandin analogues, which are usually administered as vaginal creams or hydrogels. Progesterone has been given as vaginal suppositories (pessaries) for some years, and better results are obtained in this way than after an oral dose.

Formulation of vaginal dosage forms

Many different types of formulations have been and are applied vaginally, e.g. tablets, capsules, pessaries, solutions, sprays, foams, creams and ointments. Because of the rather low moisture content under normal physiological conditions, additives are added to improve the disintegration of vaginal tablets, e.g. bicarbonate together with an organic acid, which results in CO_2 release. A good filler for vaginal tablets is lactose, since this is a natural substrate for the vaginal microflora, which convert lactose into lactic acid, resulting in a pH value of 4–4.5.

Vaginal suppositories pessaries are mostly prepared with glycerol–gelatin bases, since this mixture is well tolerated. Polyethylene glycols are less common, since they are said to promote irritation. Also fatty excipients are not very much used. Most delivery forms for vaginal application demand an auxiliary application device, in order to obtain deep insertion of the delivery system.

BIBLIOGRAPHY

de Blaey, C. J. and Polderman, J. (1980) Rationales in the design of rectal and vaginal delivery forms of drugs. In: *Drug Design*, Vol. 9 (Ed. E. J. Ariëns), pp. 237–266, Academic Press, New York.

De Boer, A. G., Molenaar, F., de Leede, L. G. J. and Breimer, D. D. (1982) Rectal drug administration: clinical pharmacokinetic considerations. *Clin. Pharmacokin.*, 7, 285–311.

Carter, S. J. (1975) Dispensing for Pharmaceutical Students, 13th edn, Pitman Medical, London.

Müller, B. (Ed.) (1986) *Suppositorien*. Wissenschaftliche Verlagsgesellschaft mbH, Stuttgart.

Senior, N. (1974) Rectal administration of drugs. In: *Advances in Pharmaceutical Sciences IV* (Eds. H. S. Bean *et al.* pp. 369–435, Academic Press, New York.

Thoma, K. (1980) Arzneiformen zur rectalen und vaginalen Applikation. *Werbe- und Vertriebsgesellschaft Deutscher Apotheker m.b.H.*, Frankfurt am Main, West Germany.

PART FOUR

Pharmaceutical microbiology

Fundamentals of microbiology

Dimorphic fungi
Filamentous fungi
Reproduction of fungi
Asexual reproduction
Sexual reproduction

Micro-organisms are ubiquitous in nature and are vital components in the cycle of life. Of all the myriads of microscopic life present in soil, water and atmosphere only a tiny fraction cause disease. Similarly, a small proportion attempt to counterbalance the debits of their colleagues by providing mankind with beneficial materials which would otherwise be difficult or impossible to synthesize. The majority are free-living organisms growing on dead or decaying matter whose prime function is the turnover of organic materials in the environment.

In order to understand micro-organisms more fully, scientists have grouped together organisms of similar characteristics into taxonomic units. The most fundamental division is between prokaryotic and eukaryotic cells which differ in a number of respects (see Table 24.1) of which the most important concerns the nuclear material. Eukaryotic cells contain chromosomes which are separate from the cytoplasm and contained within a limiting nuclear membrane, i.e. they possess a true nucleus. Prokaryotic cells do not possess a true nucleus and their nuclear material is free within the cytoplasm although it may be aggregated into discrete areas called nuclear bodies. Prokaryotic organisms make up the lower forms of life and include rickettsiae, chlamydiae, mycoplasmas, bacteria and blue/green algae. Eukaryotic cell types embrace all the higher forms of life of which only the fungi will be dealt with in this chapter.

VIRUSES

The very simplest forms of life are virus particles and it is a philosophical argument as to whether these should be considered as living organisms. They are obligate intracellular parasites with no intrinsic metabolic activities, being devoid of ribosomes and energy-producing enzyme systems. They are thus incapable of leading an independent existence and cannot be cultivated on cell-free media no matter how nutritious.

The size of human viruses ranges from the largest poxviruses measuring about 300 nm (1 nm = 10^{-9} m) to the picornaviruses such as the poliovirus which is approximately 20 nm. When one considers that a bacterial coccus measures 1000 nm in diameter it can be appreciated that only the very largest virus particles may be seen under the light microscope and electron microscopy is required for visualizing the majority.

Viruses consist of a core of nucleic acid (either DNA as in vaccinia virus or RNA as in poliovirus) surrounded by a protein shell or capsid. Most DNA viruses have linear double-stranded DNA but it is single stranded in the case of the parvovirus. The majority of RNA-containing viruses contain one molecule of single-stranded RNA although in reoviruses it is double stranded. The protein capsid comprises 50–90% of the weight of the virus and since nucleic acid can only synthesize approximately 10% its own weight of protein the capsid must be made up of a number of identical protein molecules. These individual protein units are called capsomeres and are not in themselves symmetrical but are arranged around the nucleic acid core in characteristic symmetrical patterns. Additionally, many of the larger viruses possess a lipoprotein envelope surrounding the capsid which arises from the membranes within

Table 24.1 Differences between prokaryotic and eukaryotic organisms

Structure	Prokaryotes	Eukaryotes
Cell wall structure	Usually contains peptidoglycan	Peptidoglycan absent
Nuclear membrane	Absent	Present. Possess a true nucleus
Nucleolus	Absent	Present
Number of chromosomes	One	More than one
Mitochondria	Absent	Present
Mesosomes	Present	Absent
Ribosomes	70s	80s

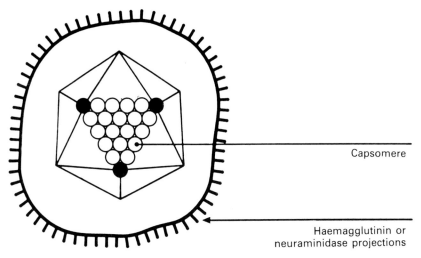

Fig. 24.1 Enveloped icosahedral virus (capsomeres shown on one face only)

the host cell. In many instances the membranes are virus-modified to produce projections outwards from the envelope which can take the form of either haemagglutinins or neuraminidase (see Fig. 24.1). The enveloped viruses are often called ether-sensitive as the membrane may be dissolved by ether and other organic solvents.

The arrangement of the capsomeres can be of a number of types:

1 Helical — the classical example is tobacco mosaic virus (TMV) which resembles a hollow tube with capsomeres arranged in a helix around the central nucleic acid core. Other examples include mumps and influenza virus.
2 Icosahedral — these often resemble spheres on cursory examination but when studied more closely they are made up of icosahedra which have 20 triangular faces each containing an identical number of capsomeres. Examples include the poliovirus and adenovirus.
3 Complex — the poxviruses and bacterial viruses (bacteriophages) make up a group whose members have a geometry which is individual and complex.

Human virus cultivation

Viruses require living cells in which to propagate and three types of system can be used:

1 Living animals — this method poses a number of problems apart from ethical or even financial considerations. The animals not only vary greatly in their response to the inoculation of virus but they may also not be entirely free from their own viruses and these may act as contaminants. Growth of the virus within the animal is determined by signs of disease or possibly death and so specific virus/cell interactions are difficult to observe with this type of model.
2 Fertile chicken eggs — viruses can be inoculated directly into fertile chicken eggs and will generally show a preference for growth in specific areas within the embryonic tissues. Poxviruses grow and produce lesions on the chorioallantoic membrane whereas influenza virus will grow on the membrane adjacent to the amniotic cavity.
3 Tissue culture — certain tissues, e.g. monkey kidney, can be enzymatically disrupted to produce individual cells which, when placed in a suitable nutrient medium, will settle and grow over the surface of the glass in a monolayer. This is called a primary cell culture and can be subcultured by treatment with trypsin and reinoculation into fresh medium producing secondary cell cultures. Repeated subculture generally results in cells of reduced vigour and eventually they will die.

Continuous cell lines usually originate from malignant cells and have the capacity to divide indefinitely. Alternatively, transformation of secondary cell cultures may occur such that the properties of the cells alter and established cell lines are formed.

Monolayers of cells can be inoculated with suspensions of virus particles and the progress of infection followed. The viruses attach to specific surface receptors whereupon the particles enter the cells usually by engulfment. The protein capsid then breaks down liberating the viral nucleic acid which enters the nucleus of the host cell. The host cell protein synthesizing machinery is then taken over for the purpose of producing viral components. New virus particles are assembled from these products and are released from the host cell either by gradual extrusion or lysis of the infected cell. The visible degeneration of a cell within the monolayer is called the cytopathic effect and can be studied microscopically. Not all viruses produce a cytopathic effect although they may be present within the cell.

RICKETTSIAE

The family Rickettsiaceae includes the genus *Rickettsia* containing organisms responsible for epidemic typhus, murine typhus, trench fever and spotted fever, and also the genus *Coxiella* which contains the organism responsible for Q fever. The rickettsiae are very small prokaryotic cells which are pleomorphic varying in shape from coccal to filamentous forms. Their cell wall composition bears similarities to that of Gram-negative bacteria (see later) and in general they stain this way. The majority of rickettsiae are obligate intracellular parasites and cannot be grown on cell-free media although, unlike many viruses, they do possess some independent enzymes. Multiplication is intracellular and is by binary fission. Rickettsiae have a range of animal and insect hosts including fleas, lice and ticks and the diseases associated with them usually accompany war, poverty and deprivation. Chemotherapy involves the use of chloramphenicol or tetracycline and is reasonably effective. Vaccines are also available but are only rarely used.

CHLAMYDIAE

These are small prokaryotic cells which have weak Gram-negative characteristics. They are obligate intracellular parasites possessing some independent enzymes but lacking an ATP generating system. Two cell forms can be identified:

1 a highly infectious, small 300 nm elementary body,
2 a larger 800–1200 nm initial body which is the replicating form of the organism.

Chlamydiae are responsible for trachoma which is the most common cause of blindness in the world and also a respiratory condition acquired as a result of handling infected birds.

Treatment involves sulphonamides and tetracycline but an increase in hygiene and social standards should be the major objective.

MYCOPLASMAS

Mycoplasmas are the smallest prokaryotic cells capable of growing on cell-free media. They were initially isolated from the pleural fluids of cattle and became grouped together with other similar organisms under the name pleuropneumonia-like organisms (PPLO). This term has now been superseded by the name *Mycoplasma*.

Mycoplasmas are pleomorphic forms resembling soft-bodied branching filaments with periodic swellings. Other species may simply grow as coccobacillary forms. Peptidoglycan (see later under Bacterial cell wall) is absent from the cell walls and the cell is limited by a double-layered plasma membrane 8–15 nm thick containing substantial amounts of phospholipids and cholesterol. The lack of peptidoglycan is the reason for the organism being completely resistant to penicillin and lysozyme. Mycoplasmas can be grown on cell-free media at 35 °C and most are aerobes or facultative anaerobes. On solid media the best known characteristic is the 'fried egg' appearance of the colonies. Bacterial spheroplasts and protoplasts often bear a striking resemblance to mycoplasmas in their cultural reactions probably due to their lack of a cell wall. Mycoplasmas cause a number of infections in animals and are of particular importance in the veterinary field. In humans they have been associated with respiratory and genitourinary infections but can generally be effectively treated using either tetracycline or erythromycin.

BACTERIA

Shape, size and aggregation

Bacteria occur in a variety of shapes and sizes (see Fig. 24.2) determined not only by the nature of the organism itself but also by the way in which it is grown. In general bacterial dimensions lie in the range 0.75 μm to 5 μm (1000 μm = 1 mm). The most common shapes are the sphere (coccus) and the rod (bacillus). Some bacteria grow in the form of rods with distinct curvature, e.g. vibrios are rod-shaped cells with a single curve resembling a comma whereas a spirillum possesses a partial rigid spiral, spirochaetes are longer and thinner and exhibit a number of turns, they are also more flexible. Rod-shaped cells occasionally grow in the form of chains but this is dependent upon growth conditions rather than a characteristic of the species. Cocci, however, show considerable variation in aggregation which is characteristic of the species. Cocci growing in pairs are called diplococci, those in four, tetrads and in groups of eight, sarcina. If a chain of cells is produced resembling a string of beads this is termed a streptococcus whereas an irregular cluster similar in appearance to a bunch of grapes is called a staphylococcus. In many cases this is sufficiently characteristic to give rise to the generic name of the organism, e.g. *Staphylococcus aureus*, *Streptococcus faecalis*. Note that the name is written in italics and that the genus name begins with a capital letter while the species name begins with a lower case letter. When italics cannot be used the name should be underlined.

Anatomy

Figure 24.3 is a diagrammatic representation of a typical bacterial cell. The various components are described below.

Capsule

A capsule is an extracellular, highly viscous slime layer which adheres firmly to the cell. It is non-living and non-essential. The composition varies considerably but is generally polysaccharide in nature although some are polypeptide and others are complexes of these. Not all bacteria produce a capsule and even those that can will only do so under certain circumstances. Many encapsulated pathogens when first isolated give rise to colonies on agar which are smooth (S) but subculturing leads to the formation of rough colonies (R). This S → R transition is due to loss in capsule production. Reinoculation of the R cells into an animal results in the resumption of capsule formation indicating that the capacity has not been irrevocably lost.

The function of the capsule is generally regarded as protective since encapsulated cells are more resistant to disinfectants, desiccation and phagocytic attack. In some organisms, however, it serves as an adhesive mechanism, *Streptococcus mutans* is an inhabitant of the mouth which metabolizes sucrose to produce a polysaccharide capsule enabling the cell to adhere firmly to the teeth. This is the initial step in the formation of dental plaque which is a complex array of microorganisms and organic matrix adhering to the teeth ultimately leading to decay. Substitution of sucrose by glucose prevents capsule formation and hence eliminates plaque.

Cell wall

Bacteria can be divided into two broad groups on the basis of their cell wall structure (Fig. 24.4). This classification is based upon their ability to retain the dye methyl violet after washing with a decolorizing agent such as absolute alcohol. (See later in this Chapter for details of the Gram-staining procedure.) Gram-positive cells retain the dye whereas Gram-negative cells are decolorized. As a *very rough* guide the majority of rod-shaped cells are Gram-negative, exceptions include the Bacillaceae and the actinomycetes, while the majority of cocci are Gram-positive with the exception of the Neisseriaceae.

Bacteria are unique in that they possess peptido-

Genus		Approximate dimensions (μm)
Staphylococcus Irregular clusters of spherical cells. Resemble bunch of grapes. Non-motile	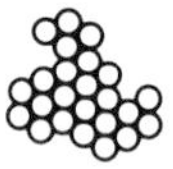	0.5–1.5
Streptococcus Spherical or ovoid cells occurring in pairs or in chains. Non-motile	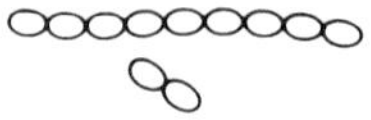	<2.0
Neisseria Small Gram negative cocci. Occur in pairs with adjacent sides flattened. Non-motile	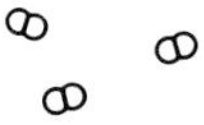	0.6–1.0
Lactobacillus Shape variable between long and slender to short coccobacillus. Non-motile, chain formation common	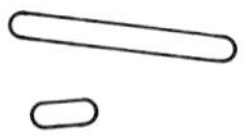	0.5–0.8 × 2–9
Escherichia Short rods, motile by peritrichous flagella	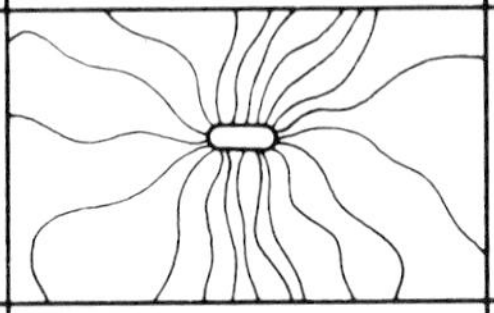	1.1–1.5 × 2–6
Bacillus Large endospore-forming rods. Motile by lateral flagella (not shown). Gram-positive	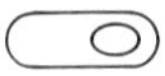	0.3–2.2 × 1.2–7.0
Vibrio Short curved or straight rods. Sometimes 'S' shaped. Motile by single polar flagellum	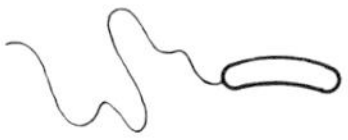	0.5 × 1.5–3.0
Spirochaeta Thin, flexible, helically coiled cells. Motile, possess axial fibrils (not shown)	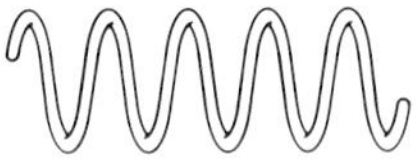	0.2–0.75 × 5–500
Spirillum Long, slender cells in rigid spirals. Number of turns varies. Motile, bipolar flagellation	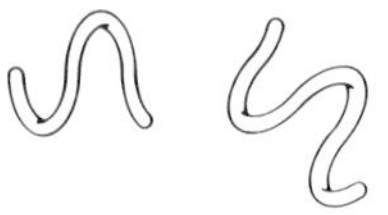	0.2–1.7 × 0.5–60
Streptomyces Slender, non-septate branching filaments. Form reproductive spores. Non-motile	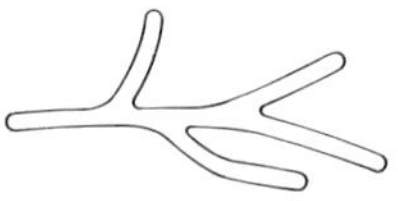	0.5–2.0 (diameter)

Fig. 24.2 Morphology of different bacterial genera

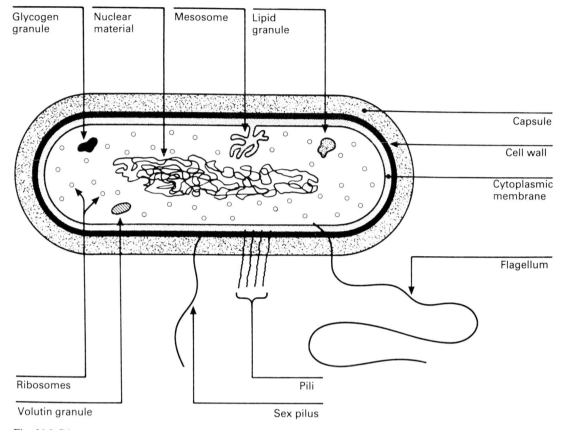

Fig. 24.3 Diagrammatic representation of a typical bacterial cell

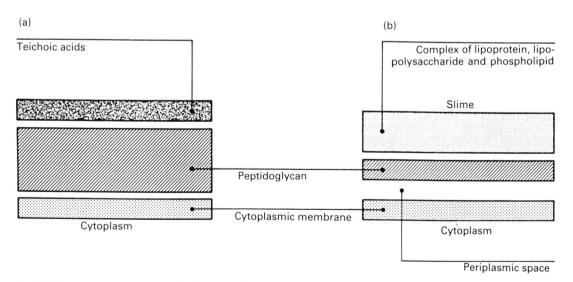

Fig. 24.4 Structural components of (a) Gram-positive, and (b) Gram-negative cell envelopes

glycan in their cell walls. This is a complex molecule with repeating units of N-acetylmuramic acid and N-acetylglucosamine. This extremely long molecule is wound around the cell and cross-linked by polypeptide bridges to form a structure of great rigidity. It imparts to the cell its characteristic shape and has principally a protective function. Peptidoglycan (also called murein or mucopeptide) is the site of action of a number of antibiotics such as penicillin, bacitracin, vancomycin and cycloserine. The enzyme lysozyme is also capable of hydrolysing the β, 1–4 linkages between N-acetylmuramic acid and N-acetylglucosamine.

Cytoplasmic membrane

The cytoplasmic membrane is composed of phospholipids and proteins and is a flexible structure with very little tensile strength. It possesses selective permeability and controls the passage of nutrients and waste products into and out of the cell. The internal hydrostatic pressure of the cell can be up to 20 bar and this forces the cytoplasmic membrane firmly against the inside of the cell wall.

Treatment of bacterial cells with lysozyme may remove the cell wall and, as long as the conditions are isotonic, the resulting cell will survive. These cells are called protoplasts and since the cytoplasmic membrane is now the limiting structure the cell assumes a spherical shape. Protoplasts of gram-negative bacteria are difficult to obtain because the layer of lipopolysaccharide protects the peptidoglycan from attack. In these cases mixtures of EDTA and lysozyme are used and the resulting cells which still retain a thin layer of cell envelope are termed spheroplasts.

Nuclear material

The genetic information necessary for the functioning of the cell is contained within a single circular molecule of double-stranded DNA. When unfolded this would be about 1000 times as long as the cell itself and so exists within the cytoplasm in a considerably compacted state. It is condensed into discrete areas called chromatin bodies which

are not surrounded by a nuclear membrane. Rapidly dividing cells may contain up to four areas of nuclear material but these are copies of the same chromosome not different chromosomes and arise because DNA replication is initiated before the previous round is completed.

Mesosomes

These are irregular invaginations of the cytoplasmic membrane which are quite prominent in Gram-positive bacteria but less so in Gram-negative bacteria. They are thought to have a variety of functions including cross-wall synthesis during cell division and furnishing an attachment site for nuclear material facilitating the separation of segregating chromosomes during cell division. They have also been implicated in enzyme secretions and may act as a site for cell respiration.

Ribosomes

The cytoplasm of bacteria is densely populated with between 10 000 and 50 000 ribosomes which are complexes of RNA and protein in discrete particles 20 nm in diameter. They are the sites of protein synthesis within the cell and the numbers present reflect the degree of metabolic activity of the cell. They are frequently found organized in clusters called polyribosomes or polysomes.

Inclusion granules

Certain bacteria tend to accumulate reserves of materials after active growth has ceased and these become incorporated within the cytoplasm in the form of granules. The most common are glycogen granules, volutin granules (containing polymetaphosphate) and lipid granules (containing poly-β-hydroxybutyric acid). Other granules such as sulphur and iron may also be found in the more primitive bacteria.

Flagella

These thread-like processes are the means by which many bacteria achieve mobility. The flagellum arises from the cytoplasmic membrane and is composed of a basal body, hook and fila-

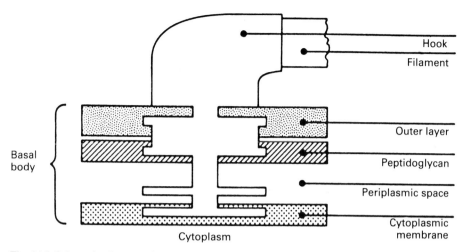

Fig. 24.5 Schematic diagram of the component parts of a bacterial flagellum

ment (Fig. 24.5). The filament is made up of parallel protein strands joined together to form a single unit. The number and arrangement of flagella depends upon the organisms and varies from a single flagellum (monotrichous) to a complete covering (peritrichous).

Pili (fimbriae)

These are smaller than flagella but also orginate in the cytoplasmic membrane. A number of different types of pili have been identified of which the most important are the common pili and the F-pili. The common pili are found all over the surface of certain bacteria and are believed to be associated with adhesiveness and pathogenicity. They are also antigenic. F-pili are larger and of a different structure to common pili and are involved in the transfer of genetic information from one cell to another. This is of major importance in the transfer of drug resistance between cell populations.

Spores

Under conditions of specific nutrient deprivation some genera of bacteria, in particular *Bacillus* and *Clostridium*, undergo a differentiation process and change from an actively metabolizing vegetative form to a resting spore form. The process of sporulation is not a reproductive mechanism as found in fungi but serves to enable the organism to survive periods of hardship. A single vegetative cell differentiates into a single spore. Subsequent encounter with favourable conditions results in germination of the spore and resumption of vegetative activities.

Spores are very much more resistant to heat, disinfectants, desiccation and radiation than vegetative cells, making them difficult to eradicate from foods and pharmaceutical products. Most vegetative bacteria would be killed by heating at 80 °C for 10 minutes whereas some spores will resist boiling for several hours. The sterilization procedures now routinely used for pharmaceutical products are thus designed specifically with reference to the destruction of the bacterial spore (see Chapter 43). The mechanism of heat resistance was at one time thought to be due to the presence of a unique spore component dipicolinic acid (DPA). This compound is found only in bacterial spores where it is associated in a complex with calcium ions. The isolation of heat-resistant DPA-less mutants led to the demise of this theory. Spores do not have water content appreciably different from vegetative cells but the distribution within the different compartments is unequal and this is thought to generate the heat resistance. The central core of the spore houses the genetic information necessary for growth after germination and this becomes dehydrated by expansion of the cortex against the rigid outer protein coats. Water is thus squeezed out of the central core. Osmotic pressure differences also help to maintain this water imbalance.

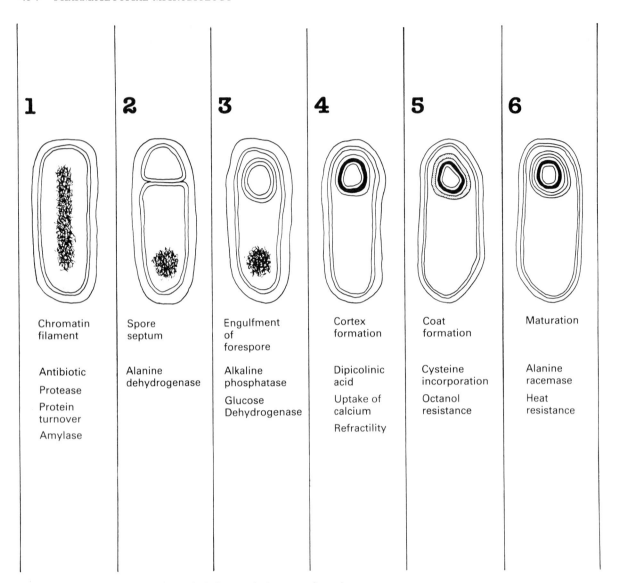

Fig. 24.6 Morphological and biochemical changes during spore formation

The sequence of events involved in sporulation is illustrated in Fig. 24.6, and is a continuous process although for convenience it is divided into six stages. The complete process take about 8 hours although this may vary depending upon the species and the conditions used. Occurring simultaneously with the morphological changes are a number of biochemical events which have been shown to be associated with specific stages and occur in an exact sequence. One important biochemical event is the production of antibiotics. Peptides possessing antimicrobial activity have

been isolated from the majority of *Bacillus* species and many of these have found pharmaceutical applications.

Microscopy and staining of bacteria

Bacterial cells contain about 80% water by weight and this results in a very low refractility, i.e. they are transparent when viewed under ordinary transmitted light. Consequently, in order to visualize bacteria under the microscope the cells must either be killed and stained with some compound which scatters the light or, if live preparations are required, special adaptations must be made to the microscope. Such adaptations are found in phase contrast, dark ground and differential-interference contrast microscopy.

The microscopical examination of fixed and stained preparations is a routine procedure in most laboratories but it must be appreciated that not only are the cells dead but they may also have been altered morphologically by the often quite drastic staining process.

The majority of stains used routinely are basic dyes, i.e. the chromophore has a positive charge and this readily combines with the abundant negative charges present both in the cytoplasm in the form of nucleic acids and on the cell surface. These dyes remain firmly adhered even after washing with water. This type of staining is called simple staining and all bacteria and other biological material are stained the same colour. Differential staining is a much more useful process since different organisms or even different parts of the same cell can be stained distinctive colours.

To prepare a film ready for staining the glass microscope slide must be carefully cleaned to remove all traces of grease and dust. If the culture of bacteria is in liquid form then a loopful of suspension is transferred directly to the slide. Bacteria from solid surfaces require suspension with a small drop of water on the slide to give a *faintly* turbid film. A common fault with inexperienced workers is to make the film too thick. The films must then be allowed to dry in air. When thoroughly dry the film is fixed by passing the back of the slide through a small bunsen flame until the area is just too hot to touch on the palm of the hand. The bacteria are killed by this procedure and also stuck onto the slide. Fixing also makes the bacteria more permeable to the stain and inhibits lysis. Chemical fixation is commonly carried out using formalin or methyl alcohol and this causes less damage to the specimen but tends to be used principally for blood films and tissue sections.

Differential stains

A large number of differential stains have been developed and the reader is referred to the bibliography for a full discourse on the subject. Only a few of those available will be discussed here.

Gram's stain By far the most important in terms of use and application is the Gram stain which was developed by Christian Gram in 1884 and subsequently modified. The fixed film of bacteria is flooded initially with a solution of methyl violet. This is followed by a solution of Gram's iodine which is an iodine–potassium iodine complex acting as a mordant fixing the dye firmly in certain bacteria and allowing easy removal in others. Decolorization is effected with either alcohol or acetone or mixtures of these. After treatment some bacteria retain the stain and appear a dark purple colour and these are called Gram-positive cells. Others do not retain the stain and appear colourless (Gram-negative). The colourless cells may be stained with a counterstain of contrasting colour such as 0.5% safranin which is red.

This method although extremely useful must be used with caution since the Gram reaction may vary with the age of the cells and on the technique of the operator. For this reason known Gram-positive and Gram-negative controls should be stained alongside the specimen of interest.

Ziehl–Neelsen's acid-fast stain *Mycobacterium tuberculosis* contains within its cell wall a high proportion of lipids, fatty acids and alcohols which render the bacterium resistant to normal staining procedures. Inclusion of phenol into the dye solution together with the application of heat enables the dye (basic fuchsin) to penetrate the cell and once attached resists vigorous decolorization by strong acids, e.g. 20% sulphuric acid. Hence these organisms are called *acid-fast*. Any unstained material can be counterstained with a contrasting colour, e.g. methylene blue.

Malachite green spore stain Spores are very refractile bodies and do not take up stain easily. Vigorous staining methods will introduce dye into the spore and once in it will resist decolorization in a way similar to that demonstrated by acid-fast bacteria. Fixed bacterial films are flooded with 5% malachite green solution and placed over a beaker of boiling water. After washing with cold water a counterstain such as 0.5% safranin is applied. On examination the spores appear green and the vegetative bacilli appear red.

Fluorescence microscopy

Certain materials, when irradiated by short wave illuminations, e.g. u.v. light become excited and emit light of a longer wavelength which is visible. This phenomenon is termed fluorescence and will persist only for as long as the material is irradiated. A number of dyes have been shown to fluoresce and are useful in that they tend to be specific to various tissues which can then be demonstrated by u.v. irradiation and subsequent fluorescence of the attached fluorochrome. Specificity can be enhanced by coupling antibodies to the fluorochromes and this technique has found wide application in microbiology. As with the staining procedures described before this technique can only be applied to dead cells. The following techniques have been developed for the examination of living organisms.

Dark ground microscopy

The usual function of the microscope condenser is to concentrate as much light as possible through the specimen and into the objective. The dark ground condenser performs the opposite task. It produces a cone of light which comes to a focus on the specimen. The rays of light in the cone are at an oblique angle such that after passing across the specimen they continue without meeting the front lens of the objective resulting in a dark background. Any objects present at the point of focus scatter the light which enters the objective to show up as a bright image against the dark background.

Specimen preparation is more critical since very dilute bacterial suspensions are required preferably with all the objects in the same plane of focus. Air bubbles must be absent both from the film and the immersion oil, if used. Dust and grease also scatter light and destroy the uniformly black background required for this technique.

Phase contrast microscopy

This technique allows us to see transparent objects well contrasted from the background in clear detail and is the most widely used image enhancement method used in microbiology. The theory is too complex to explain in detail here but in essence an annulus of light is produced by the condenser and focused on the back focal plane of the objective. Here a phase plate comprising a glass disc containing an annular depression is situated. The direct rays of the light source annulus pass through the annular groove while any diffracted rays pass through the remainder of the disc. Passage of the diffracted light through this thicker glass layer results in retardation of the light thus altering its phase relationship to the direct rays and increasing contrast.

Differential-interference-contrast microscopy

This method utilizes polarized light and has other applications which are outside the scope of this chapter such as detecting surface irregularities in opaque specimens. However, it does have some advantages over phase contrast microscopy notably the elimination of haloes around the object edges and enables extremely detailed observation of specimens. It does, however, tend to be more difficult to set up.

Electron microscopy

The highest magnification available using a light microscope is about 1500 times. This limitation is imposed not by the design of the microscope itself, since much higher magnifications are possible, but by the wavelength of light. An object can only be seen if it causes a ray of light to deflect. If a particle is very small indeed then no deflection is produced and the object is not seen. Visible light has a wavelength between 0.3 and 0.8 μm and objects less than 0.3 μm will not be clearly resolved, i.e. even if the magnification was increased no more detail could be seen. In order to increase the resolution it is necessary to use light of a shorter wavelength such as u.v. light. This has been done and resulted in some useful applications but generally, for the purposes of increased definition, electrons are now used and they can be thought of as behaving like very short wavelength light.

Transmission electron microscope (TEM)
Electrons are generated by heating a tungsten filament in an evacuated chamber and are made

to accelerate by a very high potential (-60 to -100 kV) towards a positively charged anode. Some electrons are allowed to pass through a small hole in the anode and a series of electromagnetic lenses focus the electrons into a beam. Electrons pass through the specimen which must be extremely thin and is mounted on a copper grid for support. Dense areas within the specimen scatter the electrons in a similar manner to light. Since our eyes cannot detect electrons a projector lens collects the electrons passing through the specimen and projects the image on to a screen which is capable of fluorescence. Using this mechanism magnifications up to 200 000 times are possible.

Specimen preparation for TEM Three main methods are available for the preparation of microbiological specimens for TEM.

1 Negative staining — the cells are mixed with an electron dense material such as sodium phosphotungstate, placed on a grid and allowed to dry. The micro-organism shows up as a bright object within a dark background and this technique is particularly useful for the study of virus structure.
2 Ultrathin section — an ultramicrotome can produce sections of suitably embedded specimens between 50 and 60 nm thick. As the process involves numerous drastic steps such as fixation and dehydration prior to embedding and cutting care must be taken in the interpretation of these images due to the possible formation of artefacts.
3 Freeze etching — this is a less severe process and involves shadowing the specimen with metal and making a carbon replica of the sample. The specimen is dissolved away and the carbon replica examined. In addition to causing fewer artefacts this method also allows different layers of bacterial cell walls to be examined.

Scanning electron microscope (SEM) This extremely useful instrument differs in construction from the TEM and is used to examine surface structures only. It has a very large depth of field producing images which have almost a three-dimensional quality.

Growth and reproduction of bacteria

The growth and multiplication of bacteria can be examined in terms of individual cells or populations of cells. During the cell division cycle a bacterium assimilates nutrients from the surrounding medium and increases in size. When a predetermined size has been reached a cross-wall will be produced dividing the large cell into two daughter cells. The process is known as binary fission. In a closed environment such as a culture in a test tube the rate at which the cell division occurs varies according to the conditions and this manifests itself in characteristic changes in the population concentration. When fresh medium is inoculated with a small number of bacterial cells the number remains static for a short time while the cells undergo a period of metabolic adjustment. This period is called the *lag phase* (See Fig. 24.7) and its length is dependent upon the degree of readjustment necessary. Once the cells are adapted to the environment they begin to divide in the manner described above and this division occurs at regular intervals. The numbers of bacteria during this period increase in an exponential fashion, i.e. 2, 4, 8, 16, 32, 64, 128 etc. and hence this is termed the exponential or logarithmic phase. When cell numbers are plotted on a log scale against time a straight line results for this phase.

During exponential growth (Fig. 24.7) the medium undergoes continuous change as nutrients are consumed and metabolic waste products excreted. The fact that the cells continue to divide exponentially during this period is a tribute to their physiological adaptability. Eventually, the medium becomes so changed either due to substrate exhaustion or excessive concentrations of toxic products that it is unable to support further growth. At this stage cell division slows and eventually stops leading to the stationary phase (see Fig. 24.7). During this period some cells lyse and die while others sporadically divide but the cell numbers remain more or less constant. Gradually, over a period of time, all the cells lyse and the culture enters the phase of decline.

It should be appreciated that this sequence of events is not a characteristic of the cell but a consequence of the interaction of the organisms

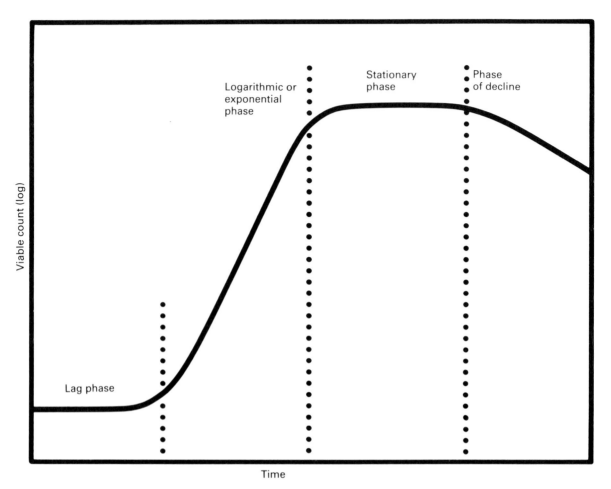

Fig. 24.7 Phases of bacterial growth

with the nutrients in a closed environment and does not necessarily reflect the way in which the organism would behave *in vivo*.

Genetic exchange

In addition to mutations bacteria can alter their genetic make-up by transferring information from one cell to another either as fragments of DNA or in the form of small, extrachromosomal elements (plasmids).

Transfer can be achieved in three ways:

1 transformation
2 transduction
3 conjugation.

Transformation   When bacteria die they lyse

and release cell fragments including DNA into the environment. Several bacterial genera (*Bacillus*, *Haemophilus*, *Streptococcus* etc.) are able to take up these DNA fragments and incorporate them into their own chromosome thus inheriting the characteristics carried on that fragment. Cells able to participate in transformation are called competent and the development of competence has been shown in some cases to occur synchronously in a culture under the action of specific inducing proteins.

Transduction   Bacteriophages are bacterial viruses which do not enter the host cell intact but inject their nucleic acid into the bacterial cytoplasm whereupon it is replicated via the host cell's enzymatic machinery. Some virulent phages result in a complete takeover of the host cell's metabolism followed by lysis and liberation of new phage progeny. Other phages are able to incorporate their nucleic acid into the host cell chromosome with the result that the viral genes are replicated along with the bacterial DNA. In many instances this is a dormant lysogenic state for the phage but sometimes it is triggered into action and lysis of the cell occurs with liberation of phage particles. These new phage particles may have bacterial DNA incorporated into the viral genome and this will infect any new host cell. On entering a new lysogenic state the new host cell will replicate the viral nucleic acid in addition to that portion received from the previous host. Bacteria in which this has been shown to occur include *Mycobacterium*, *Salmonella*, *Shigella* and *Staphylococcus*.

Conjugation Gram-negative bacteria such as *Salmonella*, *Shigella* and *E. coli* have been shown to transfer genetic material conferring antibiotic resistance by cellular contact. This process is called conjugation and is controlled by an R-factor plasmid which is a small circular strand of duplex DNA replicating independently from the bacterial chromosome. R-factor comprises a region containing resistance transfer genes controlling the formation of sex pili, together with a variety of genes which code for the resistance to drugs. Conjugation is initiated when the resistance transfer genes stimulate the production of a sex pilus and random motion brings about contact with a recipient cell. One strand of the replicating R-factor is nicked and passes through the sex pilus into the recipient cell. On receipt of this single strand of plasmid DNA the complementary strand is produced and the free ends joined. For a short time afterwards this cell has the ability to form a sex pilus itself and so transfer the R-factor further.

It should be appreciated that this is by no means an exhaustive discussion of genetic exchange in bacteria and the reader is referred to the bibliography for further information.

Bacterial nutrition

Bacteria require certain elements in fairly large quantities for growth and metabolism including carbon, hydrogen, oxygen and nitrogen. Sulphur and phosphorus are also required but not in such

large amounts while only low concentrations of iron, calcium, potassium, sodium, magnesium and manganese are needed. Some elements such as cobalt, zinc and copper are required only in trace amounts and an actual requirement may be difficult to demonstrate.

The metabolic capabilities of bacteria differ considerably and this is reflected in the form in which nutrients may be assimilated. Bacteria can therefore be classified according to their requirements for carbon and energy.

Lithotrophs (synonym: autotrophs) These utilize carbon dioxide as the main source of carbon. Energy is derived from different sources within this group thus

1 chemolithotrophs (chemosynthetic autotrophs) obtain their energy from the oxidation of inorganic compounds,
2 photolithotrophs (photosynthetic autotrophs) obtain their energy from sunlight.

Organotrophs (synonym: heterotrophs) Organotrophs utilize organic carbon sources and can similarly be divided into

1 chemo-organotrophs which obtain their energy from oxidation or fermentation of organic compounds,
2 photo-organotrophs which utilize light energy.

Oxygen requirements

As mentioned above all bacteria require elemental oxygen in order to build up the complex materials necessary for growth and metabolism but many organisms also require free oxygen as the final electron acceptor in the breakdown of carbon and energy sources. These organisms are called aerobes. If the organism will only grow in the presence of air it is called a strict aerobe but most organisms can either grow in its presence or its absence and are called facultative anaerobes. A strict anaerobe cannot grow and may even be killed in the presence of oxygen because some other compound replaces oxygen as the final electron acceptor in these organisms.

A fourth group of microaerophilic organisms has also been recognized which grow best in only trace amounts of free oxygen and usually prefer an increased carbon dioxide concentration.

Influence of environmental factors on the growth of bacteria

The rate of growth and metabolic activity of bacteria is the sum of a multitude of enzyme reactions and so it follows that those environmental factors which influence enzyme activity will also affect growth rate. Such factors include temperature, pH and osmolarity.

Temperature   Bacteria can survive wide limits of temperature but each organism will exhibit minimum, optimum and maximum growth temperatures and on this basis fall into three broad groups.

1 Psychrophils — grow best below 20 °C but have a minimum about 0 °C and a maximum of 30 °C. These organisms are responsible for low temperature spoilage.
2 Mesophils — exhibit a minimum growth temperature of 5–10 °C and a maximum of 45–50 °C. Within this group two populations can be identified — saprophytic mesophils with an optimum temperature of 20–30 °C and parasitic mesophils with an optimum temperature of 37 °C. The vast majority of pathogenic organisms are in this latter group.
3 Thermophils — can grow at temperatures up to 70–90 °C but have an optimum of 50–55 °C and a minimum of 25–40 °C.

Organisms kept below their minimum growth temperature will not divide but can remain viable. As a result very low temperatures (−70 °C) are used to preserve cultures of organisms for many years. Temperatures in excess of the maximum growth temperature have a much more injurious effect and will be dealt with in more detail later (see Chapter 25).

pH   Most bacteria grow best at around neutrality in the pH range 6.8–7.6. There are, however, exceptions such as the acidophilic organism lactobacillus, a contaminent of milk products, which grows best at pHs between 5.4 and 6.6. *Vibrio cholerae* is the causative agent of cholera and is very sensitive to acid conditions growing most effectively at pH 9.6. Yeasts and moulds prefer acid conditions with an optimum pH range of 4–6. The difference in pH optima between fungi and bacteria is used as a basis for the design of media which will permit the growth of one group of organisms at the expense of others. Sabouraud medium for example has a pH of 5.6 and is a fungal medium whereas nutrient broth which is used routinely to cultivate bacteria has a pH of 7.4. The adverse effect of extremes of pH has been used for many years as a means of preserving foods against microbial attack, for example, pickling.

Osmotic pressure   Bacteria tend to be more resistant to extremes of osmotic pressure than other cells due to the presence of a very rigid cell wall. The concentration of intracellular solutes gives rise to an osmotic pressure equivalent to between 5 and 20 bar and most bacteria will thrive in a medium containing around 0.75% w/v sodium chloride. Staphylococci have the ability to survive higher than normal salt concentrations and this has enabled the formulation of selective media such as mannitol salt agar containing 7.5% w/v sodium chloride which will support the growth of staphylococci but restrict other bacteria.

Halophilic organisms can grow at much higher osmotic pressures but these are all saprophytic and are non-pathogenic to man.

High osmotic pressures generated either by sodium chloride or sucrose have for a long time been used as preservatives. Syrup BP contains 66.7% w/w sucrose and is of sufficient osmotic pressure to resist microbial attack. This is used as a basis for many oral pharmaceutical preparations.

The handling and storage of micro-organisms

Since micro-organisms have such a diversity of nutritional requirements there has arisen a bewildering array of media for the cultivation of bacteria, yeasts and moulds. Media are produced either as liquids or solidified with agar. Agar is an extract of seaweed which at concentrations of between 1 and 2% sets to form a firm gel below 45 °C. Unlike gelatin, bacteria cannot utilize agar as a nutrient and so even after growth the gel remains firm. Liquid media are stored routinely in test tubes or flasks depending upon the volume, both secured with either loose-fitting caps or plugs of sterile cotton wool. Small amounts of solid media are stored in Petri dishes or slopes (also known as butts or slants) while larger volumes may be incorporated in Roux bottles or Carrell flasks.

Bacteria may only be maintained on agar in Petri dishes for a short period of time (days) before the medium dries out. For longer storage periods the surface of an agar slope is inoculated and after growth the culture may be stored at 4 °C for several weeks. If even longer storage periods are required then the cultures should be stored under liquid nitrogen or alternatively placed in ampoules and freeze-dried (lyophilized) before being stored at 4 °C. Vegetative cells which survive this process may retain their viability for many years in this way.

When a single cell is placed on the surface of an overdried agar plate it becomes immobilized but can still draw nutrients from the substrate and consequently grows and divides. Eventually the numbers of bacterial cells are high enough to become visible and a colony is formed. Each of the cells in that colony is a descendant from the initial single cell and so the colony is a pure culture with each cell having identical characteristics. Formation of single colonies is one of the primary aims of surface inoculation of solid media and allows the isolation of pure cultures from specimens containing mixed flora.

Inoculation of agar surfaces by streaking

The agar surface must be smooth and without moisture which may cause the bacteria to become motile and the colonies to merge together. To dry the surface of the agar the plates are inverted in an incubator or drying cabinet with the lids removed.

An inoculating loop is made of either platinum or nichrome wire twisted along its length to form a loop 2–3 mm in diameter at the end. Nichrome wire is cheaper than platinum but has similar thermal properties. The wire is held in a handle with an insulated grip and the entire length of the wire is heated in a bunsen flame to red heat to sterilize it. The first few centimetres of the holder are also flamed before setting aside the loop in a rack to cool.

When cool the loop is used to remove a small portion of liquid from a bacterial suspension and this is then drawn across the agar surface from A to B as indicated in Fig. 24.8. The loop is then resterilized and allowed to cool. At this stage the loop is not reinoculated but streaked over the surface again ensuring a small area of overlap with

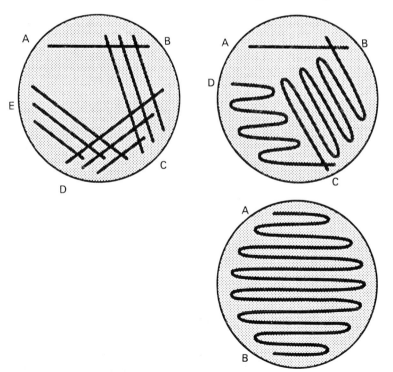

Fig. 24.8 Typical streaking methods for obtaining isolated colonies

the previous streak line. The procedure is repeated as necessary. The pattern of streaking (see other examples in Fig. 24.8) is dictated largely by the concentration of the original bacterial suspension. The object of the exercise is to thin out the culture such that, after incubation, single colonies will arise in the later streak lines where the cells were sufficiently separated. All plates are incubated in an inverted position to prevent condensate from the lid falling on the surface of the medium and spreading the colonies.

Inoculation of slopes

A wire needle may be used to transfer single colonies from agar surfaces to the surface of slopes for maintenance purposes. The needle is similar to the loop except that the wire is single and straight, not terminating in a closed end. This is flamed and cooled as before and a portion of a single colony picked off the agar surface. The needle is then drawn upwards along the surface of the slant. Before incubation the screw cap of the bottle should be loosened slightly to prevent oxygen starvation during growth. Some slopes are prepared with a shallower slope and a deeper butt to allow the needle to be stabbbed into the agar when testing for gas production.

Tranference of liquids

Graduated pipettes and Pasteur pipettes are generally used for this purpose, the latter being short glass tubes one end of which is drawn into a fine capillary. Both types of pipettes should be plugged with sterile cotton wool and filled via pipette fillers of appropriate capacity. Mouth-pipetting should *never* be permitted.

Release of infectious aerosols

During all of these manipulations two considerations must be borne in mind. First, the culture must be transferred with the minimum risk of contamination from outside sources. To this end all pipettes, tubes, media etc. are sterilized and the manipulations carried out under aseptic conditions. Second, the safety of the operator is paramount. During operations with micro-

organisms it must be assumed that all organisms are capable of causing disease and that any route of infection is possible. Most infections acquired in laboratories cannot be traced to a given incident but arise due to the inadvertent release of infectious aerosols. Two types of aerosols may be produced. The first kind produces large droplets (>5 μm), containing many organisms, which settle locally and contaminate surfaces in the vicinity of the operator. These may initiate infections if personnel touch the surfaces and subsequently transfer the organisms to eyes, nose or mouth. The second type of aerosol contains droplets less than 5 μm in size which dry instantly to form droplet nuclei remaining suspended in the air for considerable periods of time. This allows them to be carried on air currents to situations far removed from the site of initiation. These particles are so small they are not trapped by the usual filter mechanisms and may be inhaled, giving rise to infections of the lungs.

The aerosols just described may be produced by a variety of means such as heating wire loops, placing hot loops into liquid cultures, splashing during pipetting, rattling loops and pipettes inside test tubes, opening screw-capped tubes and ampoules etc. All microbiologists should have an awareness of the dangers of aerosol production and learn the correct techniques required to minimize them.

Cultivation of anaerobes

Anaerobic microbiology is a much neglected subject due principally to the practical difficulties involved in growing organisms in the absence of air. However, with the increasing implication of anaerobes in certain disease states and improved cultivation systems the number of workers in this field is growing.

The most common liquid medium for cultivation of anaerobes is thioglycollate medium. In addition to sodium thioglycollate the medium contains methylene blue as a redox indicator and it permits the growth of aerobes, anaerobes and microaerophilic organisms. When in test tubes the medium may be used after sterilization until not more than one-third of the liquid is oxidized as indicated by the colour of the methylene blue indicator. Boiling and cooling of the medium just prior to inoculation is recommended for maximum performance. In some cases the presence of methylene blue poses toxicity problems and under these circumstances the indicator may be removed.

Anaerobic jars have considerably improved in recent years making the cultivation of even strict anaerobes now relatively simple. The most common ones consist of a clear polycarbonate jar with a lid housing a cold catalyst in a mesh container and are designed to be used with disposable H_2/CO_2 generators. The agar plates, which may need to be pre-reduced prior to inoculaton, are placed in the jar together with a gas generator and an anaerobic indicator. Water is added to the gas generator sachet in a measured amount and the lid sealed. Hydrogen and carbon dioxide are evolved and the hydrogen combines with any oxygen present under the action of the cold catalyst to form a light mist of water vapour. Carbon dioxide is produced in sufficient quantities to allow the growth of many fastidious anaerobes which fail to grow in its absence.

The absence of oxygen will be demonstrated by the action of the redox indicator which in the case of methylene blue will be colourless.

Counting bacteria

Estimates of bacterial numbers in a suspension can be evaluated from a number of standpoints each equally valid depending upon the circumstances and the information required. In some cases it may be necessary to know the total amount of biomass produced within a culture irrespective of whether the cells are actively metabolizing. In other instances only an assessment of living bacteria may be required. Bacterial counts can be divided into total counts and viable counts.

Total counts

These counts estimate the total number of bacteria present within a culture, both dead and living cells. A variety of methods are available for the determination of total counts and the one chosen will depend largely upon the characteristics of the cells being studied, i.e. whether they aggregate together.

Microscopic methods Microscopic methods employ a slide counting chamber which has a flat circular platform engraved with a grid of small squares each 0.0025 mm^2 in area. The platform is depressed 0.02 mm and an optically plane glass coverslip is placed over the platform enclosing a space of known dimensions. The volume above each square is 0.5×10^{-8} ml. A bacterial suspension is fixed by adding 2–3 drops of 40% formaldehyde solution per 10 ml of culture to prevent the bacteria from moving across the field of view. A drop of the suspension is then applied to the platform and the coverslip firmly applied ensuring that liquid does not enter a trench which surrounds the platform; the liquid must fill the whole space between the coverslip and the platform. This slide is examined using phase contrast or dark ground microscopy and if necessary the culture is diluted to give 2–10 bacteria per small square. Between 100 and 1000 bacterial cells must be counted to give statistically significant results.

Another microscopic technique is Breed's method. A microscopic slide is marked with a square of known area and a known small volume of bacterial suspension is spread evenly over the square. This is allowed to dry, fixed and stained. A squared eyepiece micrometer is then used to determine the original count knowing the dilution and the size of each square.

Spectroscopic methods These methods are simple to use and very rapid but require careful calibration if meaningful results are to be obtained. Either opacity or light scattering may be used but both methods may only be used for dilute suspensions since at higher concentrations the cells obscure each other in the light path and the Beer–Lambert law is not obeyed. Simple colorimeters and nepholometers can be used but more accurate results are obtained using a spectrophotometer.

Electronic methods The instrument most widely used here is the Coulter Counter which may be adapted for counting bacterial suspensions. The Coulter Counter is described in Chapter 33.

Other methods If an organism is prone to excessive clumping or if a measure of biomass is needed rather than numbers then estimates may be made by performing dry weight or total nitrogen determinations. For dry weight a sample of suspension is centrifuged and the pellet washed free of culture medium by further centrifugation in water. The pellet is collected and dried to constant weight in a desiccator.

Total nitrogen measures the total quantity of nitrogenous material within a cell population. A known volume of suspension is centrifuged and washed as before and the pellet digested using sulphuric acid in the presence of a $CuSO_4–K_2SO_4$–selenium catalyst. This produces ammonia which is removed using boric acid and estimated either by titration or colorimetrically.

Viable counts

These are counts to determine the number of bacteria in a suspension which are capable of division. In all these methods the assumption is made that a colony arises from a single cell although clearly this is often not the case as cells frequently clump or grow as aggregates, e.g. *Staphylococcus aureus*. In these cases the count is usually given as colony forming units (c.f.u.) per ml rather than cells per ml.

Spread plates A known volume, usually 0.2 ml, of a suitably diluted culture is pipetted onto an overdried agar plate and distributed evenly over the surface using a sterile spreader made of wire or glass capillary. The liquid must all be allowed to soak in before the plates are inverted. A series of tenfold dilutions should be made in a suitable sterile diluent and replicates plated out at each dilution in order to ensure that countable numbers of colonies (50–200) are obtained per plate.

The viable count is calculated from the average colony count per plate knowing the dilution and the volume pipetted onto the agar.

Pour plates A series of dilutions of original culture is prepared as before ensuring that at least one is in the range 50–500 organisms per ml. One millilitre quantities are placed into empty, sterile Petri dishes and molten agar, cooled to 45 °C is poured onto the suspensison and mixed by gentle swirling. After setting the plates are inverted and incubated. Since the colonies are embedded within the agar they do not exhibit the characteristic morphology seen with surface colonies. In general

they assume a lens shape and are usually smaller. Since the oxygen tension is reduced below the surface this method is not suitable for strict aerobes.

Miles Misra method An overdried agar plate is divided on the back into a number of segments. A suitably diluted bacterial suspension is prepared of which 0.02 ml is placed in each segment as a discrete drop and allowed to soak in without spreading. A number of dilutions are prepared and different plates are inoculated. After incubation the colonies are counted in each segment (usually up to 20) provided they are not confluent.

Membrane filtration This method is particularly useful when the level of contamination is very low such as in water supplies. A known volume of sample is passed through a cellulose acetate/nitrate membrane filter of sufficient pore size to retain bacteria (0.2–0.45 μm). The filtrate is discarded and the membrane placed bacteria uppermost on the surface of an overdried agar plate avoiding trapped air between membrane and surface. The bacteria draw nutrients through the membrane and form colonies which can be counted.

Isolation and identification of bacteria

Mixed bacterial cultures from pathological specimens or other biological materials are isolated first on solid media to give single colonies and the pure cultures resulting can then be subjected to identification procedures. The techniques used for isolation depends upon the proportion of the species of interest compared to the background contamination.

Direct inoculation can only be used when an organism is found as a pure culture in nature. Examples include bacterial infections of normally sterile fluids such as blood or cerebrospinal fluid.

Streaking is the most common method employed and if the proportions of bacteria in the mixed culture are roughly equal then streaking on an ordinary nutrient medium should yield single colonies of all microbial types. More usually the organism of interest is present only as a very small fraction of the total microbial population necessitating the use of selective media.

A selective enrichment broth is initially inoculated with the mixed population of cells and this inhibits the growth of the majority of the background population. At the same time the growth of the organism of interest is encouraged. After incubation in these media the cultures are streaked out onto solid selective media which frequently contain indicators to further differentiate species on the basis of fermentation of specific sugars. An example of the use of enrichment and selective media is shown in Fig. 24.9 which summarizes the BP test for microbial contamination.

Having isolated a pure culture, identification can then take place. Tests used are based upon morphological, physiological, biochemical and serological characteristics. In many cases presumptive identification can be made on the basis of microscopical examination and cultural characteristics such as colonial morphology and nutritional requirements. However, it is usual to perform additional tests in order to obtain a definitive identification.

Biochemical tests

These tests are designed to examine the enzymatic capabilities of the organism. Sugar fermentation is one of the most common tests and examines the ability of the organism to ferment a range of sugars. A number of tubes of peptone water are prepared each containing a different sugar. An acid/base indicator is incorporated into the medium which also contains a Durham tube (a small inverted tube filled with medium) capable of collecting any gas produced during fermentation. After inoculation and incubation the tubes are examined for acid production as indicated by a change in the colour of the indicator and gas production as seen by a bubble of gas collected in the Durham tube.

Proteases are produced by a number of bacteria, e.g. *Bacillus* species and *Pseudomonas*, and they are responsible for the breakdown of protein into smaller units. Gelatin is a protein which can be added to liquid media to produce a stiff gel similar to agar. Unlike agar which cannot be utilized by bacteria those organisms which produce proteases will destroy the gel structure and liquefy the medium. A medium made of nutrient broth solidified with gelatin is normally incorporated in boiling tubes or small bottles and inoculated by

means of a stab wire. After incubation it is important to refrigerate the gelatin prior to examination otherwise false positives may be produced.

Proteases can also be detected using milk agar which is opaque. Protease producers form colonies with clear haloes around them where the enzyme has diffused into the medium and digested the casein.

Oxidase is produced by *Neisseria* and *Pseudomonas* and can be detected using 1% tetramethylparaphenylene diamine. The enzyme catalyses the transport of electrons between electron donors in the bacteria and the redox dye. A positive reaction is indicated by a deep purple colour in the reduced dye. The test is carried out by placing the reagent directly onto an isolated colony on an agar surface. Alternatively a filter paper strip impregnated with the dye is moistened with water and a bacterial colony spread, using a platinum loop, across the surface. A purple colour will appear within 10 seconds if positive. Note the use of iron loops may give false-positive reactions.

The indole test distinguishes those bacteria capable of decomposing the amino acid tryptophan to indole. Any indole produced can be tested by a colorimetric reaction with p-dimethylaminobenzaldehyde. After incubation in peptone water 0.5 ml Kovacs reagent is placed on the surface of the culture, shaken and left to stand. A positive reaction is indicated by a red colour. Organisms giving positive indole reactions include *E. coli* and *Proteus vulgaris*.

Catalase is responsible for the breakdown of hydrogen peroxide into oxygen and water. The test may be performed by adding 1 ml of 10 vol hydrogen peroxide directly to the surface of colonies growing on an agar slope. The presence of catalase is indicated by a vigorous frothing of the surface liquid. *Staphylococcus* and *Micrococcus* are catalase positive whereas *Streptococcus* is catalase negative.

Urease production enables certain bacteria to break down urea to ammonia and carbon dioxide.

$$NH_2-CO-NH_2 + H_2O \xrightarrow{\text{urease}} 2NH_3 + CO_2$$

This test is readily carried out by growing the bacteria on a medium containing urea and an acid/base indicator. After incubation the production of ammonia will be shown by the alkaline

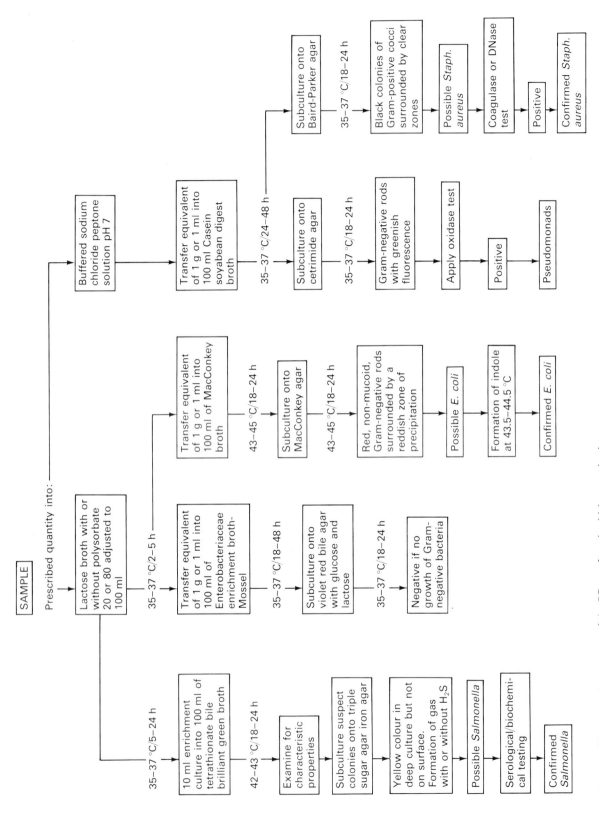

Fig. 24.9 Diagrammatic summary of the BP test for microbial contamination

reaction of the indicator. Examples of urease-negative bacteria include *E. coli* and *Streptococcus faecalis*.

Simmons citrate agar was developed to test for the presence of organisms which could utilize citrate as the sole source of carbon and energy and ammonia as the main source of nitrogen. It is used to differentiate members of the Enterobacteriaceae. The medium containing bromothymol blue as indicator is surface inoculated on slopes and citrate utilization demonstrated by an alkaline reaction and a change in the indicator colour from a dull green to a bright blue. *E. coli*, *Shigella*, *Edwardsiella* and *Yersinia* do not utilize citrate whereas *Serratia*, *Enterobacter*, *Klebsiella* and *Proteus* do and so give a positive result.

The methyl red test is used to distinguish those organisms which produce and maintain a high level of acidity from those which initially produce acid but restore neutral conditions with further metabolism. The organism is grown on glucose phosphate medium and after incubation a few drops of methyl red are added and the colour immediately recorded. A red colour indicates acid production (positive) while a yellow colour indicates alkali (negative).

Some organisms can convert carbohydrates to acetyl methyl carbinol (CH_3–CO–CHOH–CH_3). This may be oxidized to diacetyl (CH_3–CO–CO–CH_3) which will react with guanidino residues in the medium under alkaline conditions to produce a colour. This is the basis of the Voges Proskauer test which is usually carried out at the same time as the methyl red test. The organism is again grown in glucose phosphate medium and after incubation 40% KOH is added together with 5% α-naphthol in ethanol. After mixing, a positive reaction is indicated by a pink colour in 2–5 min, gradually becoming darker red up to 30 min. Organisms giving positive Voges Proskauer reactions usually give negative methyl red reactions since the production of acetylmethyl carbinol is accompanied by low acid production. *Klebsiella* is an example of an organism showing a positive Voges Proskauer reaction.

Rapid identification systems With the increasing demand for quick and accurate identification of bacteria a number of micromethods have been developed combining a variety of biochemical tests selected for their rapidity of reading and high discrimination. The API® bacterial identification system is an example of such a micromethod and comprises plastic trays containing dehydrated substrates in a number of wells. Culture is added to the wells, dissolving the substrate thus allowing the fermentation of carbohydrates or the presence of enzymes similar to those just described to be demonstrated. In some cases incubation times of 2 hours are sufficient for accurate identification. Kits are available with different reagents permitting identification of Enterobacteriaceae, Streptococcaceae, staphylococci, anaerobes, yeasts and moulds. Accurate identification is made by reference to a table of results.

Serological tests

Bacteria have antigens associated with their cell envelopes (O-antigens), with their flagella (H-antigens) and their capsules (K-antigens). When injected into an animal, antibodies will be produced directed specifically towards those antigens and able to react with them. Specific antisera are prepared by immunizing an animal with a killed or attenuated bacterial suspension and taking blood samples. Serum containing the antibodies can then be separated. If a sample of bacterial suspension is placed upon a glass slide and mixed with a small amount of specific antiserum than the bacteria will be seen to clump when examined under the microscope. The test can be made more quantitative by using the tube dilution technique where a given amount of antigen is mixed with a series of dilutions of specific antisera. The highest dilution at which agglutination occurs is called the agglutination titre.

Phage typing

Many bacteria are susceptible to lytic bacteriophages whose action is very specific. Identification may be based on the susceptibility of a culture to a set of type-specific lytic bacteriophages. This method enables very detailed identification of the organisms to be made, e.g. one serotype of

Salmonella typhi has been further subdivided into 80 phage types using this technique.

ACTINOMYCETES

This group of micro-organisms provides the link between bacteria and fungi. They are now generally accepted as bacteria being prokaryotic in nature. Four families are of pharmaceutical importance, viz. Mycobacteriaceae, Nocardiaceae, Streptomycetaceae and Actinomycetaceae.

The morphology of the actinomycetes varies from genus to genus but all show some tendency to produce hyphae and to branch. Spores, when produced, may either be endogenous e.g. *Thermoactinomyces* (in which case they bear similarities to those produced by *Bacillus* species) or occur by division of the existing hyphal strands, e.g. *Streptomyces, Nocardia*. The spores are reproductive in function and in many instances are not much more resistant to heat than vegetative cells although they are more resistant to desiccation. *Mycobacterium* including the pathogenic species *Myco. tuberculosis* and *Myco. leprae* (causative agents of tuberculosis and leprosy respectively) are acid-fast organisms showing the least tendency to branch and hyphae are never seen. The organisms are Gram-positive in nature, non-motile and do not form spores.

Nocardia contain a number of species which have been shown to be pathogenic to man but occur principally in tropical climates. They are usually aerobic organisms and are mostly acid-fast.

The Actinomycetaceae have only one human pathogen, *A. israelii*, which is an anaerobic Gram-positive micro-organism with branching filaments. Infections which occur are generally in the cervico–oro–facial region but other infections do arise in the abdomen and other organs. They are usually non-acid-fast and tend to fragment into short coccal forms.

The Streptomycetaceae contain no human pathogens and are responsible for the production of a very wide range of therapeutically useful antibiotics including streptomycin, chloramphenicol, oxytetracyline, erythromycin and neomycin. They are aerobic organisms producing a non-fragmenting branching mycelium which may bear spores.

FUNGI (EUMYCETES)

Yeasts and moulds are eukaryotic organisms possessing organized demonstrable nuclei enclosed within a nuclear membrane, a nucleolus and chromatin strands which become organized into chromosomes during cell division. Their role in nature is predominantly a scavanging one and in this respect they are vital for the decomposition and recycling of organic materials. Only a few are pathogens and most of these are facultative and not obligate parasites. In recent years however, the relative importance of fungal infections has increased as bacterial infections have been brought under more effective control by improved standards of hygiene and widespread antibiotic use. In addition, long term use of broad spectrum antibiotic allows opportunist infections by resistant organisms such as *Candida albicans* to develop.

Fungi have for many years been invaluable to man in the production of bread, cheese and fermented drinks while more recently they have been used commercially for the manufacture of organic acids, antibiotics, steroids, etc. The Eumycetes can be divided into four broad groups on the basis of their morphology.

Yeasts

These are spherical or ovoid unicellular bodies 2–4 μm in diameter which reproduce by budding. Examples include *Saccharomyces cerevisiae*, strains of which are used in baking and in the production of wines and beers. *Cryptococcus neoformans* is the only significant pathogen.

Yeast-like fungi

These organisms normally behave like a typical budding yeast but under certain circumstances the buds do not separate and become elongated. The resulting structure resembles a filament and is called a pseudomycelium. The most important member of this group is *Candida albicans* which is usually resident in the mouth, intestine and vagina. Under normal conditions *Candida* does not cause any problems but if the environment balance is disturbed then infections can arise. These include vaginal thrush (vaginitis) and oral thrush. More serious infections include bronchial and pulmonary candidiasis and also some deep seated systemic infections.

Dimorphic fungi

These grow as yeasts or as filaments depending upon the cultural conditions. At 22 °C either in the soil or in culture media filamentous mycelial forms are produced whereas at 37 °C in the body they assume a yeast-like appearance. *Histoplasma capsulatum* is the most important of the dimorphic fungi and gives rise to a range of conditions varying from asymptomatic chest infections through to a fatal generalized disease.

Filamentous fungi

This group comprises those moulds which are multicellular and grow in the form of long, slender filaments called hyphae 2–10 μm in diameter. The branching hyphae, which constitute the vegetative or somatic structure of the mould, intertwine and gradually spread over the entire surface of the available substrate extracting nutrients and forming a dense mat or mycelium. Hyphae may be non-septate (coenocytic) or septate but in each case the nutrients and cellular components are freely diffusible along the length of the filament. This is facilitated by the presence of pores within the septa. The hyphal wall is composed of poly-

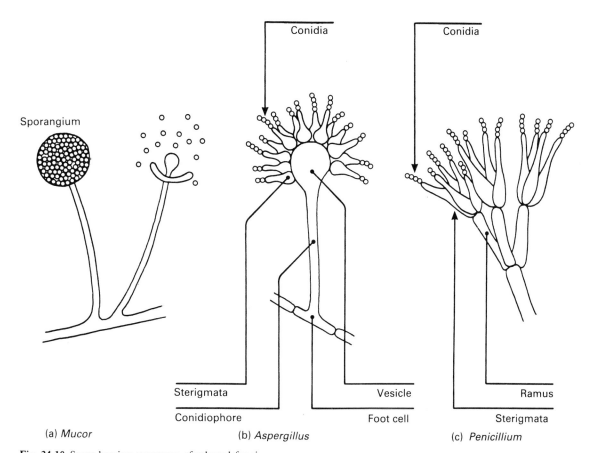

(a) *Mucor* (b) *Aspergillus* (c) *Penicillium*

Fig. 24.10 Spore-bearing structures of selected fungi

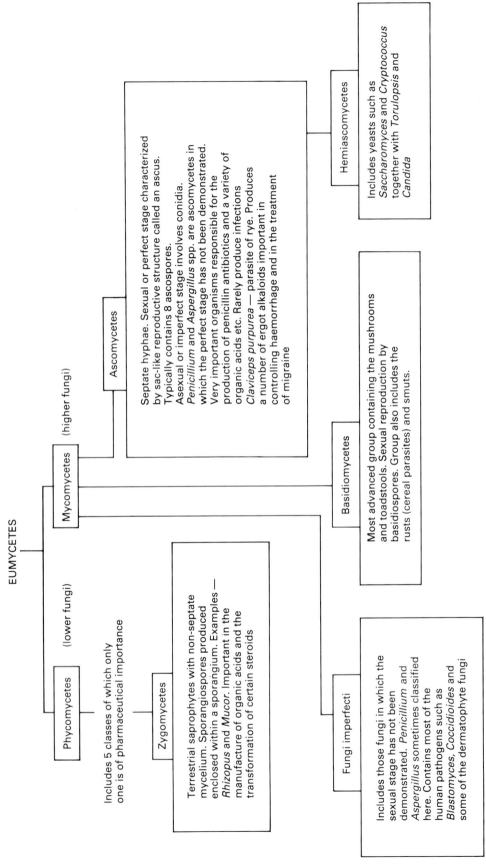

Fig. 24.11 Characteristics of some pharmaceutically important fungi

EUMYCETES

Mycomycetes

Phycomycetes — (lower fungi)

(higher fungi)

Includes 5 classes of which only one is of pharmaceutical importance

Zygomycetes

Terrestrial saprophytes with non-septate mycelium. Sporangiospores produced enclosed within a sporangium. Examples — *Rhizopus* and *Mucor*. Important in the manufacture of organic acids and the transformation of certain steroids

Fungi imperfecti

Includes those fungi in which the sexual stage has not been demonstrated. *Penicillium* and *Aspergillus* sometimes classified here. Contains most of the human pathogens such as *Blastomyces, Coccidioides* and some of the dermatophyte fungi

Ascomycetes

Septate hyphae. Sexual or perfect stage characterized by sac-like reproductive structure called an ascus. Typically contains 8 ascospores. Asexual or imperfect stage involves conidia. *Penicillium* and *Aspergillus* spp. are ascomycetes in which the perfect stage has not been demonstrated. Very important organisms responsible for the production of penicillin antibiotics and a variety of organic acids etc. Rarely produce infections *Claviceps purpurea* — parasite of rye. Produces a number of ergot alkaloids important in controlling haemorrhage and in the treatment of migraine

Basidiomycetes

Most advanced group containing the mushrooms and toadstools. Sexual reproduction by basidiospores. Group also includes the rusts (cereal parasites) and smuts.

Hemiascomycetes

Includes yeasts such as *Saccharomyces* and *Cryptococcus* together with *Torulopsis* and *Candida*

saccharide and in most moulds this is chitin mixed with cellulose, glucan and mannan.

Reproduction of fungi

In the somatic portion of most fungi the nuclei are very small and the mechanism of nuclear division is uncertain. Under the correct environmental conditions the organisms will switch from the somatic or vegetative growth phase to a reproductive form so that the fungus may propagate the species by producing new mycelia on fresh food substrates.

Two types of reproduction are found: asexual and sexual.

Asexual reproduction

Asexual reproduction is in general more important for the propagation of the species and mechanisms include fragmentation, binary fission, budding and spore formation. Each new mycelium is an exact replica of the parent and no species variation can occur. Spore formation is the most common method of asexual reproduction and the spores vary in colour, arrangement and the way they are held (see Fig. 24.10). Spores can either be borne on sporangia surrounded by a limiting membrane in which case they are called sporangiospores or they are produced as single separable cells at the tips of the hyphal threads and are called conidia. Spores arising from the fragmentation of the mycelium are called oidia, arthrospores or

chlamydospores. The latter are enveloped within a thick wall before they separate. This acts as a resting stage rich in food reserves and helps maintain the species during periods unfavourable for growth.

Flagellated zoospores are produced by the more primitive aquatic fungi but spores of the higher terrestrial fungi are usually dispersed by the wind.

It is widely accepted that vegetative growth and spore formation are mutually exclusive processes and that sporulation will only occur when certain essential nutrients have become exhausted.

Sexual reproduction

Sexual reproduction involves the union of two compatible nuclei and allows variation of the species. Some species produce distinguishable male and female sex organs on the same thallus and are thus hermaphroditic, i.e. a single thallus can reproduce by itself. Others produce thalli which are either male or female and are called dioecious.

Three stages are involved in sexual reproduction:

1 plasmogamy — the two nuclei are brought together in the same cell,
2 karyogamy — the two nuclei fuse,
3 meiosis — restoration of the original haploid state.

Figure 24.11 illustrates some of the characteristics of the pharmaceutically important fungi.

BIBLIOGRAPHY

British Pharmacopoeia (1980) and Addendum (1986) HMSO, London.
Buchanan, R. E. (1974) *Bergey's Manual of Determinative Bacteriology*, 8th edn, Williams and Wilkins, Baltimore.
Burnett, J. H. (1976) *Fundamentals of Mycology*, 2nd edn, Edward Arnold, London.
Casartelli, J. D. (1969) *Microscopy for Students*, 2nd edn, McGraw-Hill, London.
Duguid, J. P., Marmion, B. P. and Swain, R. H. A. (1978) *Medical Microbiology*, 13th edn, Churchill-Livingstone, Edinburgh.
Gottleib, D. (1973) General consideration and implications of the Actinomycetales. In *Actinomycetales: Characteristics and Practical Importance* (eds G. Sykes, and F. A. Skinner), pp. 1–10, The Society for Applied Bacteriology Symposium series No. 2, Academic Press, New York.
Gould, G. W. and Dring, G. J. (1974) Mechanisms of spore heat resistance. *Adv. Microb. Physiol.*, **11**, 137–164.
Hugo, W. B. and Russell, A. D. (1983) *Pharmaceutical*

Microbiology, 3rd edn, Blackwell Scientific Publications, Oxford.
Mandelstam, J. (1969) Regulation of bacterial spore formation. *Symp. Soc. Gen. Microbiol.*, **19**, 377–404.
Mandelstam, J., McQuillan, K. and Dawes, I. (1982) *Biochemistry of Bacterial Growth*, 3rd edn, Churchill-Livingstone, Edinburgh.
Mitruka, B. M. (1976) *Methods of Detection and Identification of Bacteria*, CRC Press, Boca Raton, Florida.
Primrose, S. B. and Dimmock, N. J. (1980) *Introduction to Modern Virology*, 2nd edn, Blackwell Scientific Publications, Oxford.
Stryer, L. (1981) *Biochemistry*, 2nd edn, W. H. Freeman and Co., San Francisco, California.
The Oxoid Manual of Culture Media, Ingredients and Other Laboratory Services, (1980) 4th Edition, Oxoid Ltd, London.
Wilson, Sir G. S. and Miles, Sir A. (1975) *Topley and Wilson's Principles of Bacteriology and Immunity*, Vols. 1 and 2., 6th edn, Edward Arnold, London.

The action of physical and chemical agents on micro-organisms

The subject of this chapter is of importance to the pharmacist because he has a responsibility for

1 the production of medicines having, as their prime function, the destruction of micro-organisms, e.g. antiseptic liquids and antibiotic formulations, or
2 the production of sterile medicaments having no living micro-organisms, e.g. injections and eye drops, and finally
3 the production of a wide range of medicines which must be effectively protected against microbial spoilage.

Thus the major pharmaceutical interest in micro-organisms is that of killing them or, at least, preventing their growth. Consequently it is necessary both to have an understanding of the physical processes, e.g. heating and irradiation, which are used to kill micro-organisms and to have a knowledge of the more diverse subject of antimicrobial chemicals.

This background knowledge must therefore include an understanding of the kinetics of cell inactivation, the calculation of parameters by which microbial destruction or growth inhibition are measured and an appreciation of the factors which influence the efficiency of the physical and chemical processes used. These aspects, together with a synopsis of the major groups of antimicrobial chemicals, are the subject of this chapter which is intended also as an introduction to subsequent chapters on the theoretical design and operation of sterilization processes (Chapters 26 and 43) and the laboratory procedures used to measure the activity of antimicrobial chemicals (Chapter 28).

THE KINETICS OF CELL INACTIVATION

The death of a population of cells exposed to heat, radiation or toxic chemicals is often found to follow or approximate to first order kinetics. In this sense it is similar to bacterial growth during the logarithmic phase of the cycle, the graphs representing these processes are similar but of opposite slope. Assuming first order kinetics (the exceptions will be considered later), an initial population of N_o cells per ml will, after a time t minutes, be reduced to N_t cells per ml according to the following equation in which k is the inactivation rate constant.

$$N_t = N_o e^{-kt} \tag{25.1}$$

$$\ln N_t = \ln N_o - kt \tag{25.2}$$

$$\log_{10} N_t = \log_{10} N_o - \frac{kt}{2.303} \tag{25.3}$$

Thus the data in Table 25.1 may be used to produce a plot of logarithm of cell concentration against exposure time (Fig. 25.1) where the intercept is log N_o and the slope is $-k/2.303$. This may be plotted with logarithm of the per cent survivors

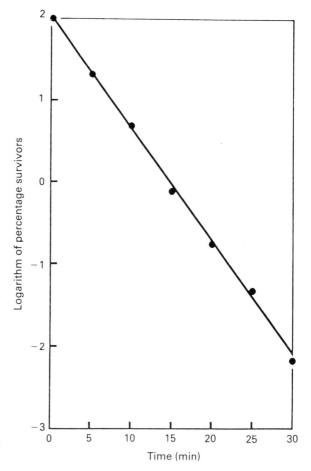

Fig. 25.1 Heat inactivation of *Bacillus megaterium* spores at 95 °C

Table 25.1 Death of *B. megaterium* spores in pH 7.0 buffer at 95 °C

Time (min)	Viable cell concentration ml^{-1}	Per cent survivors	Log$_{10}$ per cent survivors
0	2.50×10^6	100	2.000
5	5.20×10^5	20.8	1.318
10	1.23×10^5	4.92	0.692
15	1.95×10^4	0.78	-0.108
20	4.60×10^3	0.18	-0.745
25	1.21×10^3	0.048	-1.319
30	1.68×10^2	0.0067	-2.174

as the ordinate, thus the largest numerical value on this axis is 2.0. For convenience such plots are often constructed on semilogarithmic graph paper which eliminates the need to calculate logarithmic values for each point. An important feature of Fig. 25.1 is the fact that there is no lower end point to the ordinate scale, it continues indefinitely. If the initial population was 1000 cells ml^{-1} the logarithmic value would be 3.0; at 100 cells ml^{-1}, the value would be 2.0, at 10 cells ml^{-1} 1.0 and at 1 cell ml^{-1} zero. The next incremental point on the logarithmic scale would be -1 which corresponds to 0.1 cells ml^{-1}. It is clearly nonsense to talk of a fraction of a viable cell per ml, but this value corresponds to 1 whole cell in 10 ml of liquid. The next point, -2.0, corresponds to 1 cell in 100 ml, and so on. Sterility is the complete absence of life, i.e. zero cells ml^{-1} which has a log value of $-\infty$. *Guaranteed* sterility would therefore require an infinite exposure time. This has important implications in the design of sterilization processes which are considered in Chapters 26 and 43.

D value or decimal reduction time

It is characteristic of first order kinetics that the same percentage change in concentration occurs in successive time intervals. Thus in Fig. 25.1 it can be seen that the viable population falls to 10% of its initial value after 7.5 minutes: in the next 7.5 minute period the population again falls to 10% of its value at the start of that period. This time period for a 90% reduction in count is related to the slope of the line and is one of the more useful parameters by which the death rate may be indicated. It is known as the decimal reduction time or D value. It usually has a subscript showing the temperature at which it was measured, e.g. $D_{115\,°C}$ or $D_{121\,°C}$. It is quite possible to indicate the rate of destruction by the inactivation rate constant calculated from the slope of the line, but the significance of this value cannot be as readily appreciated during conversation as that of a D value so the former is less frequently used.

Z values

When designing sterilization processes it is necessary to know both the D value which is a measure of the effectiveness of heat at any given temperature and the extent to which a particular increase in temperature will reduce the D value, i.e. it is necessary to have a measure of the effect of temperature change on death rate. One such measure is the Z value which is defined as the number of degrees temperature change required to achieve a tenfold change in D value, e.g. if the D value for *B. stearothermophilus* spores at 110 °C was 20 minutes and it has a Z value of 9 °C, this means that at 119 °C the D value would be 2.0 min, and at 128 °C the D value would be 0.20 min. The relationship between D and Z values is shown in Fig. 25.2. The Z value is one of several parameters which relate change in

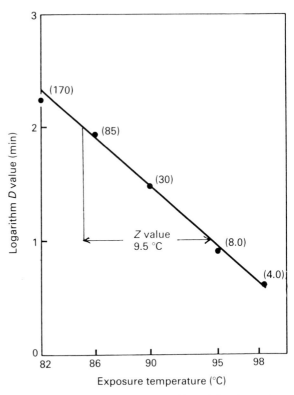

Fig. 25.2 Relationship between logarithm of D value and exposure temperature for heated *Bacillus megaterium* spores. Individual D values (minutes) are shown in parentheses

temperature to change in death rate and is probably the most commonly used and readily understood. The activation energy obtained from an Arrhenius plot (see Chapter 7) or a temperature coefficient, a Q_{10} value (change in rate for a 10 °C change in temperature), do the same but are less commonly used.

Alternative survivor plots

It was stated earlier that bacterial death often approximates to first order kinetics although exceptions do arise. Some of the more common are illustrated in Fig. 25.3. The plot labelled A is that conforming to first order kinetics which has already been described. A shoulder on the curve as in case B is not uncommon and various explanations have been offered. Cell aggregation or clumping may be responsible for such a shoulder because it would be necessary to apply sufficient heat to kill *all* of the cells in the clump, not merely

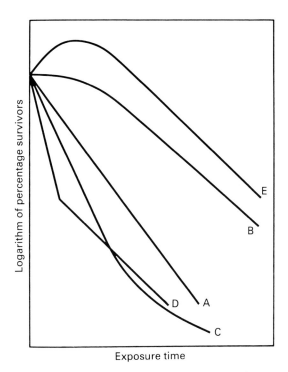

Fig. 25.3 Alternative survivor plots for cells exposed to lethal agents

there are alternative explanations, one of the most common being that the cells dying during the early exposure period release chemicals which help to protect those which are still alive.

A sharp break in the line as in D usually indicates that there are two distinct populations of cells present which have markedly different resistances. Contamination of a cell suspension or culture is a possible explanation, or it may be that a mutant has arisen naturally and the cultural conditions are such that it has a selective advantage and its numbers have increased until it is a substantial proportion of the population.

Plot E is uncommon and is usually only seen as a result of 'heat activation' of bacterial spores. This is a situation in which a significant proportion of a population of spores (usually a thermophil) remain dormant and fail to germinate and produce colonies under 'normal' conditions. If the suspension receives a heat stimulus or shock which is insufficient to kill the spores some or all of those which would otherwise remain dormant become activated, germinate and thus produce a rise in the colony count.

ANTIMICROBIAL EFFECTS OF MOIST AND DRY HEAT

Moist heat (steam) and dry heat (hot air) both have the potential to kill micro-organisms but their efficiencies and their mechanisms of action differ. In autoclaves dry, saturated steam, i.e. 100% water vapour with no liquid water present, is used at temperatures between 115 and 135 °C, at which it rapidly kills micro-organisms. An advantage of using steam is that is possesses latent heat of vaporization which it transfers on to any object upon which it condenses (see Chapter 30). It is essential to use dry saturated steam if maximal autoclaving efficiency is to be achieved. If the steam is wet, i.e. it contains liquid water, penetration of vapour phase steam into dressings may be retarded. If the steam is superheated, i.e. its temperature has been raised whilst the pressure remained constant or the pressure fell whilst the temperature remained constant, it contains less moisture and latent heat than dry saturated steam

the most sensitive, before a fall is observed in the number of colonies appearing on the agar. Under normal circumstances one single colony could arise both from one cell alone or from 100 cells aggregated together. In the latter case if sufficient heat was applied to kill only the 99 most sensitive cells in the clump the colony count would be unaltered. Clumping is not the only explanation, because substantial shoulders may arise using suspensions where the vast majority of cells exist individually. An alternative suggestion is that there is more than one sensitive site (target) in the cell which must be inactivated before the cell dies.

Tailing of survivor curves as in plot C is often observed if the initial cell concentration is high. This has been attributed to the presence of mutants which are exceptionally resistant to the lethal agent. If the proportion of mutants were 1 in 10^6 cells and the initial concentration only 10^5 cells ml^{-1} the mutant would not be detected, but an initial population of 10^9 cells ml^{-1} would permit easy detection if the inactivation plot were continued down to low levels of survivors. Again

at the same temperature. In this case the effect is similar to using a steam–air mixture at that temperature. The process by which steam kills cells is hydrolysis of essential proteins (enzymes) and nucleic acids. In contrast, dry heat causes cell death by oxidative processes although it is, again, the proteins and nucleic acids which are the vulnerable targets. Dry heat is a much less effective method of killing micro-organisms than steam at the same temperature. Exposures of not less than one hour at 170 °C (or an equivalent temperature/time combination) are recommended in the BP for sterilization by dry heat methods. The state of hydration of a cell is thus an important factor determining its resistance to heat.

Resistance of micro-organisms to moist and dry heat

Numerous factors influence the observed heat resistance of microbial cells and it is difficult to make comparisons between populations unless these factors are controlled. Not surprisingly, marked differences in resistance exist between different genera, species and strain and between the spore and vegetative cell forms of the same organism. The resistance may be influenced, sometimes extensively, by the age of the cell, i.e. lag, exponential or stationary phase, its chemical composition which, in turn, is influenced by the medium in which the cell is grown and by the composition and pH of the fluid in which the cell is heated. It is difficult to obtain strictly comparable heat resistance data for grossly dissimilar organisms but the values quoted in Table 25.2 indicate the relative order of heat resistance of the various microbial groups. Tabulation of D values at a designated temperature is perhaps the most convenient way of comparing resistance, but this is only suitable for first order kinetics. Alternative methods of comparison include the time to achieve a particular percentage kill or the time required to achieve no survivors; the latter is, of course, dependent upon the initial population level.

Bacterial endospores are invariably found to be the most heat resistant cell type and those of certain species may survive boiling water for many hours. (The term endospores refers to the spores

Table 25.2 Heat resistances of different micro-organisms

Cell type	Heat resistance — values are for fully hydrated organisms unless otherwise stated
Bacterial endospores	Little or no inactivation at <80 °C. Some species survive boiling for several hours
Fungal spores	Ascospores of *Byssochlamys* species survive 60 min at 88 °C but majority of species less resistant
Actinomycete spores	Spores of *Nocardia sebivorans* reported to survive 10 min at 90 °C but majority of species less resistant
Yeasts	Ascospores and vegetative cells show little difference in resistance. Survival for 20 min at 60 °C typical
Mycobacterium tuberculosis	May survive 30 min at 100 °C in dry state but usually killed after 20 min at 60 °C when moist
Eubacteria	D_{60} = 1–5 min typical for staphylococci and many enteric organisms. Pneumococci may survive 30 min at 110 °C when dry
Fungal mycelia and actinomycete vegetative cells	Similar to Eubacteria
Viruses	Rarely survive for >30 min at 55–60 °C. Exceptional survival of >4 h at 60 °C reported for serum hepatitis virus
Protozoa and algae	No more resistant than mammalian cells. Survival only for a few hours at >40–45 °C
Psychrophilic bacteria	D value of only 6 min at 30 °C reported for a species of *Serratia*, but majority of psychrophils probably less sensitive

produced by *Bacillus* and *Clostridium* species and is not to be confused with the spores produced by other bacteria such as actinomycetes; these do not develop within the vegetative cell.) The majority of *Bacillus* and *Clostridium* species normally form spores which survive in water for 15–30 min at 80 °C without significant damage or viability loss. Because endospores are more resistant than other cells they have been the subject of a considerable amount of research in the food and pharmaceutical industry over the last 50 years: much of this work has been reviewed by Russell (1982). Mould spores and those of yeasts and actinomycetes usually exhibit a degree of moist heat resistance intermediate between endospores and vegetative cell forms: survival at 60 °C for several hours but death at 80 °C or higher would be typical of such cells. Vegetative cells of bacteria and yeasts and mould mycelia themselves vary significantly in heat resistance. Mycobacteria, which possess a high proportion of lipid in their cell wall, tend to be more resistant than others. Protozoa and algae are, by comparison, susceptible to heat, and they, like mammalian cells, rapidly die at temperatures much in excess of 40 °C.

Information on the heat resistance of viruses is limited, but the available data suggest that whilst they may vary significantly between types, the majority of viruses are no more heat resistant than vegetative bacteria.

Resistance to dry heat by different groups of micro-organisms usually follows a similar pattern to that in aqueous environments. Again endospores are substantially more resistant than the other cell types with those of *B. stearothermophilus* and *B. subtilis* usually representing the extreme. Exposures of the order of 150–160 °C for one hour are adequate to achieve reductions in viable numbers in excess of 10^6-fold, and thus easily kill the concentrations of spores likely to be found on washed glassware and as contaminants in oils and powders. The cells of pneumococci have been reported to survive dry heat at 110 °C for 30 minutes but this represents exceptional resistance for vegetative cells most of which may be expected to die after a few minutes' heating at 100 °C or less.

Valid comparisons of dry heat resistance amongst dissimilar organisms are even less common than those for aqueous environments because there is the additional problem of distinguishing the effects of drying from those of heat. For many cells desiccation is itself a potentially lethal process even at room temperature, so that experiments in which the moisture content of the cells is uncontrolled may produce results which are misleading or difficult to interpret. This is particularly so when the cells are heated under conditions where their moisture content is changing and they become progressively drier during the experiment.

Factors affecting heat resistance and its measurement

The major factors affecting heat resistance have been listed in the previous section and will be considered in some detail here. The subject has been extensively studied, and again much of the experimental data and consequently many of the examples quoted in this section come from the field of spore research.

The measurement of heat resistance in fully hydrated cells, i.e. those suspended in aqueous solutions or exposed to dry saturated steam, does not normally represent a problem when conducted at temperatures <100 °C. Errors may occasionally arise when spore heat resistance is measured at higher temperatures. In these circumstances it is necessary to heat suspensions sealed in glass ampoules immersed in glycerol or oil baths or to expose the spores to steam in a modified autoclave. Monitoring and control of heat-up and cool-down times become important, and failure to pay adequate attention to these aspects may lead to apparent differences in resistance which may simply be due to such factors as variations in thickness of glass in two batches of ampoules.

Species and strain differences

Variations in heat resistance between the species within a genus are very common. However careful scrutiny of much of the data which apparently illustrate this fact shows that other factors may have contributed to the differences, e.g. use of different growth media or incubation temperatures. Murrell and Warth (1965) produced 20 spore crops from 13 *Bacillus* species and found a 700-fold variation in their *D* values at 100 °C. However, this was achieved using eight different culture media, three incubation temperatures and six procedures for 'cleaning' the spores and separating them from the vegetative cells and debris. Differences between strains of a single species are, not surprisingly, more limited; $D_{90\ °C}$ values ranging from 4.5 to 120 minutes have been reported for five strains of *Clostridium perfringens* spores.

Cell form

Whether or not the heated cells exist in the vegetative or spore form may in some cases be related to the age of the culture or the cell population being heated. In cultures of *Bacillus* and *Clostridium* species the proportion of spores usually increases as the incubation period is extended and the culture ages. This may be due to more and more of the vegetative cells producing spores, in which case the spore count increases. Alternatively the spore count may remain unchanged but the vegetative cell count falls due to the action of lytic enzymes produced by the cells themselves. Amongst the common mesophilic *Bacillus* species spore formation is largely complete 6–10 hours after the end of exponential growth under optimal cultural conditions. The degree of heat resistance and the concentration of spores would not be expected to rise much after this time. Conducting heat resistance studies on a mixture of spores and vegetative cells is undesirable because the likely result is a rapid initial fall in count due to killing of the vegetative cells and a subsequent slower rate due to death of spores. If necessary the vegetative cells can usually be removed by addition of the enzymes lysozyme and trypsin.

The degree of heat resistance shown by vegetative cells may also be influenced by the stage of growth from which the cells were taken. It is normally found that stationary phase cells are more heat resistant than those taken from the logarithmic phase of growth, although several exceptions have been reported.

Cultural conditions

The conditions under which the cells are grown is another factor which can markedly affect the heat resistance. Insufficient attention was paid to this potential source of variation in a substantial part of the research conducted during the first half

of this century, and the same criticism might even be made of some of that reported more recently. Not infrequently, insufficient detail of the cultivation procedures are described in the scientific reports, or materials of variable composition, e.g. tap water or soil extracts were used in media without regard to the possible differences that may have arisen between successive batches or populations of cells.

Factors such as growth temperature, medium pH and buffering capacity, oxygen availability and concentrations of culture medium components may all affect resistance.

Thermophilic organisms generally are more heat resistant than mesophils, which in turn tend to be more resistant than psychrophils. If a 'league table' of spore heat resistance were constructed it is probable that *B. stearothermophilus*, *B. coagulans* and *Cl. thermosaccharolyticum* would head the list; all three have growth optima of 50–60 °C. Variable results have arisen when single species have been grown at a variety of temperatures. *E. coli* and *Streptococcus faecalis* have both been the subject of conflicting reports on the influence of growth temperature on heat resistance whilst spores of *B. cereus* produced at temperatures between 20 and 41 °C showed maximal resistance at 30 °C.

The effects of medium pH, buffering capacity, oxygen availability and the concentrations of culture medium components are often complex and inter-related. An unsuitable pH, inadequate buffer or insufficient aeration may all limit the extent of growth, with the result that the cells which do grow each have available to them a higher concentration of nutrients than would be the case if a higher cell density had been achieved. The levels of intracellular storage materials and metal ions may therefore differ and so influence resistance to heat and other lethal agents. Cells existing in or recently isolated from their 'natural' environment, e.g. water, soil, dust or pharmaceutical raw materials, have often been reported to have a greater heat resistance than their progeny which have been repeatedly subcultured in the laboratory and then tested under similar conditions. This phenomenon has been widely recognized for many years, so much so that standardized soil preparations are regularly used in West Germany for the purpose of testing autoclave efficiency because of their content of heat resistant spores.

pH and composition of heating menstruum

It is frequently found that cells more readily survive heating when they are at neutrality (or their optimum pH for growth if this differs from neutrality). The combination of heat and an unfavourable pH may be additive or even synergistic in killing effects, thus *B. stearothermophilus* spores survive better at 110 °C in dilute pH 7.0 phosphate buffer than at 85 °C in pH 4.0 acetate buffer. Differences in heat resistance may also result merely from the presence of the buffer regardless of the pH it confers. Usually an apparent increase in resistance occurs when cells are heated in buffer rather than in water alone. A similar increase is often found to occur on addition of other dissolved or suspended solids, particularly those of a colloidal or proteinaceous nature, e.g. milk, nutrient broth, serum. Because dissolved solids can have such a marked effect on heat resistance great care must be taken in attempting to use experimental data from simple solutions to predict the likely heat treatment required to kill the same cells in a complex formulated medicine or food material. An extreme case of protection of cells from a lethal agent is the occlusion of cells within crystals. When spores of *B. subtilis var. niger* were occluded within crystals of calcium carbonate their resistance to inactivation was approximately 900 times and 9 times higher than for unoccluded spores when subjected to steam and dry heat respectively at 121 °C; an exposure period of 2.5 h at 121 °C (moist heat) was required to eliminate survivors within the crystals. It is to minimize the risk of such situations arising that there is a requirement in the DHSS *Guide to Good Manufacturing Practice* that medicines be prepared in clean conditions.

The solute concentrations normally encountered in dilute buffer solutions used as suspending media for heat resistance experiments cause no significant reduction in the vapour pressure of the solution relative to that of pure water, i.e. they do not reduce the water activity, A_w, of the solution (which has a value of 1.0 for water). If high solute concentrations are used or the cells are heated in a 'semi-dry' state the A_w is significantly lower and the resistance is increased, e.g. a 1000-fold increase in D value has been reported for *B. megatrium* spores when the water activity was reduced from 1.0 to between 0.2 and 0.4.

The recovery of heat-treated cells

The recovery conditions available to cells after exposure to heat may influence the proportion of cells which produce colonies. A heat-damaged cell may require an incubation time longer than normal to achieve a colony of any given size and the optimum incubation temperature may be several degrees lower. The composition of the medium may also affect the colony count, with nutritionally rich media giving a greater percentage survival than a 'standard' medium whereas little or no difference can be detected between the two when unheated cells are used. Adsorbents such as charcoal and starch have been found to have beneficial effects in this context. Table 25.3 illustrates the effects of adding amino acids to a minimal medium on the recovery of heated *B. stearothermophilus* spores.

Table 25.3★ The relative influence of amino acid supplements in the medium on the recovery of *B. stearothermophilus* spores after heating[†]

Recovery medium	% colony forming units
Minimal medium (mm) + 0.5% casein hydrolysate	100
mm + amino acid mixture	24
mm + L-glutamic acid 14.4 mg 100 ml^{-1}	14
mm + L-lysine 16.2 mg 100 ml^{-1}	3.7
mm alone	1.7

★ Adapted from Campbell *et al.* (1965).
[†] 12 min at 121 °C.

IONIZING RADIATIONS

Ionizing radiations can be divided into electromagnetic radiations and particulate (corpuscular) radiations. Electromagnetic radiations include gamma rays and X-rays while particulate radiation includes alpha and beta particles, positrons and neutrons.

Particulate radiation

The nuclear disintegration of radioactive elements results in the production of charged particles. Alpha particles are heavy and positively charged being equivalent to the nuclei of helium atoms. They travel relatively slowly in air and although they cause a great deal of ionization along their paths they have very little penetrating power, their range being just a few centimetres in air. Alpha particles have no application in this aspect of pharmacy and will not be considered further. Beta particles are negatively charged and have the same mass as an electron. In air the penetrating power of these particles is a few metres but they will be stopped by a thin sheet of aluminium. Beta particles resulting from radioactive decay are therefore not sufficiently penetrative for application in sterilization processes but the production of electrons from man-made machines (cathode rays) results in particles of great energy with enhanced penetrating power.

Electromagnetic radiation

Gamma radiation results when the nucleus still has too much energy even after the emission of alpha or beta particules and this energy is dissipated in the form of very short wavelength radiation which, since it has no mass or charge, travels with the speed of light penetrating even sheets of lead. Although travelling in a wave form gamma radiation behaves as if composed of discrete packets of energy called quanta (photons). A ^{60}Co source emits gamma rays with photons of 1.17 and 1.33 MeV and the source has a half-life of 5.2 years. X-rays are generated when a heavy metal target is bombarded with fast electrons and they have similar properties to gamma rays although originating from a shift in electron energy rather than from the nucleus.

Units of radioactivity

The unit of activity is the becquerel (Bq) which is equal to one nuclear transformation per second. This replaces the term curie (Ci) and 3.7×10^{10} becquerels = 1 curie. The unit of absorbed dose according to the SI system is the gray (Gy) which is equal to one joule per kilogram. However, the term rad is still widely used and is equivalent to 100 ergs per gram of irradiated material.

$$1 \text{ gray} = 100 \text{ rads}$$

The energy of radiation is measured in electron volts (eV) or millions of electron volts (MeV). An electron volt is the energy acquired by an electron falling through a potential difference of one volt.

Effect of ionizing radiations on materials

Ionizing radiations are absorbed by materials in a variety of ways, depending upon the energy of the incident photons.

1 Photoelectric effect: low energy radiation (< 0.1 MeV) is absorbed by the atom of the material resulting in the ejection or excitation of an electron.
2 Compton effect: incident photons of medium energy 'collide' with atoms and a portion of the energy is absorbed with the ejection of an electron. The remaining energy carries on impacting with further atoms and emitting further electrons until all the energy is scattered.
3 Pair production: radiations of very high energy are converted on impact into negatively charged electrons and positively charged particles called positrons. The positron has an extremely short life and quickly annihilates itself by colliding with an orbital electron.

The ionization caused by the primary radiation results in the formation of free radicals, excited atoms, etc. along a discrete track through the material. However, if secondary electrons contain sufficient energy they may cause excitation and ionization of adjacent atoms thus effectively widening the tract. Temperature rise during irradiation is very small and even high energy radiation resulting in pair production is only accompanied by an increase of approximately 2 °C but nevertheless the chemical changes which occur in irradiated materials are very widespread.

The lethal effect of irradiation on microorganisms can occur in two ways.

1 Direct effect: in this case the ionizing radiation is directly responsible for the damage by

causing a direct hit on a sensitive target molecule. It is generally accepted that cellular DNA is the principal target for inactivation and that the ability to survive irradiation is attributable to the organism's ability to repair damaged DNA rather than any intrinsic resistance of the structure. Further damage may be caused by free radicals produced within the cell but not directly associated with DNA. These radicals can diffuse to a sensitive site and react with it, causing damage.

2 Indirect effects: the passage of ionizing radiation through water causes ionization along and immediately next to the track and the formation of free radicals and peroxides.

Some of the possible reactions are as follows:

$$H_2O \xrightarrow{\text{radiation}} H_2O^+ + e^-$$
$$H_2O^+ \longrightarrow {}^{\cdot}OH + H^+$$
$$e^- + H_2O \longrightarrow OH^- + H^{\cdot}$$
$$2H^{\cdot} \longrightarrow H_2$$
$$2{}^{\cdot}OH \rightarrow H_2O_2$$

The presence of oxygen has a significant effect on the destructive properties of ionizing radiation due to the formation of hydroperoxyl radicals.

$$H^{\cdot} + O_2 \rightarrow {}^{\cdot}HO_2$$

These peroxides and free radicals can act as both oxidizing and reducing agents according to the conditions.

Factors affecting the radiation resistance of micro-organisms

Oxygen has already been mentioned as having a significant effect on radiation resistance since the increased levels of hydroperoxyl radicals leads to marked increases in sensitivity. Freezing increases the radiation resistance due to the reduction of mobility of free radicals in the menstruum preventing them from diffusing to sites of action at the cell membrane. Above the freezing point there is very little effect of temperature.

A variety of organic materials provide a protective environment for micro-organisms and comparison of radiation resistance is greatly complicated by different complexities of media

used. Sulphydryl groups have a protective effect on micro-organisms due to their interaction with free radicals. In contrast compounds which combine with –SH groups such as halogenated acetates tend to increase sensitivity.

ULTRAVIOLET RADIATION

Although u.v. radiation has a range of wavelength from approximately 15 nm to 330 nm its range of maximum bactericidal activity is much narrower (220–280 nm) with an optimum of about 265 nm. Whereas ionizing radiations cause electrons to be ejected from atoms in their path u.v. radiation does not possess sufficient energy for this and merely causes the electrons to become excited. It has much less penetrating power than ionizing radiations and tends to be used for the destruction of micro-organisms in air and on surfaces.

The bactericidal effect of u.v. light is due to the formation of linkages between adjacent pyrimidine bases in the DNA molecule to form dimers. These are usually thymine dimers although other types have been identified. The presence of thymine dimers alters the structural integrity of the DNA chain thus hindering chromosome replication. Damaged DNA can be repaired by certain cells in a variety of ways, enhancing their radiation resistance.

Exposure of u.v. damaged cells to visible light (photoreactivation) enables a light-dependent photoreactivating enzyme to split the thymine dimers into monomers. A second mechanism is not light dependent and is called dark recovery. In this case the thymine dimers are removed by a specific endonuclease enzyme which nicks the damaged DNA strand either side of the dimer. DNA polymerase then replaces the missing nucleotides and the ends are joined by a ligase enzyme.

Factors affecting resistance to u.v. light

As already mentioned u.v. light has very little penetrating power and anything which acts as a shield around the cells will afford a degree of protection. The formation of aggregates of cells will result in those cells at the centre of the aggregate surviving an otherwise lethal dose of radiation. Similarly micro-organisms suspended in water withstand considerably higher doses of radiation compared with the dry state due to lack of penetration of the radiation. Suspension of bacteria in broths containing organic matter such as proteins increases the resistance of the cells still further. The stage of growth of the culture will affect the sensitivity of the cells with maximum sensitivity being shown during the logarithmic phase.

Other factors shown to influence radiation resistance include pH, temperature and humidity although the effect of the latter parameter is still somewhat confused.

GASES

The use of gases as antimicrobial agents has been documented for centuries although it is only recently that the mechanisms of action and factors affecting activity have been elucidated. A wide variety of gaseous agents have been used for their antimicrobial properties but due to the constraints of space imposed by this chapter only a few of the major ones will be dealt with here.

Ethylene oxide

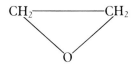

Ethylene oxide is a gas at room temperature (with a boiling point at 10.7 °C) which readily permeates a variety of materials (plastics, cardboard, cloth, etc.) but not crystals. Its odour is reported as being rather pleasant although the levels at which it is detected in the atmosphere (700 ppm) greatly exceed the maximum safety limits for humans. Toxicity problems include burns and blistering if the material comes into contact with the skin whereas inhalation results in lachrymation, headache, dizziness and vomiting. Great care must be taken to ensure removal of ethylene oxide from treated products (e.g. rubber gloves) to avoid the risk of skin reactions. Explosive mixtures are formed when ethylene oxide is mixed with air at any concentration above 3% and this is especially dangerous if the gas mixture is confined. Addition of carbon dioxide or fluorinated hydrocarbons will eliminate this risk.

Ethylene oxide is extremely effective at killing micro-organisms and its activity is related to its action as an alkylating agent. Reactive hydrogen atoms on hydroxyl, carboxyl, sulphydryl and amino groups can all be replaced with hydroxyethyl groups thus interfering with a wide range of metabolic activities. In contrast to other bactericidal agents the resistance of bacterial spores is only slightly greater than vegetative cells $(5\times)$.

Factors affecting the activity of ethylene oxide

The bactericidal activity of ethylene oxide is proportional to the partial pressure of gas in the reaction chamber, time of exposure, temperature of treatment and level and type of contamination. At room temperature the time taken to reduce the initial concentration of cells by 90% can be very slow and for this reason the *British Pharmacopoeia* recommends elevated temperatures of 60 °C which results in vastly increased rates of kill. Concentrations of ethylene oxide between 500 and 1000 mg l^{-1} are usually employed. Relative humidity has a most pronounced effect since at very high humidities ethylene oxide may be hydrolysed to the much less active ethylene glycol and this is borne out by the observation that the gas is ten times more active at 30% RH than 97% RH. The optimum value for activity appears to be between 28 and 33%. Below 28% the alkylating action of ethylene oxide is inhibited due to lack of water. The degree of dehydration of cells greatly influences activity and it may not be possible to rehydrate very dry organisms simply by exposure to increased RH.

Dadd and Daly (1980) have looked at the effect of ethylene oxide on a variety of micro-organisms and found that the spores of *B. subtilis var. niger* are among the most resistant. The heat-resistant spore former *B. stearothermophilus* and spores of *Clos. sporogenes* were no more resistant than a number of vegetative organisms such as *Staph. aureus*, *Strept. faecium* and *Micrococcus luteus*. The difference in resistance between spore formers and vegetative cells was only of the order of five to ten times compared to several thousandfold differences with other physical and chemical processes. Fungal spores exhibit the same order of resistance as vegetative cells. Micro-organisms may be protected from the action of ethylene oxide by occlusion within crystalline material or when coated with organic matter or salts. *B. subtilis var. niger* spores dried from salt water solutions are much more resistant to the gas than suspensions dried from distilled water. A similar effect was noted when broth suspensions of spores were found to be difficult to kill.

Biological indicators used to test the efficacy of ethylene oxide treatment employ spores of *B. subtilis* dried onto suitable carriers such as pieces of aluminium foil.

Formaldehyde

Formaldehyde (H.CHO) in its pure form is a gas at room temperature, with a boiling point of $-19\ °C$, but readily polymerizes at temperatures below 80 °C to form a white solid. The vapour, which is extremely irritating to the eyes, nose and throat, can be generated either from solid polymers such as paraformaldehyde or from a solution of 37% formaldehyde in water (formalin). Formalin usually contains about 10% methanol to prevent polymerization. As with ethylene oxide formaldehyde is a very reactive molecule and there is only a small differential in resistance between bacterial spores and vegetative cells. Its bactericidal powers are superior to ethylene oxide (concentrations of 3–10 mg l^{-1} are effective) but it has weak penetrating power and is really only a surface bactericide. Adsorbed gas, however, is very difficult to remove and long airing times are required. Its mechanism of action is thought to involve the production of intramolecular cross-links between proteins together with interactions with RNA and DNA. It acts as a mutagenic agent and an alkylating agent reacting with carbonyl, thiol and hydroxyl groups. In order to be effective the gas has to dissolve in a film of moisture surrounding the bacteria and for this reason relative humidities in the order of 75% are required.

β-Propiolactone

This is a colourless liquid at room temperature with a pungent odour and a boiling point of 162 °C. It has a wide spectrum of activity, the vapour being bactericidal to both Gram-positive and Gram-negative bacteria, viruses, rickettsiae, fungi and also *Mycobacterium*. It is less active against bacterial spores. It is quicker acting than formaldehyde and does not give problems with polymerization but it has feeble penetrating powers. In order to sterilize enclosed spaces concentrations between 2 and 5 mg l^{-1} of air are necessary at a relative humidity of 80% and these conditions maintained for 2 hours at 24 °C.

Unfortunately, the use of β-propiolactone has been limited by doubts raised over its safety. It has been shown to be carcinogenic in animals. It is used in liquid form for the sterilization of rabies vaccine and the sterilization of various graft tissues.

Propylene oxide

Propylene oxide is a liquid (b.p. = 34 °C) at room temperature which requires heating to volatilize. It is inflammable between 2.1 and 21.5% by volume in air but this can be reduced by mixing with CO_2. The mechanism of action is similar to ethylene oxide and involves the esterification of carbonyl, hydroxyl, amino and sulphydryl groups present on protein molecules. It is, however, less effective than ethylene oxide in terms of its antimicrobial activity and its ability to penetrate materials. Whereas ethylene oxide breaks down to give ethylene glycol or ethylene chlorhydrin both of which are toxic, propylene oxide breaks down to propylene glycol which is much less so.

Methyl bromide

Methyl bromide is a gas at room temperatures and is used as a disinfectant at concentrations of

3.5 mg l⁻¹ with a relative humidity between 30 and 60%. It has inferior antimicrobial properties to the previous compounds but has good penetrating power.

ANTIMICROBIAL EFFECTS OF CHEMICAL AGENTS

Chemical agents have been used since very early times to combat such effects of microbial proliferation as spoilage of foods and materials, infection of wounds and decay of bodies. Thus, long before the role of micro-organisms in disease and decay was recognized salt and sugar were used in food preservation, a variety of oils and resins were applied to wounds and employed for embalming, and sulphur was burned to fumigate sick rooms.

The classic researches of Pasteur, which established micro-organisms as causative agents of disease and spoilage, paved the way for the development and rational use of chemical agents in their control. Traditionally, two definitions have been established describing the antimicrobial use of chemical agents. Those used to destroy micro-organisms on inanimate objects are described as *disinfectants* and those used to treat living tissues as in wound irrigation, cleansing of burns or eye washes are called *antiseptics*. Other definitions have been introduced to give more precise limits of meaning viz.: *bactericide* and *fungicide* for chemical agents which kill bacteria and fungi respectively: *bacteriostat* and *fungistat* for those which prevent the growth of a bacterial or fungal population. The validity of drawing a rigid demarcation line between those compounds which kill and those which inhibit growth without killing is doubtful. In many instances concentration and time of contact are the critical factors. The term *preservative* is used to describe the purpose of antimicrobial agents in protecting medicines, pharmaceutical formulations, cosmetics, foods and general materials against microbial spoilage, rather than be associated with any particular compound (see Chapter 27). This means that we should say that a product 'contains X as a preservative', rather than 'contains the preservative X'.

The mechanisms whereby antimicrobial agents exert their effects have been intensively investigated and the principal sites of their attack upon microbial cells identified. These are the cell wall, the cytoplasmic membrane and the cytoplasm. Chemical agents may weaken the cell wall, allowing extrusion of cell contents, resulting in distorted shape, filament formation, or complete lysis. The cytoplasmic membrane, controlling as it does permeability, and being a site of vital enzyme activity is vulnerable to a wide range of substances which interfere with reactive groups or can disrupt its phospholipid layers. The cytoplasm, site of genetic control and protein synthesis, presents a target for those chemical agents which disrupt ribosomes, react with nucleic acids or generally coagulate protoplasm.

Principal factors affecting activity

The factors most easily quantified are temperature and concentration.

In general an increase in temperature increases the rate of kill for a given concentration of agent and inoculum size. The commonly used nomenclature is Q_{10} which is the change in activity of the agent per 10 °C rise in temperature (e.g. Q_{10} phenol = 4).

The effect of change in concentration of a chemical agent upon the rate of kill can be expressed as:

$$C_1^n t_1 = C_2^n t_2$$

Where C_1 and C_2 represent the concentrations of agent required to kill a standard inoculum in times t_1 and t_2. The concentration exponent η represents the slope of the line when log death time (t) is plotted against log concentration (C).

When values of η are greater than 1, changes of concentration will have a pronounced effect. Thus, in the case of phenol, when $\eta = 6$, halving the concentration will decrease its activity by a factor of 2^6 (64-fold) whereas for a mercurial compound, $\eta = 1$, the same dilution would only reduce activity twofold (2^1).

Other factors including pH, suspended solids and fats are discussed in Chapter 27.

The range of chemical agents

The broad categories of antibacterial chemical compounds have remained surprisingly constant

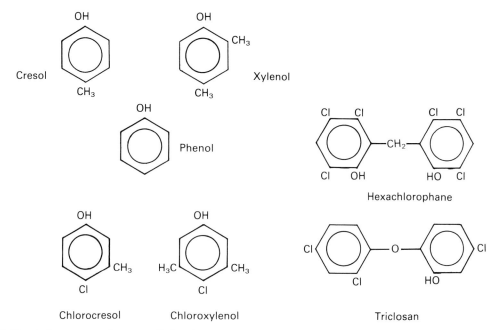

Fig. 25.4 Chemical structures of a range of phenols

over the years with phenolics and hypochlorites comprising the major disinfectants and quaternary ammonium compounds widely used as antiseptics. The compounds capable of use as preservatives in preparations for oral, parenteral or ophthalmic administration are obviously strictly limited by toxicity requirements.

Phenolics (Fig. 25.4)

Various distillation fractions of coal tar yield phenolic compounds including cresols, xylenols and phenol itself, all of which are toxic and caustic to skin and tissues. Common disinfectant formulations, the, so-called, 'black fluids' and 'white fluids', are prepared from higher boiling coal tar fractions. The former make use of soaps to solubilize the tar fractions in the form of stable homogenous solutions whereas the latter are emulsions of the tar products and unstable on dilution. Lysol (Cresol and Soap Solution BP 1968) and Roxenol (Chloroxylenol Solution BPC 1973, Dettol) are also examples of low solubility phenolic compounds solubilized by the use of soap.

Remarkable success has been achieved in modifying the phenol molecule by the intro-

duction of chlorine and methyl groups as in chlorocresol and chloroxylenol. This has the dual effect of eliminating toxic and corrosive properties whilst at the same time enchancing and prolonging antimicrobial activity. Thus, chlorocresol is used as a bactericide in injections and to preserve oil in water creams, whilst chloroxylenol finds widespread applications as a household and hospital antiseptic. Phenol may itself be rendered less caustic by dilution to 1% w/v or less for lotions and gargles or by dissolving in glycerol for use as ear drops. Bisphenols such as hexachlorophane and triclosan (Irgasan) share the low solubility and enhanced activity of the other phenol derivatives described but have a substantive effect which makes them particularly useful as skin antiseptics. Formulated as creams, cleansing lotions or soaps they have proved valuable in reducing postoperative and cross-infection. Hexachlorophane may cause brain damage in infants and for this reason all preparations of this compound should carry the cautionary label 'not to be used for babies' Phenols generally are active against vegetative bacteria and fungi, are readily inactivated by dilution and organic matter and are most effective in acid conditions. According to concentration, phenols may cause cell lysis at low concentrations or general coagulation of cell contents at higher concentrations.

Alcohols, aldehydes, acids and esters

Ethyl alcohol has long been used, usually as 'surgical spirit' for rapid cleansing of preoperative areas of skin before injection. It is rapidly lethal to bacterial vegetative cells and fungi and is most effective at concentrations of 60–70%. The effect of aromatic substitution is to produce a range of compounds which are less volatile and less rapidly active and find general use as preservatives, e.g. phenylethanol for eye drops and contact lens solutions, benzyl alcohol in injections, Bronopol (2-bromo-2-nitropropane-1,3-diol) in shampoos and other toiletries. Phenoxyethanol, which has good activity against *Ps. aeruginosa*, has been used as an antiseptic.

Formaldehyde and glutaraldehyde are both powerful disinfectants, denaturing protein and destroying vegetative cells and spores. Formaldehyde is used in sterilization procedures both as a gas and as a solution in ethyl alcohol. Glutaraldehyde solutions are also used to sterilize surgical instruments.

The organic acids, sorbic and benzoic and their esters, by virtue of their low toxicity, are well established as preservatives for food products and medicines (see Chapter 27).

Quaternary ammonium compounds (Fig. 25.5)

These cationic surface active compounds are, as their name implies, derivatives of an ammonium halide in which the hydrogen atoms are substituted by at least one lipophilic group, a long chain alkyl or aryl–alkyl radical containing C_8–C_{18} carbon atoms. In marked contrast to phenol and the cresols these compounds are mild in use and active at such high dilutions as to be virtually non-toxic. Their surface-active properties make them powerful cleansing agents, a useful adjunct to their common use as skin antiseptics and preservatives in contact lens cleansing and soaking solutions. They are also safe for formulating into eyedrops and injections and are widely used in gynaecology and general surgery. Active as cations, ambient pH is important as is interference

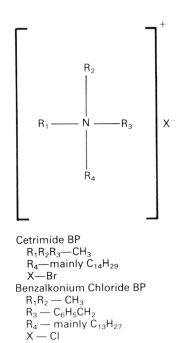

Cetrimide BP
  $R_1R_2R_3$—CH_3
  R_4—mainly $C_{14}H_{29}$
  X—Br
Benzalkonium Chloride BP
  R_1R_2 — CH_3
  R_3 — $C_6H_5CH_2$
  R_4 — mainly $C_{13}H_{27}$
  X — Cl

Fig. 25.5 Chemical structure of cetrimide and benzalkonium chloride

caused by anions. Thus, alkaline conditions promote activity and it is important that all traces of soap, being anion active, are removed from the skin prior to treatment with a quaternary ammonium compound. Foreign organic matter and grease also cause inactivation.

One effect of the detergent properties of these compounds is to interfere with cell permeability such that susceptible bacteria, mainly the Gram-positive groups, leak their contents and eventually undergo lysis. Gram-negative bacteria are less susceptible and to widen the spectrum to include these, mixtures of quaternary ammonium compounds with other antimicrobial agents such as phenoxyethanol or chlorhexidine are used.

Diguanides and amidines

Two guanidine compounds have found general use as antimicrobial agents namely chlorhexidine (Fig. 25.6) and picloxydine and of the aromatic diamidines, propamidine and dibromopropamidine are used. Chlorhexidine and the amidines are non-toxic antiseptics and the former is widely used in general surgery alone and in combination

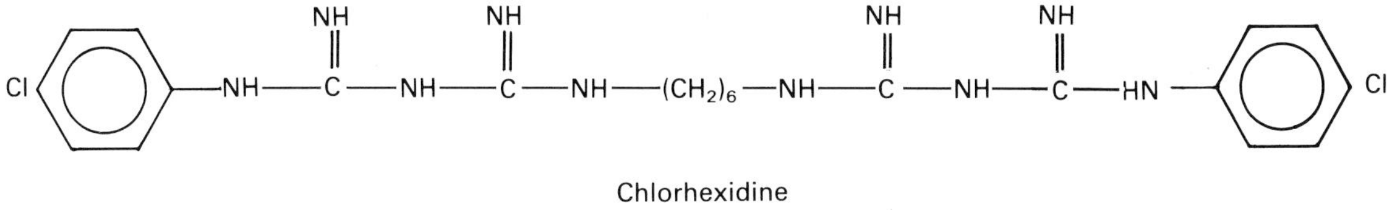

Chlorhexidine

Fig. 25.6 Chemical structure of chlorhexidine

with cetrimide, and also as a preservative in eye drops.

The halogens and their compounds

Chlorine gas is a powerful disinfectant used in the municipal treatment of drinking water and in swimming baths. Solutions of chlorine in water may be made powerful enough for use as general household bleach and disinfectant and dilute solutions are used for domestic hygiene. Well known pharmaceutical formulations are Eusol (Chlorinated Lime and Boric Acid Solution BPC 1973) and Dakin's Solution (Surgical Chlorinated Soda Solution BPC 1973) both of which are designed to provide slow release of chlorine.

An alternative method of obtaining more prolonged release of chlorine is by the use of organic chlorine compounds such as Chloramine T (sodium *p*-toluene-sulphonchloramide) and Halazone BPC 1973 (*p*-sulphondichloramide benzoic acid), the former used as a skin antiseptic and the latter for treating contaminated drinking water. The high chemical reactivity of chlorine renders it lethal to bacteria, fungi and viruses, and to some extent, spores, and this activity is optimal at acid pH levels around 5.0.

Iodine, like chlorine a highly reactive element, denatures cell proteins and essential enzymes due to its powerful oxidative effects. Traditionally it has been used in alcoholic solutions such as Tincture of Iodine (BP 1973) or complexed with potassium iodide to form an aqueous solution (Lugol's Iodine BP 1973). The staining and irritant properties of iodine have resulted in the development of 'iodophores' mixtures of iodine with surface-active agents, which hold the iodine in micellar combination from which it is released slowly. Such a preparation is Betadine (polyvinyl-pyrrolidone-iodine), used as a non-staining, non-irritant antiseptic.

Metals

Many metallic ions are toxic to essential enzyme systems, particularly those utilizing thiol (-SH) groups, but those used medically are restricted to mercury, silver and aluminium. The extreme toxicity of mercury has rendered its use obsolete apart from in organic combination. The organic compounds used in pharmacy are phenylmercuric nitrate (and acetate), as a bactericide in eyedrops and injections and thiomersal (sodium ethylmercurithiosalicylate) as a preservative in biological products and certain eyedrops.

Silver, in the form of the nitrate, is used to treat infections of the eyes, as are silver protein solutions. Aluminium foil has been used as a wound covering in the treatment of burns and venous ulcers and has been shown to adsorb micro-organisms and inhibit their growth.

The acridines

This group of compounds interferes specifically with nucleic acid function and has some ideal antiseptic properties, thus aminacrine hydrochloride is non-toxic, non-irritant, non-staining and active against Gram-positive and Gram-negative bacteria even in the presence of serum.

This brief survey has given some indication of the variety of antimicrobial compounds available. Each of these has a defined spectrum of utility and in the correct conditions of use can substantially contribute to the control of microbial proliferation and infection.

ANTIBIOTICS AND CHEMOTHERAPEUTIC AGENTS

Antibiotics may be defined as substances produced by micro-organisms or compounds derived from

Table 25.4 Routes of administration, microbial spectra and mode of action of some commonly-used antibiotics

Antibiotic	Route*	Microbial spectrum	Mode of action	Other comments
Penicillins			Bactericidal antibiotics. Interfere with the biosynthesis of cell wall peptidoglycan causing lysis of susceptible cells. Act only on growing cells and not resting ones. These antibiotics inhibit not only transpeptidase, which cross-links the linear polymer of peptidoglycan, but also carboxypeptidase which removes the terminal D-alanine group from the cross-linking decapeptide	Approximately 8% of population show hypersensitivity to penicillins. May lead to anaphylaxis which can be fatal. First line treatment for a wide range of infections.
Benzylpenicillin	I	Gram-positive bacteria (G +ve)		
Phenoxymethylpenicillin	O	G +ve		
Ampicillin	O/I	G +ve and some Gram-negative (G −ve)		
		G +ve		‡Active against beta lactamase producers
Flucloxacillin‡	O/I			ᴪActive against *Pseudomonas*
Carbenicillinᴪ	I	Some G +ve and some G −ve		
Cephalosporins		Most G +ve, some G −ve		Cephalosporins are closely related to penicillins. About 10% of penicillin-sensitive patients show sensitivity to cephalosporins also. Newer cephalosporins are more active against Gram-negative than Gram-positive bacteria and also tend to be more resistant to beta lactamases
Cephaloridine	I			
Cephradine	O	As above, inactive against *Haemophilus*		
Cefuroxime	I	As above		
Cefotaxime	I	Wider spectrum active against *Pseudomonas*		
Cephalexin	O	Some G +ve, some G −ve but not *Pseudomonas*		
Tetracyclines		G +ve and G −ve bacteria. Plus rickettsiae, chlamydiae and mycoplasmas	Bacteriostatic antibiotics. Inhibit protein synthesis by binding to 30s bacterial ribosomal subunit preventing the binding of aminoacyl transfer RNA to initial site on ribosome. Selective inhibition of bacteria arises from an active transport system involving permease enzymes which accumulate the antibiotic within the cell against a concentration gradient	Although these are broad spectrum antibiotics their usefulness has been restricted due to the development of resistance. Tetracyclines tend to be deposited in growing bone and teeth causing staining which prevents their use in children and pregnant women. Should not be given concurrently with milk, iron or antacids since these will hinder absorption
Tetracycline	O/I			
Chlortetracycline	O/I			
Oxytetracycline	O/I			
Minocycline	O/I	As above plus *Pseudomonas*		
Doxycycline	O/I	As minocycline plus *Neisseria meningitidis*		
Aminoglycosides		G +ve and some G −ve bacteria. No activity against *Clostridium* or *Pseudomonas*	The aminoglycosides are the only group of antibiotics acting upon the ribosome which have a direct bactericidal action. They bind to 30s ribosomal subunit causing misreading of the code on mRNA. They may also act by a separate action on the initiation and elongation reactions of protein synthesis	§Reserved almost entirely for the treatment of TB. Development of resistance is a major problem with 9-aminoglycoside inactivating enzymes having been isolated. Most of the aminoglycosides are inactivated by a combination of these enzymes except amikacin which is only susceptible to one. They are not absorbed from the gut. Ototoxicity and nephrotoxicity are the main side effects
Streptomycin§	I			
Gentamicin	I			
Neomycin	O/T			
Amikacin	I			
Spectinomycin	I	More limited range than above. Used almost exclusively in treatment of gonorrhoea		

* I, injection, O, oral; T, topical.

Table 25.4 (*Cont'd*)

Antibiotic	Route*	Microbial spectrum	Mode of action	Other comments
Lincomycins				
Lincomycin	O /I	G +ve bacteria	Bind to 50s ribosomal subunit of Gram-positive cells only. This action leads to the breakup of polysomes. Detailed mechanism of action is still uncertain	Both have serious side effects which tend to limit their use. Useful for staphylococcal bone and joint infections as the drug tends to concentrate in bone. Also used to treat peritonitis
Clindamycin	O			
Miscellaneous				
Chloramphenicol	O/I/T	G +ve and G −ve	Inhibits protein synthesis by binding to peptidyl transferase. Selective for 70s ribosomes only	Toxic drug used systemically only for life-threatening infections. Widely used in eyedrops and eye ointments
Cycloserine	O	Limited spectrum mainly used against *Myco. tuberculosis*	Concentrates inside cells and inhibits wall synthesis due to competitive inhibition of alanine racemase and alanine synthetase	Used to treat TB in patients who fail to respond to first line drugs. Care should be taken as this is a very toxic drug
Rifampicin	O	G +ve and G −ve plus *Myco. tuberculosis*	Acts specifically on bacterial RNA polymerase inhibiting the initial step in mRNA synthesis	Bactericidal against *Myco. tuberculosis*. Used in conjunction with other drugs, e.g. isoniazid and ethambutol to treat TB
Polymyxin B	O/I	G −ve bacteria	Binds to cell membrane causing disruption and leakage of nucleotides and pentoses.	Useful in treatment of infections due to *Ps. aeruginosa*
Novobiocin	O/I	G +ve bacteria	Inhibits DNA synthesis by interfering with DNA gyrase. Chelates Mg^{2+} ions also	Somewhat limited clinical use to development of resistance and side effects
Fusidic acid	O/T	G +ve bacteria	Binds to 50s subunit. Forms a complex with elongation factor/GDP on ribosome. Prevents normal dissociation of this complex	Used against beta-lactam producing staphylococci as in osteomyelitis. Potent topical antibacterial agent useful in treating abscesses, boils and other skin infections
Bacitracin	T	G +ve bacteria	Acts on a whole series of reactions to prevent cell wall synthesis	Not absorbed orally and nephrotoxic when given parenterally. Useful topical antibiotic
Vancomycin	O	G +ve bacteria	Has a similar but not identical mechanism of action to bacitracin	Used to treat antibiotic associated pseudomembranous colitis. Ototoxic and nephrotoxic
Antifungal agents				
Nystatin	O/T	*Candida* and dermatophytes	Both nystatin and amphotericin B bind to fungal cell membrane resulting in altered cell permeability and leakage of cell constituents	Not absorbed from gut. Toxic if given systemically. Widely used as a topical antifungal agent

* I, injection, O, oral; T, topical.

Table 25.4 (*Cont'd*)

Antibiotic	Route*	Microbial spectrum	Mode of action	Other comments
Amphotericin B	O/I	*Candida* and dermatophytes		Not absorbed from gut. Only polyene antibiotic which can be given systemically. Toxic but very useful antifungal agent
Griseofulvin	O	Dermatophytes	Fungistatic. Mechanism of action unclear. Inhibits mitosis and may have action on spindle microtubules	Becomes incorporated into keratin of nails and hair. Long term treatment (up to 1 year) of dermatophyte infections
Imidazoles	O/T	As a group these compounds have a wide range of activity against yeasts, dermatophytes, filamentous and dimorphic fungi	Mechanism of action uncertain. May bind to cell wall and membranes causing leakage of ions, amino acids and proteins. Miconazole has also been shown to inhibit demethylation of sterols	Mainly used for vaginal candidiasis and dermatophyte infections. Very useful drugs with few, mild side effects

Synthetic antibacterial agents

Antibiotic	Route*	Microbial spectrum	Mode of action	Other comments
Sulphonamides	O/I	G +ve and some G −ve	Bears structural resemblance to para-aminobenzoic acid (PABA) which is used in synthesis of folic acid therefore acts as competitive inhibitor. Also forms a complex with pteridine nucleus preventing utilization of PABA	Often used in conjunction with trimethoprim giving a synergistic effect. Usage has decreased since advent of antibiotics which are more effective and less toxic
Nalidixic acid	O	G −ve except *Ps. aeruginosa*	Inhibits DNA synthesis and breaks down pre-existing DNA. Selectively toxic for prokaryotic cells	Bacterial resistance may develop rapidly
Nitrofurantoin	O	Bactericidal to most G +ve and G −ve urinary tract organisms	The drug is activated in the cell by nitroreductase enzymes and the products cause a variety of effects including strand breakage of bacterial DNA and degradation of ribosomes and RNA	Used almost exclusively for urinary tract infections. Has greater activity against anaerobes than aerobes. *Ps. aeruginosa* usually resistant
Metronidazole	O/I	G +ve and G −ve bacteria especially anaerobes, plus protozoa and some helminths	As with nitrofurantoin the drug must be reduced in cell for activity which explains its selectivity for anaerobes. After reduction the drug binds to DNA causing strand breakage and inhibition of replication and transcription	Used in treatment of trichomoniasis of genitourinary system and infections due to anaerobes such as *Bacteroides* and *Fusobacterium*.
Trimethoprim	O	Active against a range of aerobic G +ve and G −ve bacteria. No activity against *Pseudomonas* or *Neisseria*	Inhibits dihydrofolate reductase thus interfering with nucleoprotein metabolism in microorganisms. Acts at a later stage in synthesis than sulphonamides	Used in treatment of respiratory and urinary tract infections. Synergistic with sulphonamides due to their different points of action on the synthesis of folic acid

* I, injection, O, oral; T, topical.

or structurally related to such substances which in dilute solution inhibit the growth of, or destroy, other micro-organisms. This definition does not cover materials which may be byproducts of primary metabolic processes such as acids or alkalis nor does it include enzymes or toxins which may have inhibitory characteristics. The majority of antibiotics are secondary metabolites and are therefore not of vital importance to the functioning of the cell. Most are produced after the period of active growth has ceased but they should not be looked upon as waste products since in many cases complex enzymatic processes are required for their biosynthesis coupled with the expenditure of energy.

Antibiotics are produced by spore-forming bacteria (e.g. bacitracin, polymyxin, tyrocidine), by actinomycetes notably *Streptomyces* (e.g. tetra-cycline, streptomycin), and fungi (e.g. penicillins and cephalosporins). Some antibiotics such as chloramphenicol are now produced entirely synthetically, while others are chemically modified after microbial biosynthesis.

Antimetabolites are substances which oppose the action of a metabolite or prevent its assimilation by an organism. If an antimetabolite is to be used as an antimicrobial agent it is necessary that the reaction inhibited is exclusive to micro-organisms and not the host; otherwise untoward side effects would occur with the drug being just as toxic to the host.

A number of antimetabolite and other synthetic chemotherapeutic agents are available and are listed along with some of the more commonly used antibiotics in Table 25.4.

REFERENCES AND BIBLIOGRAPHY

ABPI Data Sheet Compendium (1983–84 edn) The Association of the British Pharmaceutical Industry, London.

Campbell, L. L., Richards, G. M. and Sniff, E. E. (1965) Isolation of strains of *Bacillus stearothermophilus* with altered requirement for spore germination. In *Spores III* (eds L. L. Campbell and H. O. Halvorson pp. 55–63, America Society for Microbiology, Ann Arbor, Michigan.

Carter S. J. (1975) *Cooper and Gunn's Dispensing for Pharmaceutical Students*, 12th edn, Pitman Medical Publishing Co., London.

Dadd, A. H. and Daley, G. M. (1980) Resistance of microorganisms to inactivation by gaseous ethylene oxide. *J. app. Bacteriol.*, **49**, 89–101.

Department of Health and Social Security (1983) *Guide to Good Manufacturing Practice*, HMSO, London.

Edwards, D. I. (1980) *Antimicrobial Drug Action*, The MacMillan Press Ltd, London.

Garrod, L. P., Lambert, H. P. and O'Grady, F. (1981) *Antibiotic and Chemotherapy*, 5th edn, Churchill Livingstone, Edinburgh.

Hugo, W. B. and Russell, A. D. (1983) *Pharmaceutical Microbiology*, 3rd Edn, Blackwell Scientific Publications, Oxford, London, Edinburgh.

IAEA Technical Report Series No. 149 (1973) *Manual on Radiation Sterilization of Medical and Biological Materials*, IAEA, Vienna.

Idziak, E. S. (1973) Radiation sensitivity of microorganisms. Effect of radiations on microorganisms. *Int. J. Radiat. Steril.*, **1**, 45–59.

Murrell, W. G., and Warth, A. D. (1965) Composition and heat resistance of bacterial spores. In *Spores III* (eds L. L. Campbell and H. O. Halvorson), pp. 1–24, American Society for Microbiology, Ann Arbor, Michigan.

Phillips, C. R. (1977) Gaseous sterilization. In *Disinfection, Sterilization and Preservation* (ed. S. S. Block), 2nd edn, pp. 592–610, Lea and Febiger, Philadelphia.

Rawlins, E. A. (1977). *Bentley's Textbook of Pharmaceutics*, Baillière Tindall, London.

Russell, A. D., (1982). *The Destruction of Bacterial Spores*, Academic Press, London.

Russell, A. D., Hugo, W. B. and Ayliffe, G. A. J. (1982) *Principles and Practice of Disinfection, Preservation and Sterilization*, Blackwell Scientific Publications, Oxford.

Silverman, G. J. and Sinskey, A. J. (1977) Sterilization by ionising radiations. In *Disinfection, Sterilization and Preservation* (ed. S. S. Block), 2nd edn, pp. 542–561, Lea and Febiger, Philadelphia.

Skinner, F. A., and Hugo. W. B. (1976) *Inhibition and Inactivation of Vegetative Microbes*, Society for Applied Bacteriology, Symposium Series No. 5., Academic Press, London.

Sykes, G. (1965) *Disinfection and Sterilisation*, Chapman and Hall, London.

Principles of sterilization

The need for sterility

There exists a wide variety of materials that are required to be sterilized and to be maintained in a sterile state in order to avoid the possibility of infection arising during their usage. It is taken for granted that all dosage forms for parenteral administration, i.e. products introduced into the body directly into or through the skin, the mucous or the serous membranes, must be sterilized. A number of non-parenteral products also need to be sterile. These include non-injectable fluids such as bladder irrigation solutions and peritoneal dialysis solutions, and ophthalmic preparations. Microbiological media and equipment also require sterilization. The development of aseptic techniques in surgery have resulted in the need for sterile surgical materials and instruments.

More recently the development of complex surgical equipment, life support machines, pacemakers, etc. have presented new challenges and this together with the need to sterilize large components, e.g. spacecraft, has stimulated renewed interest in sterilization and sterilization technology. The development of new drug delivery systems and the use of modern materials for construction of containers and equipment has necessitated an expansion of our basic knowledge and has initiated new research. It is likely that these incentives will lead to new techniques of sterilization and significant improvements to existing methods. It is therefore pertinent at this stage to review the principles of sterilization. The current state of the art regarding the practice of sterilization processes and their control are described in Chapter 43.

Definitions

Sterility is defined as the absence of all viable life forms. It is therefore an absolute term and any expressions implying degrees of sterilization such as 'partially sterile', 'virtually sterile' or 'commercially sterile' are contradictions in terms and must be avoided. *Sterilization* is the process of achieving sterility and is therefore the process by which all viable life forms are removed or destroyed. The viable life forms concerned are usually micro-organisms, i.e. bacteria (including bacterial spores), yeasts, moulds, viruses, rickettsiae and mycoplasma.

It is important to distinguish between disinfection and sterilization since the same agent may be used, in different ways, to achieve both. *Disinfection* is any process, by means of which pathogenic agents are destroyed. It is therefore a process which will destroy infective vegetative agents but will not necessarily kill resistant spores. As such it is a selective process and not an absolute process and must not be confused with sterilization. In the food industry the term *appertization* is used to describe a process by which food is rendered free from pathogenic, toxigenic and spoilage organisms. This process will not necessarily kill thermophilic spores and thus products subjected to the process may not be sterile.

While it is a simple matter to define sterility it is an impossible task to achieve it in practice. This is because when a population of micro-organisms is exposed to a lethal agent they do not all die at the same time. The number of organisms decreases exponentially with the time of exposure (see Chapter 25). This exponential decline means that sterility, that is zero organisms, will only be obtained after exposure to the agent for an infinite time. Sterility is therefore never attained in practice. When viable organisms are no longer detectable a probability region is reached, i.e. region which states the probability of finding one surviving organism after a particular exposure time. This is referred to as the *area of calculated risk* (Fig. 26.1). The sterilization process will not therefore achieve sterility but can only minimize the probability of having viable organisms remaining in the product. A further problem arises from our understanding of what is a viable organism. An organism is considered dead when it is unable to form progeny. An organism which is alive but unable to reproduce to form a colony on solid medium or turbidity in liquid culture is classified as dead by this criterion.

It is clear from this discussion that sterility is an abstract concept of a negative state, and even if it was theoretically possible to achieve this state it would not be possible to demonstrate it practically.

In an attempt to equate the theoretical concept with the practical situation the *Pharmaceutical Handbook* (1980) redefined sterility as 'free from demonstrable forms of life' and considers sterilization to be the process of achieving such a state with the minimum acceptable calculated risk of viable survivors. This of course requires that the levels of acceptable risk are established and this involves principles of risk analysis that are beyond the scope of this chapter. However, a number of mathematical terms have been derived to aid calculation of the probability of achieving sterility.

Inactivation factor (IF)

This is defined as the reduction in the numbers of a given organism brought about by a defined sterilization process. This can be expressed in terms of the D value for the organism (see Chapter 25) as

$$IF = 10^{t/D}$$

where D is the D value for the organism under the sterilizing conditions and t is the time of exposure to the conditions.

If an organism with a D value of 1.5 minutes at 121 °C is exposed to the BP sterilization protocol of autoclaving at 121 °C for 15 minutes, the process will have an inactivation factor of $10^{15/1.5} = 10^{10}$ and will reduce the number of organisms by 10 log cycles or 10 decimal reductions.

The inactivation factor is often expressed simply as the exponent t/D. An example is the use of the '12 D concept' which specifies that the sterilization process is required to produce 12 decimal reductions, i.e. to have an inactivation factor of 10^{12} (Fig. 26.1).

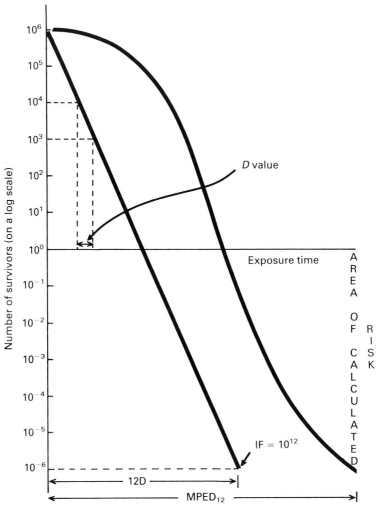

Fig. 26.1 Survivor curve — isothermal conditions

Most probable effective dose (MPED)

The calculation of IF using the D value is only justified if the survivor curve for the organism is linear over the entire exposure time range. Problems frequently arise in practice because the survivor curve exhibits a shoulder and/or a tail (Fig. 26.1). To overcome the problem of non-linear survivor curves the food industry have introduced the $MPED_n$ value. This is the Most Probable Effective Dose to achieve n decimal reductions in the number of organisms and is independent of the shape of the survivor curve. For linear survivor curves $MPED_n = IF \ 10^n = nD$.

F value

The F value is a 'unit of lethality' devised by the food industry in order to compare the relative sterilizing capacities of different heat processes. The F value is a measure of total process lethality and equates a heat treatment at any temperature to the time in minutes at a designated reference temperature that would be required to produce the same lethality in a reference organism. Thus if a process has an F value of 3 the sum of all lethal effects of the process is equivalent to the lethal effect of 3 minutes at the designated reference temperature. Since the F value compares lethal effects at different temperatures it is dependent upon the Z

value (see Chapter 25) for the reference organism and must always be quoted with this Z value.

121 °C is frequently used as a reference temperature and *Bacillus stearothermophilus* spores, which usually have a Z value of 10 °C, are often used as the reference organism. Under these conditions F becomes F_o. A process with an F_o of 8 therefore has the same lethality on the reference spore as heating at 121 °C for 8 minutes. F_o can also be derived from D_{121}, the D value of the organism at 121 °C, and the IF value since

$$F_o = D_{121} \log \text{IF}$$

Determination of sterilization protocols

It is first necessary to select a reference organism. There is considerable variation in the response of micro-organisms to the agents used in sterilization processes (see Chapter 25) but bacterial spores are generally among the most resistant. Spores are frequently found in dust particles and are common contaminants of natural and manufactured products. Ideally the sterilization protocol should be decided for each product with prior knowledge of the type and numbers of contaminating organisms and of their sensitivities. The pharmacopoeias have to give general sterilizing methods without the benefit of this knowledge and these are based on data obtained with highly resistant bacterial spores. Ease of cultivation and identification, and reproducibility of response to the sterilizing agent are important considerations in the selection of the reference organism. Ideally the survivor curve for the organism under sterilization conditions should be linear to enable meaningful D values and IF values to be determined.

Current practice is to use *B. stearothermophilus* spores as the reference organism for moist and dry heat processes, *B. pumilus* spores for ionizing radiation and *B. subtilis var. niger* spores for ethylene oxide. Atoxigenic *Clostridium tetani* has been suggested as a suitable test organism for dry heat sterilization processes and in the food industry *Cl. botulinum* is frequently used as the reference organism for heat processes.

Having selected the reference organism it is now necessary to determine its D value under defined standard conditions. Since a variety of external factors can affect the resistance of the test organism (see Chapter 25) these determinations should be carried out with the organism in an environment similar to the product being sterilized.

If a product containing 10^6 spores is exposed to a sterilization process with an IF of 10^{10} there would be a 1 in 10 000 chance of one spore remaining at the end. If, however, the spore content of the product was 10^2 spores the probability of finding one viable spore at the end of the process would be reduced to 1 in 10^8. The determination of a sterilization protocol therefore requires a knowledge of the number of organisms that may be assumed to be present in the product. This is often referred to as the *bioload*. The maximum acceptable probability of finding a viable organism remaining at the end of the process must also be defined. This will enable the IF value for the process to be established.

Knowing the IF value for the process, and the D value for the reference spore, the time of exposure to the defined conditions can be calculated. The equivalent exposure times under other conditions can then be determined.

Integrated lethality in sterilization practice

Moist and dry heat sterilization protocols define a holding time at a specific temperature. The temperature cannot be achieved instantaneously and there is always a heating-up time. Cooling of the product at the end of the sterilization cycle is also non-instantaneous. If the load has a large thermal capacity the heating-up and cooling-down stages of the cycle will be prolonged. The heat imparted to the load during these stages will have lethality and will contribute to the overall lethality of the process often resulting in significant overheating. The official sterilization protocols ignore the lethality of the heating and cooling stages and consider only the lethality of the holding time. Considerable reduction in energy consumption, processing time and product degradation can be achieved by integrating the lethality of the total heat process. For a given load the heating and cooling curves are usually reproducible. If a complete record of the load temperature during the heating, holding, and cooling stages is available the lethality of the heating and cooling stages can be calculated as an F value. The holding time can then be reduced to the minimum necessary to ensure that the predetermined F value for the sterilization process is achieved. Methods for calculating the lethal contributions of the heating and cooling stages of sterilization cycles are detailed by Davies and Hobbs (1983). The application of microprocessors to integrated lethality calculations and sterilizer control has considerable potential.

Tests for sterility of the product

As mentioned earlier, sterility is an abstract concept and as such is not capable of practical demonstration. The BP 'Test for Sterility' is therefore a misnomer. Tests performed under this heading are estimates of the probability of absence of certain types of micro-organisms and would be better called 'probability of contamination tests'. Procedures for sterility testing are laid down in the *British Pharmacopoeia* and the practical aspects of such tests are considered in Chapter 28.

Essentially in a sterility test samples of the material to be tested are added to suitable culture media which are then incubated and examined for microbial growth. The following criteria are required.

1 Since the test is destructive it is not possible to examine the whole product batch. Adequate sampling of the batch must therefore be made and the probability of contamination of the batch estimated from the state of the samples.
2 The media used in the test must be capable of initiating and maintaining the growth of a small number of micro-organisms, especially pathogens, and the more common contaminants likely to be present in the raw materials or likely to be introduced during processing. Survivors from sterilization processes will invariably be damaged and require special recovery conditions that favour repair of cellular damage and spore germination. The test is normally restricted to detecting bacteria, yeasts and moulds and will not detect viruses.
3 The effect of any antimicrobial substances in the material must be neutralized.

4 The technique of performing the test should not be such as to subject the material under test to any antimicrobial agent other than those that may already be present in the material.
5 The technique must be such that the introduction of accidental contamination is reduced to a minimum and where contamination does occur it should be detectable and measurable. It is therefore an exacting test which has to be carried out under aseptic conditions by skilled operators.

Statistical considerations of sterility testing

As it is not possible in a sterility test to test the whole of a batch of a sterile product. The sterile or non-sterile condition of the batch must be deduced from the data obtained from examining a part of the batch. The first essential is that the part of the batch, or sample, must be random, i.e. a representative sample. The sterility test is then subject to the statistics of sampling. The binomial distribution is a close approximation to the distribution which fits the sterility test.

Since the end point in the test is growth or no growth an item can either be contaminated or non-contaminated, there are no degrees of contamination. Thus if the probability of an item being contaminated is p and the probability of the item being non-contaminated is q then $p + q = 1$. The probabilities of finding $0,1,2,\ldots n$ contaminated items in a sample of n items are the successive terms of the expansion

$$(p + q)^n$$

In a sterility test the batch would be rejected if any contaminated items were found in the sample. The probability of finding n non-contaminated items in a sample of n would be q^n or $1 - p^n$ and the probability of finding one or more contaminated items would be $1 - q^n$ or p^n.

The *British Pharmacopoeia* defines the sampling procedures to be used in tests for sterility in the UK and these vary for different batch sizes. It prescribes the examination of at least four items for a batch of less than 100 items, of at least 10 items for a batch of 100–500 items, and at least 20 items for a batch of more than 500 items. The probability $P = 1 - p^n$ of accepting the batch as

Table 26.1 Probability (*P*) of accepting batches of different per cent contamination as sterile in a single BP Test for Sterility

Batch size	Sample size n	% contaminated items in the batch					
		0.1	1	5	10	20	50
<100	4	0.996	0.961	0.815	0.656	0.410	0.063
100–500	10	0.990	0.904	0.599	0.349	0.107	0.001
>500	20	0.980	0.818	0.358	0.122	0.012	<0.0001

sterile when the BP sampling scheme is applied to batches containing different percentages of contaminated items, i.e. different values of *p*, is given in Table 26.1. These values show that with low levels of contamination the probability of accepting a contaminated batch as sterile is extremely high and that only when the contamination level is high does this probability become acceptably small. It is clear that the sterility test is unable to detect low levels of contamination reliably. It can also be seen that as the sample size increases the probability of a contaminated batch being accepted as sterile decreases. Furthermore, since *P* depends only on *p* and *n*, the batch size is irrelevant.

The problems associated with sampling are even greater where it is not possible to examine the total amount of the sample. Where, for practical purposes, an aliquot only can be assessed the BP requires that this should be proportional to the total capacity of the sample, and in no case should be less than 10%. Proportionate sampling results in a dramatic increase in the probability of accepting a contaminated batch as sterile (Table 26.2). An advantage of the filtration technique in sterility testing (Chapter 28) is that it permits the examination of the total sample, irrespective of its volume, thereby eliminating the need for proportionate sampling.

In an attempt to identify contamination intro-

duced accidently during the course of the sterility test the BP allows the test to be repeated using the same sample size. Far from improving the chances of the correct decision being made the retest procedure in fact increases significantly the probability of accepting a contaminated batch as sterile (Table 26.2). The probability *P* is increased from $1 - p^n$ to $1 - p^n[2 - (1 - p^n)]$ by a single retest. The BP actually permits the test to be repeated twice. The probability of accepting a contaminated batch is increased even further by the introduction of the second retest.

It is apparent from these statistical considerations that the test for sterility by itself cannot give absolute assurance that a batch of a product is sterile. With products that are terminally sterilized by, for example, autoclaving, the contamination level would be expected to be well below 0.1% and the probability of detecting it would be extremely small. In these cases the value of the sterility test is doubtful, and where the sterilization process is the subject of reliable in-process validation, good manufacturing procedures provide a greater assurance of sterility. The sterility test will, however, detect gross contamination and total process failure, and may provide more valuable information when the product is sterilized by a less reliable method such as ethylene oxide. Sterility tests are required to be carried out on all products that are sterilized by filtration or

Table 26.2 Probability (*P*) of accepting batches of different per cent contamination as sterile in a single BP Test for Sterility using proportionate sampling, and after a single retest

	% contaminated items in the batch					
	0.1	1	5	10	20	50
Using total sample volume	0.980	0.818	0.358	0.122	0.012	<0.0001
Using 10% of sample volume	0.998	0.980	0.905	0.820	0.670	0.360
After a single retest	>0.999	0.967	0.588	0.229	0.024	<0.0001

produced by an aseptic process since with these procedures in-process validation is not possible.

No practical sterility test has yet been devised which will by itself ensure that a batch of product is sterile. Nevertheless, a carefully performed and correctly interpreted sterility test provides an additional safety check on products that require sterilization, and is an important part of quality assurance. The sterility test also has important ethical and legal implications.

REFERENCES AND BIBLIOGRAPHY

British Pharmacopoeia (1980) Pharmaceutical Press, London.

Davies, D. J. G. and Hobbs, R. J. (1983) Principles of sterilisation. In *Pharmaceutical Microbiology* (ed. W. B. Hugo and A. D. Russell), pp. 366–386, Blackwell Scientific Publications, Oxford.

Perkins J. J. (1969) Principles and methods of sterilization in health services, 2nd edn, Charles Thomas Publishers, Springfield, Illinois, USA.

Pharmaceutical Codex (1979) Pharmaceutical Press, London.

Pharmaceutical Handbook (1980) 19th edn, Pharmaceutical Press, London.

Russell, A. D., Hugo, W. B. and Ayliffe, G. A. J. (1982) *Principles and Practice of Disinfection, Preservation and Sterilisation*, Blackwell Scientific Publications, Oxford.

Microbiological contamination and preservation of pharmaceutical preparations

SOURCES AND INCIDENCE OF CONTAMINATION

Micro-organisms form an integral part of our environment. They are present in the air that we breathe, the food that we eat and the water that we drink. Some micro-organisms indigenous, to the body are present in considerable numbers; they constitute up to one-third of the dry weight of faeces. In this situation it is apparent that both raw materials and final medicines will contain micro-organisms unless specific measures are adopted to exclude them. The preparation of sterile medicaments is a skilled and expensive procedure demanding sophisticated equipment, skilled personnel and a controlled working environment. To produce all medicines to such a standard would require clear arguments to justify the considerable costs involved and the consequent expense to consumers. Factors to be considered are: the sources and incidence of micro-organisms in drugs and medical preparations, the consequences of such contamination both for the stability of medicines and for the health of the patient and, arising from these, the levels and types of micro-organism which might be tolerated.

As indicated in Table 27.1 and Fig. 27.1, there will be many factors potentially contributing to the microbial load carried by a pharmaceutical preparation at every stage of manufacture from assembling the raw materials to packaging the final product. A large number of papers have been published drawing attention to these problems following the classical investigation by Kallings and his colleagues (1966) of an outbreak of salmonellosis in Sweden attributed to contaminated

Table 27.1 Sources of microbial contaminants

Water	Low demand Gram-negative groups: *Pseudomonas, Xanthamonas, Flavobacterium, Achromobacter*
Air	Mould spores: *Penicillium, Mucor, Aspergillus* Bacterial spores: *Bacillus* spp. Yeasts Micrococci
Raw materials	
Earths	Anaerobic spore formers: *Clostridium* spp.
Pigments	*Salmonella*
Starches	Coliforms
Gums	*Actinomyces*
Animal products	*Salmonella* Coliforms
Personnel	Coliforms Staphylococci Streptococci Corynebacteria

tablets. In this instance the infection was traced to the original defatted thyroid powder imported from Hungary which was used to make the tablets. The Pharmaceutical Society of Great Britain set up a working party in 1968 to investigate microbial contamination of pharmaceutical preparations in manufacturing establishments and

in hospital and retail pharmacies (Sykes, 1971). The procedure followed, in the case of manufactured preparations, was to examine raw materials and finished products in the final packs, whilst, for hospitals and community pharmacies, products were examined as received from manufacturers and after dispensing from bulk packs. The results from this and subsequent surveys (Table 27.2) indicated that major sources of contamination are the water and the raw materials used in preparing medicines. Crude drugs of natural origin present a particular hazard. Digitalis leaf was found to contain up to 160×10^3 viable bacteria per gram and acacia 1.8×10^3 per gram. Another group of materials commonly found to be heavily contaminated is the natural earths including kaolin, chalk, talc and bentonite. In spite of the high bacterial counts often recorded and the common occurrence of moulds, *salmonella* was not detected, as was the case in Kallings' investigation and, of the *coli-aerogenes* bacteria, *E. coli* type I is rare. The usual water-borne organisms found are the *Pseudomonas–Achromobacter–Alcaligenes* types including occasionally, *Ps. aeruginosa*. Purified water has proved to be a typical source of microorganisms in that during use the ion-exchange

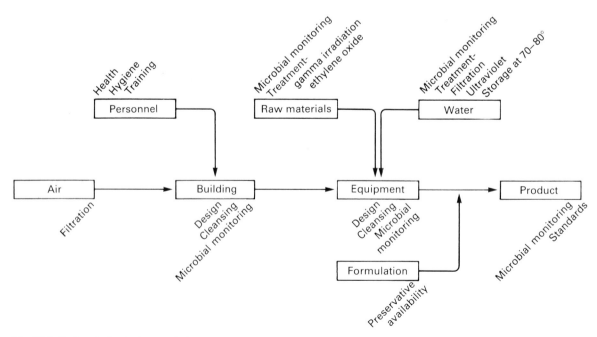

Fig. 27.1 Factors in hygienic manufacture

Table 27.2 Microbial content of drugs and medicines*

Origin	Viable count range (per g or ml)	Types of organism
Crude drugs		
Digitalis Leaf	10^2–10^3	Moulds; coliforms
Gelatin	10–10^3	Coliforms
Tragacanth	10–10^3	Moulds
Starch (potato)	10–10^2	Coliforms
Thyroid	10^2–10^6	*Salmonella*; coliforms
Earths		
Kaolin	10^2–10^6	Moulds; spore formers (Gram-positive)
Chalk	10–10^2	Moulds; spore formers (Gram-positive)
Talc	10–10^3	Moulds; spore formers (Gram-positive)
Mixtures		
Kaolin and morphine	10–10^3	Pseudomonads
Magnesium trisilicate	10–10^6	Pseudomonads; Gram-positive bacilli
Sulphadimidine paediatric	10–10^3	Pseudomonads
Tablets		
Aspirin	0–10	Moulds
Digitalis	10–10^5	Moulds; coliforms
Thyroid	10–10^3	*Salmonella*; coliforms
Miscellaneous		
Peppermint water	10^2–10^5	Pseudomonads; fungi
Syrup	10–10^3	Pseudomonads; yeasts
Liquid paraffin emulsion	10–10^2	Pseudomonads; spore formers (Gram-positive)

* Reported from various sources.

column may become contaminated from the water passing through and the entrapped organisms rapidly multiply to produce high counts in the outflowing water. Somewhat less expected has been the incidence of contamination of distilled water reported from several hospital pharmacies and a common exacerbating factor here is the multiplication of organisms in stored water. These usually gain access to distilled water by way of poor quality rubber or plastic connection tubing or inadequate closure of storage containers, whilst for purified water, as already indicated, they are shed from contaminated exchange columns. Whatever their origin it is evident that, during storage at ambient laboratory temperature, high counts of micro-organisms can be attained.

As would be anticipated medicines prepared from contaminated drugs and with contaminated vehicles will be themselves infected with the micro-organisms concerned. Further, it is important to realize that in some cases the initial bacterial count in a freshly prepared mixture can increase substantially during storage, particularly in those cases in which the formulation contains no preservative.

A major potential source of microbial contamination is that represented by the personnel preparing medicines and the patients in using them (Table 27.1). In the environment generally it is people who generate most of the airborne bacteria. Body movements, exhaling, speaking and, of course, coughing and sneezing represent significant sources of contamination. The micro-organisms which can be disseminated in this way include staphylococci, present on the skin and in the nostrils of healthy persons, streptococci, sometimes present in the throat, and a variety of Enterobacteriaceae including salmonellae and coliforms present in the intestines. Other microflora which may be found as contaminants of medicines and which are not normally associated with humans, are the airborne spores of both bacteria and moulds, including several wild yeasts, anaerobic inhabitants of soil and earths such as the clostridia and low demand, water-borne bacteria, usually Gram-negative forms (Table 27.2).

There is considerable potential for micro-organisms to enter medicines during both manufacture and use and in this situation it is not surprising that whenever non-sterile preparations and their ingredients are screened for microbial contamination, organisms are detected. As has been discussed, the incidence of microflora in medicines as issued from the dispensary or manufacturers is dictated very much by the nature of the ingredients, i.e. whether natural or synthetic, the quality of the vehicle and the care and attitude of personnel involved.

The situation is very different for sterile preparations in that detection of any micro-organisms represents an unacceptable situation usually indicative of a breakdown in the sterilization process. Thus when in 1972 infusion fluids used in a Plymouth hospital were found to be contaminated, the Secretary of State required the Medicines Commission to 'review measures which should be taken in the course of the production, distribution, storage and use of medicinal products to prevent their becoming vehicles of infection'. It is indicative of the rarity of such incidents that an inquiry was deemed to be necessary.

GROWTH AND MULTIPLICATION OF MICRO-ORGANISMS IN PHARMACEUTICAL PRODUCTS

Most raw materials and consequently the pharmaceutical preparations containing them will support some form of micro-organism. Although this ability varies considerably according to the nutritive properties and moisture content of the materials concerned, it is unwise to assume that, for instance, a dry powder or a tablet is safe from microbial spoilage. The problem can be appreciated by considering the range of habitats of micro-organisms, encompassing as they do volcanic regions to the Antarctic wastes and nutrient sources as unlikely as glass and concrete. The majority of medicines present a ready source of nutrients and moisture and there are many reports of the effects of microbial proliferation within them with attendant odours and visible spoilage. Troublesome and expensive as this obvious deterioration may be, a more serious problem is the development of micro-organisms without obvious signs or involving delayed effects. For this reason it is important to have a knowledge of the microbial content of all drugs and medicines rather than restrict attention to those required to be sterile and those shown to be particularly spoilage prone. A study of the interaction of micro-organisms within foods such as milk or meat products has shown how pioneer forms can prepare the way for later invaders by degrading complex nutrients, altering pH levels, or making more moisture available until the final spoilage population is established. The initial invaders, in either foods or medicines, can reach high levels without visible effects and furthermore when the finally spoiled product is investigated, they may have been completely displaced by a final spoilage form. Unless this chain reaction of spoilage is appreciated harmful effects of apparently stable medicines can be unresolved and the importance of some contaminants not realized. Thus, syrup or mixtures rich in sugar may become initially contaminated by osmophilic yeasts which can thrive at high sugar concentrations and create conditions by utilizing the sugars to allow secondary, less specialized organisms to become established. When such syrups are examined there may be little evidence of the yeasts which initiated the spoilage process and so their role may be overlooked.

CONSEQUENCES OF CONTAMINATION

It is now realized that the presence of micro-organisms in a pharmaceutical preparation may have a variety of consequences ranging from the negligable to the very serious. For example, spores of the mould *Mucor* may be present in a dormant form and never produce spoilage or harm the patient who takes the medicine. In complete contrast to this would be the presence of *Salmonella* in a medicine which although causing little or no visible spoilage, would represent a serious health hazard.

The instances in which there have been serious consequences attending contaminations have been, in the main, concerned with those preparations which are required to be supplied sterile. This might be anticipated since sterile preparations are usually administered parenterally or into the eyes and in these circumstances extraneous micro-organisms present a particular danger. Intravenous infusion fluids are recognized as a potential area for concern particularly since their implication in the case, previously mentioned, where contaminated fluid resulted in the death of several patients. The established practice of adding drugs to infusions, often at patient level in hospital wards, can present an additional microbiological hazard unless closely supervised by skilled staff. Preparations for ophthalmic use, including contact lens solutions, have been responsible for serious infections of the eye, some resulting in blindness, as a result of microbial contamination.

Considered against the background of the high volume of medicinal products used annually by the public, the serious consequences of contamination are very few. Where they do occur, however, the public is justifiably worried and the implications for the profession are grave.

Apart from possible infection of patients the other important effect of contamination of medicines is that of general spoilage. This may result in obvious changes such as discoloration, breakdown of emulsions and the production of gas and various odours. Such comparatively dramatic effects of deterioration do have the virtue of directing the consumer's attention to the problem and, hopefully, discouraging their use of the medicine. In other cases, however, active ingredients may be utilized by invading micro-organisms without overt visible signs of spoilage. Thus, salicylates (including aspirin), phenacetin, paracetamol, atropine, chloramphenicol and hydrocortisone can be degraded to a variety of therapeutically inactive products. Preservatives, intended to protect formulations against micro-organisms can themselves present a ready source of microbial nutrition particularly if their levels become depleted and if they are aromatic in structure.

Bacteria can produce various toxic substances which are a potential danger in contaminated products even when a sterilization procedure has been applied and only dead cells or their residues remain. In parenteral preparations pyrogenic agents, usually lipopolysaccharides, represent a particularly hazardous product released by Gram-negative bacteria. Moulds produce mycotoxins which from early times have been implicated in illnesses such as ergotism and more recently with gastroenteritis both caused by using contaminated grain. The involvement of mycotoxins, particularly aflatoxin, in cancer has added an urgency to our study of them, but as yet there is no evidence of their implication in medicines.

SCREENING FOR CONTAMINATION

A consideration of Fig. 27.1 will show that if contamination is to be minimized then a knowledge of the microbial levels associated with all aspects of the production of a medicine is required. Thus, examining prepared medicines for their contamination will not, in itself, further our efforts to reduce this unless parallel screening is done upon the manufacturing process and environment, including air, equipment, personnel and raw materials.

Methods for the detection, enumeration and identification of micro-organisms have been described in Chapter 24. Some of these methods can be applied to determine the number and type of micro-organisms at any stage in the preparation or manufacture of a medicine. The most relevant are discussed below.

Air sampling

The usual methods for sampling from air are by free fall or settling, forced air flow and filtration.

Free fall or settling

As the name implies, this involves the sampling of organisms deposited naturally from the atmosphere. This is typically carried out by exposing plates of suitable nutrient medium for selected periods in the locations to be sampled. The procedure is empirical, with the counts obtained depending upon time of exposure, the nature of any activity in the area and the siting of the plates in relation to such activity.

Forced air flow

Forced air flow samplers allow a measured volume of air to be examined by directing it on to a solid agar surface or drawing it through sterile saline or nutrient broth from which plate counts can be made. A variety of commercially available apparatus may be used to apply this method.

Filtration

Filtration involves the drawing of air through a membrane filter which is then aseptically removed, placed upon suitable nutrient agar and incubated.

Care must be taken in interpreting results obtained by these various methods and thought given to location and timing of sampling, period of exposure or volume of air examined and movement of personnel. In general, if contamination problems are likely to be due to particles settling from the air then free fall methods are adequate. If, however, contaminating particles tend to remain airborne some form of forced air sampling is essential. The actual timing of sampling will provide information upon conditions during typical busy working periods and the efficiency of any air filtration system in coping at peak times.

Sampling of surfaces and equipment

Simple techniques can be used to assess the level of contamination of surfaces, such as swabbing with sterile cotton tipped sticks, which can be transferred to suitable recovery media, or by placing a sterile agar surface in contact with the area to be sampled and, after removal, incubating. It is easier to use swabs for flexible and uneven surfaces and agar contact methods for firm flat surfaces.

Measuring contamination levels in raw materials and final preparations

The nature of raw material and final preparations will determine the method used to detect microbial contamination. Water, water-miscible liquids or soluble solids present no difficulties for conventional plate counting or filter membrane methods. Insoluble or oily materials and preparations need to be suitably dispersed and homogenized if contaminating micro-organisms are to be isolated. In every instance any antimicrobial activity of the sample under examination must be neutralized. Methods of counting micro-organisms and the inherent errors are described briefly in Chapter 24 and in more detail in standard bacteriological textbooks.

There is increasing interest in methods for the rapid detection of micro-organisms in food and drugs which can be automated and should remove much of the drudgery of traditional counting techniques. These methods are based upon the measurement of some metabolic activity or other feature of organisms and include microcalorimetry, electrophoresis and impedence determinations. In the case of sterile production, the entire system can be monitored by processing a

sterile nutrient medium (for liquid preparations) or soluble sterile powder (for solids) and examining final preparations for contamination, together with samples taken at various intermediate stages.

CONTROL OF MICROBIAL CONTAMINATION

There are essentially two strategies to be adopted in the preparation of microbiologically acceptable pharmaceutical preparations. The first, and most important, is to minimize the access of micro-organisms from the sources summarized in Fig. 27.1 and Table 27.1, and the second is to formulate the final product so as to be hostile to micro-organisms, normally by the addition of preservatives.

For sterile preparations there is either a terminal sterilization process or a closely controlled aseptic manufacturing procedure. In every case the final pack should be designed to protect the product during storage and minimize in-use contamination. The *Guide to Good Pharmaceutical Manufacturing Practice* or 'Orange Guide' provides guidance upon premises, equipment, raw materials, packaging, storage and the training of personnel.

Premises and equipment

Premises need to be purpose built to provide a logical work flow, with separation of areas of different grades of cleanliness, appropriate air supplies, construction materials which are resistant to dirt and easy to keep clean. The equipment should be as simple as possible for the purposes required with a minimum of junctions, valves and pumps, to allow cleaning in place by circulation of detergents or other chemical antimicrobial agents such as hypochlorites, followed by steam or hot water flushing. The degree of air treatment required will depend upon the type of product involved with aseptic manipulation demanding filtration efficient enough to remove particles down to 0.1 μm. For general manufacture a level of less than 100 particles per cubic foot (3.5 litres) ranging between 0.5 μm and 5.0 μm is acceptable. The 'Orange Guide' gives advice upon basic environmental standards with allowance made for people present in working areas.

Raw materials

Raw materials, particularly those of natural origin, and water are a potentially rich source of micro-organisms and may require treatment to reduce or eliminate these. It is a pharmacopoeial requirement in Great Britain, Europe and the United States that only potable water is used for pharmaceutical manufacture. This, in effect, means that the water must not contain more than 10 coliforms per 100 ml and, in addition to this, the common low demand spoilage forms should be eliminated as far as possible. Water may be treated by u.v. treatment units or filtration and stored at elevated temperature (65–80 °C) to discourage microbial growth.

For raw materials, generally, any treatment applied to remove or reduce the microbial load must be such that the materials are not adversely affected. A variety of processing procedures are available including ionizing radiations, microwaves, gassing and, of course, heat. In every case close monitoring for possible deleterious effects is essential.

Personnel

There is little doubt that however comprehensive the procedures adopted to control contamination, they will be of little avail unless the personnel involved understand and appreciate the problems and significance of microbial contamination. This requires education in hygiene to minimize introduction of micro-organisms by staff and to underline the importance of appropriate protective measures. The approach will, of course, differ depending upon the level of education of the people involved but it cannot be overemphasized that all personnel and visitors, however senior, must be required to comply with regimens of hygiene and protective clothing. A full range of appropriate clothing is commercially available, which for the manufacturer of sterile preparations, completely shields the product from body surfaces, with, for instance, hood, mask, overall, protective gloves and boots. For other manufacturing areas good quality overalls and head cover represent a minimal requirement. General dispensing requires careful attention to hygiene, provision of suitable overalls and a ban upon food consumption and smoking in the dispensary.

THE PRESERVATION OF PHARMACEUTICAL PREPARATIONS

By an understanding of the many factors involved in the microbial contamination of medicines and application of the procedures described, a range of products can be obtained which, if required, are sterile, or have an acceptable level of organisms present. Having achieved this is, in itself, not sufficient, without further steps being taken to minimize contamination and spoilage of the medicines during use. Well designed containers, usually single dose in the case of sterile preparations, and sensible storage contribute a great deal to this end but, whenever acceptable, an added safeguard is to incorporate an antimicrobial substance or preservative into the formulation.

The correct approach to preservation has as its foundation two important principles. The first of these is that the addition of a preservative to a product must not be done to mask any deficiencies in the manufacturing procedures and the second is that the preservative should be an integral part of the formulation, chosen to afford protection in that particular environment. The increasing care now being given to the hygienic preparation of pharmaceutical products is, hopefully, removing the need for preservatives to cope with high initial microbial loads but the problem remains of protecting against spoilage resulting from in-use contamination. If a preservative is to prevent such spoilage the factors affecting its efficacy must be appreciated.

Factors in preservative efficacy

The range of antimicrobial agents available is apparently very wide (see Chapter 25 and Table 27.3) until the particular requirements of a

Table 27.3 Preservatives used in pharmaceutical preparations

Preparation	Preservative	Concentration % w/v	Special factors
Injections	Phenol	0.5	Not for intraocular, intracardiac or intracisternal or over 15 ml single dose. Closures pretreated
	Cresol	0.3	
	Chlorocresol	0.1	
	Phenylmercuric nitrate	0.001	
	Benzyl alcohol	1.0	
Eyedrops	Phenylmercuric nitrate or acetate	0.002	Dropper teats pretreated.
	Chlorhexidine acetate	0.01	
	Benzalkonium chloride	0.01	Silicone rubber teats
Mixtures	Chloroform	0.25	Adsorption. Volatile
	Benzoic acid	0.1	pH (pK_a 4.2)
	Methyl paraben	0.1	Adsorption
	Alcohol	12–20	Volatile
	Sulphur dioxide	400 parts/10^6	Volatile
Creams	Parabens	0.1–0.2	⋆ K_w^o R high
	Chlorocresol	0.1	K_w^o R high
	Dichlorobenzyl alcohol,	0.05–0.2	K_w^o
	Cetyltrimethyl ammonium bromide	0.01–0.1	R high
	Phenylmercuric nitrate	0.001	
Tablets	Methylparaben	0.1	

⋆ K_w^o values	Mineral oil	Vegetable oil
Chlorocresol	1.5	117
Methylparaben	0.02	7.5
Propylparaben	0.5	80.0

R = ratio of total to free preservative in non-ionic surfactant–water system.

preservative for a formulated medicine are considered. To state that the preservative must be non-toxic, odourless, stable and compatible with other formulation components whilst exerting its effect against the wide range of potential microbial contaminants, is an oversimplification. Toxicity alone debars many antimicrobial compounds from use in preparations for parenteral, ophthalmic or oral use, whilst the increased sophistication of some modern formulations makes it difficult to avoid preservative–ingredient interactions. Any organisms which do enter a preparation will multiply in the aqueous phase or immediate interface and thus it is the prime function of the preservative to attain a protective concentration in this phase. As shown in Fig. 27.2, the major reasons for a preservative not attaining an effective concentration in the aqueous phase are its possible solubility in oil, interaction with emulgents, hydrocolloids and suspended solids, its interaction with the container or its volatility. In addition to this, the ambient pH of the formulation can have a marked influence upon preservative effectivity.

Oil–water partition

In a simple two-phase system of oil and water a preservative will partition until:

$$\frac{C_o}{C_w} = K_w^o$$

where, C_o is the concentration of preservative in oil at equilibrium, C_w is the concentration of preservative in water at equilibrium and K_w^o is the oil–water partition coefficient at the given temperature. It will be apparent from Table 27.3 that oil solubility will be an important parameter in preserving formulations containing vegetable oils such as arachis or soya; and for such preparations the esters of parahydroxybenzoic acid (parabens) are unsuitable. Faced with this problem it is necessary to change the preservative or alter the formulation and given the restricted choice of preservatives, the formulation becomes all important. Thus, it was found that by substituting liquid paraffin (mineral oil) for arachis oil (vegetable oil) in formulations of Calamine Cream,

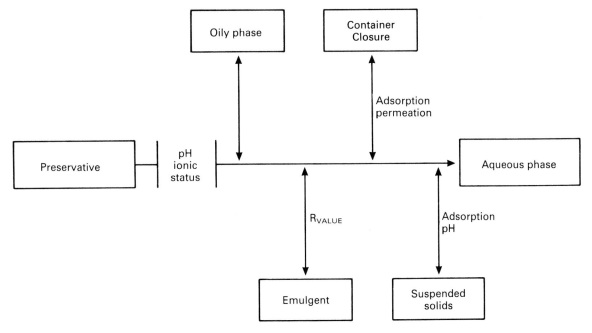

Fig. 27.2 Preservative availability

a preservative such as chlorocresol would afford better protection ($K_w^o = 117$ (arachis oil): 1.5 (liquid paraffin)). The further step of using a less oil-soluble preservative such as phenoxyethanol ($K_w^o = 0.12$ liquid paraffin) further improved the system.

Emulsions

Many emulgents are used in pharmaceutical preparations to produce elegant applications or palatable medicines (see Chapter 16). A variety of interactions will occur between preservatives and the emulsified oil phase and with emulgent molecules or micelles. Attempts have been made to quantify such interactions by measuring the proportion of free preservative in emulsions in a variety of ways including dialysis and dissolution techniques. The use of predictive data can greatly assist in the formulation, provided that the different behaviour of different emulgents, effects of temperature and influence of oil:water ratio are appreciated. A simple mathematical model has been described by Bean (1972):

$$C_w = C \, \frac{\phi + 1}{K_w^o \, \phi + 1}$$

where C_w is the concentration of preservative in total aqueous phase, C is the total concentration of preservative and ϕ is the oil:water ratio. In the presence of an emulgent the amount of free preservative can be measured and the result expressed as the factor R; then:

$$C_w = \frac{C}{R}$$

where $R = \dfrac{\text{total preservative } (C)}{\text{free preservative } (C_w)}$.

The equation becomes:

$$C_w = C \, \frac{\phi + 1}{K_w^o \phi + R}$$

Using this model it can be calculated for instance that to attain the required protective concentration of 0.2% w/v methyl paraben in a liquid paraffin/water emulsion containing 5% polysorbate 80 and 50% oil, a total concentration of some 0.5% must be used. Alterations in type and concentration of emulgent, nature of oil and oil:water ratio will all influence the concentration of preservative needed to protect the system.

Interaction with other formulation components

Many of the hydrocolloids used as dispersants or thickeners such as methylcellulose, alginates, polyvinylpyrrolidone and tragacanth can interact to some degree with preservatives and diminish their activity. In some cases this is a direct incompatibility as between alginates, which are anionic, and cation-active preservatives, whereas in other cases a variety of physicochemical interactions operate.

Therapeutically active ingredients in the form of suspended solids in mixtures, including suphadimidine, magnesium trisilicate, kaolin and rhubarb have all been shown to deplete preservative concentrations, probably by adsorption. Similarly, fillers and disintegrants cause problems in tablet preservation due to their interaction with added preservatives such as methylhydroxybenzoate.

Effects of containers

Preparations packed in traditional glass containers can be expected to retain their preservative content provided the closure is suitably airtight. The greatly increased use of plastics in packaging has brought with it a number of difficulties ranging from permeation of preservatives through the container to interaction with it. There is a great deal of published work describing the losses of preservative to plastic medicine bottles, contact lenses and their containers and plastic syringes. Given the complexity of modern plastics with their differences in thickness, surface characteristics, filler and plasticizer content it is necessary to choose the material for the pack of a preserved formulation on the basis of adequate trials.

Although rubber reacts with many preservatives it still finds use for teats and closures. These are required to be pretreated with the preservatives they are to be in contact with, in order to minimize subsequent uptake during storage (Table 27.3).

Influence of pH

An appreciation of the many obstacles which may prevent a preservative attaining an adequate protective concentration in a given preparation must be complemented by some understanding of the interaction between that preservative and any micro-organisms present as contaminants. Thus, not only must free preservative be available in a formulation but it must be present in an active form. This is particularly important when activity is related to degree of ionization, as is the case with both anion- and cation-active antimicrobial agents. An example is that of a weak acid preservative such as benzoic acid which requires to be predominantly in the undissociated form in order to exert antimicrobial activity. Since this acid has a pK_a value of 4.2, an ambient pH below this is needed for efficient preservative activity.

The relationship between degree of dissociation and pH is given by:

$$\text{Fraction of undissociated preservative} = \frac{1}{1 + \text{antilog } (pH - pK_a)}$$

In most cases more than one factor is involved, as with Kaolin Mixture Paediatric PC in which the preservative used is benzoic acid. The dual problem here is that the adsorption of the benzoic acid by the light kaolin diminishes at pH values above 5, whereas the acid preservative is most efficient at lower values. In this situation the formulator faces opposing choices. He may opt for an alternative preservative or use a mixture of preservatives. Kaolin mixture has the added interest that in order to render it attractive to children, raspberry syrup flavouring is used, presumably with disregard to possible tooth decay, producing a pH of 3.5. In this formulation about 83% of benzoic acid is present in the biologically active undissociated form but adsorption on to the kaolin is favoured. The Codex formulation incorporates chloroform as an additional preservative in an effort to adequately protect this mixture.

The majority of preservatives are less dependent upon pH, although cationic active quaternary ammonium compounds are more active at high pH values.

Preservatives in combination

The use of a single preservative to protect a pharmaceutical preparation may be unrealistic.

Increasing attention has focused upon the use of mixtures of preservatives and the addition of various potentiators to achieve better results. The justification for using mixtures of antimicrobial compounds must reside in an increased spectrum of antimicrobial activity, a synergistic effect enabling decreased levels of component preservatives to be used, an attendant decrease in toxicity, and a reduction in the emergence of resistant forms. One of the oldest examples of a preservative mixture used in pharmacy is the former vehicle for eyedrops, 'Solution for Eyedrops', which contained a mixture of methyl and propyl esters of p-hydroxybenzoic acid designed to exert antibacterial and antifungal effects. Modern formulations for eyedrops and contact lens solutions include phenylethyl alcohol and phenoxetol in conjuction with benzalkonium chloride to widen the antimicrobial spectrum and aid access to susceptible sites on the micro-organisms. The chelating agent ethylenediamine tetra-acetate (EDTA) has also been used with preservatives other than those yielding metallic ions, to enhance activity, by interfering with vital metal ion balance and associated permeability. A rather different mechanism is to increase the availability of lipophilic preservatives by reducing their loss to emulgents in the formulation, as with the addition of propylene glycol to emulsions preserved with parabens to reduce loss to micelles.

A correctly designed preservative system is the appropriate complement to hygienic manufacture. Both demand a rational approach based upon an appreciation of interacting factors. Thus, just as there is little justification in providing a high quality manufacturing environment and introducing poor quality raw materials, there is equally little point in an *ad hoc* addition of preservatives to preparations without investigation of formulation interactions involved.

MICROBIAL STANDARDS FOR PHARMACEUTICAL PREPARATIONS

The design of microbial standards for pharmaceutical preparations must be realistic in that they relate to the intended use of the preparation and can be applied without ambiguity. The types of standard used to monitor microbial content, are twofold, namely, an absolute exclusion of all micro-organisms or named organisms, and a numerical limit upon all organisms or named organisms. The first type or exclusion standard in its most severe form, is that requiring sterility, and is applied to solutions for injection, ophthalmic preparations and certain other fluids for body irrigation. In these cases no organisms can be tolerated and the role of any preservative is to maintain the sterility of the sterilized preparation during use. Although such an absolute standard is not required for medicines for oral or topical use, nevertheless certain bacteria can represent a hazard and be indicative of poor manufacturing practice and should be excluded. The *United States Pharmacopoeia* suggests an exclusion standard for *E. coli* to all solutions for oral use and for *S. aureus* and *Ps. aeruginosa* to topical preparations. In addition to this both the British and United States pharmacopoeias apply exclusion standards for named organisms from certain raw materials and final preparations (Table 27.4).

Standards based upon numerical limits usually apply more broadly and are typified by the '100 cell limit' which allows no more than 100 cells of non-specified aerobic organisms in one ml or g of a given preparation.

Compliance with these standards can only be assured by strict control of manufacture from raw materials to final preparation (Fig. 27.1). Incorporation of a product designed preservative system represents an additional safeguard.

The application of the various standards described depends in the last analysis upon the reliability of the techniques available for detection and enumeration of micro-organisms in raw materials and final preparations. The established methods of the microbiologist are time consuming and have the errors of any biological measurements. As indicated earlier a range of methods of detection and quantification based upon properties such as metabolic heat production, charge on organisms or their resistance are coming into use and should add a new dimension to the use of microbial standards.

Table 27.4 Microbial standards for pharmaceutical preparations

Requirement	Authority*
Exclusion	
1 Complete exclusion — sterility	
Injections. Ophthalmic preparations	BP, EP, USP
2 Exclusion of named organisms	
Raw materials:	
e.g. Aluminium Hydroxide —	BP
Ps. aeruginosa/1 g, *E. coli*/1 g	BP
Cochineal. Gelatin — *E. coli*/1 g	BP
Pancreatin. Thyroid —	BP
Salmonella/10 g	
Maize starch *E. coli*/1 g	
Tragacanth	
Oral dosage forms:	
Free from *E. coli*	USP
Free from *E. coli* and *Salmonella*/1 ml	EP
Topical preparations:	
Free from *Ps. aeruginosa* and *S. aureus*	USP
Free from Enterobacteria, *S. aureus*	
and *Ps. aeruginosa*	EP
Limit upon number of viable organisms	
Oral dosage forms:	USP
Limit upon total aerobic count of non-specified viable organisms, e.g. Milk of Magnesia 100 cells/ml	
Raw materials:	
$\not> 10^4$ aerobic bacteria/ml	
$\not> 10^2$ yeasts or moulds/ml	EP
$\not> 10^2$ enterobacteria/ml	
Topical preparations:	
$\not> 100$ organisms/g or ml	EP

* BP, British Pharmacopeia 1980; BP Addendum 1986; USP, United States Pharmacopeia XXI; EP, European Pharmacopeia (draft proposals).

Challenge testing

The methods and philosophy of challenge testing are dealt with in Chapter 28. In the particular case of preserved preparations the test must be designed to provide a realistic measure of the ability of the formulation to cope with normal use. Many arguments have been made for the choice of challenge organisms, their use at various concentrations, the number of challenges made and so on. The current BP test specifies all of these parameters for parenteral, ophthalmic, topical and oral liquid preparations together with the end point required. In this respect it provides general guidelines but in addition most manufacturers apply their own challenge tests based upon their experience with the particular product.

CONCLUSION

As with many areas of study that of the microbial contamination of pharmaceuticals began with an awareness that a problem existed. The consequences of this problem extended both to economy of production and to safety of the patient. The skills of the microbiologist, chemist, engineer and pharmacist have been combined to enable medicines to be prepared which are microbiologically safe. The maintaining of this situation depends upon constant vigilance over every aspect of manufacture and formulation.

REFERENCES

Bean, H. S. (1972) Preservatives for pharmaceuticals. *J. Soc. Cosmet. Chem.*, **23**, 703–720.

Guide to Good Manufacturing Practice (1983) (ed. Sharpe, J. R.), HMSO, London.

Kallings, L. O., Ringertz, O., Silverstone, L. and Ernerfeldt, F. (1966) Microbial contamination of medical preparations. *Acta Pharmaca Suecica*, **3**, 219–228.

Sykes, G. (1971) Microbial contamination of pharmaceuticals for oral and topical use: Pharmaceutical Society of Great Britain's working party report. *Pharm. J.*, **207**, 400–402.

BIBLIOGRAPHY

Baird, R. M. (1981) Drugs and cosmetics. In *Microbial Deterioration* (ed. A. H. Rose), pp. 387–429, Academic Press, London.

Beveridge, E. G. (1975) The microbial spoilage of pharmaceutical products. In *Microbial Aspects of the Deterioration of Materials* (eds R. J. Gilbert and D. W. Lovelock), pp. 213–235, Academic Press, London.

Guide to Good Manufacturing Practice (1983) (ed. Sharpe, J. R.), HMSO, London.

Parker, M. S. (1982) The preservation of pharmaceutical and cosmetic products. In *Principles and Practice of Disinfection, Preservation and Sterilisation* (eds A. D. Russell, W. B. Hugo and G. A. J. Ayliffe), pp. 285–305, Blackwell Scientific Publications, Oxford, London, Edinburgh.

Underwood, E. (1982) Good manufacturing practice. In *Principles and Practice of Disinfection, Preservation and Sterilisation* (eds A. D. Russell, W. B. Hugo and G. A. J. Ayliffe), pp. 221–243, Blackwell Scientific Publications, Oxford, London, Edinburgh.

Pharmaceutical applications of microbiological techniques

The purpose of this chapter is to bring together those microbiological laboratory methods and procedures which are relevant to the design and production of pharmaceutical dosage forms. These are methods used to determine:

1 the levels of microbial contamination in pharmaceutical materials,
2 the potency or activity of antimicrobial chemicals, e.g. antibiotics, preservatives and disinfectants, and
3 the efficiency and safety of sterilization processes.

There are several other areas of microbiology relevant to pharmacy in which micro-organisms are grown rather than killed, or they are otherwise used to provide information which is not a measure of the effectiveness of antimicrobial agents or processes. These include antibiotic biosynthesis and 'fermentation', the production of dextran, asparaginase, streptokinase and other microbial metabolites which have a medicinal application, interconversion of steroid molecules, the detection of mutagenicity by the Ames test and the toxicity screening of pharmaceutical materials using mammalian cell cultures. These topics are beyond the scope of this book although they are included in the recommended further reading.

This chapter describes experimental procedures which are unique or particularly relevant to pharmacy, rather than those procedures which are common to microbiology as a whole. In the latter category, for example, are procedures used to identify and to enumerate micro-organisms, and these, together with staining and microscopical techniques, are described earlier in Chapter 24.

Several of the methods and tests discussed here are the subject of monographs or appendices in the *British Pharmacopoeia* or they are described in *British Standards* or other recognized reference works. It is not the intention to reproduce these official testing procedures in detail here, but rather to explain the principles of the test, to draw attention to difficult or important aspects and to indicate the advantages, problems or shortcomings of the various methods.

MEASUREMENT OF ANTIMICROBIAL ACTIVITY

In most of the methods used to assess the activity of antimicrobial chemicals, an inoculum of the test organism is added to a solution of the chemical under test, samples are removed over a period of time, the chemical inactivated and the proportion of cells surviving is determined. Alternatively, culture medium is present together with the chemical, and the degree of inhibition of growth of the test organism is measured. In each case it is necessary to standardize and control such factors as the concentration of the test organism, its origin, i.e. the species and strain employed together with the culture medium in which it was grown, the phase of growth from which the cells were taken and the temperature and time of incubation of the cells after exposure to the chemical. Because such considerations are common to several of the procedures described here, e.g. antibiotic assays, preservative challenge tests and determinations of minimum inhibitory concentration (MIC), it is appropriate that they should be considered first, both to emphasize their importance and to avoid repetition.

Factors to be controlled in the measurement of antimicrobial activity

Origin of the test organism

Although two cultures may bear the same generic and specific name, i.e. they may both be called *Escherichia coli*, this does not mean that they are identical. Certainly they would normally be *similar* in many respects, e.g. morphology (appearance), cultural requirements and biochemical characteristics, but they may exhibit slight variations in some of these properties. Such variants are described as *strains* of *E. coli*, and it is desirable in experimental work to name or describe the strain of organism being used. A variety of strains of a single species may normally be obtained from a culture collection; there are, for example, five pages of the catalogue of the *National Collection of Type Cultures* describing strains of *E. coli* alone. Different strains may also occur in hospital pathology laboratories by isolation from swabs taken from infected patients, or by isolation from contaminated food, cosmetic or pharmaceutical products, and from many other sources. Strains obtained in these ways are likely to exhibit variations in resistance to antimicrobial chemicals. Strains from human or animal infections are frequently more resistant to antimicrobial chemicals, particularly antibiotics, than those from other sources. Similarly, strains derived from contaminated medicines may be more resistant to preservative chemicals than those obtained from culture collections. Therefore to achieve results which are reproducible by a variety of laboratories it is necessary to specify the strain of the organism used for the determination.

Composition and pH of the culture medium

There are several methods of assessing antimicrobial activity which all have in common the measurement of inhibition of growth of a test organism when the antimicrobial chemical is added to the culture medium. In such cases the composition and pH of the medium may influence the concentration of test chemical at which growth occurs. The medium may contain substances which antagonize the action of the test compound, e.g. high concentrations of folic acid or para-aminobenzoic acid will interfere with sulphon-amide activity.

The antimicrobial activities of several groups of chemical are influenced by the ease with which they cross the cell membrane and interfere with the metabolism of the cell. This, in turn, is influenced by the lipid solubility of the substance since the membrane contains a high proportion of lipid and tends to permit the passage of lipid-soluble substances. Many antimicrobial chemicals are weak acids or weak bases which are more lipid soluble in the unionized form. pH therefore affects their degree of ionization, hence their lipid solubility and so, ultimately, their antimicrobial effect. Benzoic acid, for example, is a preservative used in several oral mixtures which has a much greater activity in liquids buffered to an acid pH value than those which are neutral or alkaline. Conversely, weak bases such as the aminoglyco-side antibiotics, e.g. streptomycin, neomycin and gentamicin, are more active at slightly alkaline pH values. The presence of organic matter, e.g. blood, pus or serum, is likely to have a marked protective effect on the test organism and so antimicrobial chemicals may appear less active in the presence of such material.

Temperature and time of incubation

To obtain results in the shortest time period the mixture of chemical and test organism is usually incubated at the optimum growth temperature of the organism, frequently 37 °C. One factor to be considered is that certain chemicals, particularly antibiotics, may be relatively unstable and lose a significant proportion of their activity after only 1 day at 37 °C, e.g. cephaloridine at pH 7.0 is reduced by approximately 15% of its initial activity after this time. If the antibiotic does not kill the bacteria but acts merely by inhibition of growth, the possibility arises of the test organisms growing after the antibiotic has degraded. Even in the case of a stable chemical there is the possibility of the cells slowly adapting to its presence and acquiring some degree of resistance during a protracted incubation period.

Inoculum concentration and physiological state

It is, perhaps, not surprising that the concen-tration of the inoculum can markedly affect anti-microbial action with high inoculum levels tending to result in reduced activity. There are two main reasons for this. First of all there is the pheno-menon of drug adsorption on to the cell surface or absorption into the interior of the cell. If the number of drug molecules in the test tube is fixed yet the number of cells present is increased, this obviously results in fewer molecules available per cell and consequently the possibility of a dimin-ished effect. In addition to this there is the second more specialized case, again concerning anti-biotics, where it is frequently observed that certain species of bacteria can synthesize antibiotic inactivating enzymes, the most common of which are the various types of β-lactamase (those destroying penicillin and cephalosporin anti-biotics). Thus a high inoculum means a high carry-over of enzyme with the inoculum cells, or at least a greater potential synthetic capacity.

Perhaps less predictable than the inoculum concentration effect is the possibility of the inoculum history influencing the result. There is a substantial amount of evidence to show that the manner in which the inoculum of the test organism has been grown and prepared can signi-ficantly influence its susceptibility to toxic chemi-cals. Features such as the nature of the culture medium, e.g. nutrient broth or a defined glucose–salts medium, the metal ion composition of the medium and hence of the cells themselves and the physiological state of the cells, i.e. 'young' actively growing cells from the logarithmic growth phase or 'old' non-dividing cells from the stationary phase, all have the potential to influence the observed experimental values.

ANTIBIOTIC ASSAYS

Antibiotics may be assayed chemically or biologi-cally. This means the concentration of antibiotic may be determined by either conventional chemical methods, e.g. titrations, spectrophotometry or high performance liquid chromatography, or by an assay in which the biological activity, in this case bacterial growth inhibition, of the 'test' solution is compared with a reference standard. Chemical assays are to be preferred because they are usually more precise, faster and cheaper. In certain situations, however, chemical methods cannot conveniently be used, or the sophisticated and expensive equipment required is not available.

Biological assays are most likely to be employed:

1 when the antibiotic is present in a solution containing a wide variety of complex substances which would interfere with a chemical assay, e.g. fermentation broth, serum or urine,

2 when the antibiotic is present together with significant concentrations of its breakdown products from which it cannot readily be distinguished chemically,

3 when it has been extracted from a formulated medicine, for example a cream or linctus, as would be the case during stability trials; here again excipients may interfere with the assay,

4 where the commercially available product is a mixture of isomers, which have inherently different antimicrobial activities, which cannot easily be distinguished chemically and which may differ in proportion from batch to batch and

5 where the antibiotic is present at a low concentration which is not detectable by chemical means.

An account of chemical assay methods is not included in this chapter. It is sufficient to say that such methods are being increasingly used and this is certainly a desirable trend. Nevertheless, biological assays of antibiotics are still used extensively in the pharmaceutical industry, and in hospitals where modified procedures may be used for monitoring blood levels of potentially toxic antibiotics like gentamicin.

Biological antibiotic assays, or bioassays as they are frequently known, may be of two main types, agar diffusion and turbidimetric. In each case a reference material must be available of known activity. When antibiotics were in their infancy few could be produced in the pure state free from contaminating material, and specific chemical assays were rarely available. Thus the potency or activity of references standards was expressed in terms of (international) units of activity. There are few antibiotics for which dosage is still normally expressed in units; nystatin and polymyxin are

two of the remaining examples. More commonly, potencies are recorded in terms of μg per ml of solution or μg antibiotic per mg of salt, with dosages expressed in mg. Antibiotic assay results are usually in the form of a potency ratio of the activity of the unknown or test solution divided by that of the standard.

Agar diffusion assays

In this technique the agar medium in a Petri dish or a larger assay plate is inoculated with the test organism, wells are created in it by removing circular plugs of agar and these wells are filled with a solution of the chemical under test (Fig. 28.1).

The chemical diffuses through the gel from A towards B and the concentration falls steadily in that direction. The concentration in the region A to X is sufficiently high to prevent growth, i.e. it is an inhibitory concentration. Between X and B the concentration is subinhibitory and growth occurs. The concentration at X at the time the zone edge is formed is known as the *critical inhibitory concentration* (CIC). After incubation the gel between A and X is clear and that between X and B is opaque as a result of microbial growth, which, with the common test organisms is usually profuse. A zone of inhibition is therefore created (as shown in Fig. 28.1), the diameter of which will increase as the concentration of chemical in the well increases.

A graph may be constructed which relates zone diameter to the logarithm of the concentration of the solution in the well (Fig. 28.2). It is normally found to be linear over a small concentration range, but the square of the diameter must be plotted to achieve linearity over a wide range. A plot such as that in Fig. 28.2 may, quite correctly, be used to calculate the concentration of a test solution of antibiotic. In practice, however, it is found to be more convenient to obtain reliable mean zone diameters for the standard at just two or three concentrations rather than somewhat less reliable values for six or seven concentrations. There is no reason why an assay should not be based upon a two or three point line provided that those points *are* reliable and that preliminary experiments have shown that the plotted relation-

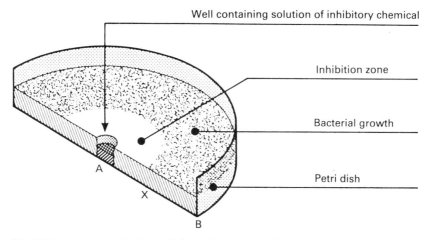

Fig. 28.1 Assessment of antimicrobial activity by agar diffusion

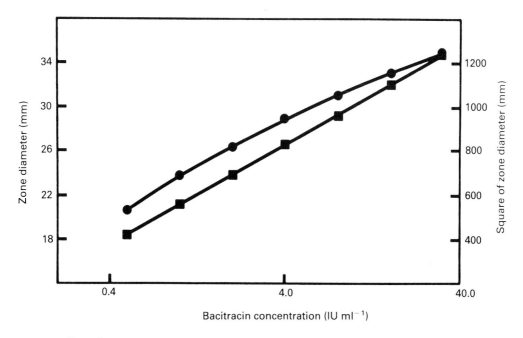

● Zone diameter
■ Square of zone diameter

Fig. 28.2 Calibration plots for agar diffusion assays

ship over the concentration range in question is linear.

Except in hospital pathology laboratories it is not common to conduct antibiotic assays in Petri dishes because too few zones may be accommodated on a standard sized dish to permit the replication necessary to obtain the required accuracy and precision. Antibiotic assays, when performed on a large scale, are more often conducted using large assay plates 300 mm or more square. The wells are created in a square design and the number that may be accommodated will depend upon the anticipated zone diameters; 36 or 64 wells are common (6 × 6 or 8 × 8 respectively). The antibiotic standard material may be used in solution at three known concentrations (frequently referred to as 'doses') and the antibiotic solution of unknown concentration treated likewise; alternatively each may be employed at two concentrations. In the latter situation there would be four separate solutions to be introduced at random into, say, 36 wells, and the plotted zone diameters would be the mean of nine values. A randomization pattern known as a latin square is used to ensure that there is a suitable distribution of the solutions over the plate thus minimizing any errors due to uneven agar thickness.

In the case of an assay based upon standard solutions used at two concentrations, the potency ratio may be calculated directly from the graph (as shown in Fig. 28.3) or by using the formula below.

$$\log X = LDR \times \frac{(UH + UL) - (SH + SL)}{(SH - SL) + (UH - UL)}$$

where X is the potency ratio, LDR is the logarithm of the dose ratio (i.e. ratio of concentrations of standard solutions), UH, UL, SH and SL are the mean zone diameters for the unknown and standard high and low doses. The derivation of

this is described in detail in the book by Kavanagh (1972) which deals extensively with the subject of antibiotic assays. The tests for acceptable limits of parallelism between the line joining the standards and that joining the test points together with confidence limits applicable to the calculated potency ratios are described in the BP appendix on antibiotic assays.

In calculating the potency ratio directly from the graph (Fig. 28.3) the zone diameter for the standard and unknown high concentrations are plotted at the same abscissa value and those for the low concentrations similarly. Two zone diameters are considered which are as widely separated on the ordinate as possible, whilst still being covered by the standard and the test lines. The ratio of the concentrations required to achieve the selected diameter is thus an estimate of the potency ratio. The mean of the two estimates taken at the extremes of the range of common zone diameters should be identical with the value by calculation from the formula. Thus, in Fig. 28.3, at a zone diameter of 23.75 mm the first estimate of potency ratio is 0.557 (antilog of 0.445 divided by antilog of 0.699); the second is 0.507 (antilog of zero divided by the antilog of 0.295). The mean value of 0.53 indicates the unknown solution to have approximately half the activity of the standard.

Practical aspects of the conduct of agar diffusion assays

The agar may be surface inoculated, or inoculated throughout whilst in the molten state prior to pouring. In the latter case zones may arise which are different in diameter at the agar surface than at the base of the Petri dish; this may complicate the recording of zone diameters. Zones which are not perfectly circular may be disregarded, although it may be appropriate to record the mean of the long and short axes. Such zones may result from non-circular wells, careless filling, or uneven drying of the agar gel due to a poorly fitting plate cover. The zones may be read directly with callipers or, more conveniently, after enlargement by projection on to a screen. Automatic zone readers incorporating a series of photocells which detect opacity changes at the zone edge are available and may be

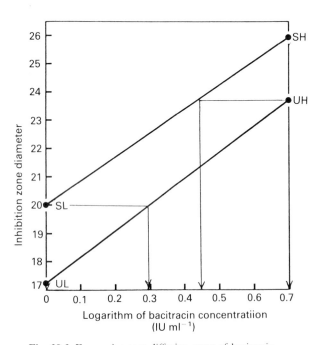

Fig. 28.3 Four-point agar diffusion assay of bacitracin

linked to a microcomputer which rapidly calculates the result together with the appropriate statistical analyses. The size of the zone is determined by the relative rates of diffusion of the drug molecule and growth of the test organism. If the assay plates are left at room temperature for 1–4 hours prior to incubation, growth is retarded whilst diffusion proceeds. This may result in larger zones with improved precision.

The zone diameter is affected by most of the factors previously stated to influence antimicrobial activity and, in addition, gel strength and the presence of other solutes in the antibiotic solution, e.g. buffer salts. If the antibiotic has been extracted from a formulated medicine, e.g. cream, lotion or mixture, excipients may be simultaneously removed and influence the diffusion of the antibiotic in the gel; sugars are known to have this effect. Because antibiotic assays involve a comparison of two solutions which are similarly affected by changes in experimental conditions, day to day variations in, for example, inoculum concentration will not have a great effect on the accuracy of the potency ratio obtained, but the precision may be affected. The volume of liquid in the well is of minimal importance; it is usually of the order of 0.1 ml and is delivered by semi-automatic pipette. As an alternative to wells the antibiotic may be introduced on to the agar using absorbent paper discs, metal cylinders or 'fish-spine' beads (beads having a hole drilled in them which contains the liquid).

The test organism is, for many antibiotics, a *Bacillus* species and the inoculum is in the form of a spore suspension which is easy to prepare, standardize and store. Alternatively frozen inocula from liquid nitrogen may be used as a means of improving reproducibility.

Careful storage and preparation of the reference standards are essential. The reference antibiotic is usually stored at low temperature in a freeze-dried condition.

Turbidimetric assays

In this case antibiotic standards at several concentrations are incorporated into liquid media and the extent of growth inhibition of the test organism is measured turbidimetrically using a nephelo-

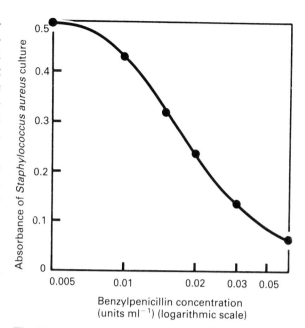

Fig. 28.4 Turbidimetric antibiotic assay calibration plot

meter or spectrophotometer. The unknown or test antibiotic preparation is run simultaneously, again at several concentrations and the degree of growth inhibition compared. A plot similar to Fig. 28.4 may be constructed. Such assays are less commonly used than agar diffusion methods because their precision is rather inferior but they do have the advantage of speed; the result may be available after an incubation period as short as 3–4 hours. They are also more sensitive than diffusion assays and consequently may be applied to low activity preparations.

The shape and slope of the calibration plot for a turbidimetric assay may be more variable than that for agar diffusion, and non-linear plots are common. The plotted points are usually the mean turbidity values obtained from replicate tubes and the assay may be conducted using a latin square arrangement of tubes incubated in a shaker which is necessary to ensure adequate aeration and uniform growth throughout the tube.

Practical aspects of the conduct of turbidimetric assays

Incubation time is critical in two respects. First it is necessary to ensure that the culture in each of the many tubes in the incubator has exactly the same incubation period, because errors of a few minutes become significant in a total of only 3–4 hours' incubation. Care must be taken therefore to ensure that the tubes are inoculated in a precise order, and that growth is stopped in the same order by addition of formalin, heating or other means.

The period of incubation must be appropriate to the inoculum level so that the cultures do not achieve maximal growth. At the concentrations used for such assays the antibiotics usually reduce growth rate but do not limit total growth. Therefore if the incubation period is sufficiently long, all of the cultures may achieve the same cell density regardless of the antibiotic concentration.

There are certain other limitations to the use of turbidimetric assays. Because it is the 'cloudiness' of the culture which is measured, standard and test solutions in which the organisms are suspended should, ideally, be clear before inoculation. Cloudy or hazy solutions which may result from the extraction of the antibiotic from a cream for example can only be determined after similarly compensating the standards or otherwise eliminating the error. Test organisms which might produce pigments during the course of the incubation period should be avoided, so too should those which normally clump in suspension.

The rate of growth of the test organism may vary significantly from one batch of medium to another. Thus it is important to ensure that all the tubes in the assay contain medium from the same batch and were prepared and sterilized at the same time. Many liquid media become darker brown on prolonged heating so samples from the same batch may differ in colour if the sterilizing time is not strictly controlled.

AMINO ACID AND VITAMIN ASSAYS

Turbidimetric methods have been used to assay these growth-promoting substances. The principle here is to develop a culture medium suitable for the test organism except for the omission of the vitamin or amino acid to be assayed. The extent of bacterial growth in the medium is thus directly proportional to the amount of vitamin or amino acid added. It is important to select a test organism which has an absolute requirement for the substance in question and is unable to obtain it by metabolism of other medium components; species of *Lactobacillus* are often used for this purpose. 'Carry-over' of the vitamin or amino acid with the inoculum culture must be avoided because this results in some growth in the system even when none of the test material has been added. Growth may be determined turbidimetrically or by acid production from sugars.

THE MEASUREMENT OF MINIMUM INHIBITORY CONCENTRATIONS (MIC)

The MIC is the lowest concentration of antimicrobial chemical found to inhibit the growth of a particular test organism. It may be applied to antiseptic, disinfectant, preservative and antibiotic chemicals in the pure state, i.e. it is particularly relevant to raw materials rather than to the final formulated medicines; the latter are usually subject to preservative efficacy (challenge) tests to assess their antimicrobial activity. MIC values are usually expressed in terms of $\mu g\ ml^{-1}$ or, less commonly, as in the case of some antibiotics, units ml^{-1}. It is important to recognize that the test organism is not *necessarily* killed at the MIC. Whether or not the cells die or merely cease growing depends upon the mode of action of the antimicrobial agent in question.

A MIC is an absolute value which is not based upon a comparison with a standard/reference preparation as in the case of antibiotic assays and certain disinfectant tests. For this reason inadequate control of experimental conditions is particularly likely to have an adverse effect on results. Discrepancies in MIC values measured in different laboratories are often attributable to slight variations in such conditions and care must be taken to standardize all the factors previously stated to influence the result. It is important also to state the experimental details concerning a MIC determination. A statement such as 'the MIC for phenol against *E.coli* is 0.1% w/v' is not, by itself, very useful. It has far more value if the strain of

E.coli, the inoculum concentration and the culture medium, etc. are also stated.

MIC test methods

The most common way of conducting MIC determination is to incorporate the antimicrobial chemical at a range of concentrations into a liquid medium, the containers of which are then inoculated, incubated and examined for growth.

Test tubes may be used, but microtitre plates (small rectangular plastic trays with, usually, 96 or 144 wells each holding approximately 0.2 ml liquid) and other miniaturized systems are becoming increasingly used. It is possible to incorporate the chemical into molten agar which is then poured into Petri dishes and allowed to set. Two advantages of using a series of agar plates are that several organisms can be tested at the same time by use of a multipoint inoculator, and there is a greater chance of detecting contaminating organisms (as uncharacteristic colonies) on the agar surface, than in liquid media. Usually the presence or absence of growth is easier to distinguish on the surface of agar than in liquid media. In tubes showing only faint turbidity it is often difficult to decide whether growth has occurred or not. Regardless of the method used the principle is the same and the MIC is the lowest concentration at which growth is inhibited.

Assuming a test tube method was used, a typical dilution scheme is shown in Table 28.1. Usually it is necessary to mix varying volumes of the test chemical with water in tubes which already contain an equal amount of double-strength growth medium. Except for the first in the series, all tubes receive a similar inoculum, the volume of which should be negligible. Final concentrations of 10^5–10^6 cells ml^{-1} are typical. The first tube checks the sterility of the medium

and the operators ability to manipulate the tubes without introducing contamination. The second tube checks the suitability of the medium for growth of the test organism and the viability of the inoculum culture.

The example in Table 28.1 shows a ten fold concentration range for the test chemical. It may be necessary to conduct a preliminary experiment to determine the *approximate* range which would be suitable for the test. In such a preliminary experiment the concentration could change by a factor of 10 from *one tube to the next*. It is also very convenient and particularly common in the case of microtitre plate methods to perform MIC determinations in which the concentration changes by a factor of two from one container to the next.

Because the incremental change in concentration is at the discretion of the operator this information should be specified, in addition to the other factors previously mentioned, when describing the experimental procedure. If, for example, a preliminary experiment is conducted with the concentrations 1, 0.1, 0.01, 0.001 and 0.0001% of the test material, and growth is observed in the three lowest concentrations, then the MIC is 0.1%. The experiment may, however, be repeated with a series ranging from 0.1 to 0.01% and a value of 0.02% be obtained for the MIC. Clearly, both are valid results but the second is much more useful.

Practical aspects of the conduct of MIC determinations

All the solutions used must be sterilized; it must not be assumed that the test chemical is self-sterilizing. Most disinfectants, antiseptic and preservative chemicals are bactericidal but they are unlikely to kill bacterial spores. Also, several antibiotics act by inhibition of growth and so

Table 28.1 A typical dilution scheme for a MIC determination in liquid medium.

Tube number	0*	0	1	2	3	4	5	6	7	8	9	10
Volume of double-strength medium (ml)	5	5	5	5	5	5	5	5	5	5	5	5
Volume of stock solution of test chemical (ml)	0	0	0.5	1.0	1.5	2.0	2.5	3.0	3.5	4.0	4.5	5.0
Volume of sterile water (ml)	5	5	4.5	4.0	3.5	3.0	2.5	2.0	1.5	1.0	0.5	0

*Uninoculated — Control.

would not necessarily *kill* vegetative cells with which they might be contaminated.

If the experiment is conducted in tubes, all the tube contents must be mixed before inoculation as well as after otherwise there is the possibility of the inoculum cells being killed by an artificially high concentration of the test chemical towards the top of the tube. If there is any risk of precipitation of the test chemical or the medium components during incubation a turbidity comparison must be available for each concentration (same tube contents without inoculum), alternatively, in the case of bactericidal chemicals, the liquid in each tube may be subcultured into pure medium to see whether the inoculum has survived.

Each of the tubes in the series may be prepared in duplicate or triplicate if it is considered desirable. This is so where the incremental change in concentration is small.

COUNTING OF MICRO-ORGANISMS IN PHARMACEUTICAL PRODUCTS

From the point of view of microbial contamination (see Chapter 27), pharmaceutical products may be considered in two categories, sterile and non-sterile; the first obviously contains no living organisms but the second will usually do so. This does not mean that non-sterile products may contain an unlimited number and that their concentration is unimportant. Those products susceptible to contamination will usually contain a preservative, the efficacy of which could be assessed by a challenge test. The levels of contamination considered acceptable are indicated by the section in the BP appendix on interpretation of challenge test results. Generally, a concentration no greater than hundreds or, exceptionally, thousands of (non-pathogenic) bacteria, yeasts or moulds per ml or gram must be achieved.

Many pharmaceutical raw materials, e.g. water, vegetable drugs and inert diluents like lactose or starch, are unpreserved yet contaminated with micro-organisms. The concentration of these contaminants would be measured during or after manufacture. Often these measurements are straightforward and the viable counting procedures described in Chapter 24 are used without modification. Occasionally the physical nature of the material or product makes counting by these techniques difficult or impossible and modifications to the procedure are necessary to reduce errors. Some of these circumstances are considered below.

Very low concentrations of micro-organisms in aqueous solutions

The reliability of calculated viable cell concentrations becomes much reduced when they are based upon colony counts much lower than about 10–15 per Petri dish. Using a surface-spread method it is rarely possible to place more than about 0.5 ml of liquid on to the agar surface in a standard Petri dish because it will not easily soak in. By a pour-plate method 1 ml or more may be used but a point is reached where the volume of sample significantly dilutes the agar and nutrients. Thus by a conventional plating technique the lowest concentration conveniently detectable is of the order of 10–50 cells ml^{-1}. When the cell concentration is below this it is necessary to pass a known quantity of the liquid, 10–100 ml or more, through a filter membrane having a pore size sufficiently small to retain bacteria. The membrane is then placed, with the organisms uppermost, on to the agar surface in a Petri dish which is incubated without inversion. As a result of diffusion of nutrients through the membrane colonies grow on the surface in the normal way. Diffusion may be assisted by the inclusion of a medium-soaked pad between the membrane and the agar. It is important to ensure that all of the membrane is in contact with the pad or agar otherwise elevated areas may become dry and no colonies will appear upon them.

Insoluble solids

It is necessary to suspend an insoluble solid in a medium which will permit uniform dispersion and adequate wetting of the suspended material. Nutrient broth, peptone water or a buffered salt solution are frequently used and a low concentration of a surfactant incorporated to promote wetting, e.g. polysorbate 80 (0.01–0.05%). Suspension in distilled water alone carries the risk of osmotic damage to sensitive cells with a consequently low count; for this reason it is best avoided. Having obtained the suspension, there are two options available depending upon the nature and concentration of the suspended material.

The first is to remove a sample of the mixed suspension, dilute if necessary, and plate in or on a suitable medium by a pour or spread plate method. If the concentration of suspended material is low it may still be possible to see clearly the developing colonies. High concentrations may obscure the colonies and make counting impossible. The alternative is to dislodge the microbial cells from the solid to which they are attached, allow the solid to sediment out then sample the supernatant. Methods of removal include vigorous manual shaking, use of a vortex mixer, or instruments designed for the purpose, e.g. Colworth 'stomacher' in which the aqueous suspension is placed in a sealed sterile bag which is repeatedly agitated by reciprocating paddles. The use of ultrasonics to dislodge the cells carries the risk of damage or lysis of the cells themselves.

Assuming the suspended material has no anti-microbial activity, plating the 'whole suspension' is probably the easiest and most reliable method. When sampling the supernatant the assumption must be made that all the cells have been removed from the solid and there is frequently no way of checking that this is so. The second method also relies upon the suspended solid sedimenting sufficiently rapidly for it to be separated from the bacteria above. If all or part of the sample has a particle size similar to that of bacteria, yeasts or mould spores, approximately 1–5 μm, then a separation cannot easily be achieved.

Oils and hydrophobic ointments

These materials are usually not heavily contaminated because they are anhydrous and micro-organisms will not multiply without water. Thus the micro-organisms contained in oily products have usually arisen by contamination from the atmosphere, equipment used for manufacture and from storage vessels. To perform a viable count the oil sample must be emulsified or solubilized without the aid of excessive heat or any other agent which may kill the cells. An oil-in-water emulsion must be produced using a suitable surfactant; non-ionic emulsifiers generally have little antimicrobial activity. Such an emulsion may be diluted in water or buffered salts solution if necessary and aliquots placed on or in the agar medium in the usual way. Alternatively the oil may be dissolved in a sterile non-toxic solvent and passed through a membrane filter. Isopropyl myristate and light liquid paraffin have been used as solvents although both may have some degree of toxicity to the microbial cells depending upon the method of sterilization used; filtration is preferable to heat sterilization in this respect.

Creams and lotions

Oil-in-water emulsions do not usually represent a problem because they are miscible with water and thus easily diluted. Water-in-oil creams, however, are not miscible and cannot be plated directly because bacteria may remain trapped in a water droplet suspended in a layer of oil on the agar surface. Such bacteria are unlikely to form colonies because the diffusion of nutrients through the oil would be inadequate. These creams are best diluted, dispersed in an aqueous medium and membrane filtered, or converted to an oil-in-water type and then counted by normal plating methods.

Addition of approximately 0.1 g of the w/o emulsion sample to 25 g of isopropyl myristate followed by membrane filtration is probably the best procedure, but dilution and emulsification of the cream in broth containing 4% Lubrol W may be satisfactory; polysorbate 80 or Triton X 100 are alternative surfactants for this purpose. These and other methods have been described in detail by Van Abbe et al. (1970).

PYROGEN TESTING

This is an aspect of microbial contamination of medicines which is not normally considered part of microbiology but it is discussed here because pyrogens are the products of microbial growth. A pyrogen is a material which will cause a rise in body temperature (pyrexia) when injected into a patient. The lipopolysaccharides and lipoproteins which comprise a major part of the cell wall of Gram-negative bacteria are called endotoxins, and it is these which are the most commonly encountered pyrogens (although any other substance which causes a rise in body temperature may be classified under the same heading). Bacterial cells may be pyrogenic even when they are dead and when they are fragmented, thus a solution or material which passes a test for sterility will not necessarily pass a pyrogen test. It follows from this that the more heavily contaminated with bacteria an aqueous injection becomes during manufacture, the more pyrogenic it is likely to be at the end of the process.

Two main procedures are used for the detection of pyrogens. The BP pyrogen test requires administration of the injection to laboratory rabbits whose body temperature is monitored for a period of time thereafter. The alternative procedure is to use the Limulus Amoebocyte Lysate Test (LAL) in which the pyrogen-containing sample causes gel formation in the lysis product of amoebocyte cells of the giant horseshoe crab *Limulus polyphemus*. This latter procedure, although unofficial, is widely used and is regarded to be more sensitive than the rabbit test.

For a more detailed account of pyrogens and their detection see Thomas *et al.* (1980).

CHALLENGE TESTS (PRESERVATIVE EFFICACY TESTS)

These are tests applied to the formulated medicine in its final container to determine whether it is adequately protected against microbial spoilage. These tests are used because it is not normally possible to predict how the activity of a preservative chemical will be influenced by the active ingredients, excipients and the container itself.

Certain products may contain no added preservative, either because the active ingredients have sufficient antimicrobial activity themselves or because they already contain high concentrations of sugar or salts which act as osmotic preservatives. Such products are, however, rare, and multidose injections or eyedrops and the majority of oral mixtures, linctuses and similar preparations together with creams and lotions all contain preservatives. They are not normally required in anhydrous products, e.g. ointments, or in single dose injections.

Again it must not be assumed that products containing antimicrobial agents as the active ingredients are self-sterilizing. It is quite possible for an antibiotic cream for example to be active against certain bacteria yet fail to restrict the growth of contaminating yeasts or moulds in the cream itself.

The basic principle of a challenge test is to inoculate separate containers of the product with known concentrations of a variety of test organisms, then remove samples from each container over a period of time and determine the proportion of the inoculum which has survived. In a very simple form the test may involve the transfer of samples into tubes of culture medium which are then incubated and examined for evidence of growth. In this case it is only possible to state that there were, or were not, survivors up to a certain time. This approach suffers from the disadvantage that growth in the tubes may result from the transfer of very few surviving cells or from many. Thus it is possible for the preservative to kill a very high proportion of the inoculum within a short period yet fail to kill a small fraction of the cells, possibly mutants, which have unusually high resistance. These few survivors may persist for several days or even longer and result in growth from all of the samples removed during that time. In this situation there is the risk that the preservative may be dismissed as insufficiently active despite the fact that it achieved a rapid and extensive initial kill. Challenge tests in which viable counts are performed on the samples are, therefore, far superior, and the benefits of their use easily outweigh the additional work involved. The tests described in the British and United States pharmacopoeias are based upon viable counts.

The BP recommends the routine use of four test organisms each at a final concentration of approximately 10^6 cells ml^{-1} or g^{-1} in the product. Counts are performed on samples removed at 0 h, 6 h, 24 h, 48 h, 7 days, 14 days and 28 days. Different criteria exist for the extent of inactivation to be achieved by preservatives in the various product types, with those for injectable and ophthalmic products being the most stringent, followed by topical and oral preparations.

Prior to the inclusion of a detailed testing procedure in the 1980 BP, there was a great deal of variation amongst the tests used by different manufacturers. Although these may still exist and manufacturers may elect to use a testing scheme which differs somewhat from that in the BP, most will adopt the BP test as a minimum standard and ensure that their own procedure incorporates and supercedes that of the BP by, for example, use of a greater variety of test organisms, heavier or repeated inocula. Various aspects of the test are considered in more detail below.

Choice of test organisms and inoculum concentration

The intention is to use organisms which are likely:

1 to arise in the raw materials used in the product,
2 to occur in the manufacturing environment,
3 to be particularly well adapted to growth in the product in question, or
4 represent a particular health hazard if they grew in the product.

The BP recommends the routine use of *Aspergillus niger*, *Candida albicans*, *Pseudomonas aeruginosa* and *Staphylococcus aureus* together with *Escherichia coli* in oral preparations, and an osmophilic yeast, *Zygosaccharomyces rouxii*, in syrups. The strains suggested are obtainable from culture collections but these may be less likely to withstand the action of preservatives than hospital isolates, or, more particularly, strains from products previously found to be contaminated. For this reason many manufacturers retain collections of such organisms to be used for testing purposes. Whilst it is desirable to use test organisms which represent a rigorous challenge to the preservative, it is widely acknowledged that 'super-resistant' strains can often be developed by adaptation and mutation. These would not be a realistic test because their resistance may far exceed that of the organisms normally found as natural contaminants of the product.

A preservative should be active against as wide a range of micro-organisms as possible hence the choice of both Gram-positive and Gram-negative bacteria, yeasts and moulds in the BP test. It may be desirable to use several examples of each of these groups together with mycobacteria, streptomycetes and anaerobes. Few preservatives actually kill dormant bacterial spores although they are effective against vegetative cells of the same species and would be likely to kill any spore which germinated; bacterial spore inocula, however, are rarely used because the probable test result would be a virtually unchanged count throughout the sampling period.

An inoculum level of approximately 10^6 cells ml^{-1} or g^{-1} is usually adopted. This is realistic in that this value would not frequently be exceeded as a result of contamination of the product via the raw materials or the patient and it allows for a fall in numbers of 10 000 fold to be easily measured. Usually the test organisms are added separately to different containers rather than as a mixed inoculum.

Sampling period and reinoculation

Usually a period of one month is adopted but this may be extended depending upon the type of product, the recommended storage conditions and shelf life. It is important to consider the possibility of the bacterial numbers dropping initially but with a few surviving cells adapting and slowly growing during later storage. If the product was kept at less than room temperature the initial killing effect and any possible regrowth would probably be slower and a longer sampling period would be required.

It is necessary to demonstrate also that the preservative will withstand repeated contamination by the user as would probably arise in the case of a cream, lotion or eyedrop, and that it will still be active at the end of its shelf life. For this reason it is common for tests to include two or three repeat inoculations of the same container at 3- or 6-monthly intervals or more, each followed by a 28-day sampling period.

Inactivation of preservative

It is quite possible for sufficient of the preservative

to be contained in, and carried over with, the sample removed from the container to prevent or retard growth of colonies on the Petri dishes. If the inoculum level of the test organism initially is about 10^6 cells ml^{-1} or g^{-1} of product, the problem of carry-over may not arise because a dilution factor of 10^3 or 10^4 would be required to achieve a countable number of colonies on a plate; at this dilution most preservatives would no longer be active. When a high proportion of the cells in the product have died, however, little or no such dilution is required, so preservative carry-over is a real problem which may artificially depress the count even more. To avoid this, preservative inhibitors or antagonists may be used. There are several of these, common examples being glycine for aldehydes, thioglycollate or cysteine for heavy metals, and mixtures of lecithin and polysorbate 80 with or without Lubrol W for quarternary ammonium compounds, chlorhexidine and para-bens. The use of these and other inactivators has been reviewed by Russell (1981). It is necessary to incorporate controls to demonstrate both that the inactivator really works and that it is not, itself, toxic. The former usually involves mixing the inactivator with the concentrations of preserv-ative likely to be carried over, then inoculating and demonstrating no viability loss. One further control is a viable count of the inoculum performed by dilution in peptone water to check the actual number of cells introduced into the product. This is necessary because even a 'zero time sample' of the product will contain cells which have been exposed to the preservative for a short period because it usually takes 15–45 seconds or more to mix the inoculum with the product and then remove the sample. Some of the cells may be killed even in such a short time and so a viable count of the inoculum culture will reflect this.

Interpretation of results

Whether or not a product passes a challenge test depends upon the extent to which the concen-tration of viable cells has been reduced. The degree of inactivation required may vary between testing procedures and product types but usually a 1000-fold drop in numbers of each bacterial

species must be achieved in a matter of 6–48 hours with no increase during the remaining test period; usually the required fall in numbers in yeasts and moulds is somewhat less, e.g. 100-fold in 7 days.

TESTS FOR STERILITY

The principle of sterility tests together with some of their fundamental deficiencies and sampling problems are described in Chapter 26. It is suffi-cient here to repeat that the test is really one of absence of gross contamination with readily grown micro-organisms, *not* a *true* sterility test.

The experimental details of these procedures are described in detail in the British and other phar-macopoeias. This section will therefore be restricted to an account of the major features of the test and a more detailed consideration of those practical aspects which are important or problematical.

It is obviously important that materials which are to be tested for sterility are not subject to contamination from the operator or the environ-ment during the course of the test. For this reason it is essential that sterility tests are conducted by competent and experienced personnel with adequate clean room and laminar flow cabinet facilities available. If contamination does arise during the test and goes undetected, there is the possibility of batches of material which were, in fact, sterile, being resterilized, or worse, discarded because they have apparently failed.

A sterility test may be conducted in two ways. The direct inoculation method involves the removal of samples from the product under test and their transfer to a range of culture media which might be expected to support the growth of contaminating organisms. After incubation the media are examined for evidence of growth which, if present, is taken to indicate that the product may not be sterile. It is not certain that the product is contaminated because the organisms responsible for the growth may have arisen from the operator or have been already present in the media to which the samples were transferred, i.e. the media used for the test were not, themselves, sterile. Thus, in conducting a sterility test it is necessary to include controls which indicate the likelihood of the contaminants arising from these sources. The size and number of the samples to be taken are described in the BP.

Again it is necessary to inactivate any antimicrobial substances contained in the sample. These may be the active drug, e.g. antibiotic, or a preservative in an eyedrop or multidose injection. Suitable inactivators may be added to the liquid test media to neutralize any antimicrobial substances, but in the case of antibiotics particularly, no such specific inactivators are available (with the exception of β-lactamases which hydrolyse penicillins and cephalosporins). This problem may be overcome using a membrane filtration technique. This, the alternative method of conducting sterility tests, is obviously only applicable to aqueous or oily solutions which will pass through a membrane having a pore size sufficiently small to retain bacteria. The membrane, and thus the bacteria retained on it, is washed with isotonic salts solution which should remove any last traces of antimicrobial substances. It is then placed in a suitable liquid culture medium. This method is certainly to be preferred to direct inoculation because there is a greater chance of effective neutralization of antimicrobial substances.

Solids may be dissolved in an appropriate solvent; almost invariably water is used because most other common solvents have antimicrobial activity. If no suitable solvent can be found the broth dilution method is the only one available. If there is no specific inactivator available for antimicrobial substances which may be present in the solid then their dilution to an ineffective concentration by use of a large volume of medium is the only course left open.

The controls associated with a sterility test are particularly important because incomplete control of the test may lead to erroneous results, e.g. a batch of material being declared non-sterile when, in fact, the contamination was introduced during the test itself. Failure to neutralize a preservative completely may lead to contaminants in the batch going undetected and subsequently initiating an infection when the product is introduced into the body.

The BP recommends three controls be incorporated. The so-called fertility or nutritive properties control simply involves the addition of low inocula (100 cells or spores per container) of suitable test organisms into the media used in the test to show that they do support the growth of the common contaminants for which they are intended. *Staphylococcus aureus* and *Bacillus subtilis* are the two aerobic bacteria used, *Clostridium sporogenes* the anaerobic bacterium and *Candida albicans* the yeast. Organisms having particular nutritional requirements such as blood, milk or serum are not included; thus they, in addition to the more obvious omissions like viruses, may not be detected in a routine sterility test because suitable cultural conditions are not provided. On the other hand it is impossible to design an all-purpose medium, and sterilization processes which kill the spore-forming bacteria and other common contaminants are likely also to eradicate the more fastidious pathogens like streptococci and *Haemophilus* species which would be more readily detected on blood-containing media. This argument does not, however, cover the possibility of such pathogens entering the product, perhaps via defective seals or packaging, after the sterilization process itself and then going undetected in the sterility test.

The second control is one intended to demonstrate that any preservative or antimicrobial substance has been effectively neutralized. This requires the addition of test organisms to containers of the various media as before, but in addition, samples of the material under test must also be added to give the same concentrations as those arising in the test itself. For the sterility test as a whole to be valid growth must occur in each of the containers in these controls.

It is necessary also to incubate several tubes of the various media just as they are received by the operator. If the tubes are not opened but show signs of growth after incubation this is a clear indication that the medium is, itself, contaminated. This should be a rare occurrence, but in view of the small additional cost or effort the inclusion of such a control is worthwhile.

A control to check the likelihood of contamination being introduced by the operator during the test has previously been required as an integral part of the test performed on surgical dressings but it is now included in the programme of regular monitoring of test facilities. Surgical dressings are probably the most difficult subjects for sterility testing because samples of known weight or area have got to be removed aseptically, which is an operation particularly susceptible to contamination.

All that is required for a control to check operator technique and the adequacy of the facilities is a quantity of material identical to that under test which has been repeatedly subjected to the sterilization process and thus has a very high probability of being sterile. This is referred to as the 'known sterile' material which is manipulated in the same way as the test items, and the tubes into which this material is placed are examined after incubation. If no contamination has arisen during the test there should, of course, be no growth in these tubes.

The difficulties in conducting a test for sterility on dressings may in some cases be circumvented by using a much larger sample rather than attempting to remove a small portion of fabric from the test item. The procedure here would be to obtain a sufficiently large clear plastic bag which has been radiation sterilized and introduce the complete roll or pack of dressing into the bag and add a sufficient quantity of culture medium to immerse the dressing. It is necessary to unravel a roll of bandage to permit free access of medium to all parts of the sample and to eliminate the possibility of aerobic bacterial spores trapped in the centre of the roll failing to grow due to insufficient diffusion of oxygen. This approach has the dual advantages of reduced risk of operator contamination and the imposition of a more rigorous test because a much larger sample is used. The volume of the dressing limits the range of materials which may be handled in this way.

The final aspect of the test which is worthy of comment is the interpretation of results. If there is evidence that any of the test samples is contaminated the batch fails the test. Under certain circumstances one, or exceptionally, two retests are permitted but this must not be misinterpreted to mean that a batch may have three opportunities to pass the test. The retests are available only to investigate the possibility that the contamination may have arisen from a source other than the test material, in which case, the test is invalid.

DISINFECTANT EVALUATION

A variety of tests have been described over a period of many years for the assessment of disinfectant activity. Those developed during the early part of this century were primarily intended for the purpose of testing phenolic disinfectants against pathogenic organisms like *Salmonella typhi*. In these respects such tests are rather outmoded because phenolic disinfectants are no longer pre-eminent, having been replaced to a certain extent by quarternary ammonium compounds or chlorhexidine for example, and *S. typhi* is no longer endemic in Britain.

Other tests of more recent date were applicable to a wider variety of disinfectant chemicals; the Berry and Bean method (1954) represented a significant scientific advance in overcoming sampling problems associated with the clumping or aggregation of cells which frequently arises with disinfectant tests.

At present there is not a universally applicable and officially recommended disinfectant testing procedure; but that which seems to have the most widespread acceptance, at least in hospital pharmacy in Britain, is the Kelsey-Sykes (Kelsey–Maurer) test (1974). This, together with certain alternative testing procedures are described below. It is important to appreciate that the procedures discussed are only selected examples from the many available, the number, variety and terminology of which may be somewhat confusing. The many aspects of disinfectants are considered in detail in the book edited by Collins *et al*, (1981). It is sufficient here to say that there are capacity methods which take into account the extent to which a disinfectant solution can withstand repeated additions of test organisms, methods developed for agents acting upon different types of micro-organism, e.g. spores, mycobacteria and fungi, and 'in-use' methods for disinfection of textiles and working surfaces.

It is quite possible and acceptable to obtain experimental data on disinfectant action by procedures which are not part of an 'official' or recognized test. Assuming adequate standardization of technique and control of the various factors which may influence the result, challenge testing type procedures may be used with a much shorter sampling period. The obvious advantage of using the recognized tests is that their faults and limitations are well documented and the significance of the test results is widely understood.

Rideal–Walker test

This was one of the first tests to become widely adopted and was designed for phenolic disinfectants. The result is expressed as a Rideal–Walker coefficient which is basically a ratio of the antimicrobial activity of the test material compared to that of phenol. A suspension of the test organism, *Salmonella typhi*, is mixed with four different concentrations of the disinfectant and solutions of phenol. Samples are removed from these mixtures at 2.5-minute intervals over a 10-minute period and transferred to a sufficient volume of sterile medium to inactivate the disinfectants by dilution. After incubation the containers are examined for growth. The phenol coefficient is the dilution of the disinfectant which permits survivors at 5 minutes but not at 7.5 minutes, divided by the dilution of phenol which does the same.

The disadvantage of this procedure and others like it is that it is susceptible to sampling errors due to cell aggregation in the presence of the disinfectant. This may occur when a sample taken at any particular time contains a small number of separate or discrete cells all of which are dead, and then a subsequent sample contains one or more aggregates of many hundreds or thousands of cells of which a few are viable. When transferred to sterile broth the second sample will show growth and the first not; on examination, the results of such a test appear, at first sight, to be illogical and erroneous. The phenomenon of 'wild plusses' (falsely positive results) may occur in any situation where samples are sequentially removed from a low concentration of surviving cells but it is more common where cell clumping or aggregation results from the disinfectant addition. Quarternary ammonium compounds possess a positive charge which tends to neutralize the negative surface charge most bacteria have at neutral pH; in such circumstances clumping is a particular problem because the mutual repulsion between cells having like charges no longer exists.

Despite its limited application and inherent faults the Rideal–Walker test is by no means obsolete. There are many formulations of phenolic disinfectants available, especially for domestic use, and it is still common for these to be subject to a Rideal–Walker test as part of the routine quality assurance process.

Testing quarternary ammonium compounds

British Standard 3286 describes procedures for testing quarternary ammonium disinfectants although the principles it embodies could equally be applied to testing other groups of disinfectant chemicals. The standard does not lay down a rigid, detailed testing scheme, but rather, it indicates the factors that must be considered in the experimental design, describes a general procedure to be adopted and recommends that such factors as the choice of organisms, contact time, number of disinfectant concentrations tested and exposure temperatures are all selected by the operator, having regard to the nature of the disinfectant formulation and its intended use.

The major advantages possessed by this test over many of those that preceded it are this flexible approach, which permits wider application, and the fact that the antimicrobial activity is based upon viable counts from which the percentage survival is calculated. This procedure therefore overcomes the defect inherent in the Rideal–Walker and several other tests that the same result, i.e. growth in a tube of broth, may arise from a single cell surviving the disinfectant exposure, or from many millions of cells doing so.

The results of the test are expressed as a plot of log percentage survivors against log concentration of disinfectant, with the intention that a minimum of three and preferably four or more concentrations of disinfectant are identified which, under the test conditions, give between 10 and 0.0001% survivors. The advantages of such a plot are that the relative activities of different compounds or of different formulations of the same compound can easily be assessed visually by the distance apart of the plotted lines on the concentration axis.

Certain of the factors identified in this standard as likely to influence the experimental results, e.g. water 'hardness' and the extent of subculturing of the test organism, are more precisely controlled in the Kelsey–Sykes test.

The Kelsey–Sykes test

Sampling problems due to clumping are not eliminated in this, currently the most important test recommended for hospital use, but their significance is diminished by the extent of replication required for a solution to pass the test. Although this procedure is not without its critics, it too represents a marked improvement upon those which preceded it. One of the major problems with older disinfectant testing procedures is the difficulty in reproducing the same experimental results when the test is performed by different operators in different laboratories, or even when performed on successive days by the same operators in a single laboratory. This is often due to variations in inoculum concentration, age or metabolic state, or the use of different diluents, suspending or recovery media. The Kelsey–Sykes test attempts to standardize all of these, and other factors.

One further interesting feature is that there is a preliminary operation to identify which of four alternative test species is the most resistant to the disinfectant and therefore to be used for the main part of the test. The four species used are *Pseudomonas aeruginosa*, *Staphylococcus aureus*, *Proteus vulgaris* and *Escherichia coli*; resistance is determined by MIC tests (see earlier in this Chapter) using doubling dilutions of the disinfectant.

Once the most resistant organism has been identified a suspension is prepared either in standard 'hard' water (containing calcium and magnesium chlorides) at a concentration between 10^8 and 10^{10} cells ml^{-1} or at the same concentration in an aqueous yeast suspension if the test is to simulate 'dirty' conditions. The disinfectant is simultaneously tested at three concentrations and each concentration is inoculated three times. After each inoculation an 8-minute exposure is allowed before replicate samples are transferred to five tubes of recovery broth. The minimum performance required for a solution to pass the test is no growth resulting in two out of the five recovery tubes following both of the first two inoculations.

REFERENCES AND BIBLIOGRAPHY

Ames, B. N., McCann, J. and Yamaski, E. (1975) Methods for detecting carcinogens and mutagens with the *Salmonella*/mammalian microsome mutagenicity test. *Mutation Res.*, **31**, 347–364.

Berry, H. and Bean, H. S. (1954) The estimation of bactericidal activity from extinction-time data. *J. Pharm. Pharmacol.*, **6**, 649–655.

British Pharmacopoeia (1980) and *Addendum* (1986) HMSO, London.

British Standards Institution (1960) British Standard Method for the laboratory evaluation of disinfectant activity of quarternary ammonium compounds by suspension test procedures. B.S. 3286, British Standards Institution, London.

Collins, C. H., Allwood, M. C., Bloomfield, S. F. and Fox, A. (1981) *Disinfectants: their Use and Evaluation of Effectiveness*. Society for Applied Bacteriology, Technical Series No. 16, Academic Press, London.

Holland, H. L., (1982). The mechanism of microbial oxidation of steroids. *Chem. Soc. Rev.*, **11**(4), 371–395.

Kavanagh, F. (ed.) (1972) *Analytical Microbiology*, Academic Press, London.

Kelsey, J. C. and Maurer, I. M. (1974) An improved Kelsey–Sykes test for disinfectants. *Pharm. J.*, **213**, 528–530.

Murray, H. C. and Maurer, I. M. (1974) An improved (1974) Kelsey-Sykes test for disinfectants. *Pharm. J.*, **528–530**.

Murray, H. C. (1976) The microbiology of steroids. In *Industrial Microbiology* (eds B. M. Miller and W. Litsky), Chapter 5, McGraw-Hill, London.

Paul J. (1975) *Cell and Tissue Culture*, 5th ed, Livingstone, London.

Russell, A. D. (1981) Neutralization procedures in the evaluation of bacterial activity. In *Disinfectants: their Use and Evaluation of Effectiveness*. (eds C. H. Collins, M. C. Allwood, S. F. Bloomfield and A. Fox). Society for Applied Bacteriology, Technical Series No. 16, Academic Press, London.

Russell, A. D. and Quesnel L. B. (Eds) (1983) *Antibiotics: Assessment of Antimicrobial Activity and Resistance*. Academic Press, London.

Thomas, W. H., Thompson, R. and Lim Kok Hui (1980) Evaluation of non-official methods of pyrogen testing of injectables. *Pharm. J.*, **224**, 259–261 and 270.

Underkofler, L. A. (1976) Microbial enzymes. In *Industrial Microbiology* (eds B. M. Millar and W. Litsky), Chapter 7, McGraw-Hill, London.

Van Abbe, N. J., Dixon, H., Hughes, O. and Woodroffe, R. C. S. (1970) The hygienic manufacture and preservation of toiletries and cosmetics. *J. Soc. Cosmet. Chem.*, **21**, 719–800.

PART FIVE

Pharmaceutical technology

Materials of fabrication and corrosion

DESIRABLE PROPERTIES AND SELECTION OF MATERIALS OF FABRICATION

In selecting materials for the construction of satisfactory plant the pharmaceutical engineer encounters problems involving chemical, physical, and economic factors. The following brief outline of these factors indicates something of the scope and limitations of his choice.

Chemical factors

Two aspects of chemical action must be considered under this heading, namely:

1 the possible contamination of the *product* by the material of the plant,
2 any effect on the *material of the plant* by the drugs and chemicals being processed.

The importance of the first of these becomes evident when it is realized that impurities often have considerable physiological effects and, also, that impurities, even in traces, may cause the product to decompose. An example of the latter is the inactivating effect of heavy metals on penicillin. The appearance of a product may also be affected by changes in colour due to contamination from the materials of the plant.

It should be remembered that contamination from some materials may be innocuous, the products being non-toxic.

Our increasing knowledge of materials of plant construction is assisting greatly in providing plant that will be resistant to attack and deterioration in use from the effects of acids, alkalis, oxidizing agents, tannins, etc. Alloys, having special physical and chemical properties, have been developed and materials such as plastics have been introduced to meet the problems encountered.

Physical factors

An ideal material of construction would satisfy all the following criteria. In practice no material is ideal and the selection must be based on compromise.

Strength   Sufficient mechanical strength is an obvious necessity and will be suited to the size of the plant and the stresses to which it will be subjected.

Weight   In most cases weight will be reduced to a minimum, other factors being satisfactory, and especially in plant that may have to be moved about from place to place. For example large filter presses may be constructed of wood to facilitate the handling of the plates and frames (see Chapter 31).

Wearing qualities   These are particularly important where there is a possibility of friction between moving parts, an extreme case in point being the material used for the grinding surfaces of mills.

Ease of fabrication   It must be possible to process the material in order to fabricate the various units of the plant. Properties that enable materials to be cast, welded, forged or machined are of prime importance.

Thermal expansion   The design of plant may be greatly complicated by the use of material that has a high coefficient of expansion. This increases the stresses and the risk of fracture with temperature changes, and the temperature range over which the plant will be operated is likely to be considerably restricted.

Thermal conductivity   In plant such as the pan and evaporator described in Chapter 30, good thermal conductivity is desirable. It must be remembered, however, that the bulk of the resistance to heat transfer may lie in the boundary layer films.

Cleansing   Smooth polished surfaces simplify cleansing processes, and materials that can be 'finished' with such surfaces are ideal when scrupulous cleanliness is necessary.

Sterilization   Where sterility is essential the material should be capable of withstanding the necessary treatment, usually steam under pressure. This factor is to some extent bound up with the previous one since cleaning is a normal preliminary to the sterilization of apparatus and plant.

Transparency   This may be a useful property where it is possible, and is one reason for the increasing use of borosilicate glass in the construction of pharmaceutical plant.

Economic factors

Cost and maintenance of plant must, of course, be economic. Here the main concern is not simply to obtain the least costly material. Better wearing qualities and lower maintenance may well mean that a higher initial cost is more economical in the long run.

MATERIALS OF FABRICATION

A brief description of materials which are suitable for the fabrication or construction of pharmaceutical apparatus and manufacturing plant is given below.

Metals

Ferrous metals — steels

The element iron is abundant in the form of its ores which are widely distributed and despite the tendency for the metal to corrode there is no practical alternative to its use in the form of steel for the fabrication of plant and equipment. Steel consists of iron with added carbon which may exist in the free state (graphite) or in chemical combination as iron carbide, Fe_3C. The phase diagram for the iron/carbon system is complex and it will not be considered in detail. It may be mentioned, however, that iron can exist in two allotropic forms. At temperatures below 940 °C the stable form is α-iron (ferrite) but the γ form (austenite) can persist at normal temperatures if other metals such as chromium and nickel are alloyed with the iron. When steel is in the molten condition, austenite is able to dissolve carbon. Various eutectics and solid solutions may form on cooling giving rise to steels of differing properties. These properties depend on the carbon content and any heat treatment that the steel may receive.

Mild steel This is the commonest form of steel for general purposes and has a carbon content between 0.15 and 0.3%. It is ductile and can be welded to give structures of high mechanical strength but the resistance to corrosion is poor.

Cast iron The effect of increasing the carbon content beyond 1.5% is to lower the melting point of iron so that it can be easily be melted and cast into sand moulds to form objects of intricate shape. Cast iron is resistant to corrosion but it reacts with materials such as phenols and tannins to give coloured compounds. Most pharmaceuticals are required to pass a limit test for iron and if they are handled in cast iron vessels they may fail to comply. Such vessels may be lined with resistant materials to take advantage of the strength of cast iron while shielding the product from the metal.

Cast iron is hard and brittle and can be welded and machined only with great difficulty. The hardness and corrosion resistance can be increased by adding silicon though such high silicon iron is extremely brittle.

Stainless steels These steels contain a proportion of nickel and chromium which confer a high degree of corrosion resistance. The stainless steels can be easily fabricated and polished to a high mirror finish. They are extensively used in the food, pharmaceutical and fermentation industries where their high cost can be fully justified.

The most common type is the so-called austenitic stainless steel where the nickel and chromium content stabilize austenite at *normal* room temperatures. As can be seen from the phase diagram (Fig. 29.1) an alloy containing 18% chromium and 8% nickel (which is more costly than chromium) is the most economical form of austenitic stainless steel. The steel is often stabilized by the addition of 1% of titanium or niobium which prevents 'weld decay'. This can result from the removal of chromium as chromium carbide along the line of any welding which may be performed. Such depleted steel is then prone to corrosion.

Stainless steel owes its resistance to a tenacious oxide layer that forms on the surface. Materials such as nitric acid which are oxidizing agents can be handled in it but chlorides can penetrate the film and stainless steel equipment should not be used for hydrochloric acid.

One minor objection to stainless steel is the low thermal conductivity when compared with other metals but this is not usually significant as the main resistance to heat transfer may reside in the boundary layers (see Chapter 30).

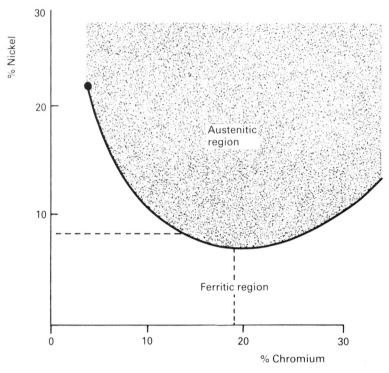

Fig. 29.1 Phase diagram for stainless steel

Stainless steels can be used for most pharmaceutical plant, including storage and extraction vessels, evaporators and fermenting vessels. Small apparatus commonly made from stainless steel includes funnels, buckets, measuring vessels, and shovels. Sinks and bench tops are also made of stainless steel where a good surface with high corrosion-resisting qualities is necessary.

The high cost often excludes its use but often the cost may be justified even on a very large scale. For example, a great deal of the plant used in the production of penicillin is of this material since it is by far the most satisfactory, being strong, corrosion-resistant, non-contaminating and readily cleansed and sterilized.

Non-ferrous metals

Copper   Copper is malleable and ductile and is, therefore, easily fabricated. It has a thermal conductivity eight times greater than steel but is corroded by a number of substances, particularly oxidizing agents. It is attacked by nitric acid in all concentrations, by hot concentrated hydrochloric

and sulphuric acids, and by some organic acids. Ammonia reacts with it readily to form blue cuproammonium compounds. Many drug constituents react with it, and for this reason copper is usually protected by a lining of tin when used for pharmaceutical plant. It was formerly used for evaporators and pans of various kinds and is still employed for pans used for sugar coating (Chapter 40). Because of its susceptibility to attack by pharmaceutical materials there is a tendency today to replace it by stainless steel where corrosion is likely.

Copper piping is easy to make because of the ductility of the metal and it is used extensively for services such as cold water, gas, vacuum, and low-pressure steam. Where necessary, copper piping may be tinned, e.g. for distilled water, but nowadays stainless steel piping can be obtained for this purpose.

Copper alloys   These include alloys with zinc, tin, aluminium, silicon and nickel, all of which have their special uses.

1 *Copper–zinc alloys (brasses):* the output of brasses exceeds that of any other copper alloy

although their use is restricted in pharmaceutical plant since their corrosion resistance is less than that of copper. They are easily worked and their tensile strength is greater than copper. Like copper, brass is often used where rusting is to be avoided.

Brasses are used for tube plates in evaporators and condensers, for tubes and valves, and extensively in making nuts, bolts, rods, etc.

2 *Copper–tin alloys* (*bronzes*): these usually contain 2–3% of tin with a small amount of phosphorus and often traces of other elements. Harder and more durable than brass they are used for filter gauzes, stirrers, valves, pumps, high pressure pipes, autoclaves, and special tablet punches and dies.

Aluminium   Aluminium has good corrosion resistance to many substances although it is attacked by mineral acids (it is resistant to strong nitric acid), caustic alkalis, mercury and its salts. Its resistance is often due to the formation of a film on the surface. For example, acetic acid forms a film of gelatinous aluminium subacetate which is then resistant to acetic acid, and pure strong ammonia solutions form a resistant film of aluminium hydroxide. It is also highly resistant to oxidizing conditions since it forms a compact oxide film.

Pure aluminium is soft but more corrosion-resistant than most of its alloys such as Duralumin. Alloys combining corrosion resistance with strength are formed with small percentages of manganese, magnesium or silicon. Plant is easily fabricated and has excellent thermal conductivity.

For plant producing medicinal substances its most valuable property is probably the non-toxicity of its salts which are, moreover, colourless. As it is also non-toxic to micro-organisms it has considerable use in biosynthetic processes such as the production of citric and gluconic acids, and of streptomycin by deep culture methods. The metal is also suitable for plant used for preparing culture media and for absorption and extraction vessels used in preparing antibiotics. Because of the formation of resistant film it is used for acetic acid plant and storage vessels for ammonia. The use of welded aluminium vessels, it has been claimed, made the nitric acid industry possible. Because of its low density it is most useful for transport containers such as drums and barrels, road and rail tankers.

Lead   Much lead is used in the chemical industry because of its remarkable resistance to corrosion and the great ease with which it can be made into complicated shapes. The lead chamber process for manufacturing sulphuric acid is one example from many in the heavy chemical industry. It is little used, however, in pharmaceutical practice because of the risk of contamination by traces of poisonous lead salts. Pharmaceutical materials must comply with a limit test for lead. Lead poisoning from lead vessels and pipes is said to have contributed to the decline of the Roman Empire.

Tin   Tin has a high resistance to a great variety of substances and, since its salts are non-toxic, it has a wide use throughout the food industry. It is, however, weak, its main use being to provide a protective coating for steel, copper, brass, etc. The coating of other metals with tin has been known for over 2000 years and today more than half the output of the metal is used for this purpose.

'Tin plate' — sheet steel coated with tin — is used for containers. Condenser tubes are often coated or 'tinned'.

Silver   Because of its high cost, silver is used only as a material of plant construction in special cases and usually silver-coated material is used rather than solid silver. It is not resistant to concentrated hydrochloric or sulphuric acids, any strength of nitric acid, and sulphur and sulphur compounds. It is resistant to organic acids and their salts.

It is even more malleable and ductile than copper and, therefore, capable of being readily worked. It has a higher thermal conductivity than all other metals.

A few examples of its special uses are: plant for the manufacture of salicylates and acetic acid; a silver-plated basket for a hydroextractor used in vitamin crystallization; a solid silver vessel in a cast-iron jacket for bromination.

Nickel   Nickel is resistant to oxidation and alkalis but is attacked slowly by dilute mineral acids and rapidly by concentrated acids. It is resistant to the weak organic acids occurring in pharmaceutical preparations, e.g. citric, tartaric, and stearic. It is also resistant to phenols. Its salts are non-toxic.

It is useful for such plant as pans, vats, tanks, mixers, valves and pumps, and nickel wire may be woven to form filter cloths. Steel may be 'clad' with a nickel coating to protect if from attack.

Monel metal, an alloy of nickel (2/3) and copper (1/3) which is harder and more resistant than nickel, may be used where corrosion resistance is essential.

Chromium   Although hard and resistant to corrosion, chromium is not normally used as a material of plant construction. It forms resistant alloys with nickel and, probably, its most important use is in the manufacture of stainless steel. It is also, like nickel, used to plate the surface of mild steel.

Non-metals

Inorganic

Glass   Glass is widely used in the laboratory and glass equipment can be obtained for operation on a larger scale.

Ordinary soda glass is used for bottles and other cheap articles but is not satisfactory for large scale plant or for containers where alkali contamination might be a serious drawback. For these purposes borosilicate glass is used. Such glass has several advantages over soda glass. It is, for example, less brittle. It has a low thermal expansion and can be used with safety over wide temperature ranges. However, its thermal conductivity is low and therefore it should be heated gradually to avoid fracturing. Pipe line may be used with pressures up to 8 bar if the pipe diameter is less than 50 mm and pipe lines with larger diameters are used with pressures up to 4 bar.

Special advantages of glass are that it can be easily cleaned and sterilized and, also, that the contents of vessels can be readily examined for colour and clarity.

A disadvantage is the difficulty of joining sections of glass plant together. Ground-glass joints are sometimes satisfactory, especially in small scale apparatus, but are rigid. Gaskets of rubber, plastics and fibre are used to form a flexible jointing but these must be chosen with care as they are normally less resistant to attack than

glass. For that reason gaskets are now often made from PTFE but careful alignment of the sections is required for their successful use.

Glass pipe line is useful for transporting liquids from stage to stage in various operations. Such pipe line is available from 15 mm to 0.3 m in diameter with fittings for the assembly of complete systems.

All-glass stills are used for preparing Water for Injections BP and other distilled preparations. Vessels up to 100 litres are used and larger tanks can be made by clamping glass plates in frames.

Glass fibres are excellent for heat insulation or refrigeration plant. Such fibre, treated with oil, is used for filtering air for asepsis rooms. Woven fibre may be used for filter cloths and glass may be sintered in the preparation of filters.

Fused silica   Fused silica (Vitreosil) has an extremely low coefficient of thermal expansion and vessels made from it can be heated to red heat and plunged into cold water without breaking. It has a high melting point and it is difficult to fuse it completely so that equipment tends to be opaque though transparent forms are available.

Glass linings and coatings   Metal may be coated with glass to give a protective lining. The dangers of such apparatus are those of uneven expansion of metal and glass, and of the glass surface accidently chipping. Great care must therefore be taken in heating and cooling and in protecting the glass lining from accidental damage.

Vessels of up to 50 000 litres capacity, pipe line and fittings, valves, condensers, columns, pumps, stirrers and mixtures are among the many glass-coated items in use.

High resistance to corrosion and ease of cleaning make it valuable for pharmaceutical use.

Stoneware   Ceramics are reasonably cheap, but their weight, low thermal conductivity and fragility give only a low resistance to mechanical and thermal shock. Corrosion resistance is usually due to a surface glaze which may become chipped.

Ceramics are used widely on a small scale but only to a limited extend on a large scale. Pipe line, tanks, vessels and filters are among the items made from it. Of special interest among ceramic products are bacteria-proof filters.

Stone, slate, brick and concrete   These have

their particular uses, among which are granite for certain types of mill, vitrefied acid-resisting bricks for tanks, drains, culverts, etc. and concrete for structural purposes and sometimes for tanks.

Organic

Plastics The range of materials known collectively as plastics is so wide that only a brief account can be given. It is convenient to group them under the following headings:

1 rigid material
2 flexible material
3 coatings and linings
4 cements and filters
5 special cases.

'Keebush' is an example of a rigid material. It is a phenolic resin with various inert fillers selected for their particular purpose. It may be machined, welded, and worked in other ways and is resistant to such an extent that it can be used for gears, bearings and similar items with a noise reduction of two-thirds compared with iron. Its weight is about one-quarter that of iron. It is resistant to corrosion except that of oxidizing substances and strong alkalis. Any item may be made from this material — vessels, pipes, fittings, valves, pumps, fans, ducts, filter presses and many others.

Polyethylene and polyvinyl chloride (PVC) are similar materials and are rigid or flexible, depending upon the amount of plasticizer added. These do not withstand high temperatures but are non-resistant only to strong oxidizing acids, halogens and organic solvents.

Rigid or semi-rigid mouldings may be used for tanks, pipes, ducts and other similar items; slightly flexible funnels, buckets and jugs are made which are almost unbreakable.

Polytetrafluoroethylene (PTFE, Teflon) is a semi-rigid plastic with extreme resistance to all agents other than fluorine or molten alkali metals. It is a slippery non-wettable material but it can be bonded to metals as a protective coating. It is also usable at temperatures above 200 °C but it is a costly material which prohibits its extensive use.

Metallic surfaces may be protected from corrosion by plastics of the polyethelene or PVC

types prepared for coating with suitable plasticizers. Perfect adhesion of plastic to metal is sometimes difficult, and other disadvantages are the differences in thermal expansion of plastic and metal and the danger of the coating accidentally chipping.

Uses of these materials include the lining of tanks and vessels and the coatings on stirrers and fans. Plastic cements are used for spaces between acid-resistant tiles and bricks, and for similar purposes.

Special cases include transparent plastic guards for moving parts of machinery and asepsis screens. Nylon and PVC fibres may be woven into filter cloths.

Rubber Hard rubber may be used for purposes similar to those mentioned under plastics. Soft rubber may be used for linings and coatings. Rubber swells in contact with oils; it is subject to oxidation and is attacked by some organic solvents. Synthetic rubbers that have greater resistance have been developed.

Timber The use of wood for tanks and vats has greatly diminished since it has the disadvantage of absorbing the contents. Its lightness is an advantage where parts have to be handled, and filter presses are sometimes made of wood for this reason.

CORROSION

Corrosion is a complex form of material deterioration as a result of a reaction with its environment. It is the destruction of a material (usually a metal) by means other than mechanical.

Most environments are corrosive. Corrosion is not restricted only to reactions with strong acids. The following have been shown to cause corrosion:

1 air and moisture,
2 rural, urban and industrial atmospheres,
3 fresh, salt and distilled water,
4 steam and gases such as chlorine, ammonia, hydrogen sulphide, sulphur dioxide,
5 mineral acids, such as hydrochloric acid, sulphuric acid, nitric acid,
6 organic acids, such as acetic, citric, formic,
7 alkalis,

8 soils,
9 organic solvents,
10 vegetable and petroleum oils.

Importance of corrosion

Corrosion is very important in the chemical and pharmaceutical process industries for a number of reasons. The possibility of any of the following occurring must be considered.

Safety

1 Loss of pharmacologically active or toxic substances.
2 Loss of inflammable or explosive chemicals.
3 Sudden loss of material being processed at high temperature or high pressure.
4 Possibility of burns from acids, etc.
5 Corroding of equipment is known to have caused fairly harmless compounds to become toxic or explosive.

Financial losses

1 Replacement of corroded parts.
2 Plant shut-down, i.e. stoppage due to unexpected corrosion failures. This leads to loss of revenue.
3 Loss of expensive chemicals.

Contamination of the product This is of particular importance in the pharmaceutical industry since the product is usually for human consumption. Metal ions can promote degradation reactions and can be toxic.

Appearance of plant This is not a minor consideration. Satisfactory factory appearance is an important aspect of good manufacturing practice.

Corrosion mechanisms

The corrosive reaction of metals is generally electrochemical in nature. The relevant points of a simple, acceptable theory of electrochemical corrosion are summarized below.

1 An anode $(-)$ and a cathode $(+)$ form a cell in conjunction with an electrically conducting environment (electrolyte). Anodic and cathodic areas can arise on a single piece of metal because of local differences in the outside environment and in the metal itself. Different stresses, nicks, scratches and impurities produce varying electrical potential. Far greater electrical potentials exist between different metals or alloys. Anodes and cathodes may be close (local cells) or far apart.

2 Direct current (d.c.) flows. The current is a flow of electrons within the metal(s) from anode to cathode. Metal ions (positive charge) travel from the anode in the electrolyte; they usually do not reach the cathode but remain in solution.

Single metal corrosion

Simple electrochemical corrosion is explained diagrammatically in Fig. 29.2. It shows the mechanism for corrosion of a single piece of steel (predominantly iron) in water (dissociated by the presence of dissolved chemicals).

The anodic reaction is

$$Fe \rightarrow Fe^{2+} + 2e$$

and the cathodic reaction is

$$2H^+ + 2e \rightarrow H_2$$

The overall reaction is therefore

$$Fe + 2H_2O \rightarrow Fe(OH)_2 + H_2$$

The important consequence of this reaction is that structurally strong metal leaves the anode as a metal ion in solution. The metal is therefore weakened and the solution contaminated with corrosion product.

Corrosion between metals

This is important because joints, flanges, seals, bolts, etc. are often constructed of different metals. A cell is set up between the metals, one becoming the anode and the other the cathode. The potential difference between the metals depends on the electrode potentials of the metals. A knowledge of the electromotive series of metals (Table 29.1) is therefore important. The following points can be noted from Table 29.1:

1 A negative sign in the third column infers that the reaction in the direction of element to ion is spontaneous, i.e. it requires negative energy to proceed in that direction.

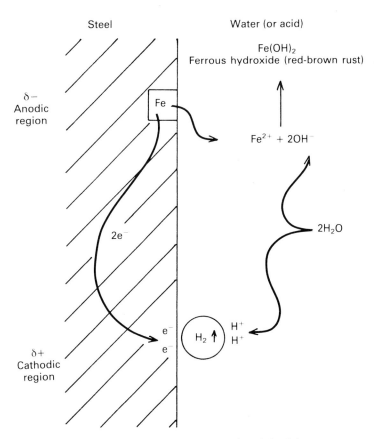

Fig. 29.2 Diagrammatic representation of the electrochemical corrosion of steel (iron) in water

Table 29.1 The electromotive series of some commonly used metals

	Element	Ion produced	Standard electrode potential (volts)
Active end	Na	Na^+	-2.71
	Mg	Mg^{2+}	-2.34
	Al	Al^{3+}	-1.67
	Zn	Zn^{2+}	-0.76
	Cr	Cr^{3+}	-0.71
	Fe	Fe^{3+}	-0.44
	Ni	Ni^{2+}	-0.25
	Sn	Sn^{2+}	-0.14
	Pb	Pb^{2+}	-0.13
Reference zero	H	H^+	0.000
	Cu	Cu^{2+}	$+0.35$
	Cu	Cu^+	$+0.52$
	Ag	Ag^+	$+0.80$
	Pt	Pt^{2+}	$+1.20$
Noble end	Au	Au^{3+}	$+1.42$

2 A metal higher in the series will be the anode and one lower will act as the cathode when two metals are coupled or in indirect contact with each other via the electrolyte.

3 Metals high in the table have less corrosion resistance. For example metals above copper readily oxidize. This also explains why gold and silver are found free in their native state whilst aluminium and iron are only found combined as oxides.

4 The greater the difference in potential between two metals, the greater will be the rate of corrosion. For example, sodium reacts violently with water, iron slowly rusts yet lead is attacked extremely slowly by water.

5 When two metals are in contact, corrosion of the anodic member of the couple is accelerated.

6 A metal will replace another metal in solution if the latter is lower in the series. This is best understood by examination of Fig. 29.3.

7 The table therefore indicates whether or not a metal is attacked by acids or water, since metals

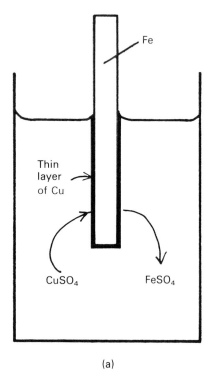

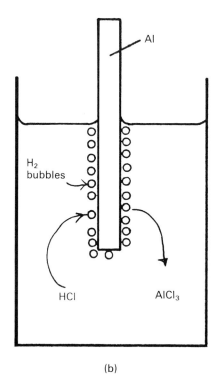

(a)   (b)

Fig. 29.3 (a) Reaction of iron in copper sulphate solution. The copper ions in solution are being replaced by iron ions (lower in table) at the same time as the copper from solution is being deposited as copper metal on the iron sheet. (b) Similarly the hydrogen in the HCl solution is replaced by aluminium ions and the hydrogen is evolved as bubbles of gas

above hydrogen are attacked because they replace hydrogen in solution, e.g.

Al + HCl (in solution) → $AlCl_3$ (in solution)
Fe + H_2O (in solution) → $Fe(OH)_2$ (in solution)

Cathodic protection This term is used to describe the technique whereby a structurally important metal is forced to become wholly cathodic (and therefore protected from corrosion) by attaching to it a more electronegative second metal. An example is galvanization in which steel is coated with a layer of zinc. The zinc becomes the anode thus protecting the steel. The advantage of this technique over normal coating is that even if the galvanized coating is scratched the exposed metal surface will remain cathodic. Metal objects can be protected in a similar way by attaching to them replaceable pieces of a more electronegative metal.

Passivity This is the phenomenon in which a metal appears in practice to be much less reactive than would be predicted by its position in the electromotive series. For example, one would expect aluminium to be extremely reactive since its electrode potential is −1.67 volts, yet aluminium is commonly used in construction because of its lack of reactivity. The explanation is that aluminium does in fact react quickly with air but an aluminium oxide coating is produced which is very resistant to further atmospheric attack. Lead, which has a small electronegativity and would therefore be expected to react at least with strong inorganic acids, is in fact used in the production of sulphuric acid (lead chamber process). In this example an impervious, unreactive layer of lead sulphate is formed on the outside of the lead sheets.

Types of corrosion

The various types of corrosion can be classified by the form in which the corrosion manifests itself. The eight most common arbitrary groups are:

1 uniform attack or general, overall corrosion,
2 galvanic or two-metal corrosion,
3 concentration-cell corrosion,
4 pitting,
5 intergranular corrosion,
6 dezincification or parting,
7 stress corrosion,
8 erosion corrosion.

Uniform attack

This is the most common form. It is normally an electrochemical reaction in which the anode and cathode move slowly over the surface of the metal. The metal becomes thinner and thinner and eventually fails e.g. sheet-iron roof, zinc in acid.

Uniform corrosion is the easiest to predict, discover and stop by means of the use of more suitable materials, inhibitors and protective coatings (paint, plastic etc.).

Galvanic corrosion

This is corrosion between two dissimilar metals (see above). An example could be the case of a concentric pipe heat exchanger in which the main structure is of steel but the heat exchange pipes are made of copper to improve heat transfer. In domestic central heating systems the commonest situation is to have steel radiators joined by copper piping.

Control of galvanic corrosion   Use only one metal if this is possible. If not:

1 Select combinations of metals as close together as possible in the electrochemical series.
2 Avoid combinations where the area of the more active metal (i.e. the anode) is small, since this increases the anodic reaction rate. It is therefore better to have the more noble metal or alloy for fastenings, bolts, etc.
3 Insulate dissimilar metals completely wherever possible.
4 Apply coatings such as paint, bitumen, plastic, but with caution. Small holes in the coating over an anodic region will result in rapid attack. Therefore, it is important to keep the coating in good repair.
5 Add chemical inhibitors to the corrosive

solution. The nature of these inhibitors depends on the specific nature of the solution to be inhibited. Particular care must be taken in their selection when the corrosive solution is the pharmaceutical product or is an intermediate for drug synthesis.
6 Avoid joining metals with threaded connections since the threads will deteriorate excessively; spilled liquids or condensates can concentrate in thread grooves. Welded joints (using welds of the same alloy) are preferred.

Concentration cell corrosion

Cells can form because of differences in the environment rather than differences in the metal itself. These are known as concentration (or solution) cells. There are two types:

1 metal ion cells and
2 oxygen cells.

Metal ion cells   These can form in areas where stagnant liquid collect. Metal ion concentration cells are caused, as their name suggests, by differences in metal ion concentration in the corroding solution. A build-up of metal ions can occur in stagnant conditions caused by holes, gaskets, lap joints, surface deposits (scale, dirt) and crevices under bolt heads and rivet heads. They can also be caused by material, such as wood, plastic, rubber etc., lying on the surface of the metal. Figure 29.4 shows the formation of a metal ion concentration cell at a lap joint.

Oxygen cells   These are similar to metal ion cells in a number of ways, but here the corrosion is caused by differences in dissolved oxygen content of the solution. The formation of an oxygen concentration cell at a lap joint is shown in Fig. 29.5.

Control of concentration cell corrosion   This can be achieved in the following ways:

1 Use welded butt joints instead of riveted or bolted joints in new apparatus.
2 Existing lap joints should be welded, sealed or soldered to close the crevices.
3 Design vessels for complete drainage, avoid sharp corners and stagnant areas.
4 Inspect and clean deposits frequently.

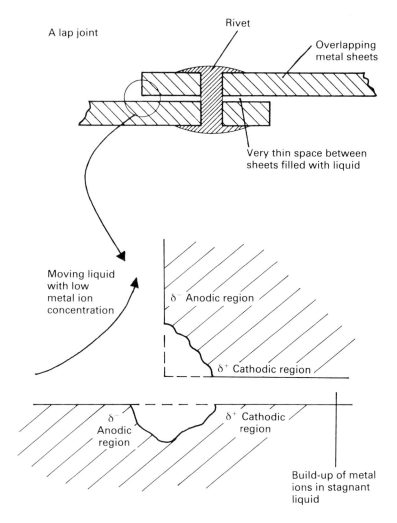

Fig. 29.4 A metal-ion concentration cell at a lap joint

5 Use solid, non-absorbent gaskets, such as Teflon, wherever possible.
6 Use welded pipes rather than the rolled-in type.

Pitting

This is a form of extremely localized attack where the anode remains as one spot. This results in rapid corrosion and deep penetration (small anode area, large cathode). Pits may be isolated or close together, the latter appear as a rough surface. The pits usually occur at impurities in the metal, grain boundaries, nicks, rough surfaces, etc.

Pitting is one of the destructive forms of corrosion. It is difficult to detect in a laboratory corrosion test because the pits are very small and there will be little loss in weight. Pitting is responsible for more unexpected plant equipment failures than any other form of corrosion.

Additionally, the liquid in the pit becomes stagnant resulting in metal ion and/or oxygen concentration cell corrosion. Furthermore, metal ions from the corrosion will accumulate in the pit. The process is therefore self-accelerating.

Control of pitting This is very difficult, but most of the points mentioned under concentration cells will help. If a test material shows the slightest signs of pitting in a laboratory test using microscopy, it must never be used.

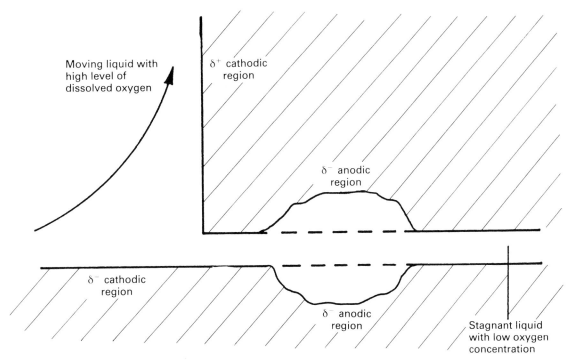

Fig. 29.5 An oxygen concentration cell at a lap joint

Intergranular corrosion

Solid metals consist of a large number of grains (actually metal crystals) and thus have a granular (or polycrystalline) structure. Localized attack at grain boundaries, with relatively little corrosion of the grains themselves, is intergranular corrosion. Due to stresses and dislocations at the grain boundaries, they are usually anodic. As corrosion proceeds, the grains fall out and the metal or alloy disintegrates. This type of corrosion occurs in stainless steel, particularly after welding (weld decay).

Control of intergranular corrosion   This can be achieved in the following ways:

1   High-temperature post-weld heat treatment (solution quenching) can be used. This involves heating the metal to about 1000 K and cooling it rapidly by quenching in water. This reduces the precipitation of carbon at the grain boundaries.
2   Add stabilizers such as columbium, tantalum or titanium. These combine strongly with free carbon to form carbides leaving no free carbon at the grain boundaries.

3   Lower the carbon content of the steel to below 0.03%. Below this figure carbon is usually completely soluble.

Parting (or dezincification)

This is a general term referring to selective corrosion of one or more components from a solid solution alloy. Removal of zinc, particularly from brass (a copper/zinc alloy), is common.

Control of parting   This is not easy. Reduction of the corrosive environment and cathodic protection are suggested. Small amounts of arsenic, antimony or phosphorous can be used as 'inhibitors'. The addition of 1% tin to brass (Admiralty brass) results in good resistance to sea water.

Stress corrosion

Generally a high stress in a piece of metal tends to make it more anodic. The greater the stress, the greater this effect. There are two main categories, as follows.

Stress accelerated corrosion   This is a

decrease in corrosion resistance due to continuous static stress such as applied stresses or residual stresses after welding.

Stress corrosion cracking This is an increase in the tendency of the metal to crack or show brittle fracture. It is usually caused by alternating stresses.

Erosion corrosion

Erosion is a mechanical process, corrosion is chemical. They combine in situations where corrosive products are eroded by mechanical wear or rapid fluid flow. This maintains a fresh metal surface in contact with the corrosive environment.

BIBLIOGRAPHY

Alexander, W. and Street, A. (1979) *Metals in the Service of Man*, 7th edn, Penguin Books Ltd, Harmondsworth.
Buckley, P. (1980) Stainless steel — strength matched with versatility. *Mfg Chem. Aerosol News*, **51**(7), 31–33.
Stafford, P. (1981) Rubber and its pharmacuetical applications. *Mfg Chem. Aerosol News*, **52**(6), 25–28.

Heat transfer and the properties of steam

Many pharmaceutical processes involve the heating of materials and this chapter will consider the methods by which heat can be transferred. The unit operation of evaporation is used to concentrate solutions by driving off some of the vapour and for this and other heating purposes steam is a most important medium for heat transfer.

SOME FUNDAMENTAL PRINCIPLES

Heat is due to the motion of molecules and a substance will have zero heat content only if it is at absolute zero (0 K). Although heat is intangible it is a form of energy and can be accurately measured and expressed in joules. The joule is a very small unit and a more practical quantity is the kilojoule (kJ) or the megajoule (MJ) which denote a thousand and a million joules respectively. It requires about 160 kJ of heat to raise 500 ml of water from room temperature to boiling point.

Many of the principles to be discussed in this chapter can be illustrated by the operation of a laboratory water bath of construction shown in Fig. 30.1. The water in the bath is heated by the gas burner and this heat raises the water in the bath to the boiling point. The heat is sensible heat — it produces an appreciable rise in temperature.

When the boiling point has been attained, further heat generates steam without any increase in temperature. This heat is termed *latent heat of evaporation* and is utilized to change the water into vapour at constant temperature. The steam rises and impinges on the dish which initially is at room temperature. The steam condenses on the

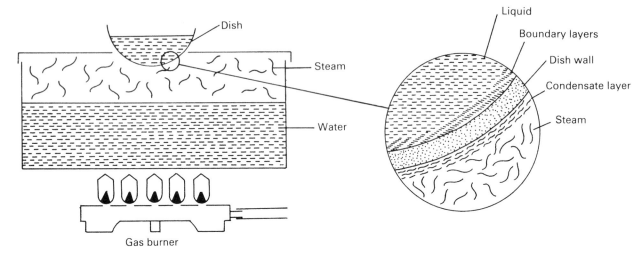

Fig. 30.1 Thermal resistances. Heat transfer from a 'water' bath to a dish

cool outer surface of the dish and in doing so it gives up the latent heat it contains thus forming a layer of condensate on the dish which runs down over the surface and drops back into the bath. Fresh condensate is continually formed to take its place so a layer of condensate will always be present. The latent heat which is liberated passes by conduction through the wall of the dish and into the contents to be heated. The term 'water bath' is a misnomer and the equipment can be described more accurately as a 'steam bath'. The steam functions as a heat transfer agent whereby the heat from the gas burner is transferred by the liberation of the latent heat into the liquid in the dish. There are advantages in this indirect heating in that the temperature can never exceed 100 °C and since the steam circulates over the whole dish surface, heating is much more uniform than it would be if the dish was heated directly over the gas flame.

Methods of heat transfer

Conduction

As explained above the latent heat from the steam must pass through the condensate layer and the wall of the dish. The wall is solid and little mixing takes place in the condensate film so the heat energy is transferred to adjacent molecules by momentum transfer. This is the process of heat transfer by conduction.

Convection

When the heat has passed by conduction in this way the cold fluid in contact with the inner wall of the dish is heated and expands. This lowers the density of the fluid and convection currents will be set up as the warm fluid rises and mixes with colder fluid. This is heat transfer by natural convection.

In industry fluids are often heated as they flow inside metal tubes in turbulent flow (see Chapter 2). Since mixing in turbulent flow is rapid, heat transfer by this 'forced convection' is more efficient than by natural convection.

Radiation

The energy emitted by the sun is transmitted in the form of electromagnetic waves through empty space. When it is absorbed by a body on which it falls it reappears as heat. All hot bodies radiate energy in this way but a consideration of this mode of heat transfer will be deferred until drying by radiant heat is discussed in Chapter 38.

Heat transfer by conduction

The insert in Fig. 30.1 shows a section of the dish wall in greater detail. If this is considered to be rotated into a vertical position and straightened slightly it would appear as in Fig. 30.2. A temperature drop occurs from the temperature of

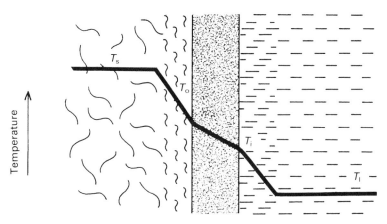

Fig. 30.2 Temperature gradients from steam through boundary layers and pan wall

the condensing steam to the lower temperature of the liquid in the dish. If this liquid is assumed to be of a lower boiling point than water, then eventually it will boil at this lower constant temperature and the temperature gradients would appear as in Fig. 30.2. T_s denotes the steam temperature, T_l the temperature of the boiling liquid and T_i, T_o are the temperatures of the inner and outer surfaces of the dish.

It is often important to know the rate at which heat can be transferred in a process. This must be carefully distinguished from the actual quantity of heat which needs to be supplied. Consider a domestic kettle brought to the boil over a low gas flame. Under such conditions it might take 20 minutes to boil while requiring perhaps 5 minutes over a full flame. Neglecting heat losses, the quantity of heat required would be the same in each case but the rate of heat transfer would be four times greater over the full flame.

Returning once more to Fig. 30.1, there are three barriers to heat flow, namely the condensate layer, the dish wall and the liquid side boundary layer adjacent to the dish wall. The origin and nature of this type of boundary layer is discussed in Chapter 2. The same quantity of heat must pass through each layer in turn so in the first instance the factors which affect the heat transfer through the dish wall alone should be considered. The quantity of heat transferred (Q joules) in time t seconds will depend on the difference in temperature between the inner and outer surfaces of the dish and the dish thickness L_d. It will also depend on the area available for heat transfer A.

Combining all these factors and introducing a proportionality constant K_d gives

$$\frac{Q}{t} = \frac{K_d A (T_o - T_i)}{L_d} \tag{30.1}$$

K_d is known as the coefficient of thermal conductivity. Putting appropriate SI units into Eqn 30.1. and rearranging shows that the units of K_d are $W\ m^{-1}\ K^{-1}$. Table 30.1 gives some typical values and it will be seen that metals are usually good conductors (high K values) though stainless steel is rather poor.

Table 30.1

Material	Thermal conductivity $W\ m^{-1}\ K^{-1}$
Copper	379
Aluminium	242
Steel	43
Stainless steel	17
Borosilicate glass	1
Water	0.6
Boiler scale	0.09–2.3
Diatomite	0.07
Glass wool	0.06
Air	0.03

Illustrative calculation   Calculate the quantity of heat passing through a stainless steel dish whose effective surface is 20 cm² and whose thickness is 1 mm in a period of 5 minutes if the temperatures at the inner and outer surfaces of the dish are 90 °C and 80 °C respectively.

Care must be taken to use correct units which are consistent.

$L_d = 1 \times 10^{-3}$ m. $A = 20 \times 10^{-4}$ m^2 and $K = 17$ W m^{-1} K^{-1} (Table 30.1)

The heat transferred per second is given by Eqn 30.1. In SI units a rate of heat transfer of one joule per second is termed 1 watt.

$$\frac{Q}{t} = \frac{KA(T_o - T_i)}{L_d} = \frac{17 \times 20 \times 10^{-4} \times 10 \text{ W}}{1 \times 10^{-3}}$$

$$= 340 \text{ W}$$

In 5 minutes (300 s) a quantity of heat $= 340 \times 300 = 102$ kJ will be transferred.

Heat transfer through films and boundary layers

Equation 30.1 for heat transfer through the wall alone can be rearranged into the following form

$$\frac{Q}{t} = \frac{T_o - T_i}{L_d/K_d A} = \frac{\Delta T}{L_d/K_d A}$$

This is an example of a very general form of equation for any rate process such as the rate of filtration (Chapter 31) or the rate of dissolution of a crystal (Chapter 5) all of which can be expressed as a driving force divided by a resistance term. In the above case the temperature *difference* ΔT is the driving force and the group $L_d/K_d A$ represents the thermal resistance of the dish wall.

The flow of heat is analogous to the flow of electricity. In the simple circuit shown in Fig. 30.3 the current I flowing in the circuit is given by

$$I = E/(R_1 + R_2 + R_3)$$

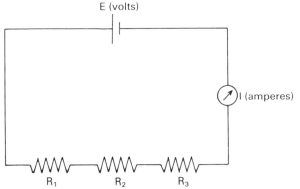

Fig. 30.3

where E is the voltage developed across the combined resistances. The total thermal resistance of layers of Fig. 30.2 can in a like manner be obtained by adding the thermal resistances together.

Total thermal resistance =
$$L_s/K_s A + L_d/K_s A + L_w/K_w A$$

The total driving force corresponding to the voltage due to the battery in Fig. 30.3 is the difference between the steam temperature and the temperature of the boiling fluid. The equation for rate of heat transfer then becomes

$$\frac{Q}{t} = \frac{(T_s - T_w)}{L_s/K_s A + L_d/K_d A + L_w/K_w A} \quad (30.2)$$

It is convenient to define a quantity U known as the overall heat transfer coefficient (OHTC), where

$$\frac{1}{U} = L_s/K_s + L_d/K + L_w/K_w \quad (30.3)$$

Making this substitution into Eqn 30.2 gives

$$\frac{Q}{t} = U.A. \, \Delta T_{total} \quad (30.4)$$

where $\Delta T_{total} = T_s - T_w$

Film heat transfer coefficients

The thicknesses of the boundary and condensate layers are not usually known and they do not remain constant when heating conditions are changed. To get over this difficulty it is customary to use film heat transfer coefficients defined by the expressions

$$\frac{1}{h_s} = \frac{L_s}{K_s} \qquad \text{and} \qquad \frac{1}{h_w} = \frac{L_w}{K_w}$$

where h_s is the steam side film heat transfer coefficient and h_w the water side coefficient. Substituting these values into Eqn 30.3 gives

$$\frac{1}{U} = \frac{1}{h_s} + \frac{L_d}{K} + \frac{1}{h_w}$$

Methods have been devised for calculating such coefficients for heat transfer under defined conditions but these lie outside the scope of this chapter.

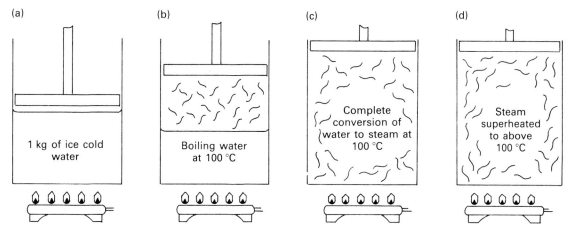

Fig. 30.4 Conversion of water to superheated steam

STEAM AS A HEATING MEDIUM

Of the various means of heating pharmaceutical materials in such operations as drying and evaporation, steam is very commonly used. As an aid to understanding the principles of heat transfer using steam the student is asked to visualize one kilogram of ice cold water contained in a cylinder closed by a leakproof piston and heated over a gas ring (Fig. 30.4). Initially all the heat supplied will be sensible heat to raise the temperature of the water to the boiling point of 100 °C. The heat required to do this is given by

mass of water × specific heat capacity × temperature rise

The heat capacity of water which is the quantity of heat required to raise 1 kg by 1 °C is 4.2 kJ. It will therefore require 420 kJ to raise the 1 kg of water to the boiling point. A graph of changes in temperature with heat input is shown in Fig. 30.5.

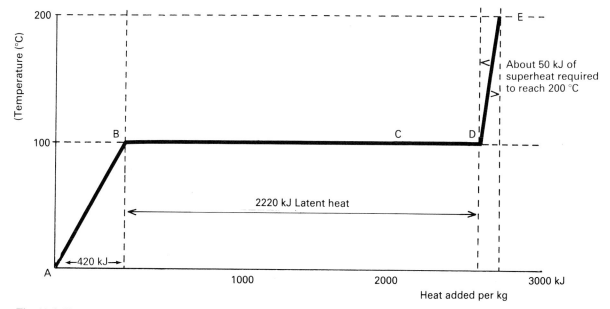

Fig. 30.5 Changes of state on addition of heat to ice cold water at atmospheric pressure

Further heat then converts some of the water into steam by supplying latent heat of evaporation at a constant temperature by 100 °C. The dryness fraction is the fraction of water converted to steam at that particular time. The latent heat of evaporation is 2240 kJ/kg so it would require $0.9 \times 2240 = 2016$ kJ of latent heat to produce a dryness fraction of 0.9 (point C, Fig. 30.5). As more heat is supplied the dryness fraction increases becoming equal to 1 at point D. At this point all the water has been converted into dry saturated steam and no liquid water remains.

If further heat is supplied there is no water left to absorb it and the temperature will rise rapidly for the absorption of a small amount of superheat. The total heat content of the steam measured from a datum temperature of 0 °C is the sum of the sensible, latent and superheat as it is termed. If superheated steam (point E, Fig. 30.5) comes into contact with a cold surface then it will lose heat in the reverse order by first cooling to the saturation temperature (point D) and giving out a small amount of superheat. Then, and only then, will the steam condense to form condensate, liberating the large amount of latent heat which it contains. It cannot be emphasized too strongly that latent heat is the 'useful' heat. Steam for process heating and sterilization procedures should ideally be dry and saturated at the point of use.

Effect of pressure

The steam could be raised under pressure by loading the piston (Fig. 30.6) with a suitable weight. If this was such that the weight exerted a pressure of a further bar above atmospheric pressure (2 bar absolute) then the saturation temperature would be raised to 120.2 °C, i.e. no steam would form until this temperature was reached. The sensible heat required would be 505 kJ and it would take 2202 kJ to convert the water into steam. Steam at this higher pressure thus contains less latent heat then steam raised at atmospheric pressure. If steam at any given pressure was led into equipment where it could condense and give up the latent heat this would occur at the saturation temperature corresponding

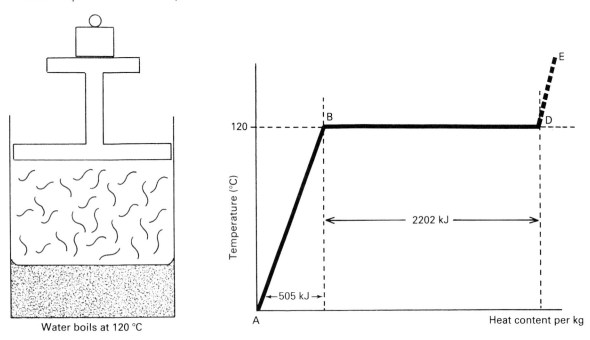

Weight sufficient to produce absolute pressure of 2 bar in cylinder

Water boils at 120 °C

Fig. 30.6 Heat content diagram from steam raised at 2 bar

to the pressure. The point is important in steriliz-ation using steam (see Chapter 43). Saturated steam will always condense at a temperature which is set by the pressure and the pressure is chosen so as to ensure that a safe temperature is attained.

Steam tables

Since steam is such a useful heat transfer agent the properties of dry saturated steam have been tabulated over a wide range of temperatures and pressures. There are also tables for superheated steam but these are mainly of interest to engineers. Steam tables give values for the sensible and latent heat content and the saturation temperature corresponding to the pressure. The specific volume, which is the volume occupied by 1 kg of steam at a given pressure is also listed.

STEAM GENERATION AND USE

In industry steam is raised under pressure in a central boiler house. Since this steam is raised in contact with liquid water it will not be super-heated and may be 'wet', i.e. it may contain suspended water droplets. The steam is led through strong steel pipes which are well lagged to prevent heat loss and subsequent condensation in the pipes. Steam may be delivered to many different locations but before use its pressure is normally lowered to give a saturation (conden-sation) temperature suitable to the process in operation.

Larger factories may generate electrical power by expanding high pressure steam in a turbine. The exhaust steam, still at a fairly high pressure is then utilized for heating. Such steam tends to be very wet unless the steam is initially super-heated.

A typical steam heated installation

The steam heated pan

This equipment is the industrial equivalent of the laboratory water bath and is shown in Fig. 30.7. It is used for the concentration of aqueous solutions by boiling off some of the water — the unit operation of evaporation. Figure 30.7 shows some of the ancillary equipment commonly

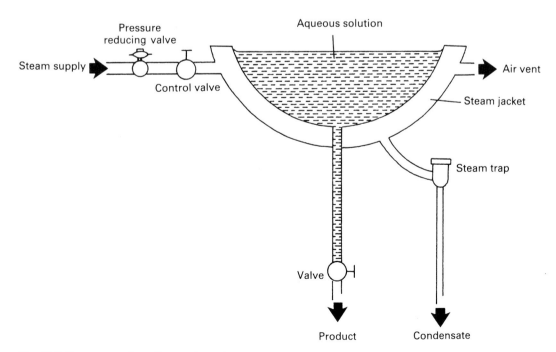

Fig. 30.7 Steam pan and auxiliary equipment

employed in steam heated installations and the function of this will be explained shortly.

If the pan was to be used for the evaporation of an aqueous liquid whose boiling point was near that of water then saturated steam at 2 bar absolute (saturation temperature circa 120 °C) would give a satisfactory temperature difference of 20 °C as the 'driving force' for heat transfer.

Steam traps

It will be recalled that the steam must condense before the latent heat content can pass into the liquid being heated. If there was no exit pipe from the jacket then this condensate would quickly fill the steam space and no more steam could enter. If, however, a drainage pipe alone was fitted to the jacket then steam would issue forth under pressure and be lost. The problem is solved by fitting a device known as a steam trap to the exit pipe. This retains the steam until it has condensed and periodically the trap opens to allow the condensate to be expelled, closing once more when steam reaches the trap.

The steam traps in common use can be divided into two main classes: *mechanical and thermostatic*. The former depend on the physical difference between steam and water, that is between vapour and liquid, while the thermostatic variety rely on the fact that condensate can lose sensible heat and so will be at a lower temperature than the steam. Mechanical traps have the advantage of possessing greater strength and the ability to operate under a greater variety of conditions than thermostatic traps; for example, if the temperature difference between the steam and the condensate is small, or if the pressure or the amount of condensate changes. On the other hand, thermostatic traps differ from mechanical traps by opening when the plant is not in use, allowing condensate to drain away and air to be swept out of the system when starting up. Thermostatic traps also vent air when operating, because of the reduction of temperature of steam when contaminated with air, whereas mechanical traps are unable to distinguish between air and steam.

Typical examples of these traps are shown in Figs 30.8–30.10. The *float trap* in Fig. 30.8 is a mechanical trap in which the outlet is opened by

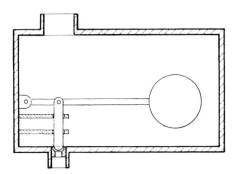

Fig. 30.8 Float type steam trap

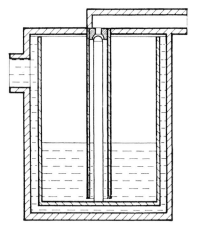

Fig. 30.9 Bucket type steam trap

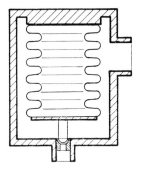

Fig. 30.10 Balanced pressure steam trap

the float as the condensate level rises. As the condensate is discharged, the float falls and the outlet closes. In the *bucket trap* (Fig. 30.9) the outlet is closed when the bucket floats in the condensate. As more condensate drains down into the trap, some overflows into the bucket until the latter sinks and opens the outlet. The condensate is blown out by the pressure of the steam until the bucket recovers its buoyancy and floats up to close the outlet once more.

Thermostatic traps can take the form of a simple thermostatic device which can be set to open at a particular temperature appropriate to the steam pressure, but this has the disadvantage that a slight variation in the steam pressure (and hence the temperature) may cause the trap to stay either open or closed until the setting has been altered to meet the new conditions.

This difficulty is overcome in the *balanced pressure expansion trap*, illustrated in Fig. 30.10. A capsule in the form of a bellows contains a liquid having a boiling point a few degrees below the boiling point of water. Thus, when surrounded by steam, the liquid in the capsule boils, causing the bellows to expand and close the outlet. Condensate cools the capsule, the liquid then ceases to boil, and the bellows contract, opening the outlet and discharging the condensate. When all the condensate is removed, steam causes the trap to close again. A particular advantage of this trap is that increase of steam pressure raises the boiling point of water, but the same pressure acts on the surface of the bellows and elevates the boiling point of the liquid by a similar amount. Hence, the title applied to this type — balanced pressure expansion trap — since it will always operate a few degrees below the saturation temperature of the steam.

Pressure reduction

In general, process plant uses steam at a pressure of 1.7–2 bar, so that a reduction from the boiler pressure (often 6–8 bar) is necessary. This is carried out by a reducing valve, the principles of which are shown in Fig. 30.11.

The pressure of a spring attempts to open the valve against the high pressure steam. The closing of the valve is caused by the low pressure steam, so that, when this reaches a predetermined value, a balance will be reached in which the low pressure steam acting on the diaphragm closes the valve against the spring pressure.

In practice, an equilibrium is set up in which the valve is open slightly, sufficient steam passing

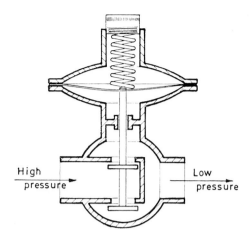

Fig. 30.11 Pressure reducing valve

through from the high pressure to maintain the desired level on the low-pressure side.

The expansion of steam

When steam is reduced in pressure by passage through a reducing valve the process is isenthalpic — that is the total heat content of the steam remains unchanged by its expansion. Suppose steam at 15 bar absolute is expanded down to a pressure of 2 bar absolute for use in a steam pan. The steam tables give the following data.

	15 bar saturated steam	2 bar saturated steam
sensible heat (h)	814 kJ kg^{-1}	505 kJ kg^{-1}
latent heat (L)	1978 kJ kg^{-1}	2202 kJ kg^{-1}
total heat (H)	2792 kJ kg^{-1}	2707 kJ kg^{-1}

There is a difference of 85 kJ/kg in the values for the total heat content and this heat must be accounted for. There are two possible ways it may be absorbed.

1 If the steam is initially wet at the higher pressure the excess heat will convert some of the free water to steam at the lower pressure and the steam will become dryer. For example, if steam of dryness fraction 0.95 is expanded as given above, the condition of the expanded steam can be calculated as follows.

The excess heat of 85 kJ will convert 85 ÷ 2202 kg of water into steam. This is 0.038 kg. The steam would improve from a dryness fraction of 0.95 to one of 0.95 + 0.038, i.e. 0.988.

It will be apparent from the above that such 'wire drawing' will not dry steam which is very wet and other means must be adopted.

2 If the steam is initially dry and saturated then there is no free water to absorb the heat. The heat will be used to raise the temperature above the saturation temperature — in other words it will become superheated. The effect is of some importance in steam sterilization since superheated steam is an inefficient sterilizing agent (Chapter 43).

Flash steam

When steam condenses in steam heated equipment the condensate produced is initially at the saturation temperature (point D in Fig. 30.5). Although the condensate may cool slightly before it is voided by a steam trap it will still be at a temperature well above 100 °C — say 117 °C or so for steam condensing at 2 bar absolute. Water at 117 °C cannot exist at atmospheric pressure so a proportion will instantly 'flash' into steam so as to absorb enough latent heat of evaporation to reduce the temperature of the remainder to 100 °C. By using steam table data it is easy to find the quantity of flash produced from 1 kg of condensate.

Sensible heat of condensate at 2 bar is 505 kJ kg^{-1} and at 1 bar (atm. pressure) it is 417 kJ kg^{-1}. The difference is therefore 88 kJ kg^{-1}. Since the latent heat of steam at 1 bar is 2258 kJ kg^{-1}, then the excess heat will produce 88 ÷ 2258, i.e. 0.039 kg of flash steam per kg of condensate.

In large installations it may well be worthwhile collecting flash and using it for space heating or other purposes. The condensate, which is still around 100 °C, may be used for space heating or returned to the boiler room as feed water.

The climbing film evaporator

The unit operation of evaporation is not now so important as it was formerly, but this evaporator is worth mentioning as another example of steam heated equipment. It is used as an alternative to the pan for the concentration of aqueous solutions. In this type of evaporator, the heating unit consists of steam-jacketed tubes, having a length to diameter ratio of about 140:1, so that a large evaporator may have tubes 50 mm in diameter and about 7 m in length.

In the commonest form, illustrated in Fig. 30.12, the liquor to be evaporated is introduced into the bottom of the tube, a film of liquid forms on the walls and rises up the tubes, hence the title *climbing film evaporator*. At the upper end, the mixture of vapour and concentrated liquor enters a separator, the vapour passing on to a condenser, and the concentrate to a receiver.

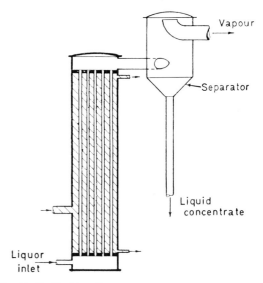

Fig. 30.12 Climbing film evaporator

The fact that the film of liquid 'climbs' up the tube through a distance of 5 or 6 metres without mechanical assistance may seem improbable, but the explanation is as follows. The various stages from start-up are illustrated in Fig. 30.13 which represents a part of the tube about one-fifth of the way from the bottom.

Cold or preheated liquor is introduced into the tube (1). Heat is transferred to the liquor from the walls, and boiling begins (2), increasing in vigour (3) and (4). Eventually, sufficient vapour has been formed for the smaller bubbles to unite to a large bubble, filling the width of the tube and trapping a 'slug' of liquid above the bubble (5). As more vapour is formed, the slug of liquid is blown up

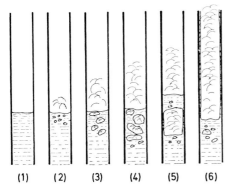

Fig. 30.13 Principles of climbing film evaporator

the tube, the tube is filled with vapour, while the liquid is spread as a film over the walls (6). This film of liquid continues to vaporize rapidly, the vapour escaping up the tube and, because of frictional (drag) between the vapour and liquid, the film also is dragged up the tube. Some idea of the rate of vaporization can be gained from the fact that the liquid film travels up the tube at velocities of the order of 6 or 7 m s⁻¹ in fully turbulant flow.

It must be emphasized that this is the sole reason why the liquor travels up the tube, and that reduced pressure, for example, does not affect this mechanism, although it is sometimes stated incorrectly that the vacuum 'draws' the liquid up the tube. While it is true that such evaporators are used commonly under reduced pressure, the climbing film evaporator will function equally well at atmospheric pressure.

The climbing film evaporator has a number of advantages over the steam heated pan.

1 The very high film velocity reduces boundary layers to a minimum giving improved heat transfer.
2 The use of long narrow tubes provides large areas for heat transfer.
3 Because of the increased efficiency of heat transfer, a small temperature difference is sufficient, with less risk of damage to thermo-labile materials.
4 The time of the contact between the liquor and the heating surface is very short. Even allowing for the preheating period, the total time a given portion of the liquor is in the evaporator is of the order of 20 seconds, of which about one

second only is occupied in climbing the tube in the boiling film. The advantage of this method for heat-sensitive materials will be realized when this time is compared with the hours of continuous boiling the liquor may receive in a pan.
5 Despite the short heating time, the evaporation rate is very high, since the film formation gives an extremely large surface area in relation to the volume of the liquid.
6 The mixture of liquid and vapour enters the separator at high velocity, which improves the separation efficiency and makes the method especially suitable for materials that foam.

The equipment has the disadvantage that it is expensive to manufacture and is difficult to clean and maintain. From the operational point of view the feed rate is critical. If too high, the liquor may be concentrated insufficiently, whereas if the feed rate is too low, the film cannot be maintained and dry patches may form on the tube wall.

Because of the rapid evaporation, minimum temperature gradient and short heating time, this method approaches most nearly the perfect method for pharmaceutical products. Even thermolabile materials can be processed in film evaporators and may have been used successfully for the concentrate of solutions such as insulin, liver extracts, and vitamins.

Adverse effects of air in steam

Water always contains dissolved air which is driven off when the water is converted to steam. Air is also present in the steam space of equipment on start-up and it may not be entirely flushed out by the incoming steam. Air is a permanent gas which remains when the steam condenses to form a condensate film and hence forms an air layer in contact with the condensate. As air is a very poor conductor (Table 30.1) it forms a formidable barrier to heat flow. It will be recalled that the value of the overall heat transfer coefficient depends on the sum of all the thermal resistances (Eqn 30.3) and the presence of as little as 1% of air in steam may result in the reduction of the value of the overall heat transfer coefficient U by half. The reduction in U as the air content of steam increases is shown in Fig. 30.14. Equip-

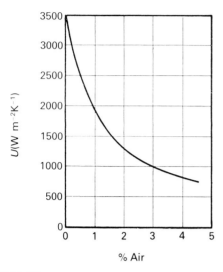

Fig. 30.14 Effect of air in steam on the coefficient of heat transfer

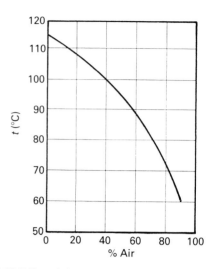

Fig. 30.15 Effect of air on steam temperature

ment which gives adequate heat transfer rates with air-free steam may therefore be undersized should the steam contain air.

Another adverse effect of air follows as a consequence of Dalton's law. The total pressure of an air/steam mixture will be due to the sum of the partial pressures of the air and steam, i.e.

$$P_T = P_A + P_S$$

If P_T, the total pressure, was 2 bar absolute and the steam contained 10% of air then P_S, the partial pressure of the steam, would be 1.8 bar with air contributing 0.2 bar. Steam tables give the saturation temperature of pure steam at 1.8 bar absolute as 117.3 °C and a mixture of air and steam at 2 bar absolute also condenses at this temperature. In other words, the partial pressure of the air contributes nothing to the saturation temperature of the mixture which is set by the partial pressure of the steam alone. Figure 30.15 shows the effect of percentage air content on the temperature of steam at a constant pressure of 1.7 bar.

Sterilization processes use steam at a specified pressure with the implicit assumption of a correct corresponding saturation temperature. This procedure is safe only if air-free steam can be guaranteed. Thermostatic traps of the balanced pressure type will void air since an air/steam mixture is at a lower temperature than pure steam

at the same pressure. Air vents based on this principle should be fitted where air is likely to be trapped, as for example, near the top of the tubes in the climbing film evaporator shown in Fig. 30.12.

Calculations

This chapter will be concluded with some illustrative calculations.

1 A steam heated pen of heated area 0.4 m² was used with steam in the jacket condensing at 115 °C. It was found that 0.8 kg of water at the boiling point was evaporated from the pan in the space of 5 minutes. Find the value of the overall heat transfer coefficient (OHTC) under these conditions. The latent heat of evaporation of water may be taken as 2.2 MJ kg⁻¹.

   The heat used to evaporate the water is $0.8 \times 2.2 \times 10^6 = 1.76 \times 10^6$ J. The rate of heat transfer was 1.76×10^6 J per 300 s or 5867 W.

   From $Q/t = UA\Delta T$ (Eqn 30.4):

   $$5867 = U \times 0.4 \times (115 - 100)$$

   and $U = 2793$ W m⁻² K⁻¹

2 A laboratory scale climbing film evaporator consists of one tube 1.6 m long and 1.27 cm outside diameter with steam condensing in the jacket at 115 °C. It was found that the vapour condensed from the separator amounted

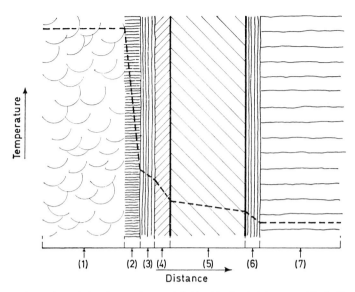

Fig. 30.16 Temperature gradients through heating surface and fluids, idealized: (1) steam, (2) air film, (3) condensate film, (4) scale, (5) metal wall, (6) liquid film, (7) liquid

to 2.4 kg when collected for 10 minutes. Find the value of the OHTC.

The heat required to form the vapour was $2.4 \times 2.2 \times 10^6$ J and the rate of heat transfer was $2.4 \times 2.2. \times 10^6/600$ J s^{-1} or 6400 W.

From $A = \pi \times D \times L$:

$A = 3.14 \times 1.27 \times 10^{-2} \times 1.6 = 0.0639$ m^2

From $Q/t = UA\Delta T$:

$$6400 = U \times 0.0639 \times (115 - 100)$$

and thus $U = 6677$ W m^{-2} K^{-1}

The data for these calculations were taken from a student laboratory notebook and the results illustrate the higher coefficient obtained from the climbing film evaporator.

3 Fig. 30.16 represents the films present in a scaled steam heated pan when air is present. Assuming the values for the thickness and conductivities of the films and a heated area of 0.5 m^2, calculate the rate of heat transfer into the boiling water.

Data

	Thickness (mm)	K (W m^{-1} K^{-1})
Air film	0.1	0.03
Condensate film	0.1	0.6
Scale	0.1	0.4
Pan wall	2.0	17
Water-side film	0.2	0.6

Using the equation $1/U = L_{air}/K_{air}$ etc., see Eqn 30.3.

$$\frac{1}{U} = \left(\frac{0.1}{0.03} + \frac{0.1}{0.6} + \frac{0.1}{0.4} + \frac{2}{17} + \frac{0.2}{0.6} \right) \times 10^{-3}$$

(The factor 10^{-3} is required to convert the thicknesses from mm to m.)

$$\frac{1}{U} = 4.200 \times 10^{-3} \text{ and}$$

$$U = 238.1 \text{ W m}^{-2} \text{ K}^{-1}.$$

Using $\dfrac{Q}{t} = UA \, \Delta T$:

$$\frac{Q}{t} = 238 \times 0.5 \times (120 - 100) = 2384 \text{ W}$$

4 Rework the above assuming the air and scale films are absent.

$$\frac{1}{U} = \left(\frac{0.1}{0.6} + \frac{2}{17} + \frac{0.2}{0.6} \right) \times 10^{-3}$$

$$\frac{1}{U} = 0.6176 \times 10^{-3} \text{ and } U = 1619 \text{ W m}^{-2} \text{ K}^{-1}$$

$$\frac{Q}{t} = 1619 \times 0.5 \times 20 = 16 \, 190 \text{ W (16.19 kW)}$$

It can be seen that in the absence of scale and air films the rate of heat transfer is increased by over sixfold.

Filtration

Definition

Definition

Filtration may be defined as the separation of an insoluble solid from a fluid by means of a porous medium that retains the solid but allows the fluid to pass. The term 'fluid' includes both liquids and gases and the removal of suspended particles from air to produce sterile air is an important operation though this chapter will deal only with the filtration of liquids.

For convenience in the later discussion, the following terms are explained here. The suspension of solid in the liquid is known as the *slurry*. The porous *filter medium* is normally contained in a suitable housing which forms the *filter*. The wet solid left on the medium forms the *filter cake* and the clear liquid passing through is the *filtrate*. Certain operations such as the extraction of vegetable drugs with a solvent may yield a turbid product with a small quantity of fine suspended colloidal matter. This is not enough to form a cake and filtration is undertaken to clarify the filtrate and produce a 'polished' clear filtrate. It is normal practice to add a filter aid prior to filtration. This is discussed later in this chapter.

FACTORS AFFECTING THE RATE OF FILTRATION

The rate of filtration may be quite slow and it is important to operate equipment so as to filter as quickly as possible whilst still ensuring an acceptable filtrate. On a small scale the laboratory Buchner funnel and flask forms a convenient example to illustrate filtration. Figure 31.1 is a sketch of this equipment. The side arm may be connected to a source of vacuum.

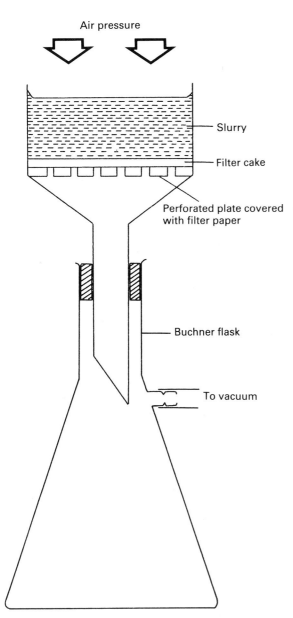

Air pressure

Slurry

Filter cake

Perforated plate covered
with filter paper

Buchner flask

To vacuum

Fig. 31.1 Buchner funnel and vacuum flask

The rate of filtration depends on the following factors:

1 the area available which is the cross-sectional area of the funnel (A).
2 the pressure difference across the filter (ΔP). This difference is due to the head of slurry and decreases as the level drops. Note that it is the *difference* which is important and this can be increased by drawing a vacuum in the flask. A proportion of the atmospheric pressure acting on the surface of the slurry would then be added to the pressure difference.
3 the viscosity of the filtrate (μ). A viscous liquid will filter more slowly than a mobile one.
4 the thickness of the cake (l). The cake will *increase* in thickness as filtration proceeds so the rate of filtration will fall.

All these factors can be combined in the Darcy equation:

$$\frac{V}{t} \text{ (volume per unit time)} = \frac{KA\Delta P}{\mu l} \quad (31.1)$$

The proportionality constant K expresses the *permeability* of the cake and it is clearly desirable that it should be large. It can be shown that K is given by

$$K = \frac{e^3}{5(1 - e)^2 \, S^2} \quad (31.2)$$

where e is the porosity of the cake and S is the specific surface area of the particles comprising the cake. If the solid material is one that forms an impermeable cake the rate may be improved by adding a filter aid (see later in this chapter). These aids form open porous cakes. There may be a contribution to filtration resistance from the filter medium but that can usually be neglected.

Cake compressibility

The filtrate percolates through the cake via a network of capillaries formed by the voids (Fig. 31.2(a)). If the pressure used is too high then the particles may deform so as to decrease the voidage (Fig. 31.2(b)). That is unlikely to happen using a Buchner funnel but may do so in commercial filters. Since the value of K is dependent on the value of e^3 (Eqn (31.2)) a small change in e greatly decreases the filtration rate. An example of a 'compressible cake' is aluminium hydroxide which precipitates as flocculent particles with little strength.

Methods to increase filtration rate

Darcy's equation suggests some ways of increasing the rate.

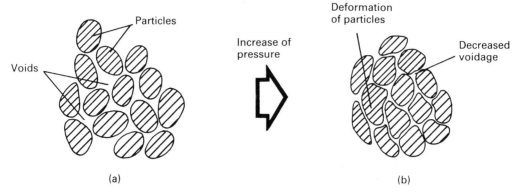

Fig. 31.2 Illustrating cake compressibility

Increase the permeability of the cake (filter aids)

The addition of filter aids to the slurry has already been mentioned. A filter aid forms a cake of an open porous nature and is commonly mixed with the slurry so that it is laid down continuously. Original colloidal particles are adsorbed on the filter aid so they are unable to form an impervious cake. Alternatively the aid may be laid down as a '*precoat*' by filtering a suspension to form a cake, following this with the slurry. A disadvantage is that the surface of the precoat may become clogged but that can be prevented in some instances (see The rotary vacuum filter later in this chapter).

Popular filter aids are diatomite (a form of diatomaceous earth) and perlite which is a type of volcanic glass. As an alternative the slurry can sometimes be 'conditioned' to produce a more desirable form. Proteins may be coagulated by heat or change of pH. Colloids can sometimes be flocculated by adding electrolytes. Flocculated suspensions may be 'thickened' by allowing the solid to settle and decanting the supernatant.

Increase area available for filtration

It will be obvious that the total volume of filtrate flowing through the filter will be proportional to the area of the filter. Hence, the rate of filtration can be increased by using larger filters, but the area can also be increased by using a number of small units in parallel (as in the filter press).

Increase pressure difference across cake

The simplest way to filter is under gravity where the liquid 'head' provides the driving force for filtration. The bag filter, which is a suspended linen bag, is still employed for small scale work but normally filtration rates are too slow for most purposes. If a vacuum is 'pulled' on the far side of the filter medium then atmospheric pressure can be utilized. The maximum pressure difference is limited to one bar and in practice it will be less. Another drawback is the boiling of hot liquids under the reduced pressure. However, despite these disadvantages vacuum is used in one important industrial filter — the rotary vacuum filter.

The most generally applicable means of obtaining a high pressure is to pump the slurry into the filter using a suitable pump. Although it is not done in practice it would be theoretically possible to do that with a Buchner funnel as shown in Fig. 31.3. Most industrial filters have positive pressure feed and the pressure is limited only by the pump and the ability of the filter to withstand the stresses. Pressures up to 15 bar are common.

Too high a pressure may be detrimental because of cake compression. There is also a danger of 'blinding' the filter medium by forcing particles into it. This is most likely in the early stages before a continuous layer of cake has formed. As a general rule filtration should start at moderate pressure which can be increased as filtration proceeds and the cake thickness builds up.

Decrease filtrate viscosity

The flow through a filter cake can be considered

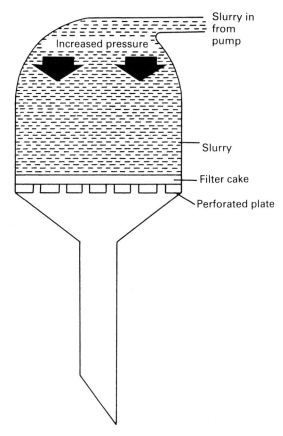

Fig. 31.3 Positive pressure filtration

as the total flow through a large number of parallel capillaries formed by the voids between the particles. The rate of flow through each is governed by Poiseuille's law in which the viscosity enters as a factor. The viscosity of the filtrate can be reduced by heating and many filters such as the filter press and metafilter (see later) can be obtained fitted with steam jackets.

Heating the slurry is normally the better procedure but if the material is thermolabile then dilution is an alternative. The viscosity falls on dilution but the total volume to be filtered is increased and there may not be an overall gain in processing time.

Decrease thickness of filter cake

Darcy's equation shows that the rate falls off as the cake increases in thickness. If a filter of large area is used then the cake thickness will be less for a given volume of filtrate passing through the filter. It is therefore doubly advantageous to have a large filtration area available.

In the rotary filter (see later) the cake thickness is kept almost constant by the action of a scraper which removes the surface layers.

MECHANISMS OF FILTRATION

The mechanisms whereby particles are retained by a filter medium are important in the early stages of the filtration of a slurry but once a layer of cake has formed this acts as its own filter medium. The process is termed autofiltration.

The pores and open spaces in a filter medium are often larger than the particles in suspension. Despite this they are held back by a number of mechanisms which are discussed below.

Straining

If the pores are smaller than the particles then these are retained. Membrane filters, as used to remove bacteria and fibres from parenteral preparations, are a good example of this type. Formerly these filters clogged too easily to be generally used but this problem has now been overcome and industrial membrane filters are discussed later.

Impingement

As a flowing fluid approaches a cylindrical object such as a fibre in the weave of a filter cloth, the flow pattern is displaced as shown in Fig. 31.4. Suspended solids may have sufficient momentum

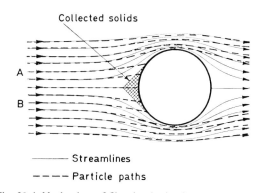

Fig. 31.4 Mechanism of filtration by impingement

to strike the fibre. If they do so they are retained but others may follow the streamlines and be trapped a little later. An accumulation of solids builds up on the fibres and eventually forms a cake over the surface.

Attractive forces

Electrostatic and other surface forces may exert sufficient hold on the particles to attract and retain them. Air can be freed from dust particles by passage over electrodes charged to a high potential in an electrostatic precipitator.

Bridging and entanglement

When using a fibrous filter cloth or filter pad the particles may entangle with the fibres and form bridges over them. Impingement is also involved as explained above.

If there is insufficient solid to form a cake then all particles must be removed by these mechanisms. There must be sufficient depth to the filter medium to ensure that they are eventually trapped with a high degree of probability. Filter sheets composed of cellulose fibres combined with

selected kieselguhrs are displacing the older woven filter cloths for use in filter presses and other filters. These sheets are 2–3 mm in thickness sufficient to trap particles from the start of the filtration. There is thus no need to recirculate any turbid first filtrate which usually resulted before the cake had formed on the older media.

Some filters such as the metafilter rely on the laying down of a precoat on a filter candle which does not require a filter medium to be incorporated. Filters having porous elements formed from sintered glass and metal or earthenware are also used on a small scale and do not require filter cloths or other media.

INDUSTRIAL FILTERS AND FILTRATION TECHNIQUES

The filter press

The majority of filter presses in current use are plate and frame type presses and a perspective view is given in Fig. 31.5. It can be seen that the assembly consists of alternate plates and frames mounted on two parallel support bars. Pressure can be applied via the screw thread so that the

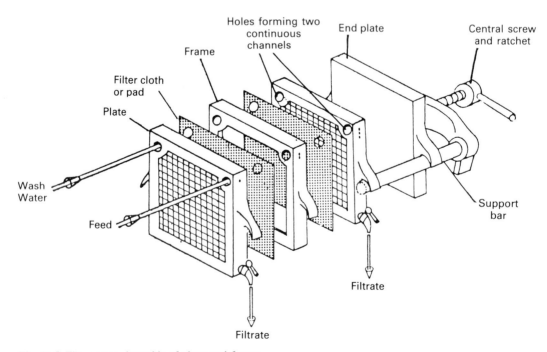

Fig. 31.5 Filter press. Assembly of plates and frames

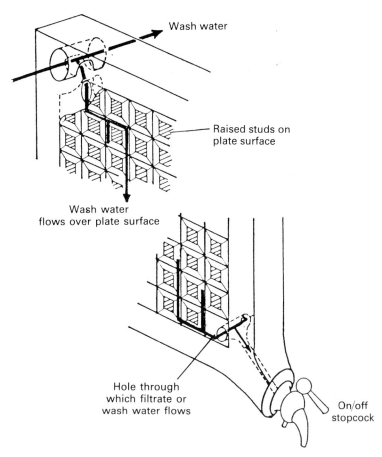

Wash water

Raised studs on
plate surface

Wash water
flows over plate surface

Hole through
which filtrate or
wash water flows

On/off
stopcock

Fig. 31.6 Filter press. Details of washing plate

plates and frames are rigidly fixed between two
end plates. The plates, shown in detail in
Fig. 31.6, are solid with a studded surface
forming the support for a filter cloth which hangs
down each side of the plate. When the press is
assembled the cloths act as a seal between the
plate and the two adjacent frames. The inlet for
the slurry is formed by eyes in the top right hand
corner of each plate and frame (Fig. 31.5) which
form a continuous channel running the length of
the press when it is assembled. The frames are
hollow and there is a connection running from the
eye into the interior of each frame.

In use the slurry is pumped in under positive
pressure which can be as high as 20 bar and fills
each frame. The filtrate passes through the cloths
on opposite sides of the frames and runs down
between the studs on the plate surfaces. Figure
31.6 shows that there is an outlet cock in the

bottom right hand corner of the frames allowing
the filtrate to discharge into a common channel.

The solids in the slurry build up to form two
cakes in each frame which will eventually meet in
the centre of the frames. When this occurs (or
earlier if the pressure required rises to a high
level) the filtration is stopped and the press
dismantled and reassembled after washing the
cake free of solute if that is desired. It is usual to
start the filtration at a low pressure and increase
this so as to keep the filtration rate nearly constant
as the cake thickness increases. This is constant
rate filtration. If the filter press is run at constant
pressure the rate of filtration will fall off as time
goes on and it may be advantageous to cease
filtration before the frames are full.

Filter presses are available in a wide variety of
sizes ranging from small laboratory presses of
plate area *circa* 100 cm^2 to large industrial types

of plate area 4–6 m². The smaller presses may be designed to use filter pads and units can be obtained which can be sterilized and are capable of retaining bacteria.

Larger presses employ filter cloths made of nylon or terylene. These are prone to leak but the press may incorporate O-ring seals between the frames and plates in the better designs. Plates and frames may be made in various materials of construction such as brass, steel and aluminium. The surface may be lacquered to minimize corrosion. Non-metals such as plastics are lighter and very large presses have been constructed of wood. These have frames which are much lighter than the corresponding metal equivalent and they are satisfactory provided they are kept wet to avoid shrinkage. Although it is not common, steam jacketed presses are available for viscous slurries which should be filtered hot.

The washing press

If it is necessary to wash the filter cake, the simple construction described so far is unsatisfactory. It is not efficient to pass wash water through the same path as the slurry since the frames will be full of cake, leaving no path for the wash water to take. To overcome this most presses have a separate wash channel which does not discharge into the frames. Instead the wash channel communicates with every alternate plate (a 'washing plate'), so that the wash water flows around the studs on each side of the plate and then through the filter cake in contact with it. Since the frame is completely filled with cake the wash water then passes through the filter cloth on the far side of the frame, finally running down the studs of the non-washing plate before leaving via the outlet on this plate. It is important to close the outlets on all the washing plates to prevent the wash water taking the path of least resistance. This is in contrast to the process of filtration where all outlets are open.

The press must be assembled in the correct sequence and the two types of plate and the frames are marked to facilitate this. The usual code is one 'dot' for a non-washing plate, two for a frame and three for a washing plate.

Assuming that the same pressure difference is used for washing as at the end of the filtration process, the rate of washing will be lower than the final rate of filtration. The reason for this is that half the outlets are closed, which has the effect of halving the area over which flow occurs. Also, the cake thickness in filtration, from the point of view of Darcy's law, is half the frame thickness. For washing, however, the water flows through the entire thickness of the frame, that is, the value of l is doubled. Hence, the effect of both factors is to reduce the washing rate to one quarter of the final filtration rate.

Advantages   These can be summarized as follows:

1 Construction is very simple and a wide variety of materials can be used, for example: cast iron, for handling common substances; bronze, for smaller units; stainless steel, where avoidance of contamination is important; hard rubber or plastics, where metals must be avoided; wood for lightness, although this must be kept wet.
2 It provides a large filtering area in a relatively small floor space.
3 It is versatile, the capacity being variable according to the thickness of the frames and the number used.
4 The sturdy construction permits the use of considerable pressure difference, and it is normal to use up to about 20 bar.
5 Efficient washing of the cake is possible.
6 Operation and maintenance is straightforward because there are no moving parts, filter cloths and pads are easily renewable and, because all joints are external, any leaks are visible and do not contaminate the filtrate.

Disadvantages   These can be summarized as follows:

1 It is a batch filter, so that there is a good deal of 'down-time', which is non-productive.
2 The filter press is an expensive filter, the emptying time, the labour involved, and the wear and tear on the cloths resulting in high costs.
3 Operation is critical, as the frames should be full; otherwise washing is inefficient and the cake is difficult to remove.
4 The filter press is used for slurries containing

less than about 5% solids; in view of the high labour costs, it is most suitable for expensive materials, many pharmaceutical substances coming into this category. Examples of the use of the filter press include the collection of bismuth salts, the collection of precipitated antitoxins, and the removal of precipitated proteins from insulin liquors.

The rotary vacuum filter

Filters such as the filter press are batch operated and can handle dilute suspensions economically. In large scale filtration, continuous operation is often desirable when it may be necessary to filter slurries containing a high proportion of solids.

The rotary filter is continuous in operation and has a system for removing the cake that is formed so that it can be run for long periods handling concentrated slurries. A rotary drum filter is shown in section in Fig. 31.7. It can be visualized as two concentric cylinders with the annular space between them divided into a number of septa by radial partitions. The outer cylinder is perforated and covered with a filter cloth. Each septum has a radial connection to a complicated rotating valve whose function is to perform the operations listed

Table 31.1 Rotary filter operation

Zone	Position	Service	Connected to:
Pick-up	Slurry trough	Vacuum	Filtrate receiver
Drainage	—	Vacuum	Filtrate receiver
Washing	Wash sprays	Vacuum	Wash water receiver
Drying	—	Vacuum	Wash receiver
Cake removal	Scraper knife	Compressed air	Filter cake conveyor

Note: in some cases, the same receiver may be used for filtrate and for wash water

in Table 31.1. The cylinder rotates slowly in the slurry which is kept agitated and a vacuum applied to the segments draws filtrate into the septa, depositing a filter cake on the filter cloth. When the deposited cake leaves the slurry bath vacuum is maintained to draw air through the cake thus aiding drainage. This is followed by wash water and further drainage in the drying zone. The cake is removed by the scraper aided by compressed air forced into the septa. It is the function of the rotary valve to direct these services into the septa where they are required.

Rotary filters may be up to 2 m in diameter and 3.5 m in length with a filtration area of around

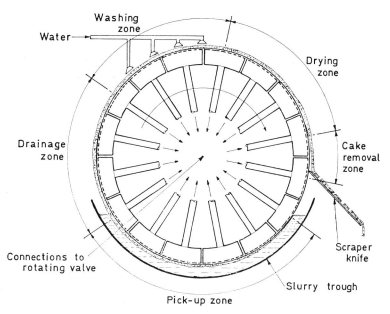

Fig. 31.7 Rotary drum filter

20 m². Special attachments may be included for particular purposes. Cake compression rollers are often fitted to improve the efficiency of washing and draining if the cake forms cracks. Difficult solids which tend to block the filter cloth need a preliminary precoat to be laid down. A filter aid is deposited on the cloth prior to filtration of the slurry. This is easily done by filtering a suspension of the aid. During the actual filtration the scraper knife is set to move slowly inwards removing the blocked outer layer of the filter aid and exposing fresh surface.

If removal of the cake presents problems, the string discharge filter may be employed. This is useful for filtration of the fermentation liquor in the manufacture of antibiotics when a felt-like cake of mould mycelia must be removed. The filter cloth in this case has a number of loops of string passing round the drum and over two additional small rollers as shown in Fig. 31.8. In operation the strings lift the cake off the filter medium and the cake is broken by the sharp bend over the rollers and collected whilst the strings return to the drum.

Advantages These can be summarized as follows:

1 The rotary filter is automatic and continuous in operation, so that labour costs are very low.
2 The filter has a large capacity.
3 Variation of the speed of rotation enables the cake thickness to be controlled, and for solids that form an impenetrable cake the thickness

may be limited to less than 5 mm. On the other hand, if the solids are coarse, forming a porous cake, the thickness may be 100 mm or more.

Disadvantages These can be summarized as follows:

1 The rotary filter is a complex piece of equipment, with many moving parts, and is very expensive. In addition to the filter itself, ancillary equipment such as vacuum pumps, vacuum receivers and traps, slurry pumps and agitators are required.
2 The cake tends to crack due to the air drawn through by the vacuum system, so that washing and drying are not efficient.
3 Being a vacuum filter, the pressure difference is limited to 1 bar and hot filtrates may boil.
4 The rotary filter is suitable only for straightforward slurries, being less satisfactory if the solids form an impermeable cake or will not separate cleanly from the cloth.

Uses of the rotary filter

The rotary filter is most suitable for continuous operation on large quantities of slurry, especially if the slurry contains considerable amounts of solids, that is, in the range 15–30%.

Examples of pharmaceutical applications include the collection of calcium carbonate, magnesium carbonate and starch, and the separation of the mycelia from the fermentation liquor in the manufacture of antibiotics.

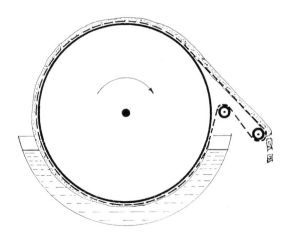

Fig. 31.8 String discharge rotary drum filter

Edge filters

A form of filter that differs markedly from those described above is the type known generally as *edge filters*. Filters such as the leaf or press act by presenting a surface of the filter medium to the slurry. Edge filters use a pack of the filter medium, so that filtration occurs on the edges. Forms using packs of media such as filter paper can be used, but in the pharmaceutical industry greatest use is made of the *metafilter*.

Metafilter

The metafilter, in its simplest form, consists of a

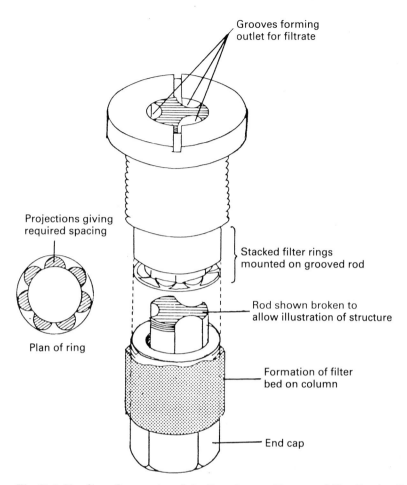

Fig. 31.9 Metafilter. Construction of the filter element. (Courtesy of Metafiltration Co. Ltd)

grooved drainage rod on which is packed a series of metal rings. These rings, usually of stainless steel, are about 15 mm inside diameter, 22 mm outside diameter and 0.8 mm in thickness, with a number of semicircular projections on one surface, as shown in Fig. 31.9. The height of the projections and the shape of the section of the ring are such that when the rings are packed together, all the same way up, and tightened on the drainage rod with a nut, channels are formed that taper from about 250 μm down to 25 μm. One or more of these packs is mounted in a vessel, and the filter may be operated by pumping in the slurry under pressure or, occasionally, by the application of reduced pressure to the outlet side.

In this form, the metafilter can be used as a strainer for coarse particles, but for finer particles a bed of a suitable material such as kieselguhr is first built up. The pack of rings, therefore, serves essentially as a base on which the true filter medium is supported.

Advantages These can be summarized as follows:

1 The metafilter possesses considerable strength and high pressures can be used, with no danger of bursting the filter medium.
2 As there is no filter medium as such, the running costs are low, and it is a very economical filter.
3 The metafilter can be made from materials that can provide excellent resistance to corrosion and avoid contamination of the most sensitive product.
4 By selection of a suitable grade of material to form the filter bed, it is possible to filter off very

fine particles; in fact, it is claimed that some grades will sterilize a liquid by filtration. Equally well, it is possible to remove larger particles simply by building up a bed of coarse substance, or even by using the metafilter 'candle' itself if the particles are sufficiently large.

5 Removal of the cake is effectively carried out by back-flushing with water. If further cleaning is required, it is not normally necessary to do more than slacken the clamping nut on the end of the drainage rod on which the rings are packed.

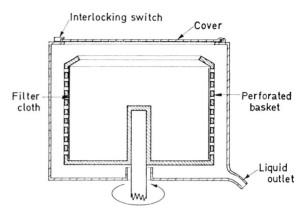

Fig. 31.10 Centrifugal dewatering filter

Uses of the metafilter

The small surface area of the metafilter restricts the amount of solid that can be collected. This, together with the ability to separate very fine particles, means that the metafilter is used almost exclusively for clarification purposes.

Furthermore, the strength of the metafilter permits the use of high pressures (up to 15 bar), making the method suitable for viscous liquids. Also, it can be constructed in materials appropriate for corrosive substances.

Specific examples of pharmaceutical uses include the clarification of syrups, of injection solutions, and of products such as insulin liquors.

Centrifugal filtration

This process finds application as a means of separating crystalline materials such as aspirin from the mother liquor. Cake washing is easy and effective and the residual moisture is often as low as 2%, greatly reducing the energy required for final drying.

A sketch of a 'dewatering' centrifuge is shown in Fig. 31.10. The construction is similar to that of a domestic spin dryer and it has a perforated rotating basket underdriven by a directly coupled electric motor. Other centrifuges have the basket suspended from the motor and are described as overdriven. The basket is lined with a filter cloth. In use the slurry enters the rotating basket through the stationary inlet pipe (omitted for clarity in Fig. 31.10) where it is held by centrifugal pressure vertically against the filter cloth.

The pressure forces the filtrate through the cloth into the space between the basket and the casing. The cake can be washed via the sprays when a suitable thickness has built up.

The centrifugal effect due to a centrifuge is defined as the number of times the centrifugal force is greater than the force due to gravity and is proportional to the product N^2D where N is the number of revolutions per second and D is the basket diameter. It is therefore advantageous to run at high speeds but as the stresses in the basket shell also increase rapidly with speed this sets a limit to the speed used in practice. Industrial centrifuges have diameters up to 2 m and are run around 20 rev s^{-1}.

Continuous centrifugation

The centrifuge described above is operated batch-wise but continuous centrifuges are available for large scale work. These have means for automatic discharge of the cake for a basket which rotates around a horizontal axis in contrast to the vertical axis. Most of the energy required to run a centrifuge is used to bring it up to operating speed and little more is needed to maintain that speed. Continuous centrifuges are therefore cheaper to run but the initial cost is considerably more.

Cross-flow microfiltration

The utility of membrane filters to remove bacteria and fibres from parenterals has been known for some time. In recent years the technology has

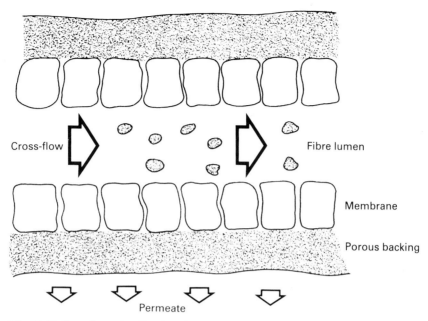

Fig. 31.11 Cross-flow microfiltration. Schematic diagram of an individual fibre

advanced so that membrane filters can be used to filter and separate many materials of pharmaceutical interest. This has been made possible by forming membrane filters within 'hollow fibres'. The membrane, of polysulphone, acrylonitrile or polyamide is laid down within a fibre which forms a rigid porous outer support (Fig. 31.11). The lumen of each fibre is small — typically 1–2 μm but a large number of them can be contained in a surrounding shell to form a cartridge which may have an effective filtration area of over 2 m².

Operation

In use the liquid to be treated is pumped through the cartridge in a circulatory system so that it passes through many times. The filtrate, which in this technique is often called the 'permeate', flows *radially* through the membrane and porous support. The great advantage of this mode of operation is that the high fluid velocity and turbulence (Chapter 2) minimizes blocking of the membranes. The energy consumption is low and at any one time there is a low volume in the circulation loop. Fresh liquid enters the system from a reservoir as filtration proceeds. Since the fluid flows *across* the surface in contrast to flow at right angles this technique is known as *cross-flow* microfiltration.

Uses

The method has been used for fractionation of biological products by first using a filter of pore size sufficient to let all the wanted molecules through and then passing the permeate through a filter which will retain them while passing smaller unwanted molecules. It is claimed that blood plasma can be processed to remove alcohol and water and prepare concentrated purified albumin. The process needs no filter aids and the filtrate is sterile. The process has been suggested for the recovery of antibiotics from fermentation media.

BILIOGRAPHY

Anon (1979) Separating out your filtration requirements. *Mfg Chem. Aerosol News*, **50**(6), 33–34.
Popp, D. M. (1983) Crossflow microfiltration of medical solutions *Filtration and Separation*, **20**(3), 118–122.
Pryoe, K. (1983) Filtration in pharmaceutical practice. *Mfg. Chem. Aerosol News*, **53**(3), 42–44.

Mixing

Mixing may be defined as a process where two or more components are treated so as to lie as nearly as possible in contact with a particle of each of the other components. The aim of the process is to produce one of the following:

1 a blend of solid particles (powder mixing),
2 a suspension of an insoluble solid in a liquid,
3 a mixture of miscible liquids,
4 a dispersion of particles in a semisolid as in the preparation of ointments or pastes.

A mixing stage is involved at some time in the preparation of practically every pharmaceutical preparation.

THEORY OF MIXING

Types of mixtures

Miscible liquids, gases and vapours will in time completely mix spontaneously by diffusion and no energy need be used for this to occur. This *positive mixing* may be contrasted with the *negative mixing* of insoluble solid particles with a liquid where the particles will separate out unless work is done by stirring to keep them dispersed. A mixture of powdered constituents is an example of a *neutral* mix. Work must be done to mix them initially but usually there is then no tendency for demixing to occur spontaneously; though demixing is possible in certain circumstances.

The mixing process

To simplify discussion the principles of mixing will be considered by reference to a system consisting of *equal* quantities of two constituents

Fig. 32.1 Powder mixing: (a) segregated particles (b) ideal mixing (c) random mixing

A and B of the same size and shape though those conditions are rarely found in practice.

The process can be represented by representing the materials as filled and open squares in Fig. 32.1. Fig. 32.1(a) shows the particles in a completely segregated state prior to mixing. As mixing proceeds it is just conceivable that a so-called *perfect* mix may be produced where each particle lies adjacent to a particle of the other component (Fig. 32.1(b)). The odds against this happening are so great that the best attainable mix will actually be a *random mix* represented by Fig. 32.1(c). A random mix may be defined as one where the probability of sampling a particular type of particle is proportional to the number of such particles on the total mix. In a large number of trials where single particles were withdrawn there would be around the same number of each type, drawn from the random mix. In a small number of trials a 'run' of a number of black or a number of white may be encountered due to chance just as a coin may fall 'heads' in three or four consecutive trials but is very unlikely to do so in a greater number of trials.

The scale of scrutiny

Figure 32.1(c) can also be viewed as a fairly large sample taken from a 50/50 bulk mix containing many thousands of particles. It contains 196 black particles and 204 white which is overall not far

(a)

(194)

20 × 20 50% RANDOM MIX

(b)

(202)

20 × 20 50% RANDOM MIX

(c)

(198)

20 × 20 50% RANDOM MIX

Fig. 32.2 Computer generated mixtures of nominal 50% active ingredient. The numbers in parentheses refer to the number of 'white' particles in the mix, theoretically 200

from the required result of 200 of each. Figures 32.2–32.4 are distribution patterns generated using a computer program simulating the taking of such samples from a *random* mix. No 'sample' in Fig. 32.2 contains exactly 200 of each but the deviation is small and acceptable.

If the proportion of one component is reduced then the variation between samples is increased. Figure 32.3 is a printout for a nominal 10% content. Fig. 32.4 shows the position when the computer was instructed to print 'samples' containing 36 particles of nominal 50% content.

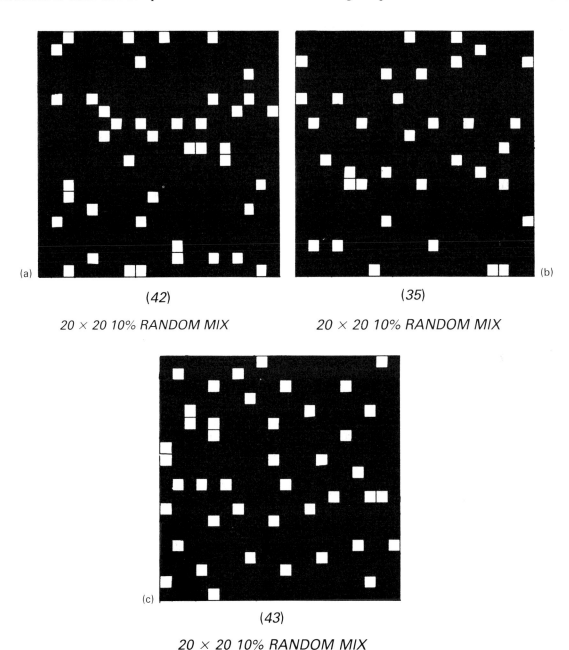

(a)   (b)

(42)   (35)

20 × 20 10% RANDOM MIX   *20 × 20 10% RANDOM MIX*

(c)

(43)

20 × 20 10% RANDOM MIX

Fig. 32.3 Computer generated mixtures of nominal 10% active ingredient. The numbers in parentheses refer to the number of 'white' particles in each mix, theoretically 40

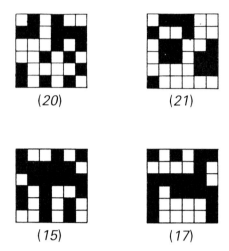

(20)   *(21)*

(15)   *(17)*

6 × 6 50% RANDOM MIX

Fig. 32.4 Computer generated mixtures of nominal 50% active ingredient showing the effect of small sample size. The numbers in parentheses refer to the number of 'white' particles in each mix, theoretically 18

Table 32.1 Results of computer simulation of sampling from a 1:1000 powder mix

Trial Number	Scale of scrutiny (no. of particles)		
	1000	10 000	100 000
1	0	8	101
2	0	6	89
3	1	10	104
4	0	5	101
5	0	4	96
6	1	14	115
7	0	8	92
8	0	10	104
9	1	9	96
10	0	15	104

The figures are the numbers of particles of minor constituent in the samples.

None has the mean number (18) of each component and the sample with only 15 particles is 16% deficient. These diagrams illustrate the important fact that 'low dose' preparations with scattered particles of the minor ingredient will show greater variation in their samples.

Consider a large weight of powder mix which may be subsequently converted into a batch of tablets. The number of particles present in each tablet will depend on the correct weight and particle size of the ingredients and the distribution of the drug should be judged on this unit weight as the sample weight or 'scale of scrutiny'.

It is of little consequence how the drug is dispersed within this weight but it is important that the scale of scrutiny should contain enough particles to avoid undue variation between tablets. The ingredients should therefore be of small particle size though decreasing this unduly may lead to aggregation where the fine particles adhere together to form agglomerates scattered throughout the mix.

The importance of the scale of scrutiny is well illustrated by the results given in Table 32.1 which were obtained from a computer simulation of sampling from a mix containing one part in one thousand of the minor constituent. The largest

sample size has an acceptable 'composition' with the content clustered around the expected mean of 100 per sample. The variation in the samples containing 10 000 particles would be unacceptably large for a real product such as a tablet or capsule.

Degree of mixing

It should be stressed that there is always some variation in the composition of samples drawn from a random mix and the standard deviation in the composition of a large number of such samples can be determined if an accurate assay method is available. A random mix, which is the best possible mix, will give samples with a *lower* standard deviation (S) than mixes of the same components which have not been mixed completely to the random state. This fact can be used to define a mixing index.

$$M = \frac{S_r}{S_{act}}$$

Where S_r is the standard deviation of samples drawn from a fully random mix and S_{act} is the actual standard deviation determined on the partially mixed system. As S_{act} is larger than S_r the mixing index approaches 1 as the mix becomes random. Several other more complicated mixing indices have been proposed but they all depend on similar principles.

THE MIXING OF POWDERED MATERIALS

The mixing of powders is often difficult especially if a small quantity of a potent substance whose dose may be measured in μg is to be mixed with a much larger quantity of diluent to form the dose weight of a tablet or capsule. The particles of drug and diluent may differ in size and shape, adding to the difficulty.

Mechanisms of powder mixing — convective, shear and diffusive mixing

If a spatula is inserted into a heap of powder on a tile then a small pile may be withdrawn on the blade and deposited elsewhere — convective mixing. At the same time an unstable shear plane is created which then collapses and produces some further mixing in the heap. Such shear and convective mixing will occur whenever a blade or ribbon moves through a powder mass and several industrial mixers operate on this principle.

There is a third mixing mechanism which is known as diffusive mixing. It can occur, for instance, in a drum mixer. In its simplest form this is a rotating cylinder in which the mix is lifted past its angle of repose (Chapter 36) so that the particles tumble over each other. There is a difference in velocity with the fastest layers near to the surface and individual particles can migrate from layer to layer in a number which is in some respects similar to the diffusion of molecules in liquids and gels.

Since diffusive mixing involves individual particles, it can in time produce a truly random mix. Shear and convective mixing can quickly produce a *rough* mix but local groups of particles may remain unseparated unless subjected to diffusive mixing. Care must be taken to allow sufficient time of mixing but for many purposes a non-random mix may be quite satisfactory.

Influence of powder aggregates on mixing

Although theory suggests that fine powders should form better mixes by increasing the number of particles in a given sample weight there is a complication caused by the increase in cohesion as the particle size decreases. The effect has been extensively investigated by Orr *et al.* (1980) who found marked variation between commercial samples of ethinyloestradiol tablets of the same nominal dose which was due to this cause. Vigorous convection and shear mixing are required to break up aggregates and disperse the particles into the bulk.

Segregation (demixing)

Powder mixes met in practice will not be composed of unisize spherical particles and certain factors may then operate when a degree of mixing has taken place which causes segregation (demixing) at the same rate as mixing occurs. If that is the case then a random mix will not be formed no matter how long mixing is continued.

The main factors promoting segregation are differences in particle size, shape and density. Smaller particles may fall through the voids between larger particles and thus make their way towards the bottom of the mass. The same effect can be caused by a difference in density even if particles are of equal size but particle size difference is the main cause of segregation.

Segregation may occur on discharge of a mixed powder for handling elsewhere. In recent years equipment which can perform both mixing and other operations in the same vessel has become popular. This avoids handling the mass between operations.

Types of segregation

Percolation segregation This is the name given to the movement of particles through the voids in the powder bed. It will occur in a static bed if the percolating particles are so small that they can fall into the void spaces between the larger particles. The percolation also takes place for a short distance on either side of shear planes formed during the mixing process and for this to occur there need be very little difference in particle diameters. This is because of dilatation along the planes which separate the particles sufficiently for smaller particles to move downwards.

Trajectory segregation During mixing particles are set in motion and kinetic energy is imparted to them. Larger particles have larger energies and tend to move a greater distance into the powder mass before they are brought to rest. This may result in preferential separation and it can occur in horizontal as well as vertical planes.

Densification segregation   Segregation due to density differences between particles may cause segregation if the mass is subject to vibration. This can occur, for instance, in the hopper of a tablet machine and it is actively promoted in vibratory sieving (Chapter 35) so as to place smaller particles directly over the mesh. It is found that large dense particles move upwards through the mass. One explanation for this is that the smaller particles beneath a dense large particle are slightly compacted, supporting the large particle. On vibration the smaller particles move beneath it and raise it upwards in the bed — the process being repeated as time goes on. For a more detailed account of this and other mixing phenomena the reader is referred to an excellent review by Staniforth (1982).

Effect of mixing time on segregation

Non-segregation mixes will continue to improve with an extended mixing time but the reverse may be true for segregating mixes. Cook and Hersey (1974) studied the mixing of fenfluramine and quinalbarbitone with various diluents in a Nauta mixer and found that the mixes worsened after 8–10 minutes. That was because the factors promoting segregation require a longer time to establish a segregation mix than is needed to produce a reasonable degree of mixing. It is therefore disadvantageous to prolong the mixing time beyond an optimum point.

Ordered mixing

If one of the constituents of a powder mix is added in a fine, often micronized form, then on mixing the *larger* particles — termed carrier particles — may adsorb some of these very small particles on to active sites on their surface and these are held tenaciously. The effect was first noticed during the mixing of micronized sodium bicarbonate with sucrose crystals when the mixture was found to be markedly stable towards segregation (Travers and White, 1971). Cook and Hersey (1974) termed

such mixes 'ordered' since in contrast to random mixes, the constituent particles are not independent of each other and sampling a host particle necessitates removing some of the adsorbed particles with it.

The practical importance of ordered mixing

It appears that the mixing of powders routinely met with in pharmaceutical processing is rarely purely random in that some interaction and cohesion will occur between constituents leading to a mix which is partly ordered and partly random. That is so regardless of the relative particle sizes of the constituents.

Johnson (1979) for example found that in the mixing of tetracyline with lactose the mix was partially ordered with some tetracyline absorbed on the surface of the crystalline and spray-dried lactose which he used as (separate) diluents while some remained free and randomly distributed. It is now recognized that ordered mixing is an important factor preventing the segregation of mixes of a drug with one or other of the direct compression bases that are discussed in Chapter 39.

Segregation of ordered mixes

Notwithstanding the above, it is possible for segregation to occur in an ordered mix in certain circumstances which are discussed below.

Ordered unit segregation   This may occur if there are size differences between particles of the carrier constituent since the larger particles are usually associated with more adsorbed material than the smaller particles. Segregation of the carrier particles can then result in drug-rich areas in the mix — resulting in ordered unit segregation.

Johnson in the work referred to above found that this could occur when coarse crystalline lactose was used as diluent and it could be avoided with finer grades which acted as carriers of uniform particle size.

Displacement segregation   The addition of another constituent to an ordered mix may result in competition for the available sites on the carrier particles and some adsorbed particles may be

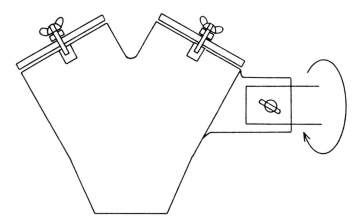

Fig. 32.5 A Y-cone blender

displaced. Magnesium stearate is commonly added as a lubricant to granulates and Lai and Hersey (1979) have demonstrated that this can displace adsorbed drugs under certain circumstances.

Saturation segregation As there are only a certain number of sites on the carrier particles any excess material will rapidly segregate by percolation if too much is added. There is some evidence that certain sites are stronger than others and particles held on the weaker sites may become dislodged if the mix is vibrated vigorously.

Industrial powder mixers

Tumbling mixers

Free-flowing material can be mixed in tumbling mixers which are rotating vessels of various shapes so that the charge flows with the vessel when the angle of repose is exceeded.

The Y-cone mixer is a good example of this type (Fig. 32.5). On rotation the charge flows into the two top arms of the Y and then back into the third arm. Mixing by shear and diffusion takes place when the streams mingle. The mixer is often used to blend in lubricant with tablet granules prior to compression when the gentle action is an advantage. Time must be allowed for the mix to flow into the arms and there is an optimum speed of rotation. Other tumbling mixers have the mixer vessel in the shape of a cube or double cone and prongs may be fixed in the vessel to increase convective mixing.

Agitator mixers

These mixers depend on the motion of a blade or paddle through the charge producing a high degree of convective mixing. The ribbon mixer (Fig. 32.6) is a common type. The helical blades rotate in a hemispherical trough but 'dead spaces' are difficult to eliminate and the shearing action of the ribbon may be insufficient to break up aggregates.

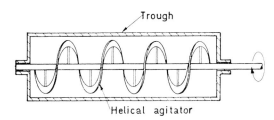

Fig. 32.6 Agitated powder mixer

A more recent type of agitator mixer is the Nautamixer (Fig. 32.7). It consists of a conical vessel fitted at the base with a rotating screw which is fastened to the end of a rotating arm at the upper end. The screw conveys material to near the top where it cascades back into the mass. The mixer thus combines diffusive, shear and convective mixing with an avoidance of dead spots since the screw visits each part of the interior in each revolution as the arm rotates.

High speed granulators

As stated earlier, there has been a trend towards

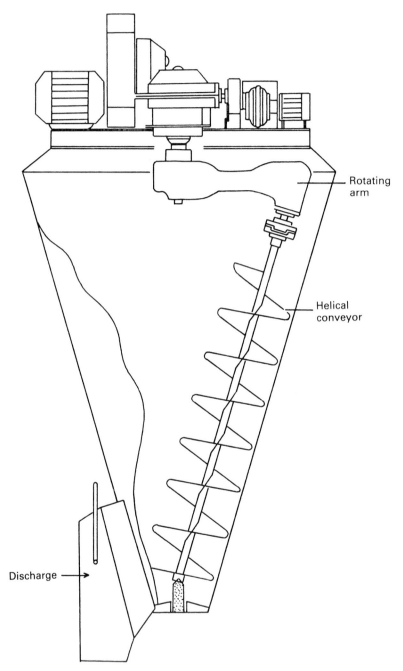

Fig. 32.7 A Nautamixer. (Courtesy of Nautamixer Ltd)

the use of composite equipment in the pharmaceutical industry. A good example is the high speed mixer/granulator combining both these operations (Fig. 32.8).

One type has a central impeller mounted as shown in Fig. 32.9. When the mix is rotated, the mixer acts to fluidize it without the need to blow air through the mass as in a fluidized bed drier (Chapter 38). When thoroughly mixed the granulating agent can be added and distributed at a

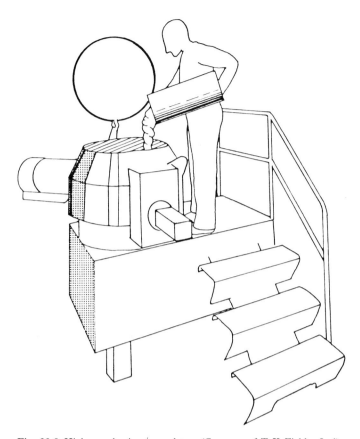

Fig. 32.8 High speed mixer/granulator. (Courtesy of T K Fielder Ltd)

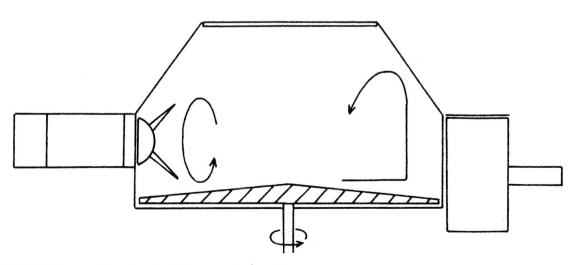

Fig. 32.9 Diagrammatic section of a high speed mixer/granulator

slower speed. The damp mass is reduced to granules by the side entering chopper blade.

The Diosna mixer/granulator (Chapter 37) is another example of this type.

Scale-up of powder mixing

Development work on a new product must of necessity be on a bench scale. There is then no guarantee that a mixing process will be satisfactory on a manufacturing scale even if a larger mixer of the same type can be used. This point was illustrated by the work of Delonca *et al* (1982) who examined the homogeneity of a sulphaguanidine/lactose mix prepared in plough mixers of different size. The bench size (5 litre) mixer yielded a poor mix but a 20 litre model gave better mixes comparable in quality to those obtained from a large (130 litre) model. In that instance the mix improved in scale-up. In another case drug deficiency in a production scale mix was traced to adsorption of the minor constituent on the mixer wall which did not occur on bench scale working.

That example illustrates the need for testing and validation at every stage in the manufacture of a new product.

THE MIXING OF MISCIBLE LIQUIDS AND SUSPENSIONS

Mobile liquids with a low coefficient of viscosity are easily mixed with each other. Solid particles are also readily suspended though these particles will settle rapidly when mixing is discontinued. More viscous liquids are difficult to stir but suspended particles will settle slowly through at a lower rate than predicted by Stokes' law because of 'hindering' by other particles.

Propeller mixers

A common arrangement for medium scale fluid mixing is a propeller type stirrer which is often used clamped to the edge of a vessel. A propeller has angled blades which cause the circulation of the fluid in both an axial and radial direction. The off-

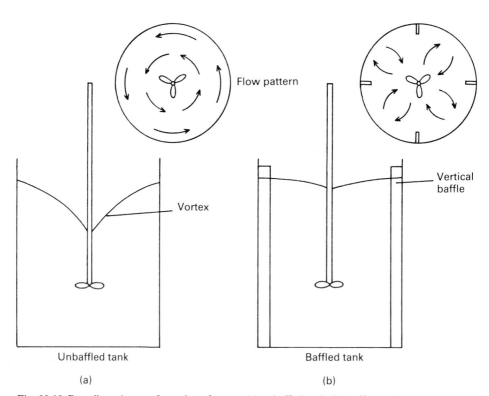

Fig. 32.10 Propeller mixer — formation of vortex (a) unbaffled tank (b) baffled tank

centre mounting discourages the formation of a vortex which may form when the stirrer is mounted centrally. A vortex forms when the circumferential motion imparted to the liquid by the propeller causes it to back up round the sites of the vessel and form a depression around the shaft. As the speed of rotation is increased air may be sucked into the fluid with frothing and possible oxidation (Fig. 32.10(a)). Another method of suppressing a vortex is to fit vertical baffles into the vessel. These divert the rotating fluid from its circular path into the centre of the vessel where the vortex would otherwise form (Fig. 32.10(b)).

Turbine mixers

The propeller stirrer depends for its action on a satisfactory axial and radial flow pattern and this will not occur if the fluid is viscous. The ratio of the diameter of a propeller stirrer to the diameter of the vessel is commonly 1 : 10 to 1 : 20 and it operates at speeds of $1-20$ rev s^{-1}. There must be a fast flow of fluid towards the propeller which can only occur if the fluid is mobile.

A turbine mixer may be used for more viscous fluids and a typical construction is given in Fig. 32.11. The impeller has four flat blades surrounded by perforated inner and outer diffuser rings. The rotating impeller forces the liquid through the perforations with considerable radial velocity sufficient to overcome the viscous drag of the bulk of the fluid. One drawback is the absence of an axial component but a different head with the perforations pointing upwards can be fitted if this is desired.

The high shear forces as the liquid is forced through the orifices also enable such mixers to produce emulsions of immiscible liquids. Turbine type mixes will not deal with liquids of very high viscosity which are best treated as semisolids and handled in the same equipment as used for such materials.

In-line mixers

As an alternative to mixing fluids in vessels mobile miscible components may be fed through an 'in-line' mixer designed to create turbulence in the stream.

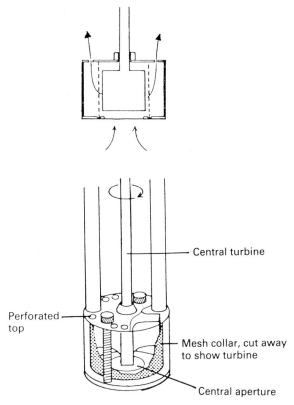

Fig. 32.11 Turbine mixer. (Courtesy of Silverson Mixers Ltd)

THE MIXING OF SEMISOLIDS

The problems which arise during the mixing of semisolids (ointments and pastes) stem from the fact that unlike powders and liquids, semisolids will not flow easily. Material that finds its way to 'dead' spots will remain there. For that reason suitable mixers must have rotating elements with narrow clearances between the mixing vessel and they must produce a high degree of shear mixing since diffusion and convective mixing cannot occur.

Mixers for semisolids

The planetary mixer

This type of mixer is commonly found in the domestic kitchen (Kenwood mixers) and larger machines which operate on the same principle are used in industry.

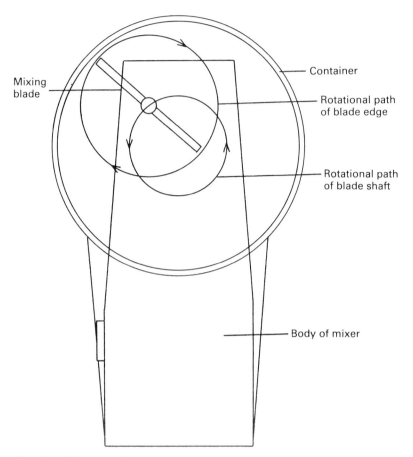

Fig. 32.12 Planetary mixer — top view showing path of paddle

The mixing paddle is set off centre and is carried on a rotating arm. It therefore travels round the circumference of the mixing bowl while simultaneously rotating around its own axis (Fig. 32.12). A small clearance between the vessel and the paddle gives shear but 'scraping down' several times is necessary to mix the contents well since some materials are forced to the top of the bowl.

The sigma blade mixer

This robust mixer will deal with stiff pastes and ointments and depends for its action on the close intermeshing of the two blades which resemble the Greek letter Σ in shape. The clearance between the blades and the mixing trough is kept small by the shape shown in Fig. 32.13.

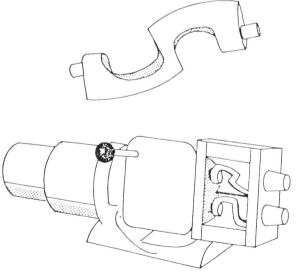

Fig. 32.13 Sigma- arm mixer

It is very difficult using primary mixers to completely disperse powder particles in a semi-solid base so that they are invisible to the eye. The mix is usually subjected to the further action of a roller mill or colloid mill so as to 'rub out' these particles by the intense shear generated by rollers or cones set with a very small clearance between them.

REFERENCES AND BIBLIOGRAPHY

Cook, P. and Hersey, J. A. (1974) Powder mixing in the tabletting of fenfluramine hydrochloride; evaluation of a mixer. *J. Pharm. Pharmacol.*, **26**, 298–303.

Delonca, H., Jeannin, C., Joachim, J., Romier, G. and Verain, A. (1982) Scaling tests on plough mixers. *Int. J. pharm. Tech prod. Mfr*, **3**(3), 87–92.

Johnson, M. C. R. (1979) Powder mixing in a direct compression formulation by ordered and random processes. *J. Pharm. Pharmacol.*, **31**, 273–276.

Lai, F. K. and Hersey, J. A. (1979) A cautionary note on the use of ordered mixtures in pharmaceutical dosage forms. *J. Pharm. Pharmacol.*, **31**, 800.

Orr, N. A., Hill, E. A. and Smith, J.F. (1980) Dosage uniformity in hydrocortisone ointment BP. *J. Pharm. Pharmacol.*, **32**, 766–772.

Rothman, H. (1981) High speed mixing in the pharmaceutical industry. *Mfg. Chem. Aerosol News*, **52**(4), 47–49.

Staniforth, J. N. (1982) advances in powder mixing and segregation in relation to pharmaceutical processing. *Int. J. pharm. Tech. prod. Mfr*, **3**(Suppl), 1–12.

Travers, D. N. and White, R. C. (1971) The mixing of micronized sodium bicarbonate with sucrose crystals. *J. Pharm. Pharmacol.*, **23** Suppl., 260S–261S.

Particle size analysis

PARTICLE SIZE AND THE LIFETIME OF A DRUG

The dimensions of particulate solids are of importance in achieving optimum production of efficacious medicines. Figure 33.1 shows an outline of the lifetime of a drug; during stages 1 and 2 when a drug is synthesized and formulated, the particle size of drug and other powders is determined and influences the subsequent physical performance of the medicine and the pharmacological performance of the drug.

Particle size influences the production of formulated medicines (stage 3, Fig. 33.1) as solid dosage forms. Both tablets and capsules are produced using equipment which controls the mass of drug and other particles by volumetric filling. Therefore, any interference with the uniformity of fill volumes may alter the mass of drug incorporated into the tablet or capsule and thus reduce the content uniformity of the medicine. Powders with different particle sizes have different flow and packing properties which alter the volumes of powder during each encapsulation or tablet compression event. In order to avoid such problems the particle sizes of drug and other

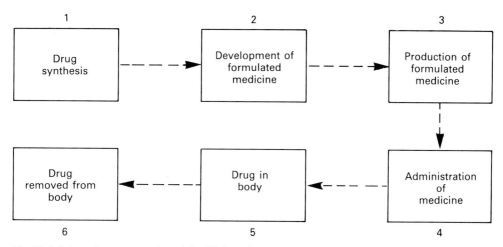

Fig. 33.1 Schematic representation of the lifetime of a drug

powder may be defined during formulation so that problems during production are avoided.

Following administration of the medicine (stage 4, Fig. 33.1), the dosage form should release the drug into solution at the optimum rate. The rate of solution depends on several factors, one of which will be the particle size of drug as predicted from the following theoretical considerations. Noyes and Whitney first showed that the rate of solution of a solid was related to the law of diffusion and proposed that the following equations could be used to predict the rate of solution of a wide variety of solutes.

$$\frac{dx}{dt} = c(C_s - C) \tag{33.1}$$

$$c = \frac{1}{t} \log_e \frac{C_s}{C_s - C} \tag{33.2}$$

where C is the concentration of solute in solution at time, t; C_s is the solubility of solute and c is a constant which can be determined from a knowledge of solute solubility. The constant c was more precisely defined by Danckwerts, who showed that the mean rate of solution per unit area under turbulent conditions was given by

$$\frac{dx}{dt} = D\sigma (C_s - C) \tag{33.3}$$

where D is a diffusion coefficient and σ is the rate of production of fresh surface. $D\sigma$ can be interpreted as a liquid film mass transfer coefficient which will tend to vary inversely with particle

size, since a reduction in size generally increases the specific surface area of particles. Thus, particles having small dimensions will tend to increase the rate of solution. For example, the drug griseofulvin has a low solubility by oral administration but is rapidly distributed following absorption; the solubility of griseofulvin can be greatly enhanced by particle size reduction, so that blood levels equivalent to, or better than, those obtained with crystalline griseofulvin can be produced using a microcrystalline form of the drug. Similar examples of a reduction in particle size improving the rate of solution include tetracycline, aspirin and some sulphonamides. A reduction of particle size to improve rate of solution and hence bioavailability is not always beneficial. For example, small particle size nitrofurantoin has an increased rate of solution which produces toxic side effects because of its more rapid absorption.

It is clear from the lifetime of a drug outlined above that a knowledge and control of particle size is of importance both for the production of medicines containing particulate solids and in the efficacy of the medicine following administration.

PARTICLE SIZE

Dimensions

When determining the size of a relatively large solid it would be unusual to measure fewer than three dimensions, but if the same solid was broken up and the fragments milled, the resulting fine particles would be irregular with different numbers of faces and it would be difficult or impractical to determine more than a single dimension. For this reason a solid particle is often considered to approximate to a sphere which can then be characterized by determination of its diameter. Because measurement is then based on a hypothetical sphere which represents only an approximation to the true shape of the particle, the dimension is referred to as the equivalent diameter of the particle.

Equivalent diameters

It is possible to generate more than one sphere which is equivalent to a given irregular particle shape. Figure 33.2 shows the two-dimensional projection of a particle with two different diameters constructed about it. The projected area diameter is based on a circle of equivalent area to that of the projected image of a solid particle; the projected perimeter diameter is based on a circle having the same perimeter as the particle. Unless the particles are unsymmetrical in three dimensions then these two diameters will be independent of particle orientation. This is not true for Feret's and Martin's diameters (Fig. 33.3) the values of which are dependent on both the orientation and the shape of the particles. These are statistical diameters which are averaged over many different orientations to produce a mean value for each particle diameter. Feret's diameter is determined from the mean distance between two

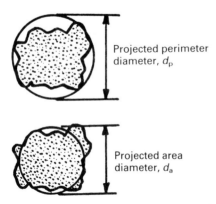

Fig. 33.2 Different equivalent diameters constructed around the same particle

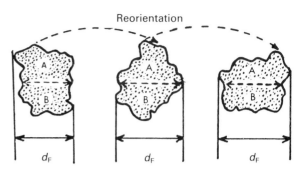

Fig. 33.3 Influence of particle orientation on statistical diameters. The change in Feret's diameter is shown by the distances, d_F; Martins diameter d_M corresponds to the dotted lines in the mid-part of each image

parallel tangents to the projected particle perimeter. Martin's diameter is the mean chord length of the projected particle perimeter, which can be considered as the boundary separating equal particle areas (A and B in Fig. 33.3).

It is also possible to determine particle size based on spheres of, for example, equivalent volume, sedimentation volume, mass or sieve mass of a given particle. In general, the method used to determine particle size dictates the type of equivalent diameter which is measured although interconversion may be carried out and this is sometimes done automatically as part of the size analysis.

Particle size distribution

A particle population which consists of spheres or equivalent spheres with uniform dimensions is monosized and its characteristics can be described by a single diameter or equivalent diameter.

However, it is unusual for particles to be completely monosized; most powders contain particles with a large number of different equivalent diameters. In order to be able to define a size distribution or compare the characteristics of two or more powders consisting of particles with many different diameters, the size distribution can be broken down into different size ranges which can be presented in the form of a histogram plotted from data such as that in Table 33.1. Such a histogram presents an interpretation of the particle size distribution and enables the percentage of particles having a given equivalent diameter to be determined. A histogram representation allows

Table 33.1 Frequency distribution data

Equivalent particle diameter (μm)	Number of particles in each diameter range (frequency)	Per cent particles in each diameter range (per cent frequency)
2	1	4.5
4	2	9.1
6	4	18.2
8	8	36.4
10	4	18.2
12	2	9.1
14	1	4.5

Table 33.2 Cumulative frequency distribution data

Equivalent particle diameter (μm)	Per cent frequency (from Table 33.1)	Cumulative per cent frequency	
		Undersize	Oversize
2	4.5	4.5	100
4	9.1	13.6	95.5
6	18.2	31.8	86.4
8	36.4	68.2	68.2
10	18.2	86.4	31.8
12	9.1	95.5	13.6
14	4.5	100	4.5

different particle size distributions to be compared; for example, the size distribution shown in Fig. 33.4(b) contains a larger proportion of fine particles than the powder in Fig. 33.4(a) in which the particles are normally distributed. The peak frequency value, known as the *mode*, separates the normal curve into two identical halves, because the size distribution is fully symmetrical. Not all particle populations are characterized by symmetrical normal size distributions and the frequency distributions of such populations exhibit skewness (Fig. 33.4(b)). A frequency curve with an elongated tail towards higher size ranges is positively skewed (Fig. 33.4(b)), the reverse case exhibits negative skewness. These skewed distributions can sometimes be normalized by replotting the equivalent particle diameters using a logarithmic scale and are thus usually referred to as log normal distributions. In some size distributions, more than one mode occurs; Fig. 33.4(c) shows bimodal frequency distribution for a powder which has been subjected to milling. Some of the coarser particles from the unmilled population remain unbroken and produce a mode towards the highest particle size, whereas the frac-

tured particles have a new mode which appears lower down the size range.

An alternative to the histogram representation of a particle size distribution is obtained by sequentially adding the per cent frequency values as shown in Table 33.2, to produce a cumulative per cent frequency distribution. If the addition sequence begins with the coarsest particles, the values obtained will be cumulative per cent frequency undersize; the reverse case produces a cumulative per cent oversize. Figure 33.5 shows two cumulative per cent frequency distributions. Once again it is possible to compare two or more particle populations using the cumulation distribution representation. For example, the size distribution in Fig. 33.5(a) shows that this powder has a larger range or spread of equivalent diameters in comparison with the powder represented in Fig. 33.5(b). The particle diameter corresponding to the point which separates the cumulative frequency curve into two equal halves, above and below which 50% of the particles lie (point *a* in Fig. 33.5(a)). Just as the median divides a symmetrical cumulative size distribution curve into two equal halves, so the lower and upper

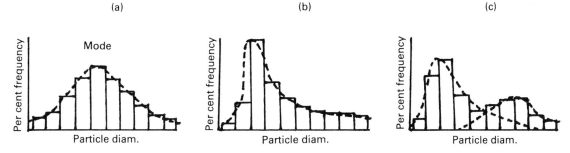

Fig. 33.4 Frequency distribution curves corresponding to (a) a normal distribution, (b) a positively skewed distribution and (c) a bimodal distribution

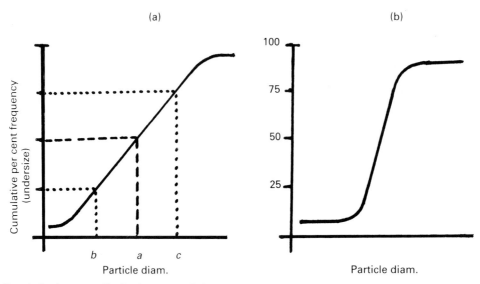

Fig. 33.5 Cumulative frequency distribution curves. Point *a* corresponds to the median diameter; *b* is the lower quartile point and *c* is the upper quartile point

quartile points at 25% and 75% divide the upper and lower ranges of a symmetrical curve into equal parts (points *b* and *c* in Fig. 33.5(a)).

Statistics to summarize data

Although it is possible to describe particle size distributions qualitatively it is always more satisfactory to compare particle size data quantitatively. This is made possible by summarizing the distributions using statistical methods.

In order to quantify the degree of skewness of a particle population, the interquartile coefficient of skewness (IQCS) can be determined

$$IQCS = \frac{(c - a) - (a - b)}{(c - a) + (a - b)} \qquad (33.4)$$

where *a* is the median diameter and *b* and *c* are the lower and upper quartile points (Fig. 33.5).

The IQCS can take any value between -1 and $+1$. If the IQCS is zero then the size distribution is practically symmetrical between the quartile points. To ensure unambiguity in interpreting values for IQCS a large number of size intervals is required.

To quantify the degree of symmetry of a particle size distribution a property known as kurtosis can be determined. The symmetry of a distribution is based on a comparison of the height or thickness of the tails and the 'sharpness' of the peaks with those of a normal distribution. 'Thick' tailed, 'sharp' peaked curves are described as leptokurtic whereas 'thin' tailed, 'blunt' peaked curves are platykurtic and the normal distribution is mesokurtic.

The coefficient of kurtosis, *k* (shown below), has a value of 0 for a normal curve, a negative value for curves showing platykurtosis and positive values for leptokurtic size distributions

$$k = \frac{n \, \Sigma(x - \bar{x})^4}{(\Sigma(x - \bar{x})^2)^2} - 3 \qquad (33.5)$$

where *x* is any particle diameter, $\bar{x}$ is mean particle diameter and *n* is number of particles.

Again, a large number of data points is required to provide an accurate analysis.

The mean of the particle population referred to above in Eqn 33.5, together with the median (Fig. 33.5) and the mode (Fig. 33.4) are all measures of central tendency and provide a single value near the middle of the size distribution which represents a central particle diameter. Whereas the mode and median diameters can be obtained for an incomplete particle size distribution, the mean diameter can only be determined when the size distribution is complete and the upper and lower size limits are known. It is also possible to define and determine the mean in

Table 33.3 Hatch–Choate relationships

$\ln d_n = \ln M + 0.5 \ln^2 \sigma_g$

$\ln d_s = \ln M + \ln^2 \sigma_g$

$\ln d_v = \ln M + 1.5 \ln^2 \sigma_g$

$\ln d_{sv} = \ln M + 2.5 \ln^2 \sigma_g k^1$

$\ln M = \ln d_g + 2.5 \ln^2 \sigma_g k^1$

$\ln d_n = \ln d_g - 2.5 \ln^2 \sigma_w$

$\ln d_s = \ln d_g - 2.0 \ln^2 \sigma_w$

$\ln d_v = \ln d_g - 1.5 \ln^2 \sigma_w$

$\ln d_{sv} = \ln d_g - 0.5 \ln^2 \sigma_w$

Key: M, geometric mean diameter by number (see Eqn 33.6); d_n, number mean diameter; d_s, surface mean diameter; d_v, volume diameter; d_{sv}, surface volume or surface weighted diameter; d_g, geometric mean diameter by weight.

several ways and, for log-normal distributions, a series of relationships known as Hatch–Choate equations link the different mean diameters of a size distribution (Table 33.3).

In a log-normal distribution, the frequency, f, of the occurrence of any given particle of equivalent diameter d is given by

$$f = \frac{\Sigma n}{2\pi \ln\sigma_g} \cdot \exp\left[-\frac{(\ln d - \ln M)^2}{2\ln^2\sigma_g}\right] \quad (33.6)$$

where M is the geometric mean diameter (Chapter 20) and σ_g is the geometric standard deviation.

Influence of particle shape

The techniques discussed above for representing particle size distribution are all based on the assumption that particles could be adequately represented by an equivalent circle or sphere. In some cases particles deviate markedly from circularity and sphericity and the use of a single equivalent diameter measurement may be inappropriate.

For example, a powder consisting of monosized fibrous particles would appear to have a wider size distribution according to statistical diameter measurements. However, use of an equivalent diameter based on projected area would also be misleading. Under such circumstances, it may be desirable to return to the concept of characterizing a particle using more than one dimension. Thus, the breadth of the fibre could be obtained using a projected circle inscribed within the fibre and the fibre length could be measured using a

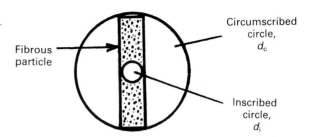

Fig. 33.6 A simple shape factor is shown which can be used to quantify circularity. The ratio i/c of two different diameters is unity for a circle and falls for acicular particles

projected circle circumscribed around the fibre (Fig. 33.6).

The ratio of inscribed circle to circumscribed circle diameters can also be used as a simple shape factor to provide information about the circularity of a particle. The ratio i/c will be 1 for a circle and diminish as the particle becomes more acicular. Such comparisons of equivalent diameters determined by different methods offer considerable scope for both particle size and particle shape analysis. For example, measurement of particle size to obtain a projected area diameter, a, and an equivalent volume diameter, v, provides information concerning the surface:volume (a/v) ratio or bulkiness of a group of particles which can also be useful in interpreting particle size data.

PARTICLE SIZE ANALYSIS METHODS

In order to obtain equivalent diameters with which to interpret the particle size of a powder it is necessary to carry out a size analysis using one or more different methods. Particle size analysis methods can be divided into different categories based on several different criteria: size range of analysis; wet or dry methods; manual or automatic methods; speed of analysis. A summary of the different methods is presented below based on the salient features of each.

Sieve methods

Equivalent diameter

Sieve diameter, d_s – the particle dimension x which passes through a square aperture as shown on the next page.

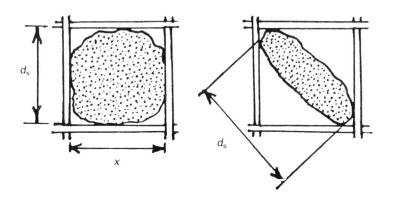
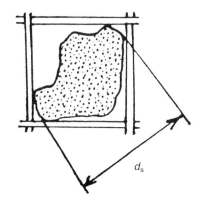

Range of analysis (as shown below)

The International Standards Organization (ISO) sets a lowest sieve diameter of 45 μm and since powders are usually defined as having a maximum diameter of 1000 μm, this could be considered to be the upper limit. In practice sieves can be obtained for size analysis over a range from 5 to 125 000 μm.

Sample preparation and analysis conditions

Sieve analysis is usually carried out using dry powders although, for powders in liquid suspension or which agglomerate during dry sieving, a process of wet sieving can be used.

Principle of measurement

Sieve analysis utilizes a woven, punched or electroformed mesh often in brass, bronze or stainless steel with known aperture diameters which form a physical barrier to particles. Most sieve analyses utilize a series, stack or nest of sieves which have the smallest mesh above a collector tray followed by meshes which get progressively coarser towards the top of the series. A sieve stack usually comprises 6–8 sieves with a progression based on a $\sqrt{2}$ or $2\sqrt{2}$ change in diameter between adjacent apertures. Powder is loaded on to the coarsest sieve of the assembled stack and the nest is subjected to mechanical vibration for, say, 20

minutes. After this time, the particles are considered to be retained on the sieve mesh with an aperture corresponding to the minimum or sieve diameter. A sieving time of 20 minutes is arbitrary and BS 1796 recommends sieving to be continued until less than 0.2% material passes a given sieve aperture in any 5 minute interval.

Alternative techniques

Another form of sieve analysis, called air-jet sieving, uses individual sieves rather than a complete nest of sieves. Starting with the finest aperture sieve and progressively removing the undersize particle fraction by sequentially increasing the apertures of each sieve, particles are encouraged to pass through each aperture under the influence of a partial vacuum applied below the sieve mesh. A reverse air jet circulates beneath the sieve mesh blowing oversize particles away from the mesh so as to prevent blocking. Air-jet sieving is often more efficient and reproducible than using mechanically vibrated sieve analysis, although with finer particles, agglomeration can become a problem.

Automatic methods

Sieve analysis is still largely a non-automated process, although an automated wet sieving technique has been described.

Range of analysis

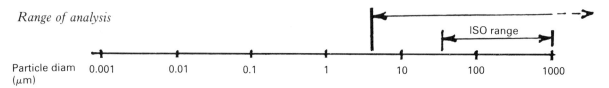

Particle diam
(μm)

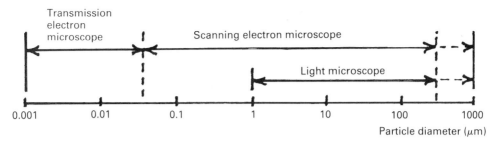

Microscope methods

Equivalent diameters

Projected area diameter, d_a; projected perimeter diameter d_p; Feret's diameter d_F and Martin's diameter d_M (see above).

Range of analysis (see above)

Sample preparation and analysis conditions

Specimens prepared for light microscopy must be adequately dispersed on a microscope slide to avoid analysis of agglomerated particles. Specimens for scanning electron microscopy are prepared by fixing to aluminium stubs or planchettes before sputter coating to produce a film of gold a few nm in thickness. Specimens for transmission electron microscopy are often set in resin and sectioned by microtome before metallic coating on a supporting metal grid.

Principle of measurement

Size analysis by light microscopy is carried out on the two-dimensional images of particles which are generally assumed to be randomly oriented in three-dimensions. In many cases this assumption is valid, although for dendrites, fibres or flakes it is very improbable that the particles will orient with their minimum dimensions in the plane of measurement. Under such conditions, size analysis is carried out accepting that they are viewed in their most stable orientation.

The two-dimensional images are analysed according to the desired equivalent diameter. Using a conventional light microscope, particle size analysis can be carried out using a projection screen with screen distances related to particle dimensions by a previously derived calibration factor using a graticule. A graticule can also be used which has a series of opaque and transparent circles of different diameters, usually in a $\sqrt{2}$ progression [BS 3406]. Particles are compared with the two sets of circles and are sized according to the circle most closely corresponding to the equivalent particle diameter being measured. The field of view is divided into segments to facilitate measurement of different numbers of particles.

Alternative techniques

Alternative techniques to light microscopy include scanning electron microscopy (SEM) and transmission electron microscopy (TEM). Scanning electron microscopy is particularly appropriate when a three-dimensional particle image is required; in addition the very much greater depth of field of a SEM in comparison with a light microscope may also be beneficial. Both SEM and TEM analysis allow the lower particle sizing limit to be greatly extended over that possible with a light microscope.

Automatic methods

Semi-automatic methods of microscope analysis use some form of precalibrated, variable distance to split particles into different size ranges. One technique, called a particle comparator, utilizes a variable diameter light spot projected onto a photomicrograph or electron photomicrograph of a particle under analysis. The variable iris controlling the light spot diameter is linked electronically to a series of counter memories each corresponding to a different size range (Fig. 33.7). Alteration of the iris diameter causes the particle count to be directed into the appropriate counter memory following activation of a switch by the operator.

A second technique uses a double prism

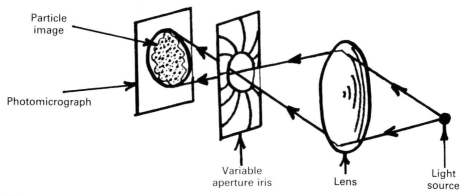

Fig. 33.7 Particle comparator

arrangement mounted in place of the light micro-scope eyepiece. The image from the prisms is usually displayed on a video monitor. The double prism arrangement allows light to pass through to the monitor unaltered where the usual single particle image is produced. When the prisms are sheared against one another a double image of each particle is produced and the separation of the split images corresponds to the degree of shear between the prisms (Fig. 33.8). Particle size analysis can be carried out by shearing the prisms until the two images of a single particle make

touching contact. The prism shearing mechanism is linked to a precalibrated micrometer scale from which the equivalent diameter can be read directly. Alternatively, a complete size distri-bution can be obtained more quickly by subjecting the prisms to a sequentially increased and decreased shear distance between two preset levels corresponding to a known size range. All particles whose images separate and overlap sequentially under a given shear range are considered to fall in this size range and are counted by operating a switch which activates the appropriate counter

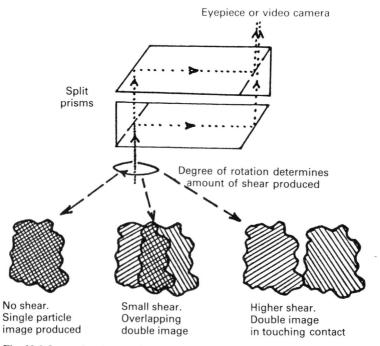

Fig. 33.8 Image-shearing eyepiece

memory. Particles whose images do not overlap in either shear sequence are undersize and particles whose images do not separate in either shear mode are oversize and will be counted in a higher size range.

Although semi-automatic size analysis methods remove some of the objectivity and fatigue associated with manual microscopic analysis, fully automatic size analysis has the advantage of being more objective, very much faster and also enables a much wider variety of size and shape parameters to be processed.

Automatic microscopy is usually associated with microprocessor-controlled manipulation of an analogue signal derived from some form of video monitor used to image particles directly from a light microscope or from photomicrographs of particles. Alternatively, the signal from an electron microscope can in some cases be processed directly without an intermediate video imaging system.

Automatic microscopy allows both image analysis and image processing to be carried out.

Electrical stream sensing zone method (Coulter counter)

Equivalent diameter

Volume diameter, d_v.

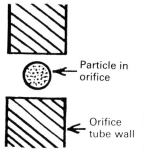

Particle in orifice

Orifice tube wall

Sample preparation and analysis conditions

Powder samples are dispersed in an electrolyte to form a very dilute suspension. The suspension is usually subjected to ultrasonic agitation for a period to break up any particle agglomerates. A dispersant may also be added to aid particle deagglomeration.

Principle of measurement

The particle suspension is drawn through an aperture accurately drilled through a sapphire crystal set into the wall of a hollow glass tube. Electrodes, situated on either side of the aperture and surrounded by an electrolyte solution, monitor the change in electrical signal which occurs when a particle momentarily occupies the orifice and displaces its own volume of electrolyte. The volume of suspension drawn through the orifice is determined by the suction potential created by a mercury thread rebalancing in a convoluted U-tube (Fig. 33.9). The volume of electrolyte fluid which is displaced in the orifice by the presence of a particle causes a change in electrical resistance between the electrodes which is proportional to the volume of the particle. The change in resistance is converted into a voltage pulse which is amplified and processed electronically. Pulses falling within precalibrated limits or thresholds are used to split the particle size distribution into many different size ranges. In order to carry out size analysis over a wide diameter range it will be necessary to change the orifice diameter used, to prevent coarser particles blocking a small diameter orifice. Conversely, finer particles in a large diameter orifice will cause too small a relative change in volume to be accurately quantified.

Range of analysis

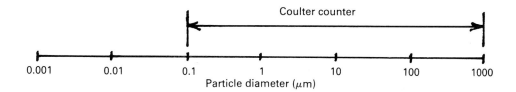

Coulter counter

0.001   0.01   0.1   1   10   100   1000

Particle diameter (μm)

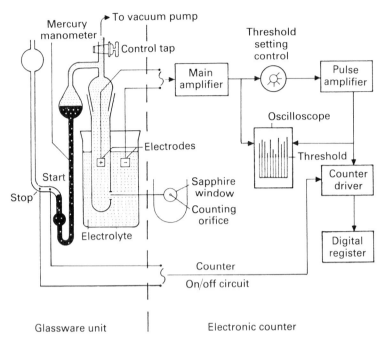

Fig. 33.9 Diagram of Coulter counter

Alternative techniques

Since the Coulter principle was first described there have been some modifications to the basic method such as use of alternative orifice designs and hydrodynamic focusing, but in general the particle detection technique remains the same.

Another type of stream sensing analyser utilizes the attenuation of a light beam by particles drawn through the sensing zone. Some instruments of this type use the change in reflectance whilst others use the change in transmittance of light. It is also possible to use ultrasonic waves generated and monitored by a piezoelectric crystal at the base of a flowthrough tube containing particles in fluid suspension.

Laser light scattering methods

Equivalent diameters

Area diameter, d_a; volume diameter d_v following computation in some instruments.

Range of analysis (as shown below).

Sample preparation and analysis conditions

Depending on the type of measurement to be carried out and the instrument used, particles can be presented either in liquid or air suspension.

Principles of measurement

Both the large-particle and small-particle analysers are based on the interaction of laser light with

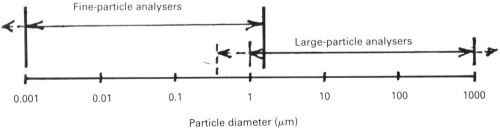

particles. For particles which are much larger than the wavelength of light, any interaction with particles causes light to be scattered in a forward direction with only a small change in angle. This phenomenon is known as Fraunhofer diffraction and produces light intensity patterns which occur at regular angular intervals and are proportional to the particle diameter producing the scatter (Fig. 33.10). The composite diffraction pattern produced by different diameter particles may be considered to be the sum of all the individual

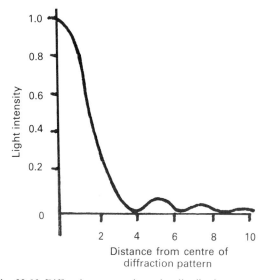

Fig. 33.10 Diffraction pattern intensity distribution

patterns produced by each particle in the size distribution.

Light emitted by a helium–neon laser is incident on the sample of particles and diffraction occurs. In some cases the scattered light is focused by a lens directly on to a photodetector which converts the signals into an equivalent area diameter. In other cases the scattered light is directed by a lens on to a rotating filter which is used to convert equivalent area diameters into volume diameters which are quantified by final focusing on to a photodetector using a second lens. The light flux signals occurring on the photodetector are converted into electrical current which is digitized and processed into size distribution data using a microprocessor (Fig. 33.11).

Analysis of small particle sizes can be carried out based on diffraction of light or by photon correlation spectroscopy.

In the former case, Fraunhofer diffraction theory is still useful for the particle fraction which is significantly larger than the wavelength of laser light. As particles approach the dimension of the wavelength of the light, some light is still scattered in the forward direction, according to Mie scatter theory, but there is also some side scatter at different wavelengths and polarizations. Use of the Mie theory requires a knowledge of the refractive index of the sample material for calculation of particle size distributions.

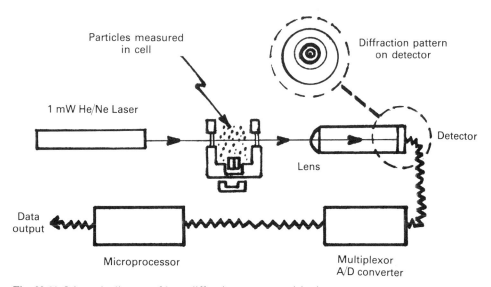

Fig. 33.11 Schematic diagram of laser diffraction pattern particle sizer

In the case of photon correlation spectroscopy (p.c.s.), the principle of Brownian motion is used to measure particle size. Brownian motion is the random movement of a small particle or macromolecule caused by collisions with the smaller molecules of the suspending fluid. It is independent of external variations except viscosity of fluid and temperature and as it randomizes particle orientations, any effects of particle shape are minimized. Brownian motion is independent of the suspending medium and while increasing the viscosity does slow down the motion, the amplitude of the movements is unaltered. Since the suspended small particles are always in a state of motion, they undergo diffusion. Diffusion is governed by the mean free path of a molecule or particle which is the average distance of travel before diversion by collision with another molecule. P.c.s. analyses the constantly changing patterns of laser light scattered or diffracted by particles in Brownian motion and monitors the rate of change of scattered light during diffusion.

Particle movement during Brownian diffusion, D, is a three-dimensional random walk where the mean distance travelled, $\bar{x}$, does not increase linearly with time, t, but according to the following relationship:

$$\bar{x} = \sqrt{Dt}$$

A basic property of molecular kinetics is that each particle or macromolecule has the same average thermal or kinetic energy, E, regardless of mass, size or shape:

$$E = kT$$

where k is Boltzmann's constant and T is absolute temperature (Kelvin).

Thus at $T = 0K$, molecules possess zero kinetic energy and therefore do not move. E can also be equated with the driving force, F, of particle motion:

$$F = \frac{E}{x}$$

At equilibrium $F = F_D$

where F_D is the drag force resisting particle motion. According to Stokes' theory, discussed below,

$$F_D = 3\pi \, d_h \, . \, \eta \, . \, v_{st}$$

where d_h is the hydrodynamic diameter, v_{st} the Stokes velocity of the particle and η is the fluid viscosity, i.e.

$$E = F\bar{x} = 3\pi \, d_h \, . \, \eta \, . \, v_{st}$$

but

$$\bar{x}^2 = Dt$$

and

$$v_{st} = \bar{x}/t$$

Substituting, $E = 3\pi \, d_h \, . \, \eta \, . \, D$

Since $E = kt$,

$$D = \frac{kT \times 10^7}{3\,\pi\,\eta\,d_n}$$

or

$$D = \frac{1.38 \times 10^{-12}\,T}{3\,\pi\,\eta\,d_n} \quad m^2\,s^{-1}$$

This equation is known as the Stokes–Einstein equation and is the basis for calculation of particle diameters using photon correlation spectroscopy.

Alternative techniques

There is a wide variety of different instruments based on laser Doppler anemometry or velocimetry, and diffraction measurements. The instruments vary according to their ability to characterize different particle size ranges, produce complete size distributions, measure both solid and liquid particles, determine molecular weights, diffusion coefficients, zeta potential or electrophoretic mobility.

Automatic methods

Most of the instruments based on laser light scattering produce a full particle size analysis automatically. The data are often presented in graphical and tabular form but in some instruments only a mean diameter is produced.

Sedimentation methods

Equivalent diameters

d_{fd}, frictional drag diameter, a sphere having an equivalent drag force to a particle of the same diameter in the same fluid at the same velocity; d_{st}, Stokes diameter, the diameter of a particle measured during sedimentation at constant rate in laminar flow conditions.

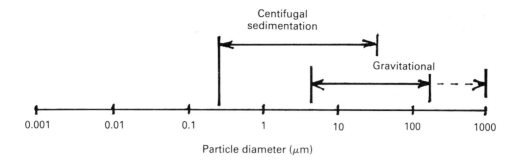

Particle diameter (μm)

Range of analysis (see above).

Sample preparation and analysis conditions

Particle size distributions can be determined by examining the powder as it sediments out. In cases where the powder is not uniformly dispersed in a fluid it can be introduced as a thin layer on the surface of the liquid. If the powder is lyophobic, e.g. hydrophobic in water, it may be necessary to add a dispersing agent to aid wetting of the powder. In cases where the powder is soluble in water it will be necessary to use non-aqueous liquids or carry out the analysis in a gas.

Principles of measurement

Techniques of size analysis by sedimentation can be divided into two main categories according to the method of measurement used. One type is based on measurement of particles in a retention zone, a second type uses a non-retention measurement zone.

An example of a non-retention zone measurement method is known as the pipette method. In this method, known volumes of suspension are drawn off and the concentration differences are measured with respect to time.

One of the most popular of the pipette methods was that developed by Andreasen and Lundberg and commonly called the Andreasen pipette (BS 3406, Part 2) (Fig. 33.12). The Andreasen fixed-position pipette consists of a 200 mm graduated cylinder which can hold about 500 ml of suspension fluid. A pipette is located centrally in the cylinder and is held in position by a ground glass stopper so that its tip coincides with the zero level. A three-way tap allows fluid to be drawn into a 10 ml reservoir which can then be emptied

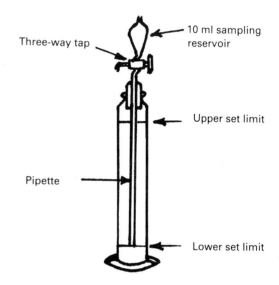

Fig. 33.12 Diagram of Andreasen pipette

into a beaker or centrifuge tube. The amount of powder can be determined by weight following drying or centrifuging; alternatively chemical analysis of the particles can be carried out. The largest size present in each sample is then calculated from Stokes' equation. Stokes' law is an expression of the drag factor in a fluid and is linked to the flow conditions characterized by a Reynolds number. Drag is one of three forces acting on a particle sedimenting in a gravitational field. A drag force, F_d, acts upwards, as does a buoyancy force, F_b, a third force is gravity, F_g, which acts as the driving force of sedimentation. At the constant terminal velocity, which is achieved rapidly by sedimenting particles, the drag force becomes synonymous with particle motion. Thus for a sphere of diameter d and density ρ_s, falling in a fluid of density ρ_f, the equation of motion is:

$$F_d = \frac{\pi}{6} (\rho_s - \rho_s)F_g.d^3$$

According to Stokes:

$$F_d = 3\pi \, d \, \eta \, v_{st}$$

where v_{st} is the Stokes terminal velocity, i.e. sedimentation rate. That is,

$$v_{st} = \frac{(\rho_s - \rho_s)F_g \, d^2}{18\eta}$$

since $v_{st} = h/t$ where h is sedimentation height or distance and t is sedimentation time. By rearrangement, Stokes' equation is obtained:

$$d_{st} = \frac{18\eta h}{(\rho_s - \rho_f)F_g \, t}$$

Stokes' equation for determining particle diameters is based on the following assumptions — near spherical particles; motion equivalent to that in a fluid of infinite length; terminal velocity conditions; low settling velocity so that inertia is negligible; large particle size relative to fluid molecular size, so that diffusion is negligible; no particle aggregation; laminar flow conditions, characterized by particle Reynolds numbers ($\rho u d_{particle}/\eta$) of less than approximately 0.2.

The second type of sedimentation size analysis, using retention zone methods, also uses Stokes' law to quantify particle size. One of the most common retention zone methods uses a sedimentation balance. In this method, the amount of sedimented particles falling on to a balance pan, suspended in the fluid, is recorded. The continual increase in weight of sediment is recorded with respect to time.

Alternative techniques

One of the limitations of gravitational sedimentation is that below a diameter of approximately 5 μm, particle settling becomes prolonged and is subject to interference due to convection, diffusion and Brownian motion. These effects can be minimized by increasing the driving force of sedimentation by replacing gravitational forces by a larger centrifugal force. Once again, sedimentation can be monitored by retention or non-

retention methods, although the Stokes equation requires modification because particles are subjected to different forces according to their distance from the axis of rotation. To minimize the effect of distance on the sedimenting force, a two-layer fluid system can be used. A small quantity of concentrated suspension is introduced on to the surface of a bulk sedimentation liquid known as spin fluid. Using this technique of disc centrifugation, all particles of the same size are in the same position in the centrifugal field and hence move with the same velocity.

Automatic methods

In general, gravity sedimentation methods tend to be less automated than those using centrifugal forces. However, an adaptation of a retention zone gravity sedimentation method is known as a Micromerograph and measures sedimentation of particles in a gas rather than a fluid. The advantages of this method are that sizing is carried out relatively rapidly and the analysis is virtually automatic.

SELECTION OF A PARTICLE SIZE ANALYSIS METHOD

The selection of a particle size analysis method may be constrained by the instruments already available in a laboratory, but wherever possible the limitations on the choice of method should be governed by the properties of the powder particles and the type of size information required. For example, size analysis over a very wide range of particle diameters may preclude use of a gravity sedimentatiion method; alternatively size analysis of aerosol particles would probably not be carried out using an electric sensing zone method. As a general guide it is often most appropriate to determine the particle size distribution of a powder in an environment which most closely resembles the conditions in which the powder will be processed or handled. There are many different factors which influence selection of an analysis method and these are summarized in Table 33.4 and may

Table 33.4 Summary of particle size analysis instrument characteristics

Analysis method			Sample measurement environment				Other functions	Rapid analysis	Size data printout available	Approximate size range (μm)				Initial cost	
			Gas	Aqueous liquid	Non-aqueous liquid	Replica				0.001–10	1–10	10–100	100–1000	High	Low
Sieve			√	√	√							√	√		√
Microscope	Light	Manual	√	√	√						√	√	√		√
		Semi-automatic	√	√	√						√	√	√		√
		Automatic	√	√	√		√		√		√	√	√	√	
	Electron					√			√	√	√			√	
Electrical stream sensing zone				√	√			√	√		√	√	√	√	
Laser light scattering	Diffraction		√	√	√		√	√	√		√	√	√	√	
	Doppler anemometry		√	√	√		√	√	√	√	√			√	
Sedimentation	Gravitational		√	√	√			√ ×	√ ×		√	√			√
	Centrifugal			√	√			√ ×	√ ×	√	√			√	

be used together with information from a preliminary microscopic analysis and any other known physical properties of the powder such as solubility, density, cohesivity, in addition to analysis requirements such as speed of measurement, particle size data processing or the physical separation of different particle size powders for subsequent processing.

BIBLIOGRAPHY

Allen, T. (1981) *Particle Size Measurement*, 3rd edn, Chapman and Hall, London and New York.

Barnett, M. I. and Nystrom, C. (1982) Coulter counters and microscopes for the measurement of particles in the sieve range. *Pharm. Tech.*, **6** (Mar.), 49–50.

Carstensen, J. T. (1977) *Pharmaceutics of Solids and Solid Dosage Forms*, John Wiley & Sons, New York and Chichester.

Felton, P. G. (1978) In stream measurement of particle size distribution, presented at *Int. Symp. on In Stream Measurements of Particle Solid Properties, Bergen, Norway*.

Groves, M. J. (ed.) (1978) *Particle Size Analysis*, Heyden, London, Philadelphia and Rheine.

Kay, B. H. (1981) *Direct Characterization of Fine Particles*, John Wiley & Sons, New York and Chichester.

Stanley-Wood, N. G. (1978) Pharmaceutical powder characterisation. *Pharm. Ind.*, **40**, 73–77.

Swithenbank, J., Beer, J. M., Taylor, D. S., Abbot, D. and McCreath, G. C. (1977) A laser diagnostic technique for the measurement of droplet and particle size distribution. In *Progress in Astronautics and Aeronautics*, (ed. B. T. Zinn), Vol. 53.

Thompson, D. H. and Stevenson, W. H. (1978) *Laser Velocimetry and Particle Sizing*, Hemisphere Publishing Corp., Washington, New York and London.

Particle size reduction

Objectives of size reduction

The significance of particle size has been discussed in Chapter 33 and some of the reasons for carrying out a size reduction operation will already have been noted. In addition, the function of size reduction may be to aid efficient processing of solid particles by facilitating powder mixing or production of suspensions. There are also some special functions of size reduction such as exposing cells prior to extraction or reducing the bulk volume of a material to improve transportation efficiency.

INFLUENCE OF MATERIAL PROPERTIES ON SIZE REDUCTION

Crack propagation and toughness

Size reduction or comminution is carried out by a process of crack propagation whereby localized stresses produce strains in the particles which are large enough to cause bond rupture and thus propagate the crack. In general, cracks are propagated through regions of a material which possess the most flaws or discontinuities and is related to the strain energy in specific regions according to Griffith's theory. The stress in a material is concentrated at the tip of a crack and the stress multiplier can be calculated from an equation developed by Inglis:

$$\sigma_{\kappa} = 1 + 2\left(\frac{L}{2r}\right)$$

where σ_{κ} is the multiplier of the mean stress in a material around a crack, L is the length of the crack and r is the radius of curvature of the crack tip. For a simple geometric figure such as a circular discontinuity $L = 2r$ and the stress multiplier σ_κ will have a value of 3. In the case of the thin disc-shaped crack shown in cross-section in Fig. 34.1 the crack was considered to have occurred at molecular level between atomic surfaces separated by a distance of 2×10^{-10} m for a crack 3 μm long which gives a stress multiplier of approximately 245. The stress concentration diminishes towards the mean stress according to the distance from the crack tip (Fig. 34.1). Once a crack is initiated the crack tip propagates at a velocity approaching 40% of the speed of sound in the solid. This crack propagation is so rapid that excess energy from strain relaxation is dissipated through the material and concentrates at other discontinuities where new cracks are propagated. Thus a cascade effect occurs and an almost instantaneous brittle fracture occurs.

Not all materials exhibit this type of brittle behaviour and can resist fracture at much larger stresses. This occurs because these tougher materials can undergo plastic flow which allows strain energy relaxation without crack propagation. When plastic flow occurs, atoms or molecules slip over one another and this process of deformation requires energy. Brittle materials can also exhibit plastic flow and Irwin and Orowan suggested a modification of Griffiths' crack theory to take this into account; the new relationship has a fracture stress which varies inversely with the square root of crack length:

$$\sigma = \frac{Ep}{C}$$

where Ep is the energy required to form unit area of double surface.

It can therefore be seen that the ease of comminution depends on the brittleness or plasticity of the material and their relationship with crack initiation and propagation.

Surface hardness

In addition to the toughness of the material described above, size reduction may also be influenced by surface hardness. The hardness of a material can be described by its position in a scale devised by a German mineralogist called Mohs.

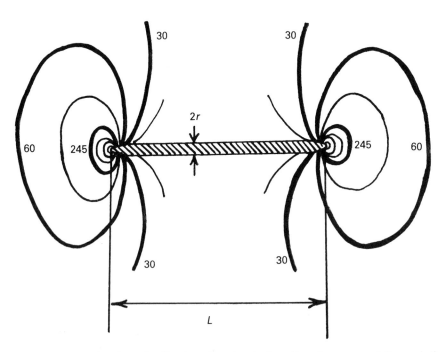

Fig. 34.1 Stress concentrations at the edges of a disc-shaped crack; r is the radius of curvature of the crack tip; L is the crack length

Mohs' scale is a table of materials, at the top of which is diamond with Mohs hardness >7 which has a surface so hard that it can scratch anything below it, at the bottom of the table with Mohs hardness <3 is talc which is soft enough to be scratched by anything above it.

A more quantitative measurement of surface hardness was devised by Brinell; such determinations of hardness may prove useful as a guide to the ease with which size reduction can be carried out — in general harder materials are more difficult to comminute and can lead to abrasive wear of metal mill parts which then cause product contamination. Conversely materials with a large elastic component such as rubber are extremely soft yet difficult to size reduce.

Materials such as rubber which are soft under ambient conditions, waxy substances such as stearic acid which soften when heated and 'sticky' materials such as gums are capable of absorbing large amounts of energy through elastic and plastic deformation without crack initiation and propagation. This type of polymeric material which resists comminution at ambient or elevated temperatures can be more easily size reduced by lowering the temperature below the glass transition point of the material. When this is carried out the material undergoes a transition from plastic to brittle behaviour and crack propagation is facilitated.

Other factors which influence the process of size reduction include the moisture content of the feed material. In general, a moisture content below 5% is suitable for dry grinding and greater than 50% if wet grinding is to be carried out.

Energy requirements of size reduction process

Only a very small amount of the energy put into a comminution operation actually effects size reduction. This has been estimated to be as little as 2% of the total energy consumption, the remainder being lost in many ways including elastic deformation of particles, plastic deformation of particles without fracture, deformation to initiate cracks which cause fracture, deformation of metal machine parts, interparticle friction, particle-machine wall friction, heat, sound and vibration.

A number of hypotheses and theories have been proposed in an attempt to relate energy input to the degree of size reduction produced. Rittinger's hypothesis is usually interpreted according to the energy, E, used in a size reduction process which is proportional to the new surface area produced, S_n, or:

$$E = \kappa_R (S_n - S_i)$$

where S_i is the initial surface area and κ_R is Rittinger's constant of energy per unit area.

Kick's theory states that the energy used in deforming or fracturing a set of particles of equivalent shape is proportional to the ratio of the change in size, or:

$$E = \kappa_K \log \frac{d_i}{d_n}$$

where κ_K is Kick's constant of energy per unit mass, d_i is the initial particle diameter and d_n the new particle diameter.

Bond's theory states that the energy used in crack propagation is proportional to the new crack length produced which is often related to the change in particle dimensions according to the following equation:

$$E = 2\kappa_B \left(\frac{1}{d_n} - \frac{1}{d_i} \right)$$

κ_B is known as Bond's work index and represents the variation in material properties and size reduction methods with dimensions of energy per unit mass.

Walker proposed a generalized differential form of the energy–size relationships which can be shown to link the theories of Rittinger and Kick and in some cases that of Bond:

$$\partial E = -\kappa \frac{\partial d}{d^n}$$

where d is a size function which can be characterized by an integrated mean size or by a weight function, n is an exponent — when $n = 1$ for particles defined by a weight function, integration of Walker's equation corresponds to a Kick-type theory; when $n = 2$, a Rittinger-type solution results and when $n = 3/2$ Bond's theory is given.

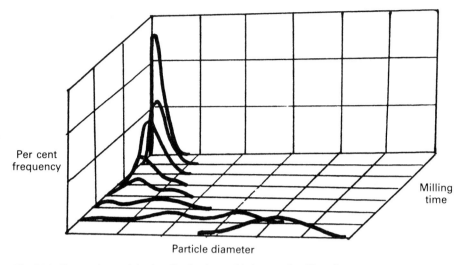

Fig. 34.2 Changes in particle size distributions with increased milling time.

When designing a milling process for a given particle, the most appropriate energy relationship will be required in order to calculate energy consumptions. It has been considered that the most appropriate values for n are 1 for coarse particles >1 μm where Kick-type behaviour occurs, 2 for Rittinger-type milling of particles <1 μm. The third value of $n = 3/2$ is the average of these two extremes and indicates a possible solution where neither Kick's nor Rittinger's theory is appropriate.

Other workers have found that n cannot be assumed to be constant, but varies according to a particle size function, so that

$$n = f(d)$$

or

$$E = -\kappa \, \frac{d}{d^{f(d)}}$$

As the particle size increases, $f(d)$ tends to 1 and as the size reduces, $f(d)$ tends to 2.

INFLUENCE OF SIZE REDUCTION ON SIZE DISTRIBUTION

In Chapter 33, several different size distributions were discussed and these were based on either a normal or log-normal distribution of particle sizes. During a size reduction process, the particles of feed material will be broken down and particles in different size ranges undergo different amounts of breakage. This uneven milling leads to a change in the size distribution which is superimposed on the general movement of the normal or log-normal curve towards smaller particle diameters. Changes in size distributions which occur as milling proceeds were demonstrated experimentally by Heywood, who showed that an initial normal particle size distribution was transformed through a size-reduced bimodal population into a much finer powder with a positively skewed, leptokurtic particle population (Fig. 34.2) as milling continued. The initial, approximately normal, size distribution was transformed into a size-reduced bimodal population through differences in the fracture behaviour of coarse and fine particles (Fig. 34.3). If milling is continued, a unimodal population reappears since the energy input is not

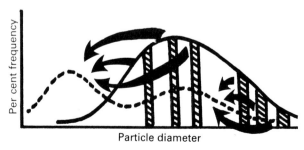

Fig. 34.3 Transformation of approximate normal particle size distribution into finer bimodal population following milling

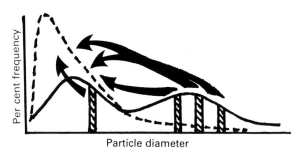

Fig. 34.4 Transformation of a fine bimodal particle population into a finer unimodal distribution following prolonged milling

great enough to cause further fracture of the finest particle fraction (Fig. 34.4). The lower particle size limit of a milling operation is dependent on the energy input and on material properties. Below particle diameters of approximately 5 μm, interactive forces generally predominate over comminution stresses which are distributed over increasing surface areas and particle agglomeration then opposes particle fracture and size reduction ceases. In some cases, particle agglomeration occurs to such a degree that subsequent milling actually causes size enlargement.

SIZE REDUCTION METHODS

There are many different types of size reduction techniques but the milling equipment used can be classified according to the principal method employed to produce size reduction. Examples of each type of milling method will be given and the approximate size reduction range will be provided although it should be remembered that the extent of size reduction is always related to milling time.

Cutting methods

Size reduction range

Principle of operation

A cutter mill (Fig. 34.5) consists of a series of knives attached to a horizontal rotor which act against a series of stationary knives attached to the mill casing. During milling, size reduction occurs by fracture of particles between the two sets of knives which have a clearance of a few millimetres. A screen is fitted in the base of the mill casing and acts to retain material in the mill until a sufficient degree of size reduction has been effected.

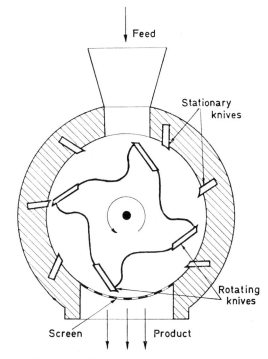

Fig. 34.5 Cutter mill

The high shear rates present in cutter mills are useful in producing a coarse degree of size reduction of dried granulations prior to tableting and of fibrous crude drugs such as roots, peels or barks prior to extraction.

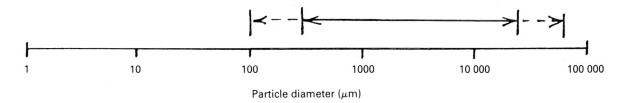

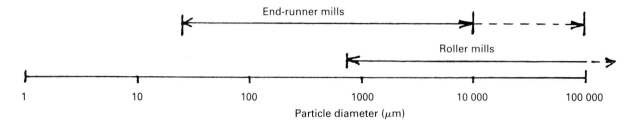

Compression methods

Size reduction range (as shown above)

Principle of operation

Size reduction by compression can be carried out on a small scale using a mortar and pestle. End-runner and edge-runner mills are mechanized forms of mortar and pestle-type compression comminution (Fig. 34.6). In the end-runner mill a weighted pestle is turned by the friction of material passing beneath it as the mortar rotates under power; the edge-runner mill has the pestle equivalent mounted horizontally and rotating against a bed of powder so that size reduction occurs by attrition as well as compression.

Alternative techniques

Another form of compression mill uses two cylindrical rolls mounted horizontally and rotated about their long axes. In roller mills, one of the rolls is driven directly while the second is rotated by friction as material is drawn through the gap between the rolls. This form of roller mill should not be confused with the type used for milling ointments where both rolls are driven but at different speeds, so that size reduction occurs by attrition.

Impact methods

Size reduction range

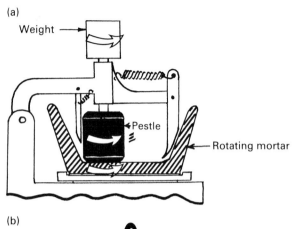

(a)

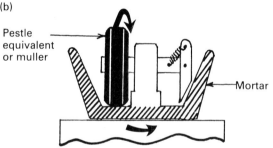

(b)

Fig. 34.6 (a) End-runner mill (b) edge-runner mill

Principle of operation

Size reduction by impact is carried out using a hammer mill (Fig. 34.7). Hammer mills consist of a series of four or more hammers, hinged on a central shaft which is enclosed within a rigid metal case. During milling the hammers swing out radially from the rotating central shaft. The

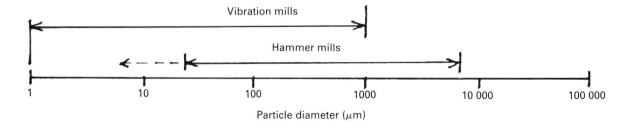

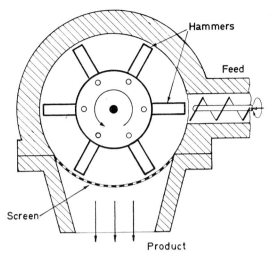

Fig. 34.7 Hammer mill

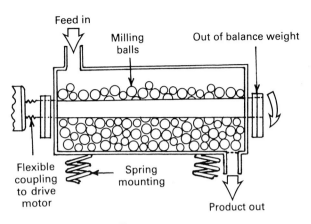

Fig. 34.8 Vibration mill

angular velocity of the hammers produces strain rates up to 80 s^{-1} which are so high that most particles undergo brittle fracture. As size reduction continues, the inertia of particles hitting the hammers reduces markedly, and subsequent fracture is less probable, so that hammer mills tend to produce powders with narrow size distributions. Particles are retained within the mill by a screen which only allows adequately comminuted particles to pass through. Particles passing through a given mesh can be much finer than the mesh apertures, since particles are carried around the mill by the hammers and approach the mesh tangentially. For this reason, square, rectangular or herring-bone slots are often used. According to the purpose of the operation, the hammers may be square-faced, tapered to a cutting edge or have a stepped form.

Alternative techniques

An alternative to hammer milling which produces size reduction is vibration milling (Fig. 34.8). Vibration mills are filled to approximately 80% total volume with porcelain or steel balls. During milling the whole body of the mill is vibrated and size reduction occurs by repeated impaction. Comminuted particles fall through a screen at the base of the mill. The efficiency of vibratory milling is greater than that for conventional ball milling described below.

Attrition methods

Size reduction range (as shown below)

Principle of operation

Roller mills use the principle of attrition to produce size reduction of solids in suspensions, pastes or ointments. Two or three porcelain or metal rolls are mounted horizontally with an adjustable gap which can be as small as 20 μm. The rollers rotate at different speeds so that the material is sheared as it passes through the gap and is transferred from the slower to the faster roll, from which it is removed by means of a scraper.

Combined impact and attrition methods

Size reduction range (as shown on next page)

Principle of operation

A ball mill is an example of a comminution method which produces size reduction by both

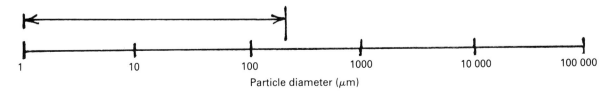

Particle diameter (μm)

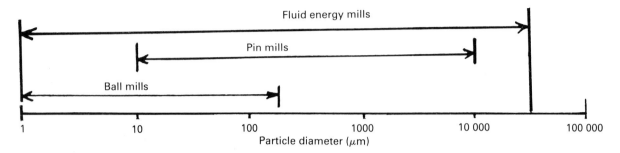

impact and attrition of particles. Ball mills consist of a hollow cylinder mounted such that it can be rotated on its horizontal longitudinal axis (Fig. 34.9). Cylinder diameters can be greater than 3 m although much smaller sizes are used pharmaceutically. The cylinder contains balls that occupy 30–50% of the total volume, ball size being dependent on feed and mill size, for example a mill 1 m in diameter might contain balls with a diameter of 75 mm. Mills usually contain balls with many different diameters due to self-attrition and this helps to improve the product since the large balls tend to break down the coarse feed materials and the smaller balls help to form the fine product by reducing void spaces between balls.

The amount of material in a mill is of considerable importance, too much feed produces a cushioning effect and too little causes loss of efficiency and abrasive wear of the mill parts. The factor of greatest important in the operation of the ball mill is the speed of rotation. At low angular velocities (Fig. 34.9(a)), the balls move with the drum until the force due to gravity exceeds the frictional force of the bed on the drum and the balls then slide back *en masse* to the base of the drum. This sequence is repeated producing very little relative movement of balls so that size reduction is minimal. At high angular velocities (Fig. 34.9(b)) the balls are thrown out on to the mill wall by centrifugal force and no size reduction occurs. At about $\frac{2}{3}$ of the critical angular velocity where centrifuging occurs (Fig. 34.9(c)), a cascading action is produced. Balls are lifted on the rising side of the drum until their dynamic angle of repose is exceeded. At this point the balls fall or roll back to the base of the drum in a cascade across the diameter of the mill. By this means, the maximum size reduction occurs by impact of the particles with the balls and by attrition. The optimum rate of rotation is dependent on mill diameter but is usually of the order of 0.5 s^{-1}.

Alternative techniques

Fluid energy milling is another form of size reduction method which acts by particle impaction and

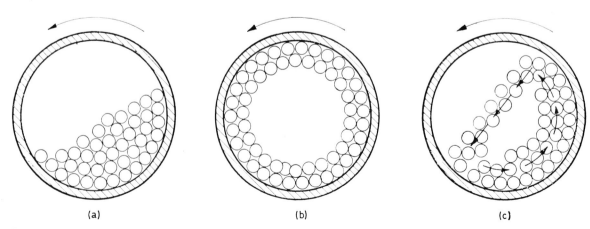

Fig. 34.9 Ball mill in operation, showing correct cascade action

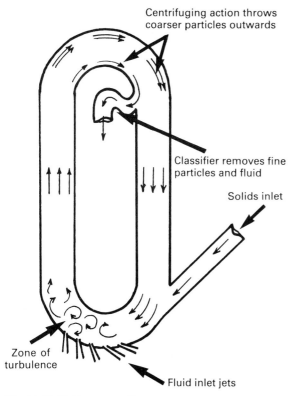

Fig. 34.10 Fluid energy mill

attrition. A typical form of fluid energy or jet mill is shown in Fig. 34.10. This type of mill or 'micronizer' consists of a hollow toroid which has a diameter of 20–200 mm, depending on the height of the loop which may be up to 2 m. A fluid, usually air, is injected as a high pressure jet through nozzles at the bottom of the loop. The high velocity of the air gives rise to zones of turbulence into which solid particles are fed. The high kinetic energy of the air causes the particles to impact *with other particles* with sufficient momentum for fracture to occur. Turbulence ensures that the level of particle–particle collisions is high enough to produce substantial size reduction by impact and some attrition. A particle size classifier is incorporated in the system so that particles are retained in the toroid until sufficiently fine and remain entrained in the air stream which is exhausted from the mill.

Other types of fluid energy mill replace the turbulence zone technique with horizontally opposed air jets through which the feed material is forced; alternatively a single air jet is used to feed particles directly on to a target plate where impaction causes fracture.

In addition to ball mills and fluid energy mills, there are other methods of comminution which act by producing particle impact and attrition. These include pin mills in which two discs with closely spaced pins rotate against one another at high speeds (Fig. 34.11). Particle size reduction occurs by impaction with the pins and by attrition between pins as the particles travel outwards under the influence of centrifugal force.

SELECTION OF PARTICLE SIZE REDUCTION METHOD

Different mills give differing products from the same starting material; for example, particle shape may vary according to whether size reduction occurs as a result of impact or attrition. In

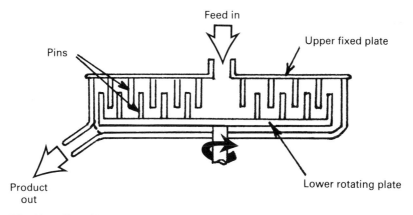

Fig. 34.11 Pin mill

Table 34.1 Selection of size reduction mills according to particle properties and product size required

Mohs' hardness'	Tough	Sticky	Abrasive	Friable
(a) Fine powder product (< 50 μm)				
1–3 (soft)	Ball, vibration (under liquid nitrogen)	Ball, vibration		Ball, vibration, pin, fluid energy
3–5 (intermediate)	Ball, vibration			Ball, vibration, fluid energy
5–10 (hard)	Ball, vibration, fluid energy		Ball, vibration, fluid energy	
(b) Coarse powder product (50–1000 μm)				
1–3	Ball, vibration, roller, pin, hammer, cutter (all under liquid nitrogen)	Ball, pin		Ball, roller, pin, hammer, vibration
3–5	Ball, roller, pin, hammer, vibration, cutter			Ball, roller, pin, vibration, hammer
5–10	Ball, vibration		Ball vibration, roller	
(c) Very coarse product (> 1000 μm)				
1–3 (soft)	Cutter, edge runner	Roller, edge runner, hammer		Roller, edge runner, hammer
3–5 (intermediate)	Edge runner, roller, hammer			Roller, hammer
5–10 (hard)	Roller		Roller	

addition, the proportion of fines in the product may vary so that other properties of the powder will be altered.

The use to which a powder will be put usually controls the degree of size reduction, but in some cases the precise particle size required is not critical. In these circumstances, the important factor is that in general the cost of size reduction increases as particle size decreases, so that it is economically undesirable to mill particles to a finer degree than necessary. Once the particle size required has been established the selection of mills capable of producing that size may be modified from a knowledge of the particle properties, such as hardness, toughness etc. The influences of various process and material variables on selection of a size reduction method are summarized in Table 34.1.

BIBLIOGRAPHY

Austin, L. G. and Brame, K. (1983) A comparison of the bond method for sizing wet tumbling ball mills with a size-mass balance simulation model. *Powder Technol.*, **34**, 261–274.

Lachman, L., Lieberman, H. A. and Kanig, J. L. (1976) In *Theory and Practice of Industrial Pharmacy*, 2nd edn, Lea and Febiger, Philadelphia.

Mecham, W. J., Jardine, L. J., Reedy, G. T. and Steindler, M. J. (1983) General statistical description of the fracture particulates formed by mechanical impacts of brittle materials. *Ind. Engng Chem. Fund.*, **22**, 384–391.

Paramanathan, B. K. and Bridgwater, J. (1983) Attrition of solids, Pts I & II. *Chem. Engng Sci.*, **38**, 197–224.

Parrott, E. L. (1974) Milling of pharmaceutical solids. *J. pharm. Sci.*, **63**, 813–829.

Voller, V. R. (1983) A note on energy–size reduction relationships in comminution. *Powder Technol.*, **36**, 281–286.

Wheeler, D. A. (1982) Size reduction. *Processing* (Dec), 55–58.

Particle size separation

The significance of particle size and the principles involved in differentiating a powder into fractions of known particle size and in reducing particle dimensions have been considered previously (Chapter 33 and 34). In this chapter, the methods by which size separation can be achieved will be discussed, together with the standards that are applied to powders for pharmaceutical purposes.

Objectives of size separation

Solid separation is a process by which powder particles are removed from gases or liquids and has two main aims:

1 to recover valuable products or byproducts,
2 to prevent environmental pollution.

Although size separation uses many similar techniques to those used in solid separation it has a different aim which is to classify powders into separate particle size ranges or 'cuts', and is therefore linked to particle size analysis. However, an important difference exists between size separation and size analysis: following size separation, powder in a given particle size range is available for separate handling or subsequent processing. This means that whereas a particle size analysis method such as microscopy would be of no use as a size separation method, the principle of sieving could be used for both purposes.

Size separation efficiency

The efficiency with which a powder can be separated into different particle size ranges is related to the particle and fluid properties and the separation method used. Separation efficiency is determined as a function of the effectiveness of a given process in separating particles into oversize and undersize fractions.

In a continuous size separation process, the production of oversize and undersize powder streams from a single feed stream can be represented by the following equation:

$$f_F = f_o + f_u$$

where f_F, f_o and f_u are functions of the mass flow rates of the feed material, oversize product and undersize product streams. If the separation process is 100% efficient, then all oversize material will end up in the oversize product stream and all undersize material will end up in the undersize product stream. Invariably, industrial separation processes produce an incomplete size separation so that some undersize material is retained in the oversize stream and some oversize material may find its way into the undersize stream.

Considering the oversize material, a given powder feed stream will contain a certain proportion of true oversize material, δ_F; the oversize product stream will contain a fraction, δ_o, of true oversize particles and the undersize stream will contain a fraction, δ_u, of true oversize material (Fig. 35.1)

The efficiency of the separation of oversize material can be determined by considering the relationship between mass flow rates of feed and product streams and the fractional contributions of true size grade in the streams. For example, the efficiency E_o of a size separation process for oversize material in the oversize stream is given by:

$$E_o = \frac{f_o \cdot \delta_o}{f_F \cdot \delta_F}$$

and the separation efficiency for undersize material in the undersize stream is given by:

$$E_u = \frac{f_u (1 - \delta_u)}{f_F (1 - \delta_F)}$$

The total efficiency, E_t, for the whole size separation process is given by:

$$E_t = E_u \cdot E_o$$

Separation efficiency determination can be applied to each stage of a complete size classification and is often referred to as 'grade efficiency'. In some cases, a knowledge of grade efficiency is insufficient; for example, where a precise particle size cut is required. A 'sharpness index' can be used to quantify the sharpness of cut-off in a given

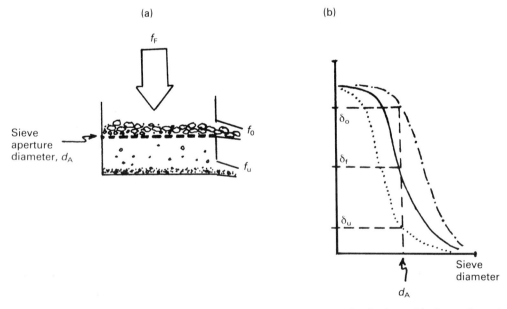

(a)

f_F

Sieve aperture diameter, d_A

f_o

f_u

(b)

δ_o

δ_f

δ_u

d_A

Sieve diameter

Fig. 35.1 Size separation efficiency determination. (a) Separation operation, (b) size distributions of feed, oversize and undersize material to obtain values for δ_o, δ_f and δ_u

size range. A sharpness index, S, can be determined in several different ways; for example, by taking the percentage values from a grade efficiency curve at the 25 and 75% levels (L):

$$S_{25/75} = \frac{L_{25}}{L_{75}}$$

or at other percentile points such as the 10 and 90% levels:

$$S_{10/90} = \frac{L_{10}}{L_{90}}$$

SIZE SEPARATION METHODS

Size separation by sieving

Separation ranges (as shown below)

Principles of operation

The principles of sieving for particle size analysis purposes have been described previously in Chapter 33. There may be some differences in the methods used to achieve size separation rather than size analysis. The wire mesh used for the construction of British Standard sieves should be of uniform circular cross-section, the sieve mesh should possess an adequate strength to avoid distortion and should also be resistant to chemical action with any of the material to be sifted. Commonly used materials for the construction of test sieve meshes for size analysis are brass and bronze, but it is probably more common and more suitable to use stainless steel meshes in process sieves used for size separation.

The use of sieving in size separation usually requires processing of larger volumes of powder than commonly found in size analysis operations. For this reason, the sieves used for size separation are often larger in area than those used for size analysis. There are several techniques for encouraging particles to separate into their appropriate size fractions efficiently. In dry sieving processes, these are based on mechanical disturbances of the powder bed and include the following.

Agitation methods Size separation is achieved by electrically induced oscillation or mechanically induced vibration of the sieve meshes or alternatively by gyration, in which sieves are fitted to a flexible mounting which is connected to an out-of-balance flywheel. The eccentric rotation of the flywheel imparts a rotary movement of small amplitude and high intensity to the sieve and causes the particles to spin, thereby continuously changing their orientation and increasing their potential to pass through a given sieve aperture. The output from gyratory sieves is often considerably greater than that obtained using oscillation or vibration methods.

Agitation methods can be made continuous by inclination of the sieve and the use of separate outlets for the undersize and oversize powder streams.

Brushing methods A brush is used to reorientate particles on the surface of a sieve and prevent sieve apertures becoming blocked. A single brush can be rotated about the midpoint of a circular sieve or for large scale processing, a horizontal cylindrical sieve is employed, with a spiral brush rotating about the longitudinal axis of the sieve.

Centrifugal methods Particles are thrown outwards on to a vertical cylindrical sieve under the action of a high speed rotor inside the cylinder. The current of air created by the rotor

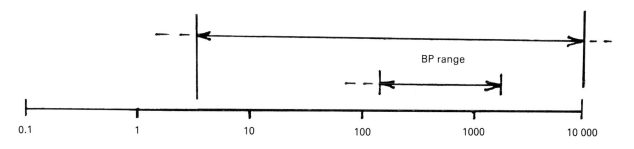

Particle diameter (μm)

movement also assists in sieving, especially where very fine powders are being processed.

Wet sieving can also be used to effect size separation and is generally more efficient than dry sieving methods.

Standards for powders based on sieving

Standards for powders used pharmaceutically are provided in the *British Pharmacopoeia* and in the *Pharmaceutical Codex*. The BP states that 'the degree of coarseness or fineness of a powder is differentiated and expressed by reference to the nominal mesh aperture size of the sieves used'. Five grades of powder are specified and defined in the BP and these are shown in Table 35.1.

Table 35.1 Powder grades specified in *British Pharmacopoeia*

Description of grade of powder	Coarsest sieve diameter (μm)	Sieve diameter through which no more than 40% of powder must pass (μm)
Coarse	1700	355
Moderately coarse	710	250
Moderately fine	355	180
Fine	180	—
Very fine	125	—

In addition to the grades of powder specified by the BP, the *Pharmaceutical Codex* defines another size fraction, known as 'ultra-fine powder'. In this case, it is required that the maximum diameter of at least 90% of the particles must be no greater than 5 μm and that none of the particles should have diameters greater than 50 μm.

It should be noted that the term 'sieve number' is used as a method of quantifying particle size in both the *British Pharmacopoeia* and the *Pharmaceutical Codex*. However, the two monographs use the term differently and in order to avoid confusion it is always advisable to refer to particle sizes according to the appropriate equivalent diameters expressed in micrometres.

The BP makes two statements with regard to the different particle size fractions:

1 It is required that when the fineness of a powder is described by a number, *all* particles of the powder must pass through a sieve mesh with aperture diameters in μm equal to that number.

2 When a vegetable drug is being ground and sifted, *none* must be rejected.

The reason for this will be apparent if the character of a drug of vegetable origin is compared to that of a chemically synthesized drug. The synthesized drug is a homogeneous material so that, if a certain quantity of a given size range is required, an excess may be milled and the desired amount of product in the size range removed by sieving, the excess oversize particles, known as tailings, being discarded. In contrast, a vegetable drug consists of a variety of tissue with different milling properties, so that softer tissues will be size reduced first, leaving tailings obtained by sifting which contain a higher proportion of harder tissues. In many cases, drug constituents are not distributed uniformly through vegetable tissues; for example, in digitalis the glycosides are concentrated in the mid-rib and veins. Hence, if tailings are discarded following milling and sifting it is possible that a high proportion of the active constituent will be lost. The Pharmacopoeia does, however, allow tailings to be withheld from a batch of vegetable drug provided that an approximately equal amount of tailings from a preceding batch of the same drug is added prior to size reduction. The object of this is to allow a batch mill to be used efficiently. Without this concession it would be necessary to mill a batch of raw material completely, and any tailings, even if the quantity were very small, would have to be ground so that the mill would eventually only contain tailings and would be operating for long periods well below a capacity suitable for efficient milling throughout its cycle.

Size separation by fluid classification

Sedimentation methods

Separation ranges (as shown on next page)

Principles of operation

The principles of liquid classification using sedimentation methods have been described previously in Chapter 33. Size separation by sedimentation utilizes the differences in settling velocities of particles with different diameters and these can be

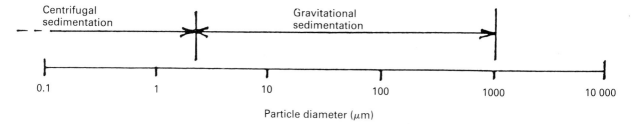

Particle diameter (μm)

related according to Stokes' equation, derived in Chapter 33.

One of the simplest forms of sedimentation classification uses a chamber containing a suspension of solid particles in a liquid, which is usually water. After predetermined times, particles less than a given diameter can be recovered using a pipette placed a fixed distance below the surface of the liquid. Size fractions can be collected continuously using a pump mechanism in place of a pipette.

Alternatively, a single separation can be carried out simply by removing the upper layer of suspension fluid after the desired time. Disadvantages of these simple methods are that they are batch processes and discrete particle fractions cannot be collected since samples contain every particle diameter up to the limiting diameter and not specific size ranges.

Alternative techniques

An alternative technique is to use a continuous settling chamber so that particles in suspension enter a shallow container as shown in Fig. 35.2. The particle Reynolds' number of the system ($\rho u d_{particle}/\eta$) is below approximately 0.2 so that

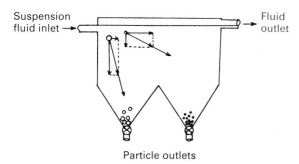

Fig. 35.2 Continuous settling chamber showing vectors of particle movement for different sizes

streamline flow occurs. Particles entering at the top of the chamber are acted upon by a driving force which can be divided into two components: a horizontal component of particle velocity which is equal to the suspension fluid velocity and a vertical component which corresponds to Stokes' settling velocity and is different for each particle size. These two components are constant for each particle so that the settling path will be given by a curve whose slope depends on particle diameter. The coarsest particles will have the steepest settling paths and will sediment closest to the inlet, whereas the finest particles with low Stokes velocity component will have the shallowest settling paths and will sediment furthest from the fluid suspension feed stream (Fig. 35.2). Particles separated into the different hopper-type discharge points can be removed continuously.

Very fine particles will not sediment efficiently under the influence of gravity due to Brownian diffusion. In order to increase the driving force of sedimentation, centrifugal methods can be used to separate particles of different sizes in the submicrometre region.

Simple cylindrical centrifuges can be used to remove single size cuts from a fluid stream, but where separation is required over a wider number of size ranges multiple-chamber centrifuges can be used. In this type of centrifuge there are a number of spinning cylinders of different diameters set inside a closed chamber (Fig. 35.3). Fine particles in liquid suspension are fed in through the top of the inner or central cylinder. As in continuous flow gravity sedimentation, the particles are acted on by two component forces — one due to fluid flow and, in this case, one due to centrifugal force. The coarsest particles will have the shallowest trajectories and will be carried to the walls of the inner cylinder (Fig. 35.4); all other particles remain entrained in the liquid and flow out at the

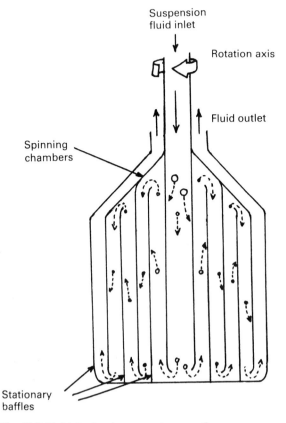

Fig. 35.3 Multiple chamber separation centrifuge

base of the cylinder and via a baffle or weir into the top of the next cylinder out where the centrifugal force is higher. This sequence continues so that only the finest particles reach the outermost spinning cylinder.

Another type of sedimentation method is based on separation from particles dispersed in air and is known as *mechanical air classification.*

Standards for powders based on sedimentation separation

There are no general pharmacopoeial standards for size separation based on sedimentation. However, tests are applied to Light Kaolin BP in order to limit the coarseness of the powder. Light Kaolin BP must consist of fine particles, partially because it is used in the form of a suspension, but also because it is used therapeutically for its adsorptive properties which are dependent on surface area and therefore on particle size. The test described fully in the *British Pharmacopoeia* uses an adaptation of the batch sedimentation chamber method described above.

Elutriation methods

Separation ranges (as shown on next page)

Principles of operation

In sedimentation methods, the fluid is stationary and the separation of particles of various sizes depends solely on particle velocity. Therefore, the division of particles into size fractions depends on the *time* of sedimentation.

Elutriation is a technique in which the fluid flows in an opposite direction to the sedimentation

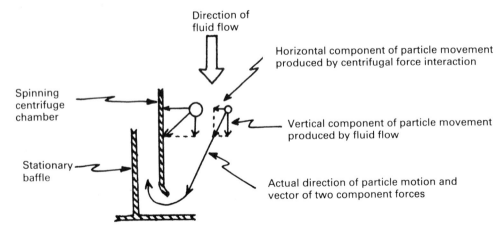

Fig. 35.4 Influence of particle size on particle movement in multiple chamber centrifuge

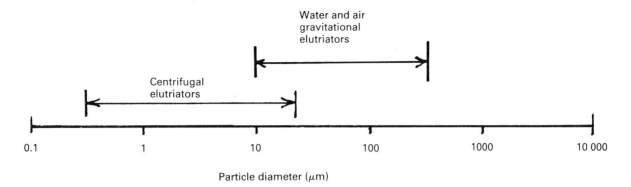

Particle diameter (μm)

movement, so that in gravitational elutriators particles move vertically downwards while the fluid travels vertically upwards. If the upward velocity of the fluid is less than the settling velocity of the particle, sedimentation occurs and the particle moves downwards against the flow of fluid. Conversely, if the settling velocity of the particle is less than the upward fluid velocity, the particle moves upwards with the fluid flow. Therefore, in the case of elutriation, particles are divided into different size fractions depending on the *velocity* of the fluid. Elutriation and sedimentation are compared in Fig. 35.5 where the arrows are vectors, that is, they show the direction and magnitude of particle movement. This figure indicates that if particles are suspended in a fluid moving up a column, there will be a clear cut into two fractions of particle size. In practice this does not occur since there is a distribution of velocities across the tube in which a fluid is flowing — the highest velocity is found in the centre of the tube and the lowest velocity at the tube walls. Therefore, the size of particles that will be separated

depends on their position in the tube, the largest particles in the centre, the smallest towards the outside. In practice, particles can be seen to rise with the fluid and then to move outwards to the tube wall where the velocity is lower and they start to fall. A separation into two size fraction occurs, but the size cut will not be clearly defined. Assessing the sharpness of size cuts is discussed in more detail above.

Separation of powders into several size fractions can be effected by using a number of elutriators connected in series. The suspension is fed into the bottom of the narrowest column, overflowing from the top into the bottom of the next widest column and so on (Fig. 35.6). Since the mass flow remains the same, as the column diameter increases, the fluid velocity decreases and therefore particles of decreasing size will be separated.

Alternative techniques

Air may be used as the counterflow fluid in place of water for elutriation of soluble particles into different size ranges. There are several types of air elutriator which differ according to the air flow patterns used. An example of an upward air flow elutriator is shown in Fig. 35.7. Particles are held on a supporting mesh through which air is drawn. Classification occurs within a very short distance of the mesh and any particles remaining entrained in the air stream are accelerated to a collecting chamber by passage through a conical section of tube. Further separation of any fine particles still entrained in the air flow may be carried out subsequently using different air velocities.

It may be required to separate finer particles than can be achieved using gravitational elutri-

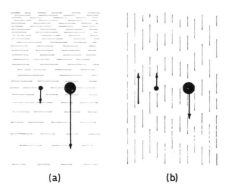

(a)   (b)

Fig. 35.5 Comparison of (a) sedimentation and (b) elutriation

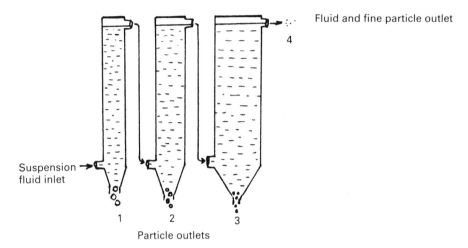

Fluid and fine particle outlet

4

Suspension fluid inlet →

1   2   3

Particle outlets

Fig. 35.6 Multistage elutriator. Particle outlets 1 to 4 collect fractions of decreasing particle size

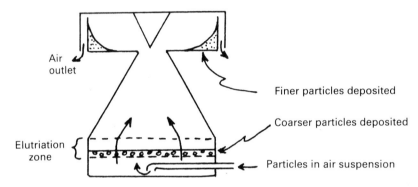

Air outlet

Finer particles deposited

Coarser particles deposited

Elutriation zone

Particles in air suspension

Fig. 35.7 Upward airflow elutriator

ation and in these cases, counterflow centrifugal methods can be used. Particles in air suspension are fed into a rotating hollow torus at high speed, tangential to the outer wall. Coarse particles move outwards to the walls against the inwardly spiralling air flow which leaves the elutriator in the centre. The desired particle size fraction can be separated by selecting the appropriate air flow rate and rotor speed.

Cyclone separation methods

Separation range

Principle of operation

Cyclone separation can take the form of a centrifugal elutriation process similar to the one described above or a centrifugal sedimentation process in which particles sediment out of a helical gas or liquid stream.

Probably the most common type of cyclone used to separate particles from fluid streams is the reverse-flow cyclone (Fig. 35.8). In this system, particles in air or liquid suspension are often introduced tangentially into the cylindrical upper section of the cyclone where the relatively high

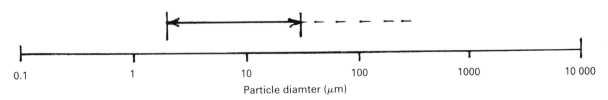

0.1   1   10   100   1000   10 000

Particle diamter (μm)

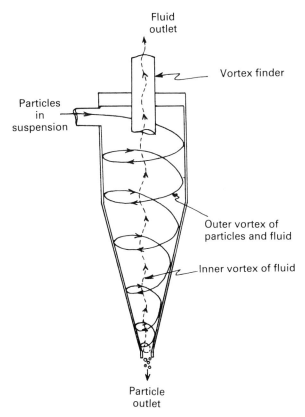

Fluid outlet

Vortex finder

Particles in suspension

Outer vortex of particles and fluid

Inner vortex of fluid

Particle outlet

Fig. 35.8 Reverse-flow cyclone separator

fluid velocity produces a vortex which throws solid particles out on to the walls of the cyclone. The particles are forced down the conical section of the cyclone under the influence of the fluid flow — gravity interactions are a relatively insignificant mechanism in this process. At the tip of the conical section the vortex of fluid is above the critical velocity at which it can escape through the narrow outlet and forms an inner vortex which travels back up the cyclone and out through a central outlet or vortex finder. Coarser particles separate from the fluid stream and fall out of the cyclone through the dust outlet whereas finer particles remain entrained in the fluid stream and leave the cyclone through the vortex finder. In some cases, the outer vortex is allowed to enter a collector connected to the base of the cyclone, but the coarser particles still appear to separate from the fluid stream and remain in the collector. A series of cyclones having different flow rates or different dimensions could be used to separate a powder into different particle size ranges.

SELECTION OF A SIZE SEPARATION PROCESS

Selection of a specific size separation may be limited by pharmacopoeial requirements, but for general cases the most efficient method should be selected based on particle properties. Of these, size is particularly important as each separation method is most efficient over a particular size range, as indicated in the foregoing text.

Particles which have just undergone size reduction will already be in suspension in a fluid whether air or water and can be separated quickly by elutriation or cyclone separation methods, so that oversize material can be returned to the mill.

Alternatively, many powders used pharmaceutically are soluble in water and size separation may have to be restricted to air classification methods.

BIBLIOGRAPHY

Allen, T. (1981) Particle Size Measurement, 3rd edn, Chapman and Hall, London and New York.

Svarovsky, L. (1981) Solid Gas Separation (Handbook of Powder Technology, Vol. 3), Elsevier, Amsterdam.

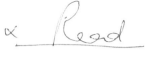
Powder flow

Powders are generally considered to be composed of solid particles of the same or different chemical compositions having equivalent diameters less than 1000 μm. However, the term 'powder' will also be used here to describe groups of particles formed into granules which may have overall dimensions greater than 1000 μm.

The largest use of powders pharmaceutically is to produce tablets and capsules. Together with mixing and compression properties, the flowability of a powder is of critical importance in the production of pharmaceutical dosage forms. Some of the reasons for producing free-flowing pharmaceutical powders include:

1 uniform feed from bulk storage containers or hoppers into the feed mechanisms of tableting or capsule-filling equipment, allowing uniform particle packing and a constant volume-to-mass ratio which maintains tablet weight uniformity;
2 reproducible filling of tablet dies and capsule dosators which improves weight uniformity and allows tablets to be produced with more consistent physicomechanical properties;
3 uneven powder flow can result in excess entrapped air within powders which in some high speed tableting conditions may promote capping or lamination;
4 uneven powder flow can result from excess fine

particles in a powder which increase particle-die wall friction, causing lubrication problems, and increase dust contamination risks during powder transfer.

There are many industrial processes which require powders to be moved from one location to another and this is achieved by many different methods such as gravity feeding, mechanically assisted feeding, pneumatic transfer, fluidization in gases and liquids and hydraulic transfer. In each of these examples, powders are required to flow and as with other operations described earlier, the efficiency with which powders flow is dependent on both process design and particle properties.

PARTICLE PROPERTIES

Adhesion and cohesion

The presence of molecular forces produces a tendency for solid particles to stick to themselves and to other surfaces. Adhesion and cohesion can be considered as two parts of the same phenomenon: cohesion occurs between like surfaces such as component particles of a bulk solid whereas adhesion occurs between two unlike surfaces, for example, between a particle and a hopper wall.

Cohesive forces acting between particles in a powder bed are composed mainly from short-range non-specific van der Waal's forces which increase as particle size decreases and vary with changes in relative humidity. Other attractive forces contributing to interparticle cohesion may be produced by surface tensional forces between adsorbed liquid layers at the particle surfaces and electrostatic forces arising from contact or frictional charging, which may have short half-lives but increase cohesion through improving interpar-

ticle contacts and hence increasing the quantity of van der Waal's interactions. Cohesion provides a useful method of characterizing the drag or frictional forces acting within a powder bed to prevent powder flow.

Measurement of adhesive/cohesive properties

Adhesive/cohesive forces acting between a single pair of particles or a particle and substrate surface can be accurately determined using a specially adapted ultracentrifuge to apply very high forces strong enough to separate the two surfaces.

However, it is more usual when studying powder flow to characterize adhesion/cohesion in a bed of powder.

Shear strength Cohesion can be defined as the stress (force per unit area) necessary to shear a powder bed under conditions of zero normal load. Using this criterion, the shear strength of a powder can be determined from the resistance to flow caused by cohesion or friction and can be measured using a shear cell.

The shear cell (Fig. 36.1) is a relatively simple piece of apparatus which is designed to measure shear stress, τ, at different values of normal stress, σ. There are several types of shear cell such as the Jenike shear cell and the Portishead shear cell which use different methods of applying the stresses and measuring the shear strengths. In order to carry out a shear strength determination, powder is packed into the two halves of the cell. Weights are placed on the lid of the assembled cell, or some other method may be used to apply the normal stress. A system of a cord connected from the lid of the cell, by a pulley, to weights, or other means are used to apply a shearing stress across the two halves of the cell. The shear stress is found by dividing the shear force by the cross-

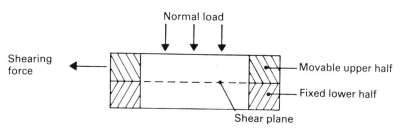

Fig. 36.1 Diagrammatic representation of Jenike shear cell

sectional area of the powder bed and will increase as the normal stress increases. One of the most convenient, informative and widely used methods of presenting this stress inter-relationship is provided by plotting a Mohr diagram.

A Mohr diagram is constructed by plotting the normal stress, τ, as the ordinate and the shear stress, σ, as the abscissa. For two values of shear stress on the abscissa, at which failure occurs and the cell is sheared, σ_1 and σ_2 are used as the diameter of a Mohr circle with radius $\dfrac{\sigma_1 + \sigma_2}{2}$ (Fig. 36.2). A series of Mohr semicircles can be

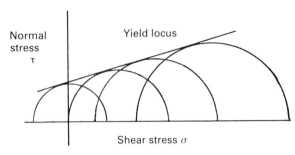

Fig. 36.3 Mohr diagram

constructed in this way with different pairs of shear stresses causing failure (Fig. 36.3). A line is constructed to touch all of the Mohr semicircles and define the critical combinations of normal and shearing stresses at which failure occurs. The line is called the yield locus and is a characteristic of the powder under given conditions. Several different properties of the powder can be obtained from the complete Mohr diagram and some of these are shown in Table 36.1.

In order to calculate the cohesion in a powder bed using the shear cell method, the yield locus

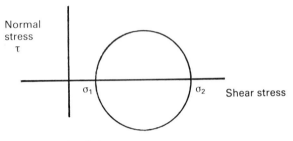

Fig. 36.2 Mohr circle

Table 36.1 Some properties relating to powder cohesion and flowability which can be obtained from Mohr diagrams

Measurement	Property measured	Powder characteristics
1 Acute angle of the extrapolated yield locus at the shear stress axis	Angle of internal friction, ϕ	Difficulty of maintaining constant volume flow
2 Tan ϕ or slope of the yield locus	Coefficient of friction	Indirect measurement of powder flowability
3 Diameter of circle with tangent to t linking minor stress at $\sigma = 0$ to major unconfined yield stress σ_u	Stress equilibrium in powder arch when no flow occurs	Minimum opening dimensions to prevent arching
4 Extrapolation of yield locus to cut normal stress axis	σ_a, apparent tensile strength of powder bed	Resistance to failure in tension
5 Shear stress, t_e, at zero normal stress, σ_o	Cohesion coefficient	Cohesion, when powder is non-cohesive, yield locus passes through origin and shear stress = 0

is extrapolated back to zero normal stress; the shear stress at zero normal stress is, by definition, equal to the cohesion of the powder. For a non-cohesive powder, the extrapolated yield locus will pass through the origin, equivalent to zero shear stress. In rheological terms, the stress due to cohesion along the yield locus may be called the yield stress and the powder termed a plastic solid.

Tensile strength   The tensile strength of a powder bed is a characteristic of the internal friction or cohesion of the particles, but unlike shear strength determinations, the powder bed is caused to fail in tension, by splitting, rather than failing in shear, by sliding. The powder is packed into a split plate, one half of which is fixed and the other half free to move by means of small wheels or ball bearings which run in tracks in a table (Fig. 36.4). The table is then tilted towards the vertical, until the angle is reached at which the powder cohesion is overcome and the mobile half-plate breaks away from the static half-plate. The tensile strength, σ_t, of the powder can then be determined from Eqn 36.1:

$$\sigma_t \frac{M \sin \theta}{A} \times 10^5 \text{ Pa} \qquad (36.1)$$

where M is the mass of the mobile half plate + powder; θ, the angle of the tilted table to the horizontal at the point of failure and A is the cross-sectional area of the powder bed.

The tensile strength values of different powders have been found to correlate reasonably well with another measurement of powder cohesion, angle of repose.

Angle of repose   From the previous discussion it will be realized that an object, such as a particle, will begin to slide when the angle of inclination is large enough to overcome frictional forces. Conversely, an object in motion will stop sliding when the angle of inclination is below that required to overcome adhesion/cohesion. This balance of forces causes a powder poured from a container on to a horizontal surface to form a heap: initially the particles stack until the approach angle for subsequent particles joining the stack is large enough to overcome friction and they slip and roll over each other until the gravitational forces balance the interparticle forces. The sides of the heap formed in this way make an angle with the horizontal which is called the angle

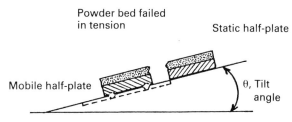

Powder bed failed in tension

Static half-plate

Mobile half-plate

θ, Tilt angle

Fig. 36.4 Measurement of tensile strength of a powder bed using tilting table method

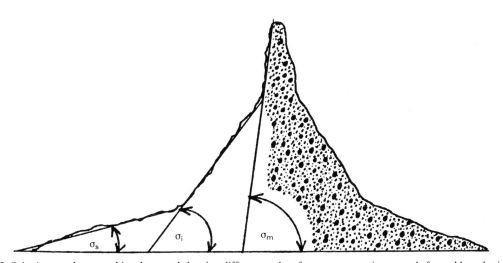

Fig. 36.5 Cohesive powder poured in a heap and showing different angles of repose: σ_m maximum angle formed by cohesive particles, σ_s shallowest angle formed by collapse of cohesive particle heap, resulting in flooding. In some cases a third angle, σ_i is identifiable as an intermediate slope produced by cohesive particles stacking on flooded powder

of repose and is a characteristic of the internal friction or cohesion of the particles. The value of the angle of repose will be high if the powder is cohesive and low if the powder is non-cohesive. If the powder is very cohesive, the powder heap may be characterized by more than one angle of repose. Initially, the interparticle cohesion causes a very steep cone to form but on addition of further powder this tall stack may suddenly collapse causing air to be entrained between particles, partially fluidizing the bed, making it more mobile. The resulting heap has two angles of repose: a large angle remaining from the initial heap and a shallower angle formed by the powder flooding from the initial heap (Fig. 36.5).

In order to overcome this problem, it has been suggested that determinations of angles of repose be carried out using different concentrations of very cohesive powders and non-cohesive powders. The angles of repose are plotted against mixture concentration and extrapolated to 100% cohesive powder content so as to obtain the appropriate angle of repose (Fig. 36.6).

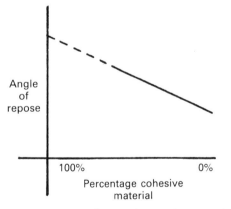

Fig. 36.6 Determination of angle of repose for very cohesive powders

Particle properties and bulk flow

In the preceding discussion concerning adhesion/cohesion it has become clear that an equilibrium exists between forces responsible for promoting powder flow and those preventing powder flow, i.e. at equilibrium:

$$\Sigma f(\text{driving forces}) = \Sigma f(\text{drag forces}) \qquad (36.2)$$

that is, Σf(gravitational force, particle mass, angle of inclination of powder bed, static head of powder, mechanical force. . . .) $= \Sigma f$(adhesive forces, cohesive forces, other surface forces, mechanical interlocking . . . .) $\qquad (36.3)$

Some of these forces are modified or controlled by external factors related to particle properties.

Particle size effects

Since cohesion and adhesion are phenomena which occur at surfaces, particle size will influence the flowability of a powder. In general, fine particles with very high surface to mass ratios are more cohesive than coarser particles which are influenced more by gravitational forces. Particles greater than 250 μm are usually relatively free-flowing, but as the size falls below 100 μm, powders become cohesive and flow problems are likely to occur. Powders having a particle size less than 10 μm are usually extremely cohesive and resist flow under gravity except possibly as large agglomerates.

Particle shape

Powders with similar particle sizes but dissimilar shapes can have markedly different flow properties due to differences in interparticle contact areas. For example, a group of spheres has minimum interparticle contact and generally optimal flow properties, whereas a group of particle flakes or dendritic particles have a very high surface-to-volume ratio and poorer flow properties.

Particle density (*true density*)

Since powders normally flow under the influence of gravity, dense particles are generally less cohesive than less dense particles of the same size and shape.

Packing geometry

A set of particles can be filled into a volume of space to produce a powder bed which is in static equilibrium due to the interaction of gravitational and adhesive/cohesive forces. By slight vibration of the bed, particles can be mobilized so that if the vibration is stopped, the bed is once more in static equilibrium but occupies a different spatial volume than before. The change in bulk volume has been produced by rearrangement of the packing geometry of the particles. In general, such geometric rearrangements result in a transition from loosely packed particles to more tightly packed particles so that the equilibrium balance moves from left to right in Eqn 36.2 and cohesion increases. This also means that more tightly packed powders require a higher driving force to produce powder flow than more loosely packed particles of the same powder.

Characterization of packing geometry

Porosity and bulk density A set of monosize, spherical particles can be arranged in many different geometric configurations. At one extreme, when the spheres form a cubical arrangement the particles are most loosely packed and have a porosity of 48% (Fig. 36.7(a)). At the other extreme, when the spheres form a rhombohedral arrangement they are most densely packed and have a porosity of only 26% (Fig. 36.7(b)). The porosity used to characterize packing geometry is linked to the bulk density of the powder. Bulk density, ρ_B, is a characteristic of a powder rather than individual particles and is given by the mass, M, of powder occupying a known volume, V, according to the relationship:

$$\rho_B = \frac{M}{V} \text{ kg m}^{-3} \qquad (36.4)$$

The bulk density of a powder is always less than the true density of its component particles, because the powder contains interparticle pores or voids. This statement reveals that whilst a powder can only possess a single true density it can have many different bulk densities, depending on the way in which the particles are packed and the bed porosity. However, a high bulk density value does not necessarily imply a close-packed, low porosity bed since bulk density is directly proportional to true density.

Bulk density α true density

i.e. bulk density $= k \cdot$ true density (36.5)

or

$$k = \frac{\text{bulk density}}{\text{true density}} \qquad (36.6)$$

The constant of proportionality, k, is known as the *packing fraction* or *fractional solids content*. For example, the packing fraction for dense, randomly packed spheres is approximately 0.63, whereas the packing fraction for a set of dense, randomly packed discs is 0.83.

Also:

$$1 - k = e \qquad (36.7)$$

where e is the fractional voidage of the powder bed, which is usually expressed as a percentage and termed the bed porosity. Another way of

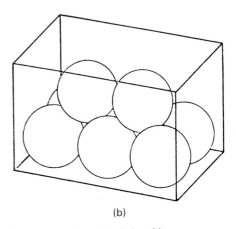

Fig. 36.7 Different geometric packings of spherical particles: (a) cubical packing (b) rhombohedral packing

expressing fractional voidage is to use the ratio of particle volume V_p to bulk powder volume V_B, i.e.

$$e = \frac{1 - V_p}{V_B} \qquad (36.8)$$

A simple ratio of void volume V_v to particle volume V_p represents the voids ratio:

$$\frac{V_v}{V_p} = \frac{e}{(1 - e)} \qquad (36.9)$$

The voids ratio provides information about the stability of the powder mass.

For powders having comparable true densities, an increase in bulk density causes a decrease in porosity. This increases the number of inter-particle contacts and contact areas and causes an increase in cohesion. In very coarse particles this may still be insufficient to overcome the gravi-tational influence on particles. Conversely, a decrease in bulk density may be associated with a reduction in particle size and produce a loose-packed powder bed, which although porous is unlikely to flow because of the inherent cohesive-ness of the fine particles. The use of porosity as a means of characterizing packing geometrics can sometimes be misleading. For example, monosize cubic crystals could be considered to be loosely packed with a porosity of 20%, since the closest packed cubic arrangement would have a porosity close to 0%. By comparison, a system of spher-onized crystals of the same size with a porosity of 30% could be considered to be more closely packed since the closest packed spherical arrange-ment has a porosity of 26%. In this example the powder with the higher porosity is relatively more closely packed than the powder with the lower porosity.

In powders where the particle shape or cohesiveness promotes arch or bridge formation, two equilibrium states could have similar porosi-ties but widely different packing geometries. In such conditions, interparticle pore size distri-butions can be useful for comparing packing geometry.

For example, Fig. 36.8(a) shows a group of particles in which arching has occurred and Fig. 36.8(b) shows a similar group of particles in which arch formation is absent. The total porosity

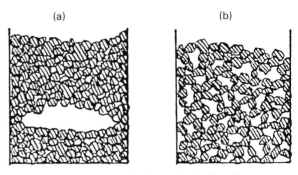

Fig. 36.8 Two equidimensional powders having the same porosity but different packing geometries

of the two systems can be seen to be similar but the pore size distributions (Fig. 36.9) reveal that the powder in which arch formation has occurred is generally more tightly packed than the powder in which arching is absent.

Factors affecting packing geometry

1 Particle size and size distribution: void spaces between coarse particles may become filled with finer particles in a powder with a wide size range, resulting in a more closely packed cohesive powder.
2 Particle shape and texture influence the minimum porosity of the powder bed. Arches or bridges within the powder bed will be formed more readily through the interlocking of non-isometric, highly textured particles.

This tendency for irregular particles to produce open structures supported by small or large powder arches causes them to have a larger difference in porosity between loose

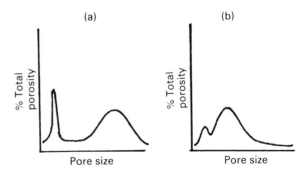

Fig. 36.9 (a) Interparticle pore size distribution corresponding to close-packed bed containing a powder arch. (b) Interparticle pore size distribution corresponding to loosely packed bed

packing and tight packing geometries than more regularly shaped particles.

3 Surface properties: the presence of electrostatic forces can add to interparticle attractions and promote closer particle packing, resulting in increased cohesion.

4 Handling and processing conditions: the way in which a powder has been handled prior to flow or packing influences the type of packing geometry.

PROCESS CONDITIONS: HOPPER DESIGN

Flow through an orifice

There are many examples of this type of flow to be found in the manufacture of pharmaceutical solid dosage forms. For example, when granules or powders flow through the opening in a hopper or bin used to feed powder to tableting machines, capsule-filling machines or sachet-filling machines. Because of the importance of such flow in producing unit doses containing the same or very

similar powder masses, and the importance of flow behaviour in other industries, the behaviour of particles being fed through orifices has been extensively studied.

A hopper or bin can be modelled as a tall cylindrical container having a closed orifice in the base and initially full of a free-flowing powder which has a horizontal upper surface (Fig. 36.10 (a)). When the orifice at the base of the container is opened, flow patterns develop as the powder discharges. (Fig. 36.10(a)–(f)).

The observed sequence is as follows.

1 On opening the orifice there is no instantaneous movement at the surface, but particles just above the orifice fall freely through it (Fig. 36.10(b)).

2 A depression forms at the upper surface and spreads outwards to the sides of the hopper (Fig. 36.10(c) and (d)).

3 Provided that the container is tall and not too narrow, the flow pattern illustrated in Fig. 36.10(e) and shown schematically in

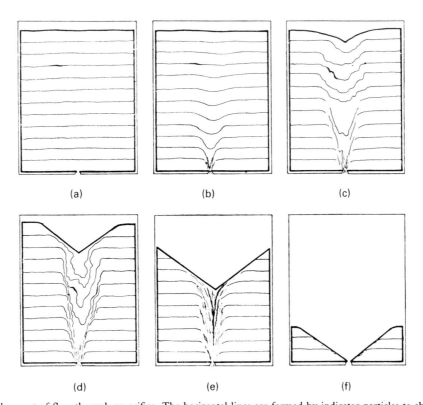

(a) (b) (c)

(d) (e) (f)

Fig. 36.10 Development of flow through an orifice. The horizontal lines are formed by indicator particles to show the course of the discharge

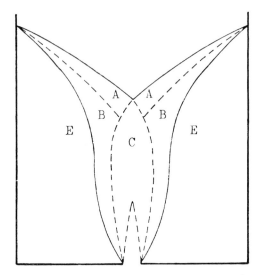

Fig. 36.11 Fully developed flow of a free-flowing powder

Fig. 36.11 is rapidly established. Particles in zone A move rapidly over the slower moving particles in zone B, whilst those in zone E remain stationary. The particles in zone A feed into zone C where they move quickly downwards and out through the orifice. The more slowly moving particles in zone B do not enter zone C.

4 Both powder streams in zone B and C converge to a 'tongue' just above the orifice where the movement is most rapid and the particle packing is least dense. In a zone just above the orifice, the particles are in free flight.

Important practical consequences of this flow pattern are that if a square-bottomed hopper or bin is repeatedly refilled and partially emptied, the particles in a zone towards the base and sides of the container (Fig. 36.10(f)) will not be discharged and may degrade; alternatively, this static zone may provide a segregation potential for previously homogeneous powders.

Factors affecting flow rates through orifices

The flow patterns described above, together with powder flow rates through orifices are dependent on many different factors, some of which are particle related and some process related. Particle-related effects, notably particle size, have been discussed above. Process-related effects include the following.

Orifice diameter   Flow rate α D_o^A. The rate of powder flow through an orifice is proportional to a function of orifice diameter, D_o (A is a constant with a value of approx. 2.6). Provided that the height of the powder bed, called the head of powder, remains considerably greater than the orifice diameter, flow rate is virtually independent of powder head. This situation is unlike that relating to liquid flow through an orifice, where the flow rate falls off continuously as the head diminishes. The constant rate of flow for powders is a useful property since it means that if a bulk powder is filled into dies, sachets, capsules or other enclosures, they will receive equal weights, if filled for equal times.

Hopper width   At different positions within a powder bed, the consolidating stresses and shear or tensile strengths are different (Fig. 36.12(b)). If the bed strength at a given point in the hopper is great enough to resist the driving forces promoting flow, then a stable arch will be formed. At all other points in the powder, the bed strength will not be high enough to support an arch against the stresses within it and flow will occur. The stresses acting on a stable arch are proportional to the width of the container and vary with diameter as exemplified in Fig. 36.12(a) and (b). The relationship between the stress on the arch and the arch strength, resulting in part from consolidating pressures at different points in the hopper (Fig. 36.12(c)), shows that with the exception of a region close to the hopper outlet and another at the point where the cylindrical section meets the conical section of the hopper, powder arches are weaker than the stresses on them. This suggests that powder flow will occur in all other regions (Fig. 36.12(d)) and allows the hopper design to be adjusted so that the minimum hopper widths are always large enough to produce arch stresses greater than arch strengths and thereby ensure continuous, uniform powder flow.

Head size   Figure 36.12(b) shows the way in which solids' pressure changes with powder head size (powder depth). The pressure increases below the upper free surface to a constant governed by frictional factors. The pressure again falls off towards the hopper outlet and drops below atmos-

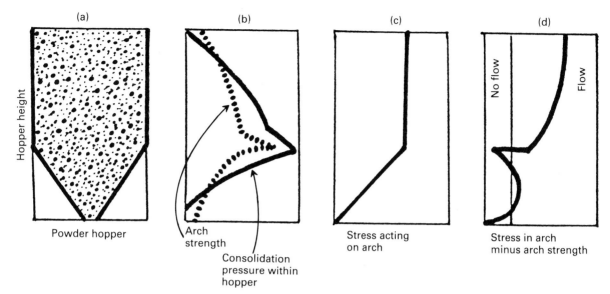

Fig. 36.12 Influence of stress interactions within a hopper on powder flow

pheric at the orifice causing air to be drawn up into the region close to the base so as to equalize this negative pressure and allow flow to continue.

Hopper wall angle It was noted above in the description of flow through an orifice, that a flat-bottomed bin retains a certain volume of powder in the form of a drained cone centred on the orifice. In order to prevent this behaviour and to ensure that all the powder is discharged from a hopper, the walls are frequently angled inwards as the outlet is approached. The wall angle which is required to ensure that powder empties freely is determined by the particle–wall adhesion component of friction within powders and is characterized by a wall-friction angle, φ. Powders with very low wall-friction angles will empty freely, even from hoppers with very shallow slopes, whereas powders with very high wall-friction angles will empty poorly even from steep-walled hoppers. In between these two extremes, powder discharge characteristics will be determined by the relationship between wall friction and hopper angle as shown in Fig. 36.13.

Mass flow and funnel flow

Powder which discharges freely from a hopper is said to undergo mass flow when particles which enter the hopper first leave it first. This first

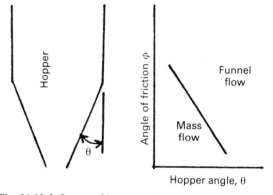

Fig. 36.13 Influence of hopper wall angle and particle–wall friction on powder flow

in–first out sequence holds throughout the bed so that powder can be considered to leave in near-horizontal bands which move down the hopper *en masse* (Fig. 36.14(a)).

Powders which do not discharge freely, either due to high adhesion/cohesion or to hopper angles which are too shallow, may undergo funnel flow (Fig. 36.14(b)). Particles which are loaded into the hopper last are among the first to leave, forming a 'pipe', 'rat-hole' or 'funnel' extending from the upper free powder surface to the hopper outlet and producing uneven erratic flow. Another problem associated with funnel flow may occur when the rat-hole collapses. This produces a

(a) (b)

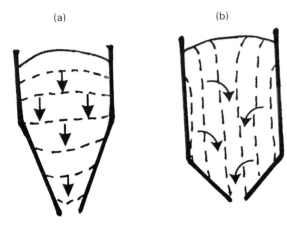

Fig. 36.14 (a) Mass flow hopper (b) funnel flow hopper

sudden, rapid discharge of powder which can entrain relatively large volumes of air causing the particles to partially fluidize and flood out of the hopper. This 'flooding' or 'flushing' may be succeeded by periods when the bed is quiescent and flow is slow or interrupted.

In general, most powders will discharge by mass flow from hoppers with θ angles of approx. 20° and by funnel flow from hoppers with angles of approximately 50°.

Mass flow rate

Throughout this section, it has been shown that specific particle properties and individual design criteria influence powder flow. However, in a given practical situation, powder flowability is the resultant of the relative influences of all these factors. An equation has been derived which relates some particulate properties, such as bulk density, ρ_B, and angle of repose, α, and hopper design criteria such as orifice diameter, D_o, and a discharge coefficient, C, to mass flow rate of powder, M:

$$M = \pi/4 \; C\rho_B\rho \; [(g \; D_o^5)/2 \tan \alpha]^{\frac{1}{2}} \quad (36.10)$$

where g is acceleration due to gravity.

CHARACTERIZATION OF POWDER FLOW

When examining the flow properties of a powder it is useful to be able to quantify the type of

behaviour and many different methods have been described, either directly, using dynamic or kinetic methods, or indirectly, generally by measurements carried out on static beds.

Indirect methods

Angle of repose

Angles of repose have been used as indirect methods of quantifying powder flowability, because of their relationship with interparticle cohesion. There are many different methods of determining angles of repose and some of these are shown in Table 36.2. The different methods may produce different values of angle of repose for the same powder, although these may be self-consistent. It is also possible that different angles of repose could be obtained for the same powder, due to differences in the way the samples were handled prior to measurement. For these reasons, angles of repose tend to be variable and are not always representative of flow under specific conditions.

As a general guide, powders with angles of repose greater than 50° (5/18 π rad) have unsatisfactory flow properties, whereas minimum angles close to 25° (5/36 π rad) correspond to very good flow properties.

Shear cell determinations

It is possible to characterize flowability indirectly from the behaviour of powder in a shear cell. A flow factor, f.f., can be obtained by determining the reciprocal slope of a curve or tangent to a curve of unconfined yield stress σ_u, plotted against the maximum normal stress on a yield locus, σ_m (Fig. 36.15(a)). The unconfined yield stresses are those in Mohr semicircles constructed through the origin; the maximum normal stresses have a semicircle passing through the largest normal stress (Fig. 36.15(b)). By plotting a series of different yield loci, several values can be obtained for σ_u and σ_m.

The relationship between flow factors and powder flowability is shown in Table 36.3.

Table 36.2 Methods of measuring angle of repose

Apparatus	Method	Angle defined	Apparatus	Method	Angle defined
	Fixed height cone	Angle of repose		Ledge	Drained angle of repose
	Fixed base cone	Angle of repose		Crater	Drained angle of repose
	Tilting table	Angle of repose		Platform	Drained angle of repose
	Rotating cylinder	Dynamic angle of repose			

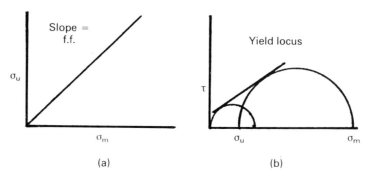

Fig. 36.15 (a) Plot of unconfined yield stress, σ_u, against maximum stress, σ_m, with a slope corresponding to the flow factor, f.f. (b) Example of Mohr diagram used to obtain one pair of values for σ_u and σ_m

Table 36.3 Relationship between flow factors (f.f.) and powder flowability

f.f. value	Flow descriptor
>10	Free flowing
4–10	Easy flowing
1.6–4	Cohesive
<1.6	Very cohesive

Bulk density measurements

The bulk density of a powder is dependent on particle packing and changes as the powder consolidates. A consolidated powder is likely to have a greater arch strength than a less consolidated powder and may therefore be more resistant to powder flow. The case with which a powder consolidates can be used as an indirect method of quantifying powder flow.

Figure 36.16 shows a mechanical tapping device or jolting volumeter which can be used to follow the change in packing volume which occurs when void space diminishes and consolidation occurs. The powder contained in the measuring cylinder is mechanically tapped by means of a constant velocity rotating cam and increases from an initial bulk density D_o (also known as fluff or poured bulk density) to a final bulk density D_f (also known as equilibrium, tapped or consolidated bulk density) when it has attained its most stable, i.e. unchanging arrangement.

Hausner found that the ratio D_f/D_o was related to interparticle friction and as such could be used to predict powder flow properties. Hausner showed that powders with low interparticle fric-

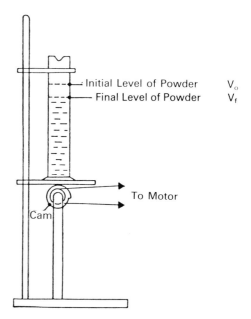

Fig. 36.16 Mechanical tapping device

tion, such as coarse spheres, had ratios of approximately 1.2, whereas more cohesive, less free-flowing powders such as flakes have Hausner ratios greater than 1.6.

Another indirect method of measuring powder flow from bulk densities was developed by Carr. The percentage compressibility of a powder is a direct measure of the potential powder arch or bridge strength and stability and is calculated according to Eqn 36.11:

$$\% \text{ compressibility} = \frac{D_f - D_o}{D_f} \times 100 \qquad (36.11)$$

Table 36.4 Relationship between powder flowability and % compressibility

% Compressibility range	Flow description
5–15	Excellent (free-flowing granules)
12–16	Good (free flowing powdered granules)
18–21	Fair (powdered granules)
23–28	Poor (very fluid powders)
28–35	Poor (fluid cohesive powders)
35–38	Very poor (fluid cohesive powders)
>40	Extremely poor (cohesive powders)

Table 36.4 shows the generalized relationship between descriptions of powder flow and % compressibility, according to Carr.

Critical orifice diameter

In order to carry out measurements of critical orifice diameter, powder is filled into a shallow tray to a uniform depth with near-uniform packing. The base of the tray is perforated with a graduated series of holes which are blocked either by resting the tray on a plane surface or by the presence of a simple shutter. The critical orifice diameter is the size of the smallest hole through which powder discharges when the tray is lifted or the shutter removed. In some cases, repetition of the experiment produces different critical orifice diameters, and in these cases maximum and minimum values are sometimes quoted.

Critical orifice diameter is a direct measure of powder cohesion and arch strength since:

$$\tan \alpha = \frac{r}{x} \qquad (36.12)$$

where r is the particle radius and x is the orifice radius, and

$$\tan F' = \frac{\tan \phi}{1 - \tan \phi \dfrac{r}{x} - \dfrac{r^2}{x^2}} \qquad (36.13)$$

where F' is the angle of form which is the obtuse angle between the contracting powder dome and the horizontal and $\tan \phi$ is a coefficient of friction.

An alternative critical orifice method for determining powder flowability uses a cylinder with a series of interchangeable base plate discs having different diameter orifices. Using this system, flowability indices related to orifice diameters have been used as a method of specifying materials for use in filling given capsule sizes or producing particular tablet sizes at a specified production rate.

Direct methods

Hopper flow rate

The simplest method of determining powder flowability directly is to measure the rate at which powder discharges from a hopper. A simple shutter is placed over the hopper outlet and the hopper is filled with powder. The shutter is then removed and the time taken for powder to discharge completely is recorded. By dividing the discharged powder mass by this time, a flow rate is obtained which can be used for quantitative comparison of different powders.

Hopper or discharge tube outlets should be selected to provide a good model for a particular flow application. For example, if a powder discharges well from a hopper into a tablet machine feed frame, but does not flow reproducibly into the tablet die, then it is likely that more useful information will be generated by selecting experimental conditions to model those occurring in flow from the feeder to the die rather than in flow from the hopper to the feeder.

Recording flow meter

A recording flow meter is essentially similar to the method described above except that powder is allowed to discharge from a hopper or container on to a balance.

In the case of analogue balances, a chart recorder is used to produce a permanent record of the increase in powder mass with time. In some systems the signal from the balance is digitized and processed by a microcomputer. Recording flow meters allow mass flow rates to be determined and also provide a means of quantifying uniformity of flow.

IMPROVEMENT OF POWDER FLOWABILITY

Alteration of particle size and size distribution

Since coarse particles are generally less cohesive than fine particles and an optimum size for free flow exists, there is a distinct disadvantage in using a finer grade of powder than is necessary.

The size distribution can also be altered to improve flowability by removing a proportion of the fine particle fraction or by increasing the proportion of coarser particles such as occurs through granulation.

Alteration of particle shape or texture

In general, for a given particle size, more spherical particles have better flow properties than more irregular particles. The process of spray drying can be used to produce near spherical excipients such as spray-dried lactose. Under certain circumstances, drug particles which are normally acicular can be made more spherical by temperature cycling crystallization.

The texture of particles may also influence powder flowability since particles with very rough surfaces will be more cohesive and have a greater tendency to interlock than smooth-surfaced particles. The shape and texture of particles can also be altered by control of production methods such as crystallization conditions.

Alteration of surface forces

Reduction of electrostatic charges can improve powder flowability and this can be achieved by alteration of process conditions to reduce frictional contacts. For example, where powder is poured down chutes or conveyed along pipes pneumatically, the speed and length of transportation should be minimized. Electrostatic charges in powder containers can be prevented or discharged by efficient earth connections.

Moisture content of particles is also of importance to powder flowability since adsorbed surface moisture films tend to increase bulk density and reduce porosity. In cases where moisture content is excessive, powders should be dried and, if hygroscopic, stored and processed under low humidity conditions.

Formulation additives: flow activators

Flow activators are commonly referred to pharmaceutically as 'glidants', although some also have lubricant or anti-adherent properties. Flow activators improve the flowability of powders by reducing adhesion and cohesion.

Some commonly used glidants include talc, maize starch and magnesium stearate which may have their effect by reducing or altering electrostatic interactions. A flow activator with an exceptionally high specific surface area is colloidal silicon dioxide which may act through reducing the bulk density of tightly packed powders. Colloidal silicon dioxide also improves flowability of formulations, even those containing other glidants, although in some cases, colloidal silicon dioxide can cause flooding.

Where powder flowability is impaired through increased moisture content, a small proportion of very fine magnesium oxide may be used as a flow activator. Used in this way, magnesium oxide appears to disrupt the continuous film of adsorbed water surrounding the moist particles.

The use of silicone-treated powder, such as silicone-coated talc or sodium bicarbonate, may also be beneficial in improving the flowability of moist or hygroscopic powder.

Alteration of process conditions

Use of vibration-assisted hoppers

In cases where the powder arch strength within a bin or hopper is greater than the stresses in it, due to gravitational effects, powder flow will be interrupted or prevented. If the hopper cannot be redesigned to provide adequate stresses and if the physical properties of the particles cannot be adjusted or the formulation altered, then extreme measures are required. One method of encouraging powder flow where arching or bridging has occurred within a hopper, is to add to the stresses due to gravitational interactions, by vibrating the hopper mechanically. Both the amplitude and frequency of vibration can be altered to produce the desired effect and may vary from a single cycle or shock produced by a compressed air device or hammer, to higher frequencies produced, for example, by out-of-balance electric motors mounted on a hopper frame.

Use of force feeders

The flow of powders which discharge irregularly or flood out of hoppers can be improved by fitting vibrating baffles, known as live-bottom feeders, at the base of the conical section within a hopper.

The outflowing stream from a hopper can be encouraged to move towards its required location using a slightly sloping moving belt, or in the case of some tableting machines, the use of mechanical force feeders. Force feeders are usually made up of a single or two counter-rotating paddles at the base of the hopper just above the die table in place of a feed frame. The paddles presumably act by preventing powder arching over dies and thereby improve die filling especially at high turret speeds.

Caution!

In most pharmaceutical technology operations, it is difficult to alter one process without adversely influencing another. For example, increasing compression pressure to produce stronger tablets may also impair disintegration and prolong dissolution; increasing mixing times of drugs with excipients in the presence of magnesium stearate, to improve homogeneity may also impair tablet strength.

In the case of alterations made in order to improve powder flow, relative particle motion will be promoted and can lead to demixing or segregation. *In extremis*, improving powder flow to improve weight uniformity may reduce content uniformity through increased segregation.

BIBLIOGRAPHY

Brown, R. L. and Richards, J. C. (1970) *Principles of Powder Mechanics*, Pergamon Press, Oxford and London.
Gioia, A. (1980) Intrinsic flowability. A new technology for powder-flowability classification. *Pharm. Techn.*, **4** (Feb.), 65–68.
Lieberman, H. A. and Lachman, L. (eds) (1981) *Pharmaceutical Dosage Forms*, Volume 2, Marcel Dekker Inc., New York and Basel.
McNaughton, K. (ed.) (1981) *Solids Handling*, McGraw-Hill Publications Co., New York.
Sadek, H. M., Olsen, J. L., Smith, H. L. and Onay, S.

(1982) A systematic approach to glidant selection. *Pharm. Tech.*, **6** (Feb.), 42–44, 46, 50, 52, 54, 56, 59–60, 62.
Shahinpoor, M. (ed.) (1983) *Advances in the Mechanics and the Flow of Granular Materials*, Volumes 1 and 2. Gulf Publishing Co., Houston and London.
Singley, M. E. and Chaplin, R. V. (1982) Flow of particulate materials, *Trans. ASAE*, **25**, 1360–1373.
Taubmann, H. J. (1982) The influence of flow activators on the flow behaviour of powders. *Aufbereitungs-Technik*, **23**, 423–428.

Granulation

INTRODUCTION TO GRANULATION

Granulation is the process in which powder particles are made to adhere to form larger particles called granules. In the majority of cases this will be undertaken in the production of tablets or capsules, when granules will be made as an intermediate product, but granules may also be used as a dosage form (see Chapter 17). Granulation will commence after mixing the necessary powdered ingredients so that a uniform distribution of each ingredient through the mix is achieved. After granulation, the granules will be packed when used as a dosage form or they may be mixed with other excipients prior to tablet compression or capsule filling.

Reasons for granulation

The reasons why granulation is often necessary are as follows.

To prevent segregation of the constituents in the powder mix

Segregation is primarily due to differences in the size or density of the components, the smaller particles concentrating at the base of a container with the large particles above them. An ideal granulation will contain all the constituents of the mix

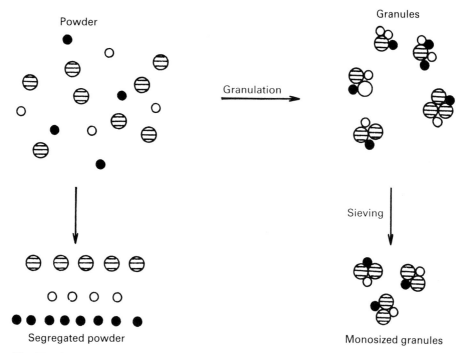

Powder

Granules

Granulation →

Sieving

Segregated powder

Monosized granules

Fig. 37.1 Granulation to prevent powder segregation

in each granule and segregation of the ingredients will not occur (Fig. 37.1).

It is also important to control the particle size distribution of the granules because, although the individual components may not segregate, if there is a wide size distribution, the granules themselves may segregate. If this occurs in the hoppers of sachet filling machines, capsule filling machines or tablet machines, products having large weight variations will result. This is because these machines fill by volume rather than weight and if different regions in the hopper contain granules of different sizes (and hence bulk density), a given volume in each region will contain a different weight of granules. This will lead to an unacceptable distribution of the drug content within the batch of finished product even though the drug is evenly distributed weight per weight, through the granules.

To improve the flow properties of the mix

Many powders, because of their small size or surface characteristics, are cohesive and do not flow well. Poor flow will often result in a wide weight variation within the final product due to variable fill of tablet dies, etc. Granules produced from such a cohesive system will be larger and more isodiametric, both factors contributing to improved flow properties.

To improve the compression characteristics of the mix

Some powders are difficult to compress even if a readily compressed adhesive is included in the mix but granules of the same formulation are often more easily compressed and produce stronger tablets. This is associated with the distribution of the adhesive within the granule and is a function of the method employed to produce the granule (Seager et al., 1979).

Other reasons

These are the primary reasons for the granulation of pharmaceutical products but there are other reasons which may necessitate the granulation of powdered material:

1 The granulation of toxic materials will reduce

the hazard of the generation of toxic dust which may arise when handling powders. Suitable precautions must be taken to ensure that such dust is not a hazard during the granulation process.

2 Materials which are slightly hygroscopic may adhere and form a cake if stored as a powder. Granulation may reduce this hazard as the granules will be able to absorb some moisture and yet retain their flowability because of their size.

3 Granules, being denser than the parent powder mix, occupy less volume per unit weight. They are therefore more convenient for storage or shipment.

Methods of granulation

Granulation methods can be divided into two types: wet methods which utilize a liquid in the process and dry methods in which no liquid is used.

In a suitable formulation a number of different excipients will be needed in addition to the drug. The common types used are diluents, to produce a unit dose weight of suitable size and disintegrating agents which are added to disintegrate the granule in a liquid medium, e.g. on ingestion by the patient. Adhesives in the form of a dry powder may also be added, particularly if dry granulation is employed. These ingredients will be mixed before granulation.

Dry granulation

In the dry methods of granulation the powder particles are aggregated using high pressure. There are two main processes. Either a large tablet (known as a 'slug') is produced in a heavy duty tableting press (a process known as 'slugging') or squeezed between two rollers to produce a sheet of material ('roller compaction'). In both cases these are broken using a suitable milling technique to produce granular material which is usually sieved to separate the desired size fraction. The unused fine material may be recycled to avoid waste. This dry method may be used for drugs which do not compress well after wet granulation or those which are sensitive to moisture.

Wet granulation (or wet massing)

Wet granulation involves the massing of the powder mix using a solvent. The solvents used must be volatile, so that they can be removed by drying, and non-toxic. Typical solvents include water, ethanol and isopropanol either alone or in combination. The solvent may be used alone or it may contain a dissolved adhesive (also referred to as binder or binding agent) which is used to cause particle adhesion. The disadvantages of water as a solvent are that it may adversely affect drug stability, causing hydrolysis of susceptible products and it needs a longer drying time than organic solvents. This long drying time increases the length of the process and again may affect stability because of the extended exposure to heat. The primary advantage of water is that it is non-flammable which means that expensive safety precautions such as the use of flame-proof equipment need not be taken. Organic solvents are used when water-sensitive drugs are processed, as an alternative to dry granulation, or when a rapid drying time is required.

In the traditional wet granulation method the wet mass is forced through a sieve to produce wet granules which are then dried. A subsequent sieving stage breaks agglomerates of granules and removes the fine material which can be recycled. Variations of this traditional method are dependent upon the equipment used but the general principle of initial particle adhesion using a liquid remains in all of the processes.

Effect of granulation method on granule structure

The type and capacity of granulating mixers significantly influences the work input and time necessary to produce a cohesive mass, adequate liquid distribution and intragranular porosity of the granular mass. The method and conditions of granulation affect intergranular and intragranular pore structure by changing the degree of packing within the granules. Seager et al. (1979) investigated the structure of granules prepared by various granulation methods. They showed that precompressed granules, consisting of compressed drug and binder particles, were held together by simple bonding during compaction. Granules prepared by the wet massing consisted of intact drug particles held together in a sponge-like matrix of binder. Fluidized bed granules were similar to granules prepared by the wet massing process, but possessed greater porosity, and the granule surface was covered by a film of binding agent. With spray-dried systems, the granules consisted of spherical particles composed of an outer shell with an inner core of particles. This study graphically indicates that the properties of the granule are influenced by the manufacturing process.

PARTICLE BONDING MECHANISMS

To form granules, bonds must be formed between powder particles so that they adhere and these bonds must be sufficiently strong to prevent breakdown of the granule to powder in subsequent handling operations.

Rumpf (1962) distinguished five primary bonding mechanisms between particles:

1 adhesion and cohesion forces in immobile liquid films,
2 interfacial forces in mobile liquid films,
3 solid bridges,
4 attractive forces between solid particles,
5 interlocking bonds.

Different types of mechanism were identified in each group and the ones discussed below are those which are of relevance to pharmaceutical granulations.

Adhesion and cohesion forces in immobile films

If sufficient liquid is present in a powder to form a very thin, immobile layer, there will be an effective decrease in interparticulate distance and increase in contact area between the particles. The bond strength between the particles will be increased because of this, as the van der Waals forces of attraction are proportional to the particle diameter and inversely proportional to the square of the distance of separation.

This situation will arise with adsorbed moisture and accounts for the cohesion of slightly damp powders. Although such films may be present as residual liquid after granules prepared by wet granulation have been dried, it is unlikely that they contribute significantly to the final granule strength. In dry granulation, however, the pressures used will increase the contact area between the adsorption layers and decrease the interparticulate distance and this will contribute to the final granule strength.

Thin, immobile layers may also be formed by highly viscous solutions of adhesives and so the bond strength will be greater than that produced by the mobile films discussed below. The use of starch mucilage in pharmaceutical granulations may produce this type of film.

Interfacial forces in mobile liquid films

During wet granulation liquid is added to the powder mix and will be distributed as films around and between the particles. Sufficient liquid is usually added to exceed that necessary for an immobile layer and produce a mobile film. Newitt and Conway-Jones (1958) distinguished three states of water distribution between particles which are illustrated in Fig. 37.2.

At low moisture levels, termed the pendular state, the particles are held together by lens-

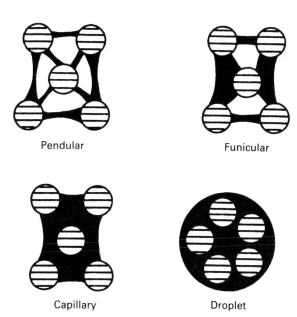

Pendular   Funicular

Capillary   Droplet

Fig. 37.2 Water distribution between particles

shaped rings of liquid. These cause adhesion because of the surface tension forces of the liquid–air interface and the hydrostatic suction pressure in the liquid bridge. When all the air has been displaced from between the particles the capillary stage is reached and the particles are held by capillary suction at the liquid–air interface which is now only at the granule surface. The funicular state represents an intermediate stage between the pendular and capillary states. Moist-granule tensile strength increases about three times from the pendular to capillary state.

It may appear that the state of the powder bed is dependent upon the total moisture content of the wetted powders but the capillary state may also be reached by decreasing the separation of the particles. In the massing process during wet granulation, continued kneading/mixing of material originally in the pendular state will densify the wet mass, decreasing the pore volume occupied by air and eventually producing the funicular or capillary state without further liquid addition.

In addition to these three states, a further state, the droplet, is illustrated in Fig. 37.2. This will be important in the process of granulation by spray drying of a suspension. In this state, the strength of the droplet is dependent upon the surface tension of the liquid used.

These wet bridges are only temporary structures in wet granulation because the moist granules will be dried. They are, however, a prerequisite for the formation of solid bridges formed by adhesives present in the liquid or by materials which dissolve in the granulating liquid.

Solid bridges

These can be formed by:

1 partial melting,
2 hardening binders,
3 crystallization of dissolved substances.

Partial melting

Although not considered to be a predominant mechanism in pharmaceutical materials, it is possible that the pressures used in dry granulation methods may cause melting of low melting point materials where the particles touch and high pressures are developed. When the pressure is relieved, crystallization will take place and bind the particles together.

Hardening binders

This is the common mechanism in pharmaceutical wet granulations when an adhesive is included in the granulating solvent. The liquid will form liquid bridges, as discussed above, and the adhesive will harden or crystallize on drying to form solid bridges to bind the particles. Adhesives such as polyvinylpyrrolidone, the cellulose derivatives (such as carboxymethylcellulose) and starch (added as a mucilage) all function in this way.

Crystallization of dissolved substances

The solvent used to mass the powder during wet granulation may dissolve one of the powdered ingredients. When the granules are dried, crystallization of this material will take place and the dissolved substance then acts as a hardening binder. Any material soluble in the granulating liquid will function in this manner; e.g. sucrose incorporated into dry powders granulated with water.

The size of the crystals produced in the bridge will be influenced by the rate of drying of the granules; the slower the drying time, the larger the particle size. It is therefore important that the drug does not dissolve in the granulating liquid and recrystallize because it may adversely affect the dissolution rate of the drug if crystals larger than that of the starting material are produced.

Attractive forces between solid particles

In the absence of liquids and solid bridges formed by binding agents, there are two types of attractive force which can operate between particles in pharmaceutical systems.

Electrostatic forces may be of importance in causing powder cohesion and the initial formation of agglomerates, e.g. during mixing. In general they do not contribute significantly to the final strength of the granule.

Van der Waals forces, however, are about four

orders of magnitude greater than electrostatic forces and contribute significantly to the strength of granules produced by dry granulation. The magnitude of these forces will increase as the distance between adjacent surfaces decreases and in dry granulation this is achieved using pressure to force the particles together.

MECHANISMS OF GRANULE FORMATION

In the dry methods, adhesion of particles takes place because of applied pressure. A compact or sheet is produced which is larger than the granule size required and therefore the required size can be attained by milling and sieving.

In wet granulation methods, liquid added to dry powders has to be distributed through the powder by the mechanical agitation produced in the granulator. The particles adhere to each other because of liquid films and further agitation and/or liquid addition causes more particles to adhere. The precise mechanism by which a dry powder is transformed into a bed of granules is probably different for each type of granulation equipment but the mechanism discussed below, originally proposed for pan granulators, serves as a useful broad generalization of the process. The Freund granulator discussed later in this chapter utilizes a principle similar to that of a pan granulator and the mechanism will therefore be of direct relevance to granulation in this type of equipment.

The proposed granulation mechanism can be divided into three stages (Barlow, 1968):

Nucleation

Granulation starts with particle–particle contact and adhesion due to liquid bridges. A number of particles will join to form the pendular state illustrated in Fig. 37.2. Further agitation densifies the pendular bodies to form the capillary state and these bodies act as nuclei for further granule growth.

Transition

Nuclei can grow by two possible mechanisms: either single particles can be added to the nuclei by pendular bridges or two or more nuclei may combine. The combined nuclei will be reshaped by the agitation of the bed.

This stage is characterized by the presence of a large number of small granules with a fairly wide size distribution. Providing that the size distribution is not excessively large, this point represents a suitable end-point for granules used in capsule and tablet manufacture as relatively small granules will produce a uniform tablet die or capsule fill. Larger granules may give rise to problems in small diameter dies due to bridging across the die and uneven fill.

Ball growth

Further granule growth produces large, spherical granules and the mean particle size of the granulating system will increase with time. If agitation is continued, granule coalescence will continue and produce an unusable, overmassed system although this is dependent upon the amount of liquid added and the properties of the material being granulated.

Although ball growth produces granules which may be too large for pharmaceutical purposes, some degree of ball growth will occur in planetary mixers and it is an essential feature of some spheronizing equipment.

The four possible mechanisms of ball growth have been summarized by Sastry and Fuerstenau (1973) and are illustrated in Fig. 37.3.

Coalescence

Two or more granules join to form a larger granule.

Breakage

Granules break into fragments which adhere to other granules forming a layer of material over the surviving granule.

Abrasion transfer

Agitation of the granule bed leads to attrition of material from granules. This abraded material adheres to other granules, increasing their size.

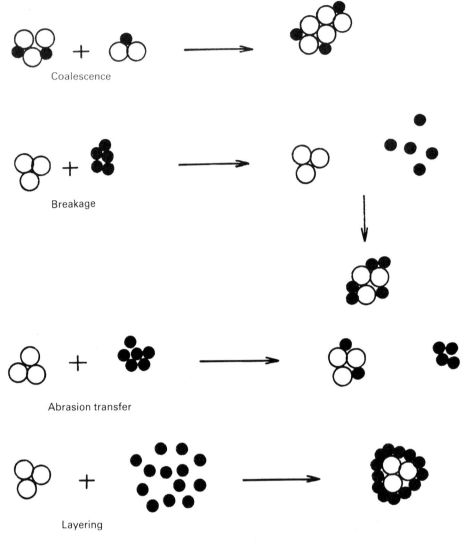

Fig. 37.3 Mechanisms of ball growth during granulation

Layering

When a second batch of powder mix is added to a bed of granules, the powder will adhere to the granules forming a layer over the surface increasing the granule size. This mechanism is only of relevance to the production of layered granules using spheronizing equipment.

There will be some degree of overlap between these stages and it will be very difficult to identify a given stage by inspection of the granulating system. For end-product uniformity it is desirable to finish every batch of a formulation at the same stage and this may be a major problem in pharmaceutical production.

Using the slower processes such as the planetary mixer, there is usually a sufficient length of time to stop the process before overmassing. In faster granulation equipment, the duration of granulation can only be used as a control parameter when the formulation is such that granule growth is slow and takes place at a fairly uniform rate. In many cases, however, the transition from a non-granulated to an overmassed system is very rapid and monitoring equipment is necessary to stop the granulation at a predetermined point. Although the topic of granulation end-point control is beyond the scope of this chapter, useful references are given in the bibliography.

PHARMACEUTICAL GRANULATION EQUIPMENT

Wet granulators

There are three main types of granulator used within the pharmaceutical industry for wet granulation.

Shear granulators

In the traditional granulation process a planetary mixer is often used for wet massing of the powders, e.g. Hobart, Collette, Beken (Fig. 37.4). Powder mixing usually has to be performed as a separate operation using suitable mixing equipment. With some formulations, such as those containing two or three ingredients in approximately equal quantities, however, it may be possible to achieve a suitable mix in the planetary mixer without a separate stage.

The mixed powders are fed into the bowl of the planetary mixer and granulating liquid added as the paddle of the mixer agitates the powders. The planetary action of the blade when mixing is similar to that of a household mixer.

The moist mass has then to be transferred to a granulator such as an oscillating granulator (Fig. 37.5). The rotor bars of the granulator oscillate and force the moist mass through the sieve screen, the size of which determines the granule size. The mass should be sufficiently moist to form discrete granules when sieved. If excess liquid is added, strings of material will be formed and if the mix is too dry the mass will be sieved to powder and granules will not be formed. The granules can be collected on trays and transferred to a drying oven although tray drying suffers from three major disadvantages:

1 There is a long drying time.
2 Migration of dissolved material to the upper surface of the bed of granules can take place as the solvent is only removed from the upper surface of the bed on the tray.
3 Granules may aggregate due to bridges formed at the points of contact of the granules.

To deaggregate the granules and remix them, a sieving stage is necessary after drying.

An alternative method is to dry the granules using a fluidized bed drier. This is a quicker method and as it keeps the individual granules separated during drying, it reduces the problems of aggregation and intergranular solute migration, reducing the need for a sieving stage after drying

The disadvantages of this traditional granulation process are its long duration, the need for

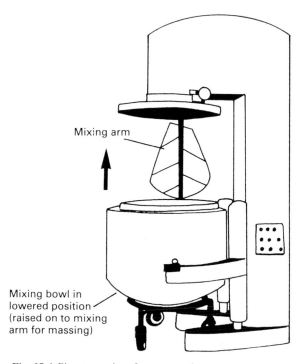

Fig. 37.4 Planetary mixer for wet massing

Mixing arm

Mixing bowl in lowered position (raised on to mixing arm for massing)

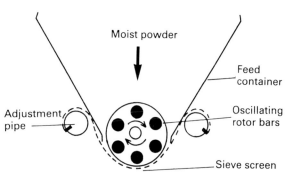

Moist powder

Feed container

Adjustment pipe

Oscillating rotor bars

Sieve screen

Fig. 37.5 Oscillating granulator

several pieces of equipment and the high material losses which can be incurred because of the transfer stages. Advantages are that the process is not very sensitive to changes in the characteristics of the granule ingredients (e.g. surface area variations in different batches of an excipient) and the end-point of the massing process can often be determined by inspection.

High speed mixer/granulators (e.g. Diosna, Fielder)

This type of granulator was originally designed solely for mixing purposes but is now used extensively for granulation. The machines have a stainless steel mixing bowl containing a three-bladed impeller which revolves in the horizontal plane and a three-bladed auxiliary chopper which revolves in the vertical plane (Fig. 37.6).

The unmixed powders are placed in the bowl and mixed by the rotating impeller. Granulating liquid is then added via a port in the lid and this is mixed into the powders by the impeller. The chopper is usually switched on when the moist mass is formed because its function is to break up

the mass to produce a bed of fine, granular material. This granular product is usually sieved as it is being discharged into the bowl of a fluid bed driver simply to remove large aggregates.

The advantage of the process is that mixing, massing and granulation are all performed in a short period in the same piece of equipment. Granulation progresses so rapidly that a usable granule can be transformed very quickly into an unusable, overmassed system and it is often necessary to use a suitable monitoring system to indicate the end of the granulation process, i.e. when a granule of the desired properties has been attained. The process is also sensitive to variations in raw materials but this may be minimized by using a suitable end-point monitor.

A variation of the Diosna/Fielder design is the Collette-Gral mixer (Fig. 37.7). Based on the bowl and overhead drive of the planetary mixer, the single paddle is replaced with two mixing shafts. One of these carries three blades which rotate in the horizontal plane at the base of the bowl and the second carries smaller blades which act as the chopper and rotate in the horizontal plane in the upper regions of the granulating mass.

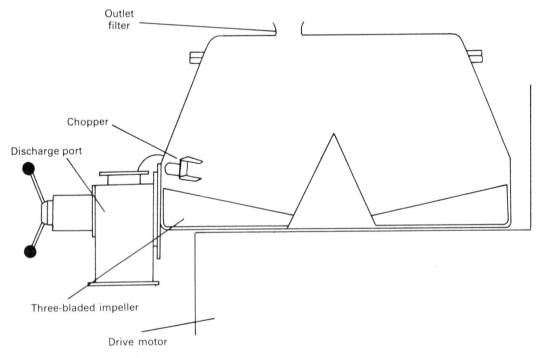

Fig. 37.6 High speed mixer/granulator

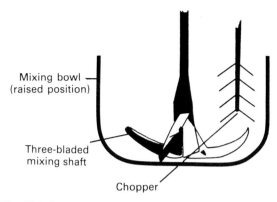

Fig. 37.7 Collette-Gral granulator: mixing shafts and bowl

Fluidized bed granulators (e.g. Aeromatic, Glatt)

The same principle utilized in fluidized bed drying, i.e. the fluidization of powder particles in a stream of air, is utilized for granulation in equipment of this type.

Heated air is blown or sucked through a bed of unmixed powders to fluidize the particles and mix the powders. Granulating liquid is pumped through a spray nozzle over the particles and this liquid causes them to adhere when they collide. Escape of material from the granulation chamber is prevented by exhaust filters which are periodically agitated to reintroduce the collected material into the fluidized bed (Fig. 37.8). Sufficient liquid is added to produce granules of the required size which are then dried in the heated fluidizing air stream.

All the processes which normally need separate equipment in the traditional method are performed in one unit, saving labour costs, transfer losses and time although the equipment is initially expensive. Other advantages of the process are that units are available with in-line condensers for solvent recovery, the production of layered granules is possible and automation of the process can be achieved once the conditions affecting the granulation have been optimized.

The optimization of process (and product) parameters affecting granulation needs extensive development work not only during initial formulation work but also during scale-up from devel-

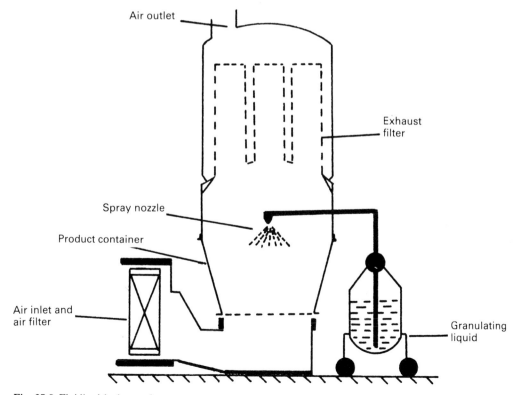

Fig. 37.8 Fluidized bed granulator

opment to production scale. Similar development work for the traditional process and that using high-speed granulators is not as extensive. The parameters affecting the quality of the final granule include such variables as the adhesive concentration used in the granulating solution, the type of adhesive, the velocity and temperature of the fluidizing air and the air pressure used to atomize the granulating liquid. A useful summary of the effects of these variables is given by Aulton and Banks (1978).

The above are the three methods most commonly used in pharmaceutical processes but for more specialized applications other equipment can be utilized.

Spray driers

A suspension of drug and excipients in adhesive solution can be dried in a spray drier (see Chapter 38). The resultant granules are free-flowing hollow spheres and the distribution of adhesive in such granules results in good compression properties (Seager et al., 1979).

This process can be used to make tablet granules although it is probably economically justified for this purpose only when used almost continuously or when suitable granules cannot be produced by the other methods. The primary advantages of the process are the short drying time and the minimal exposure of the product to heat due to the short residence time in the drying chamber. This means that little deterioration of heat-sensitive materials takes place and it may be the only process suitable for this type of product.

Spheronizers/pelletizers

For some applications it may be desirable to have a dense, spherical pellet of the type difficult to produce with the equipment above, and spheronizing or pelletizing equipment is used, e.g. Caleva Spheroniser, Freund CF Granulator. Such pellets could be used, for example, for capsule filling when coated and non-coated drug-containing pellets would give some degree of programmed drug release after the capsule disintegrates.

In the Freund granulator, the powder mix is added to the bowl and wetted with granulating liquid (Fig. 37.9). The base plate rotates at high speed and centrifugal force keeps the moist mass at the edges of the rotor where the velocity difference between the rotor and static walls causes the mass to roll and break up, forming discrete spherical pellets. These are dried by the heated inlet air from the air chamber which also acts as a positive-pressure seal during granulation.

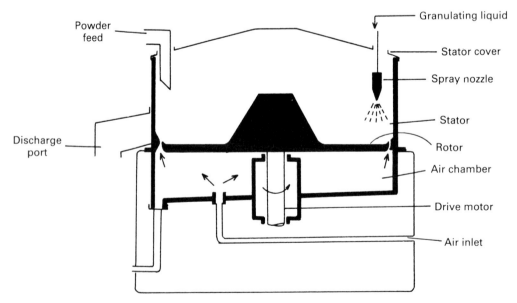

Fig. 37.9 Freund granulator

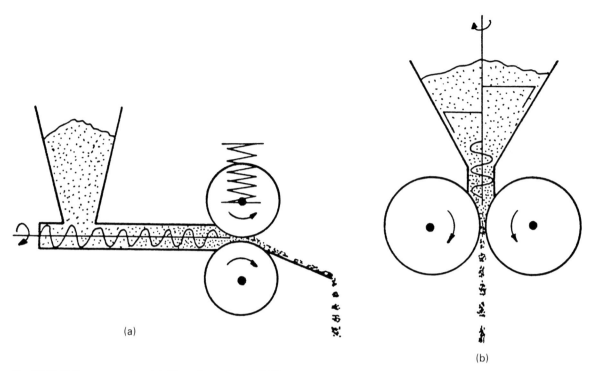

Fig. 37.10 Roller compaction: (a) Alexanderwerk and (b) Hutt types

Using this technique it is possible to coat the pellets by spraying coating solution on to the rotating pellets and layered pellets can be produced by using the pellets as nuclei in a second granulation with a powder mix of the coating ingredients.

The rotating base plate is a common feature of spheronizing equipment but some utilize a feed of pregranulated material which has been massed and extruded into short strings. Extrusion is a similar process to granulation in an oscillating granulator but requires a more moist mass than granulation processes and a more robust screen than that normally used in an oscillating granulator. For extrusion the wet mass can be fed through a perforated plate by an auger feed, a principle similar to that of the household mincer. The strings are fed on to a grooved or smooth rotating base plate and a velocity difference created by having static walls at the edge of the rotating plate breaks the material and rolls it into spheres. The spheres have then to be transferred to a fluidized bed drier for the drying process.

Dry granulators

The necessary pieces of equipment for dry granulation are first a machine for processing the dry powders and second a mill for breaking the compacts so produced.

Sluggers

The dry powders can be compressed using a tablet machine or, if higher pressures are required, a heavy duty rotary press can be used. This process is often known as 'slugging', the tablet made in the process being termed a 'slug'. See Chapter 39 for more details.

Roller compactors

Roller compaction is an alternative method, the powder mix being fed between rollers to form a compressed sheet (Fig. 37.10).

A hammer mill is suitable for breaking the compacts or sheets.

REFERENCES

Aulton, M. and Banks, M. (1978) The factors affecting fluidised bed granulation. *Mfg Chem. Aerosol News*, **49**, 50.

Barlow, C. G. (1968) The granulation of powders. *The Chemical Engineer*, **220**, CE196.

Newitt, D. M. and Conway-Jones, J. M. (1958). A contribution to the theory and practice of granulation. *Trans. Inst. Chem. Engrs*, **36**, 422.

Rumpf, H. (1962) The strength of granules and agglomerates. In *Agglomeration* (ed. W. A. Knepper), p. 379, Interscience, New York.

Sastry, K. V. S. and Fuerstenau, D. W. (1973) Mechanism of agglomerate growth in green pelletisation. *Powd. Tech.*, **7**, 97.

Seager, H., Burt, I., Ryder, J., Rue, P., Murray, S., Beal, N. and Warrack, J. K. (1979) The relationship between granule structure, process of manufacture and the tabletting properties of a granulated product. *Int. J. Pharm. Tech. Prod. Mfr.*, **1**, 36.

BIBLIOGRAPHY

Granulation: mechanisms

Capes, C. E. and Danckwerts, G. C. (1965) Granule formation by the agglomeration of damp powders. Part 1: The mechanism of granule growth. *Trans. Inst. Chem. Engrs*, **43**, T116.

Linkson, P. B., Glastonbury, J. R. and Duffy, G. J. (1973) The mechanism of granule growth in wet pelletising. *Trans. Inst. Chem. Engrs*, **51**, 251.

Granulation: equipment

Gergely, G. (1981) Granulation — a new approach. *Mfg Chem. Aerosol News*, **52**, 43.

Strutt, B. (1976) New mixer/granulator. *Mfg Chem. Aerosol News*, **47**, 47.

Wood, R. (1975) Getting to grips with granulation. *Mfg Chem. Aerosol News*, **46**, 23.

Granulation: general

There are a large number of published papers and only a very limited number are listed below.

Das, S. and Jarowski, C. I. (1979) Effect of granulating method on particle size distribution of granules and disintegrated tablets. *Drug Dev. Ind. Pharm.*, **5**, 479.

Doelker, E. and Shotton, E. (1977) The effect of some binding agents on the mechanical properties of granules and their compression characteristics. *J. Pharm. Pharmac.*, **29**, 193.

Ganderton, D. and Hunter, B. M. (1971) A comparison of granules prepared by pan granulation and massing and screening. *J. Pharm. Pharmac.*, **23** (Suppl), 1S.

Hunter, B. M. and Ganderton, D. (1973) The influence on pharmaceutical granulation of the type and capacity of mixers. *J. Pharm. Pharmac.*, **25** (Suppl), 71P.

Jaiyeoba, K. T. and Spring, M. S. (1980) The granulation of ternary mixtures: the effect of the solubility of the excipients. *J. Pharm. Pharmac.*, **32**, 1.

Granulation: end-point control

Kay, D. and Record, P. C. (1978) Automatic wet granulation end-point control system. *Mfg Chem. Aerosol News*, **49**, 45.

Leuenberger, H., Bier, H. -P. and Sucker, H. (1979) Theory of the granulating-liquid requirement in the conventional granulation process. *Pharm. Tech. Int.*, **2**, 35.

Lindberg, N.-O. and Leander L. (1977) Studies on granulation in a small planetary mixer. *Acta Pharm. Suecica*, **14**, 191, 197.

Lindberg, N.-O. and Leander, L. (1982) Instrumentation of a Kenwood major domestic-type mixer for studies of granulation. *Drug Dev. Ind. Pharm.*, **8**, 775.

Drying

Drying is an important operation in pharmaceutical practice since it is usually the last stage of manufacturing before packaging and it is important that the residual moisture is rendered low enough to prevent product deterioration and ensure free-flowing properties. This chapter is concerned with drying to the solid state starting with either a wet solid or a solution of the solutes which will form the dry final product. Formerly such solutions were first concentrated by evaporation of much of the liquid before drying the 'soft' extract so formed. Equipment such as spray and drum driers (see later in this chapter) are now capable of producing a dry product in one operation. Most pharmaceutical materials are not 'bone dry' but contain some residual moisture that may vary with the condition of the ambient air to which they are exposed. This is discussed in more detail later in this chapter.

Some crystalline materials may be freed from much of their residual moisture by treatment in a 'dewatering' centrifuge which is similar in construction to a domestic spin drier. For the purpose of this chapter, however, drying is defined as the removal of all or most of the liquid by supplying latent heat to cause thermal vaporization. In the majority of cases the 'liquid' will be water but volatile solvents such as isopropanol may also need to be removed in a drying process. The physical principles are similar regardless of the nature of the liquid though volatile solvents are normally recovered and may pose problems of safety.

THE DRYING OF WET SOLIDS

An understanding of this operation requires some preliminary explanation of the following important terms.

Moisture content

The moisture content of a wet solid is expressed as kg of moisture associated with one kg of the moisture-free or 'bone-dry' solid. A moisture content of 0.4 means that 0.4 kg of removable water is present per kg of the dry solid which will remain after complete drying. It is sometimes expressed as a *per cent* moisture content.

Equilibrium moisture content

The drying process may not remove all the possible moisture present and some moisture may be regained from the atmosphere if the 'dry' solid is exposed to air. The moisture content present is termed the equilibrium moisture content under the ambient conditions and it will change if those conditions are altered.

Part of the moisture present in crude drugs may be contained in cells or adsorbed on surfaces which prevent it from developing its full vapour pressure. Such moisture is described as 'bound' and is more difficult to remove than unbound water which exerts its full vapour pressure.

Relative humidity (RH) of air

Air at a given temperature is capable of taking up water vapour until it is saturated (at 100% RH). If the temperature is raised then the air will be able to take up more moisture and the RH falls. It should be noted that in convective drying where warm air is passed over the surface of a wet solid, the RH may rise from two separate factors namely:

1 The cooling of the air as it supplies heat to the wet solid,

2 Uptake of water vapour from the wet solid.

If the cooling is excessive the temperature of the air may fall to a value known as the *dew point* when liquid water will be deposited.

The per cent RH may be defined as

$$\frac{\text{Vapour pressure of water vapour in the air}}{\text{Vapour pressure of water vapour in air saturated at the same temperature}} \times 100$$

This is approximately equal to the ratio:

$$\frac{\text{Quantity of vapour present per kg of dry air}}{\text{Quantity required to saturate the air at the same temp}} \times 100$$

Absolute humidity

Relative humidity (RH) should be carefully distinguished from the absolute humidity which is the moisture content expressed as kg of water per kg of bone-dry air. This is *not* altered by change of temperature unless further moisture is taken up by the air.

Relationship between equilibrium moisture content and relative humidity

The equilibrium moisture content of a solid exposed to moist air varies with the relative humidity as shown in some typical plots (Fig. 38.1). Ordinary atmospheric conditions are of the order of 20 °C and 70–75% relative humidity, so that if exposed to the atmosphere a substance such as kaolin will contain about 1% moisture while crude drugs may have as much as 30% or more. Materials exposed to humid conditions will regain moisture so there is no advantage in drying to a moisture content lower than that which the material will have under the conditions of use.

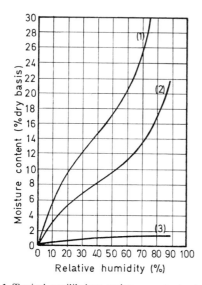

Fig. 38.1 Typical equilibrium moisture contents at 20 °C (1) crude drugs, such as leaves (2) textile fibres (3) inorganic substance, such as kaolin

Wet bulb and dry bulb temperature

If two similar thermometers are set up, one with its bulb kept moist by a wick immersed in a water reservoir, then this wet bulb thermometer will register a lower temperature than its dry bulb neighbour (Fig. 38.2). This is due to the evapo-

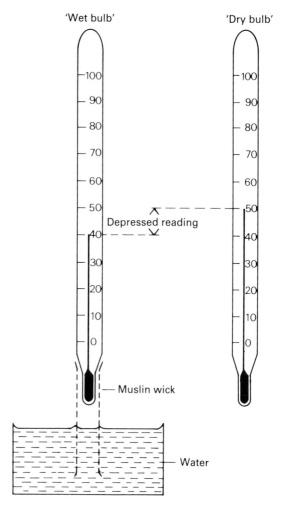

Fig. 38.2 Wet bulb and dry bulb temperatures

rative cooling as the latent heat of evaporation (Chapter 30) is partly taken from the sensible heat of the water surrounding the bulb.

In a similar way the temperature of a wet solid is kept low while free water remains but rises towards the temperature of the drying air as drying proceeds. Fortunately many materials can withstand higher temperatures when in the dry state.

CONVECTIVE DRYING OF WET SOLIDS

Fixed (or static) bed convective drying

The factors affecting drying in this manner can be illustrated by reference to the construction and use of a simple form of drier — the tray (shelf or compartment) drier.

Tray drier

An efficient type of tray drier is the directed circulation form shown in Fig. 38.3. Air flows in the direction of the arrows over each shelf in turn. The wet material may be spread directly on the shelves or on shallow trays resting on the shelves. Electrical elements or steam-heated pipes are positioned as shown so that the air is periodically reheated after it has cooled by passage over the wet material on one shelf before it passes over the material on the next. The required latent heat of evaporation is convectively transferred from the air and the rate of heat transfer may be written

$$\text{Rate} = h_c \, A \, \Delta \, T$$

where h_c is a heat transfer coefficient (Chapter 30) for convective heat transfer. The value of h_c is commonly around 10–$20 \text{ W m}^{-2} \text{ K}^{-1}$ which is much lower than the coefficients involved in heat transfer from condensing steam (Chapter 30). Convective drying is therefore slow and wet materials may take more than a day to dry.

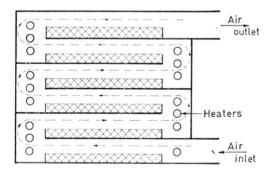

Fig. 38.3 Directed-circulation tray drier

There is another important factor controlling the rate of drying. The water vapour must pass through the boundary layers present at the surface into the turbulent air stream. For this to occur the relative humidity must be kept well below the saturation level and the boundary layers kept small (Chapters 2 and 30). These conditions are achieved by having a brisk turbulent air flow over

the surface and by the periodic reheating of the air as the temperature falls so that it can pick up further moisture.

Rate of drying in fixed beds

The rate at which drying occurs has been found to show certain phases, which are illustrated in Fig. 38.4, where the change in moisture content is plotted against time. From A to B the relationship is linear, which is known as the *constant rate period*, while from B to C the rate of loss of moisture decreases and is known as the *falling rate period*. The end of the constant rate period, B, is referred to as the *critical moisture content*.

An alternative method of representing the drying process is given in Fig. 38.5 which shows the variation of drying rate as the moisture content changes. From the graphs it can be seen that there is considerable variation in the behaviour of

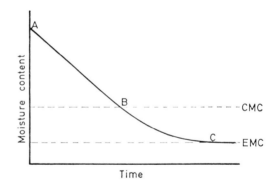

Fig. 38.4 Drying curve. CMC, critical moisture content; EMC, equilibrium moisture content

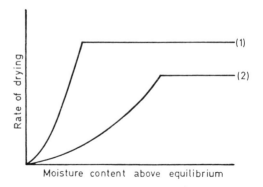

Fig. 38.5 Rate of drying curves: (1) sand (2) soap

different materials. The critical moisture content may vary also being low with non-porous materials (sand has a value of less than 10%) while colloidal organic substances may have a critical moisture content in excess of 100%.

The curves for the falling rate period may have different shapes, so that for a material such as soap (curve 2) the falling rate of drying shows a continuous decrease. In other substances, sand is a typical example, the falling rate period shows two phases. The *first falling rate period* has a linear relationship, that is, the decrease in rate is uniform, while in the *second falling rate period* there is a continuous decrease until the equilibrium moisture content is reached.

Each of these periods will be considered in more detail.

Constant rate period   For given conditions of temperature and humidity, most substances dry at a similar rate in the constant rate period. It is found that the evaporation rate is similar to that from a free liquid surface under the same conditions, indicating that the evaporation takes place from the wet surface of the solid and that the liquid is replaced from below as fast as it is vaporized.

Controlling factors in this period are the rate of which heat can be transferred and the removal of the vapour as explained earlier.

First falling rate period   As moisture is removed from the surface, a point will be reached when the rate of vaporization is insufficient to *saturate* the air in contact with the surface. Under these conditions, the rate of drying will be limited by the transfer of liquid to the surface and, since this becomes increasingly difficult, the rate decrease continuously.

For some substances with a complex structure such as gels or vegetable drugs, the rate of movement can be described by expressions resembling the diffusion equation, so that it is dependent on a moisture concentration gradient.

In packed beds of particulate materials, other factors are involved and capillary forces have a controlling effect. The liquid in the pores exerts a *suction potential* (due principally to the surface tension of the liquid) and the value of the suction potential increases as pore size decreases. Pore size will vary according to particle size and the packing

of the particle, cubical pores being larger than rhombohedral pores. Higher values of the suction potential make removal of the water from the pore more difficult, so that larger pores near the surface open first, followed by smaller pores. During drying, moisture will be drawn from the lower pores, moving to smaller pores near the surface that have been emptied, or to the surface, according to the relative values of the suction potential. Moisture movement may cause the 'migration' of soluble drugs which is discussed later in this chapter.

Eventually, the suction potential of the pores still containing moisture is so great that movement cannot occur and drying at the surface will end. As the drying rate decreases, less heat is used as latent heat of vaporization, so that the heat transfer coefficient should be reduced.

Second falling rate period   Any moisture that remains at the end of the first falling rate period is unable to move, so that drying cannot take place on the surface. Hence, the plane of vaporization retreats from the surface into the body of the solid, and the drying rate depends on the movement of the vapour through the pores to the surface, in general, by molecular diffusion.

In both cases, minimum humidity of the atmosphere above the solid will assist in maintaining the maximum vapour pressure gradient. In addition, the thermal conductivity of the solid decreases as it becomes dry; if the solid is thermostable it is safe to allow temperature gradients to increase to maintain the rate of heat transfer, but if the material is thermolabile the heating must be decreased.

In the operation of a tray drier it is usual to remove the dry material on the trays near the air inlet and replace them with the trays with partially dry material further from the inlet. Trays with fresh wet material are placed on the empty shelves. In this way the outgoing air contacts the wettest material.

Dynamic convective driers

Tunnel drier

Such counter-current movement of air and drying solids is arranged much more conveniently in the *tunnel drier*, where the drying method resembles the compartment drier, but takes the form of a long tunnel, with heated air entering at one end and some means of moving the material to be dried at the opposite end. The tunnel drier can be of any size, and the movement can be effected in a very simple manner; for example, the solids may be placed on trays on rails and, at suitable intervals, a tray may be pushed into the inlet, thereby displacing a tray from the dry end. On the other hand, a more sophisticated arrangement is a mechanical conveyor that has an automatic speed control and temperature and humidity control, including reheaters if necessary.

Compared with the compartment drier, the tunnel drier has the advantage of being semi-continuous or continuous in operation; applications are similar, but more suitable for large scale production.

Rotary drier

If powdered or granular substances are dried in the tunnel drier (see above) on the usual form of conveyor, the drying takes place from a static bed of the solid. The *rotary drier* is a modified form of the tunnel drier in which the particles are passed through a rotating cylinder, countercurrent to a stream of heated air. Due to the rotation of the cylinder, the material is turned over and drying takes place from individual particles and not from a static bed.

As indicated in the section in Fig. 38.6, the cylindrical shell (which may be as much as 10 m in length) is mounted with a slight slope, of the order of 1 in 20, so that the material will move

through the shell as it is slowly rotated at about 10 rev min^{-1}. To improve contact, the shell contains baffles or *flights* which lift the solids and spill the particles through the air stream. This gives rapid drying, so that outputs of 4 tonnes h^{-1} can be obtained with larger versions.

The rotary drier is used for continuous drying on a large scale of any powdered or granular solid.

Fluidized bed drier

Another method of obtaining good contact between hot air and particles is used in the *fluidized bed drier*; the technique of *fluidization* is used widely for fluid/solid contacting operations of all types and the general principles will be summarized before the applications to drying.

Consider the situation in which particulate matter is contained in a vessel, the base of which is perforated, enabling a fluid to pass through the bed of solids from below. The fluid can be liquid or gas, but air will be assumed for the purposes of this description, as it is most relevant to the drying process.

If the air velocity through the bed is increased gradually and the pressure drop through the bed is measured, a graph of the operation shows several distinct regions, as indicated in Fig. 38.7. At first, when the air velocity is low, A, flow takes place between the particles without causing disturbance, but as the velocity is increased a point is reached, B, when the pressure drop has attained a value where the frictional drag on the particle is equal to the force of gravity on the particle. Rearrangement of the particles occurs to offer least resistance, C, and eventually they are

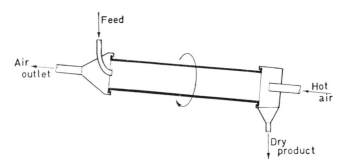

Fig. 38.6 Rotary drier

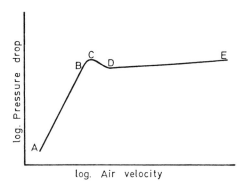

Fig. 38.7 Effect of air velocity on pressure drop through a fluidized bed

suspended in the air and can move; pressure drop through the bed decreases slightly because of the greater porosity, *D*. Further increase in the air velocity causes the particles to separate and move freely, and the bed is *fully fluidized*. Any additional increase in velocity separates the particles further, that is, the bed expands, without appreciable change in the pressure drop, until *E* when the velocity is sufficient to entrain the solids and cause transport of the particles.

In the region *D-E*, fluidization is irregular, much of the air flowing through in bubbles, the term *boiling bed* being commonly used to describe it. The important factor is that it produces conditions of great turbulence, the particles mixing, with good contact between air and particles.

Hence, if hot air is used, the turbulent conditions lead to high heat and mass transfer rates, the fluidized bed technique therefore offering a means of rapid drying. The arrangement of such a drier is shown in Fig. 38.8 and sizes are available with capacities up to 200 kg.

Advantages of fluidized bed drying

1 Efficient heat and mass transfer give high drying rates, so that drying times are shorter than static bed convection driers. A batch of tablet granules, for example, can be dried in 20–30 minutes, whereas a compartment drier would require several hours. Apart from obvious economic advantages, the heating time of thermolabile materials is minimized.

2 The fluidized state of the bed gives drying from individual particles and not from the entire bed.

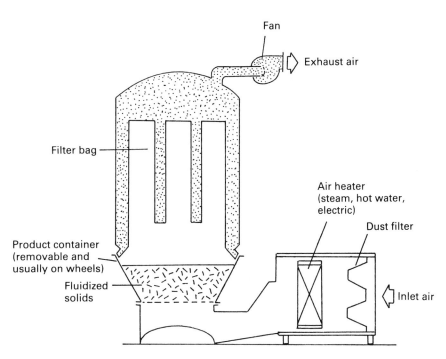

Fig. 38.8 Fluidized bed drier

Hence, most of the drying will be at constant rate and the falling rate period (when the danger of overheating is greatest) is very short.

3 The temperature of a fluidized bed is uniform and can be controlled precisely.

4 The fluidized state produces a free-flowing product.

5 The free movement of individual particles eliminates the risk of soluble materials migrating, as may occur in static beds.

6 The containers can be mobile, making handling simple, and reducing labour costs.

7 Short drying times mean that the unit has a high output from a small floor space.

Disadvantages of fluidized bed drying

1 The turbulence of the fluidized state may cause attrition of some materials, with the production of fines.

2 Fine particles may become entrained and must be collected by bag filters, with care to avoid segregation and loss of fines.

3 The vigorous movement of particles in hot dry air can lead to the generation of charges of static electricity, and suitable precautions must be taken.

A mixture of air with a fine dust of organic materials such as starch and lactose can explode violently if ignited by sparking caused by static charges. The danger is increased if the fluidized material contains a volatile solvent such as isopropanol. Simon (1979) has considered how risks may be minimized. For instance volatile solvents may be removed using an inert gas instead of air. The solvent vapour can be recovered and the gas recirculated.

CONDUCTIVE DRYING OF WET SOLIDS

In this process the wet solid is in thermal contact with a hot surface and the bulk of heat transfer occurs by conduction (Chapter 30).

Vacuum oven

This equipment is a good example of a conduction drier though it is not used so entensively as it formerly was. The vacuum oven (Fig. 38.9) consists of a jacketted vessel sufficiently stout in construction to withstand vacuum within the oven and steam pressure in the jacket. In addition, the supports for the shelves form part of the jacket, giving a larger area for conduction heat transfer. The oven can be closed by a door that can be locked tightly to give an airtight seal. The oven is connected through a condenser and receiver to a vacuum pump, although if the liquid to be removed is water and the pump is of the ejector type that can handle water vapour, the pump can be connected directly to the oven.

Operating pressure is usually about 0.03–0.06 bar, at which pressures water boils at 25–35 °C. Some ovens may be large, and continuous forms have been devised, but for pharmaceutical purposes an oven of about 1.5 m cube and with 20 shelves is commonly used, this giving an area of about 45–50 m² for heating.

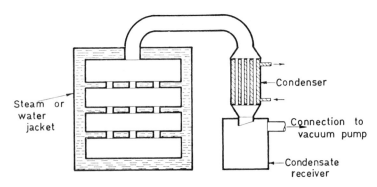

Fig. 38.9 Vacuum oven

In an alternative design there are a number of small compartments rather than one large one. This simplifies construction and operation by avoiding the need for one large and heavy door, which is replaced by small doors to each compartment. If the compartments are used in sequence, the pumping load is spread and semicontinuous operation is achieved.

The main advantage of the oven is that drying takes place at a low temperature and there is no risk of oxidation. The temperature of the dry solid will rise to the steam or water temperature at the end of the drying but this is not usually harmful. A serious drawback is the limited capacity and high labour costs of operation.

Vacuum tumbling drier

Vacuum tumbling drying finds greater application in the pharmaceutical industry. One design of tumbler drier resembles a large Y-cone mixer (discussed in Chapter 32). The vessel is steam jacketted and is connected to vacuum. It is used for drying tablet granules which tumble over the heated surface as the vessel slowly revolves. Heat transfer rates in this equipment are much higher than can be attained in a vacuum oven where the material is static.

RADIATION DRYING OF WET SOLIDS

Radiant heat transmission

Heat transmission by radiation differs from heat transfer by conduction or convection in that no medium, solid, liquid or gaseous, need be present. Heat energy in the form of radiation can cross empty space or travel through the atmosphere virtually without loss. If it falls on a body capable of absorbing it then it appears as heat but a proportion may be reflected or transmitted. All materials radiate heat over a range of wavelengths lying between 1 and 10 μm (Fig. 38.10) which lie in the infrared (above the visible red) region of the electromagnetic spectrum. The quantity of energy emitted is proportional to the fourth power of the absolute temperature. Consequently the emission of energy goes up very rapidly with an increase in

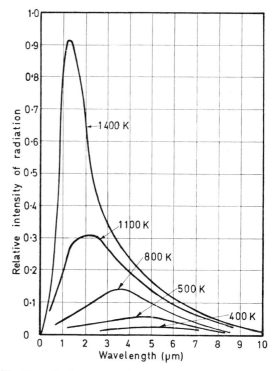

Fig. 38.10 Radiant energy distributions

the temperature of the emitter. As shown in Fig. 38.10 the energy is emitted over a range of wavelengths but there is a peak wavelength which is displaced towards the shorter wavelengths as the temperature of the emitter rises. The area under the curves in Fig. 38.10 is a measure of the total energy emitted at the relevant temperature and this rises rapidly with increase in temperature.

Use of radiant heat in drying

Infrared radiation can be used as a heat source to provide the required latent heat in drying. The wet material must be able to 'see' the source which is usually an electrically heated element operated at temperatures between 500 and 1000 K. The element can be mounted above the wet solid and placed within a reflector to direct the radiation on to the wet surface.

Infrared heating has been used to dry pharmaceutical products such as wet granules but it suffers from the disadvantage that it is absorbed very quickly and does not penetrate far into the wet mass. The surface layers dry quickly and the absorption of further energy then raises the dry material to a high value which is often detrimental to the product. For that reason infrared radiation is now seldom used as a heat source.

The use of microwave radiation

Although energy in the infrared region is more easily generated there are other longer wavelengths which can generate heat when the radiation is absorbed in a wet solid. Microwave radiation in the range of wavelength of 10 mm to 1 m penetrates much better than i.r. radiation and microwave ovens are now a common feature of a modern kitchen. Microwave driers are currently finding some appplication in the pharmaceutical industry.

Generation and action of microwaves

Microwaves are produced by an electronic device known as a magnetron which was developed for use in wartime radar. Microwave energy can be reflected down a rectangular duct (termed a waveguide) or simply beamed through a transparent window into the drying chamber. To avoid interference with radio and television it is permitted to operate only at certain frequencies which are 960 and 2450 MHz in the UK. When

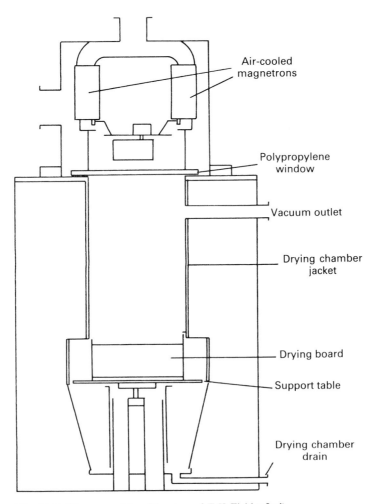

Fig. 38.11 Microwave drier. (Courtesy of T K Fielder Ltd)

microwaves fall on substances of suitable electronic structure (water is one of these) the electrons in the molecule attempt to resonate in sympathy with the radiation and the resulting molecular 'friction' results in the generation of heat. The penetration is good so that heat is generated uniformly within the solid. Dry solids may not resonate as well as water so further heating may be avoided when the water is removed.

A microwave drier for granulates

Figure 38.11 is a sketch of a microwave drier marketed for use for drying granulates. It is designed to operate under vacuum though that is not essential for the use of microwaves. The radiation is generated by ten magnetrons each producing 0.75 kW at 2450 MHz. The radiation passes through the polypropylene window into the drying chamber where it is absorbed in the wet granules contained on a tray. The heat generated in the mass drives off the moisture at a low temperature set by the vacuum in the chamber. The evolved vapour is pumped away as it is formed. When drying is nearly complete the field intensity will rise since the dry solids do not absorb as readily as water. This rise is sensed and made to turn off the magnetrons progressively so as to give an accurate control of the final moisture content.

Advantages of microwave drying   The following advantages are claimed for microwave drying.

1 It provides rapid drying at fairly low temperatures.
2 The thermal efficiency is high since the drier casing and the air remain cool. Most of the microwave energy is absorbed in the wet material.
3 The bed is stationary avoiding problems of dust and attrition.
4 Solute migration is reduced as there is uniform heating of the wet mass.

Disadvantages of microwave drying

1 The batch size (typically 25 kg) is smaller than the batch size in fluidized bed drying.
2 Care must be taken to shield operators from the microwave radiation which can cause heating of organs such as the eyes and testes. This is ensured by 'fail safe' devices preventing generation of microwaves until the drying chamber is sealed.

DRIERS FOR DILUTE SOLUTIONS AND SUSPENSIONS

The objective of these driers is to spread the liquid to a large surface area for heat and mass transfer and to provide an effective means of collecting the dry solid. Two main types are used, the first spreading the liquid to a thin film and the second dispersing the liquid to a spray of small droplets.

Drum drier

Shown in section in Fig. 38.12, the *drum drier* consists of a drum 0.75–1.5 m in diameter and 2–4 m in length, heated internally, usually by steam, and rotated on its longitudinal axis. The liquid is applied to the surface and spread to a film; this may be done in various ways, but the simplest method is that shown in the diagram, where the drum dips into a *feed pan*. Drying rate is controlled by using a suitable speed of rotation and drum temperature. The product is scraped from the surface of the drum by means of a *doctor knife*.

Advantages of the drum drier

1 The method gives rapid drying, the thin film spread over a large area resulting in rapid heat and mass transfer.
2 The equipment is compact, occupying much less space than the spray drier, for example.

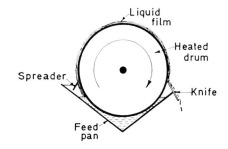

Fig. 38.12 Drum drier

3 Heating time is short, being only a few seconds.
4 The drum can be enclosed in a vacuum jacket, enabling the temperature of drying to be reduced.
5 The product is obtained in flake form, which is convenient for many purposes.

The only *disadvantage* is that operating conditions are critical and it is necessary to impose careful control on feed rate, film thickness, speed of rotation and temperature difference.

The drum drier can handle a variety of materials, either as solutions or suspensions; substances that are dried by this method include milk products, starch products, ferrous salts and suspensions of kaolin or zinc oxide.

Spray drier

The *spray drier* provides a large surface area for heat and mass transfer by atomizing the liquid to small droplets. These are sprayed into a stream of hot air, so that each droplet dries to a solid particle.

There are many forms of spray drier and Fig. 38.13 is a typical design, in which the *drying chamber* resembles a cyclone ensuring good circulation of air, to facilitate heat and mass transfer,

and that dried particles are separated by the centrifugal action.

The character of the particles is controlled by the droplet form, hence the type of atomizer is important. Jet atomizers are easily blocked and the droplet size is likely to vary, but this is not so with rotary types. One form of *rotary atomizer* is shown in Fig. 38.14. Liquid is fed on to the disc, which is rotated at high speed (up to 20,000 rev/min); a film is formed and spreads from the small disc to a larger, inverted hemispherical bowl, becoming thinner, and eventually being dispersed from the edge in a fine, uniform spray. In addition, the rotary atomizer has the advantage of being equally effective with suspensions of solids and it can operate efficiently at various feed rates.

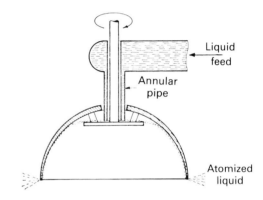

Fig. 38.14 Rotary atomizer

For crude products, drying can be effected by direct use of furnace gases, but for pharmaceutical purposes it is usual to filter the air and to heat it indirectly by means of a heat exchanger. Dust carried over in the air stream may be recovered by a cyclone separator or filter bag; in some cases the air may be scrubbed in a tower by means of the feed liquid. This has the advantage that underize particles are dissolved and cycled back to the drier and that the feed is preheated, reducing the heat requirements.

Spray-dried products are easily recognizable, being uniform in appearance and, if examined by means of a hand lens, the particles have a characteristic shape, in the form of hollow spheres with

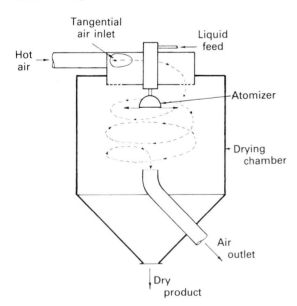

Fig. 38.13 Spray drier

a small hole. This arises from the drying process, since the droplet enters the hot air stream, and dries on the outside to form an outer crust with liquid still in the centre. This liquid then vaporizes, the vapour escaping by blowing a hole in the sphere.

It has been suggested that this method of drying allows a dry product to retain some properties of the feed; for example, a droplet from an emulsion dries with the disperse phase inside and a layer of the continuous phase on the outside. When reconstituted, the emulsion is easily reformed.

The method has been used for the microencapsulation of an oily solution of vitamins A and D by spray drying a gelatin-based emulsion. The bitter taste of certain drugs can be masked in a similar way by incorporating an organic polymer to coat the dried particles.

Advantages of the spray drying process

1 The droplets are small, giving a large surface area for heat and mass transfer, so that evaporation is very rapid. The actual drying time of a droplet is only a fraction of a second, and the overall time in the drier only a few seconds.
2 Because evaporation is very rapid, the droplets do not attain a high temperature, most of the heat being used as latent heat of vaporization.
3 The characteristic particle form gives the product a high bulk density and, in turn, ready solubility.
4 Provided that a suitable atomizer is used, the powder will have a uniform and controllable particle size.
5 The product is free-flowing, with almost spherical particles, and is especially convenient for tablet manufacture.
6 Labour costs are low, the process yielding a dry, free-flowing powder from a dilute solution, in a single operation with no handling.

Disadvantages of the spray drying process

1 The equipment is very bulky and with the ancillary equipment (fans, heaters, separators, etc.) is expensive. In a large installation, the drying chamber alone may be as much as 15 m in height and 6 m in diameter.
2 The thermal efficiency is rather low, since the air must still be hot enough when it leaves the drier to avoid condensation of moisture.

The spray drier can be used for drying almost any substance, in solution or in suspension. It is most useful for thermolabile materials, and particularly if handled continuously and in large quantities; outputs of 2000 kg h^{-1} can be attained, although pharmaceutical plants are usually somewhat smaller.

Examples of substances that are spray dried include borax, citric acid, hexamine, sodium phosphate, gelatin, acacia and extracts, while starch, barium sulphate and calcium phosphate are typical of insoluble materials. In addition, the method is widely used for products of indirect pharmaceutical interest, such as milk, soap, and detergents.

It is possible to operate driers aseptically using heated filtered air to dry products such as serum hydrolysate. Some driers operate in a closed circuit mode with an inert gas to minimize oxidation of the product. Volatile solvents can be recovered from such systems.

FREEZE DRYING

The phase diagram for water

The theory of sublimation (freeze) drying is based on an understanding of the phase diagram for the water system which is shown sketched in Fig. 38.15. The diagram consists of three separate plots which show:

1 the boiling point of water as it is lowered by reduction of the external pressure above the water (BO in Fig. 38.15),
2 the variation of the melting point of ice on reduction of the external pressure above it. There is a very slight rise in the melting point (AO),
3 the reduction of the vapour pressure exerted by ice as the temperature is reduced (CO Fig. 38.15).

Each of the areas enclosed by these plots represents a single phase either ice, water or vapour. Two phases can coexist along a line under the conditions of temperature and pressure defined by any point on the line. The point O is the one unique point where all three phases can coexist

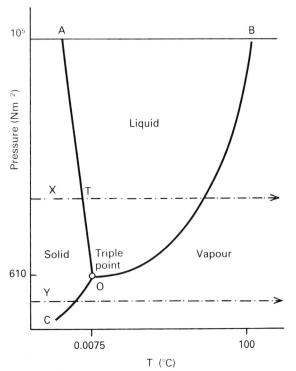

Fig. 38.15 The phase diagram for water (not to scale). For explanation see text

and known as the *triple point*. Its coordinates are a pressure of 610 N m^{-2} and a temperature of 0.0075 °C.

Suppose that solid ice exists under conditions of pressure and temperature defined by the point X. On heating the ice at constant pressure it will melt when the temperature rises to T. The ice will then change to water at this constant temperature and pressure. If, however, solid ice is maintained at a point below the triple point pressure (point Y) then on heating the ice will sublime and pass directly to water vapour without passing through the liquid phase and it will do so at a temperature which is well below 0 °C. This will only be the case if the pressure is prevented from rising above the triple point pressure and, to ensure that this is so, the vapour evolved must be removed as fast as it is formed. It is often thought that as the process takes place at a low temperature the heat required to sublime the ice will be small. In fact the latent heat of sublimation of ice at 2900 kJ kg^{-1} is appreciably larger than the latent heat of evaporation of water at atmospheric pressure and this heat must be supplied for the process to take place.

Application to freeze drying

The freeze drying of products such as blood plasma, though simple in theory, presents a number of practical problems.

1 The lowering of the freezing point by the solutes means that the solution must be frozen to well below the triple point temperature for pure water and it is usual to work in the range −10 to −30 °C.
2 Sublimation can only occur at the frozen surface and is a slow process. The surface must therefore be increased for all but very small volumes.
3 At low pressures large volumes of water vapour are produced which must be rapidly removed to prevent the pressure rising above the triple point pressure.
4 The dry material must usually be sterile and it must also be prevented from regaining moisture prior to final packing.

Stages of the freeze drying process

Freezing

The liquid material is frozen before the application of vacuum to avoid frothing and several methods are used to produce a large frozen surface.

Shell freezing This is employed for fairly large volumes such as blood products. The bottles are rotated slowly and almost horizontally in a refrigerated bath. The liquid freezes in a thin shell around the inner circumference of the bottle. Freezing is slow and large ice crystals form which is a drawback of this method.

In vertical spin freezing the bottles are spun individually in a vertical position so that centrifugal force forms a circumferential layer of solution which is cooled by a blast of cold air. The solution supercools and 'snap' freezes rapidly with the formation of small ice crystals.

Centrifugal evaporative freezing This is a similar method where the solution is spun in small containers within a centrifuge. This prevents foaming when a vacuum is applied. The vacuum causes boiling at room temperature and this removes so much sensible heat that the solutions snap freeze. About 20% of the water is removed prior to freeze drying and there is no need for refrigeration. Ampoules are usually frozen in this way, a number being spun in a vertical position in a special centrifuge head so that the liquid is thrown outwards and freezes as a wedge.

Vacuum application

The containers and the frozen material must be connected to a source of vacuum sufficient to drop the pressure below the triple point and remove the large volumes of low pressure vapour formed during drying. Heat of sublimation must be supplied. Under those conditions the ice slowly sublimes leaving a porous solid which still contains about 0.5% moisture after primary drying.

The apparatus may resemble a vacuum oven (see above) when the frozen material is introduced as a shallow layer on a tray. More commonly a number of bottles or vials are attached to individual outlets of a manifold which is connected to vacuum.

Primary drying

Primary drying can reduce the moisture content of a freeze-dried solid to around 0.5%. Further reduction can be effected by secondary drying. During the primary drying, the latent heat of sublimation must be provided and the vapour removed.

Heat transfer Heat transfer is critical; insufficient heat prolongs the process, which is already slow, and excess heat will cause melting.

Prefrozen bottles, of blood for example, are placed in individually heated cylinders or are connected to a manifold when heat can be taken from the atmosphere.

Shelf-frozen materials are heated from the drier shelf while ampoules may be left on the centrifuge head or may be placed on a manifold, but in either case heat from the atmosphere is sufficient.

In all cases, the heat transfer must be controlled, since only about 5 W m^{-2} K^{-1} is needed and overheating will lead to melting.

Vapour removal The vapour formed must be removed continually to avoid a pressure rise that would stop sublimation. To reduce the pressure sufficiently it is necessary to use efficient vacuum pumps, usually two-stage rotary pumps on the small scale, and ejector pumps on the large scale. On the small scale, vapour is absorbed by a desiccant such as phosphorus pentoxide, or is cooled on a small condenser with solid carbon dioxide. Condensation may be used on the large scale, but mechanically refrigerated condensers are used. Accumulation of ice decreases heat transfer, and for very large installations the condenser can be scraped, the ice compressed to a solid block and ejected through a special pressure lock.

For vapour flow to occur the vapour pressure at the condenser must be less than the vapour pressure at the frozen surface and a low condenser temperature is necessary. On the large scale, vapour is commonly removed by pumping but the pumps must be of large capacity and must not be affected by moisture. The extent of the pumping capacity needed will be realized from the fact that, under the pressure conditions used during primary drying, 1 g of ice will form 1000 litres of vapour. Ejector pumps are most satisfactory for this purpose.

Rate of drying The rate of drying in freeze drying is very low, the ice being removed at a rate of about 1 mm depth per hour. The drying rate curve illustrated in Fig. 38.16 shows a similar shape to the normal drying curve, the drying being at constant rate during most of the time. The two curves are not really comparable, however, since the mechanism of freeze drying resembles the falling rate period of the normal drying process. A constant rate is shown because the rate of sublimation is so slow that it is the controlling factor, whereas in the normal drying process the rate is limited by vapour diffusing through the pores. Any attempt to increase sublimation involves raising the heat transfer coefficient and would only lead to melting.

In recent years the advent of cheap microprocessor control has enabled the drying cycle to be monitored. There is an optimum vapour pressure for a maximum sublimation rate and the heat input and other variables are adjusted to maintain this value. Continuous freeze drying is

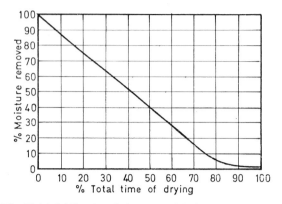

Fig. 38.16 Sublimation drying: rate of drying curve

possible in modern equipment where the vacuum chamber is fitted with a belt conveyor and vacuum locks. The frozen material is introduced in small batches and the belt is vibrated to turn the frozen granules. Despite these advances the overall drying rate is still slow.

Secondary drying

The removal of residual moisture at the end of primary drying is performed by raising the temperature of the solid to as high as 50 or 60 °C. In this secondary drying the vapour pressure of the remaining moisture is very low and the use of a desiccant such as silica gel or phosphorus pentoxide is also necessary to absorb the vapour evolved. A high temperature is permissible because the small amount of moisture remaining at the end of primary drying is not sufficient to cause spoilage.

Packaging

Attention must be paid to packaging freeze-dried products to ensure protection from moisture. Containers should be closed without contacting the atmosphere, if possible, and ampoules, for example, are sealed on the manifold while still under vacuum. Otherwise, the closing must be carried out under controlled atmospheric conditions.

Freeze drying in practice

Advantages

Freeze drying, as a result of the character of the process, has certain special advantages:

1 Drying takes place at very low temperatures, so that enzyme action is inhibited and decomposition, particularly hydrolysis, is minimized.
2 The solution is frozen such that the final dry product is a network of solid occupying the same volume as the original solution. Thus, there is no case-hardening and the product is light and porous.
3 The porous form of the product gives ready solubility.
4 There is no concentration of the solution prior to drying. Hence, salts do not concentrate and denature proteins as occurs with other drying methods.
5 Under high vacuum, there is no contact with the air, and oxidation is minimized.

Disadvantages

There are two main disadvantages of freeze drying:

1 The porosity, ready solubility and complete dryness yield a very hygroscopic product. Unless dried in the final container and sealed in situ, packaging requires special conditions.
2 The process is very slow and uses complicated plant, which is very expensive. It is not a general method of drying, therefore, but is limited to certain types of valuable products that cannot be dried by any other means.
3 It is difficult (but not impossible) to adapt the method for solutions containing non-aqueous solvents.

Uses

The method is applied only to biological products; for example, antibiotics (other than penicillin), blood products, vaccines (such as BCG, yellow fever, smallpox), enzyme preparations (such as hyaluronidase) and microbiological cultures.

SOLUTE MIGRATION DURING DRYING

Intergranular migration

Many drugs and binding agents are soluble in the granulating fluid (see Chapter 37). During the convective drying of granulates in shallow beds these solutes will move towards the bed surface and be deposited there when the fluid evaporates. This intergranular migration, where the solutes move from granule to granule, may result in gross maldistribution of active drug. When the granules are compressed the tablets may have a deficiency or an excess of drug. This was demonstrated by Chaudry and King (1972) who found that only 12% of tablets made from a tray-dried warfarin granulate were within the USP limits for drug content.

Intragranular migration

Drying methods based on fluidization and vacuum tumbling separate the granules during drying and so prevent the intergranular migration that may occur in fixed beds. Intragranular migration, where the solutes move towards the periphery of each granule, may take place. This can result in a number of problems.

Consequences of solute migration

Loss of active drug

The periphery of each granule may become enriched with the interior suffering a depletion. This will be of no consequence unless the enriched outer layer is abraded as may happen during fluid-

ized bed drying when the fine dust will be eluted. The granules suffer a net loss of drug.

Mottling of compressed coloured tablets

Coloured tablets can be made by adding soluble colour during wet granulation. Intragranular migration of the colour may give rise to dry granules with a highly coloured outer zone and colourless interior (Fig. 38.17). On compression granule fracture and rebonding take place and the colourless interior is exposed. The eye then sees the coloured fragments against a colourless background and the tablets appear mottled.

Migration may be reduced by using the insoluble aluminium 'lake' of the colouring material in preference to the soluble dyestuff itself. Armstrong and March (1978) who have made a detailed study of mottling, point out this is not the complete answer and factors such as an unfavourable pH can allow lakes to migrate. They suggest that small granules, which do not fracture so readily, are preferable to larger ones if mottling is troublesome.

The migration of soluble binders

Intragranular migration may deposit a soluble binder at the periphery of the granules and so confer a 'hoop stress' resistance making the granules harder and more resistant to abrasion. Work

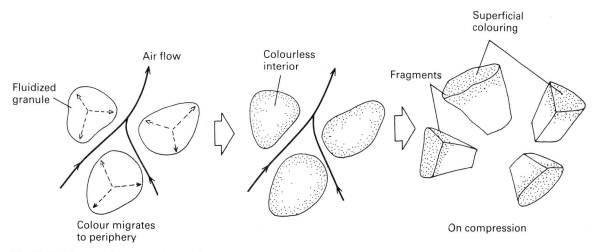

Fig. 38.17 Diagram of intergranular and intragranular migration (mottling)

by Seager and others (1979) has shown that this migration can aid the bonding process and is therefore sometimes beneficial.

Many other factors such as drying method and granulate formulation and moisture content have been shown to affect solute migration. For further details the student is referred to a review by Travers (1983).

REFERENCES AND BIBLIOGRAPHY

Armstrong, N. A. and Marsh, G. A. (1978) *Drug Dev. Ind. Pharm.*, **4**, 511.

Chaudry, I. A. and King, R. L. (1972) *J. pharm. Sci.*, **6**, 1121.

Nielson, F. (1983) Spray drying of pharmaceuticals. *Mfg Chem. Aerosol News*, **53**(7), 38–41.

Norhebel, G. and Moss, A. A. H. (1971) *Drying of Solids in the Chemical Industry*, Butterworth and Co. (Publishers) Ltd, Sevenoaks, Kent.

Powell, M. (1983) Developments in freeze drying. *Mfg Chem. Aerosol News*, **53**(7), 47–50.

Seager, H., Burt, I. Ryder, J., Rue, P., Murray, S., Beal, N. and Warrack, J. K. (1979) *Int. J. Pharm. Tech. Prod. Mfr.*, **1**, 36.

Simon, E. (1979) Containment of hazards in fluid bed technology. *Mfg Chem. Aerosol News*, **49**(1), 23–25.

Travers, D. N. (1983) Problems with solute migration. *Mfg Chem. Aerosol News*, **53**(3), 67–71.

Tableting

INTRODUCTION TO TABLETING

The earliest reference to a dosage form resembling the tablet is to be found in arabic medical literature, in which drug particles were compressed between the ends of engraved ebony rods, force being applied by means of a hammer. However details of the tableting process as it is now known were first published in 1843, when Thomas Brockedon was granted a patent for 'manufacturing pills and medicinal lozenges by causing materials when in a state of granulation, dust or powder, to be made into form and solidified by pressure in dies'. In this case too, force was applied by a hammer.

The use of the tablet rapidly increased, especially in the USA, where the demand for large quantities of medical supplies during the civil war spurred its development. Powder-driven presses replaced Brockedon's hammer, and by 1874, there existed both rotary and eccentric presses which in their mode of operation were fundamentally similar to those in use at the present time.

A monograph for Glyceryl Trinitrate Tablets was included in the *British Pharmacopoeia* of 1885. No other tablet monograph appeared until 1945; this, however, was due to the absence of acceptable quality control standards rather than lack of popularity of the dosage form itself. Despite this, the tablet did not meet with the unqualified approval of the pharmaceutical profession. 'Apprentice', writing in the *Pharmaceutical Journal* asked what his future would be if after 3 years' training, his duties would consist chiefly of counting factory-made tablets, whilst in 1895, an editorial in the *Pharmaceutical Journal* predicted that 'tablets have had their day and will pass away to make room for something else'. Notwithstanding these predictions, the 1980 Pharmacopoeia has nearly 300 monographs for tablets, far in excess of any other dosage form.

The reason for the popularity of the tablet is that it provides advantages for all those involved in the production and consumption of medicinal products. For the manufacturer, though initial capital outlay is high, tablets can be produced at a much greater rate than any other dosage form. Furthermore the fact that the tablet is a dry dosage form promotes stability, and in general, tablets have shelf lives measured in years.

From the viewpoint of the pharmacist, tablets are easy to dispense, whilst the patient receives a concentrated and hence readily portable and consumed dosage form. Furthermore if properly prepared, tablets provide a uniformity of dosage greater than, for example, a liquid medicine, and appropriate coating can mask unpleasant tastes and improve patient acceptability.

The tablet also provides a versatile drug delivery system. Whilst most tablets are intended to be swallowed intact, the same basic manufacturing process, associated with appropriate formulation, provides dosage forms for sublingual, buccal, rectal and vaginal administration, lozenges and solution tablets.

Naturally, tablets only possess these advantages if they are properly formulated and manufactured. It thus becomes possible to specify the qualities which a well prepared tablet should possess.

1 It should contain the stated dose of drug within permitted limits.
2 It should be sufficiently strong to withstand the stresses of manufacture, transport and handling, so as to reach the patient intact.
3 It should deliver its dose of drug at the site and at the speed required.
4 Its size and appearance should not detract from its acceptability by the patient.

Tablets as a dosage form are considered in detail in Chapter 18.

Processes of tablet production

Though the detailed operation of tablet presses will be considered later, the basic principle of manufacture is common to all types. The tablet ingredient, in particulate form, is fed into a die, and is then compressed between punches. Following this, the compacted mass is ejected from the die. Thus for a particulate system to be made into tablets, three vital properties are demanded.

1 The particles must be sufficiently free-flowing that they will uniformly flow into the relatively small volume in the die in a very short time.
2 The particles, when subjected to a force from the punches, cohere to form a compact of adequate strength.
3 Whilst the particles must cohere, adhesion by the tablet to the punches and dies must be avoided, otherwise damage to both tablet and press will ensue when attempts are made to remove the tablet from the die.

Unfortunately, relatively few substances possess these essential properties without some preliminary treatment. Thus two major stages of tableting are considered in this chapter:

1 preliminary (precompaction) treatment of powders,
2 compression of this material into tablets.

The assessment of the quality of the finished tablets follows.

Tablet formulation

The formulation of a tablet is governed by a number of factors:

1 the drug substance involved, its chemical and physical propertes and route of administration,
2 the manufacturing process to be employed,
3 the method by which the tablet is to be used, i.e. swallowed whole, chewed, dissolved in water, etc.

These three factors are inter-related.

The drug substance

This must be the most important consideration. Properties of the drug substance which are relevant in this context are as follows.

Site and extent of absorption of drug in the gastrointestinal tract If the drug is satisfactorily absorbed in the stomach or intestine, then a tablet can be designed which is to be swallowed and which disintegrates in the stomach. If absorption is dissolution-controlled, then the particle size of the drug may need to be reduced, or dissolution promoted in some other way. If the drug is unstable in any of the fluids of the gastrointestinal tract, then either some form of protection must be afforded, e.g. by enteric coating, or a tablet formulated for buccal or sublingual absorption. A similar solution may be adopted for substances which undergo extensive first-pass hepatic metabolism, e.g. glyceryl trinitrate.

Stability of the drug to heat or moisture Substances which would undergo appreciable hydrolysis in the conditions of the wet granulation process obviously cannot be made into tablets by this means, and alternatives such as precompression or direct compression must be used, or another dosage form chosen.

Compatibility of the drug The compatibility of the drug with other tablet ingredients in the solid state, for example magnesium stearate, lactose, microcrystalline cellulose and starch, must be considered, since this will govern those additives which can be used in the production of the tablet.

Dose of the drug The dose of the drug will decide the necessity of the filler. If a filler is not used, then there is little possibility of the direct compression method of tablet preparation being available.

Solubility of the drug The solubility of the drug, together with the proportion of drug in each tablet, will govern the need for a disintegrating agent.

The method of production

This may well be governed by the drug substance, but where a choice is available, economic factors will play an important role. The process of direct compression with its savings in time, apparatus, energy costs and space is obviously attractive, but against this must be set higher material costs.

The type of tablet

Having decided on a route of administration and method of production, a formulation must now be designed which will enable the manufacturer to produce tablets which satisfy pharmacopoeial and 'in-house' standards for performance and appearance. Thus for a tablet designed to disintegrate after swallowing, and to be made by a wet granulation process then:

1 A granulating agent must be chosen with adequate adhesive properties, and giving a granule which compresses to form tablets of acceptable strength and friability.
2 A lubricant is chosen so as to enable ejection from the die to occur without unacceptably prolonging the disintegration time or reducing tablet strength.
3 A sufficient concentration of disintegrant is used.

It must be stressed that these points are all inter-related. Thus, for example, disintegration time is not only governed by disintegrant concentration, but also by the lubricant, the compression pressure and the solubility of drug and diluent. Whilst many tablets are formulated on an *ad hoc* basis, optimum levels of additives can be determined using factorially designed experiments and computer-assisted analysis of the resulting data. The reader is referred to Schwartz (1979) for a detailed discussion of this approach.

If the tablet is not to be swallowed intact, then other formulation considerations arise. For example, if the tablet is to be dissolved in water before use, then all ingredients must be soluble. A variety of solution tablet is the effervescent tablet in which an acid (usually tartaric or citric acid) reacts with a bicarbonate (usually sodium or potassium) on the addition of water to produce carbon dioxide. In addition to solubility considerations, this type of preparation cannot be prepared with an aqueous-based granulating agent. A non-aqueous granulation or a totally dry method of tablet production is mandatory.

There are other types of tablet designed for oral administration but which are not to be swallowed. Chewable tablets are often used for children and geriatric patients who have difficulty in swallowing tablets. Since the disintegrated tablet is present in the mouth, the taste of the preparation is important in this case. Taste masking can be achieved by choice of diluent but obviously this problem becomes more acute with drugs of unpleasant taste, after-taste and high dose. A frequently used diluent is mannitol, which has a pleasant cooling sensation in the mouth, effectively disguising many taste problems.

The lozenge and the sublingual or buccal tablet are also designed to be kept in the mouth but pose opposite formulation problems. The lozenge, often containing a small amount of antibacterial substance, is designed to be kept in the mouth for long periods. Hence it should remain intact and dissolve slowly, since the patient will have difficulty in retaining fragments in the mouth. Flavour is also important, and a mixture of lactose and sucrose is often used as filler. The sublingual tablet also should not disintegrate but in this case it must dissolve rapidly. Hence a highly soluble formulation must be selected.

Further consideration of the formulation of tablets is given in Chapter 18.

PRECOMPACTION TREATMENT

Tablet production via wet massing and screening

This is the traditional method of giving a particulate solid those properties needed for it to produce satisfactory tablets. The process essentially consists of sticking the particles together using an adhesive material, thereby increasing the particle size and improving flow properties. These enlarged particles are termed granules. Other additives are also usually incorporated at some stage of the process.

The process is represented in Fig. 39.1, and each stage will be discussed in some detail.

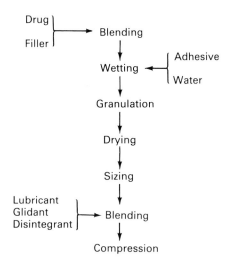

Fig. 39.1 Flow sheet of the wet granulation process of tablet production

Initial powder blending

In this stage, the drug substance is mixed, if needed, with the diluent or filler. Tablets weighing much less than 50 mg are so small as to be difficult to pick up and manipulate with the fingers, yet many drug substances are active in far lower doses. Accordingly it is necessary to dilute the drug to make a tablet of reasonable size. The ideal diluent should be inert, both chemically and pharmacologically, pose no problems on compression and should be cheap. Commonly used diluents are given in Chapter 18. The powders are blended in a powder mixer, the design and size of which is governed by the masses of powder involved. The aim is to produce a uniform dispersion of the drug in the filler. A detailed description of powder mixers, and of methods of assessing the uniformity of a powder blend is given in Chapter 32.

Wetting

The mixture of powders is now wetted and it is at this stage that the adhesive is introduced, usually as an aqueous solution or dispersion. A wide variety of adhesives (also known as binders or granulating agents) are available and some details are given in Chapter 18. The choice of granulating agent will often be governed by the intended use of the tablet. Though the more obvious role of the adhesive is to form granules, it also plays an important role in the compressive behaviour of the formulation. This point is discussed later in this chapter.

Though size enlargement takes place primarily with the adhesion of particles by a film of granulating agent, a second mechanism is available if the solid particles are soluble in the granulating fluid. Partial dissolution occurs, yielding a saturated solution of the solid. On subsequent drying, recrystallization occurs and the resultant crystal bridges between particles can contribute significantly to granule strength (see Chapter 37).

In the case of drugs which are unstable in the presence of water, a small number of non-aqueous systems, notably polyvinyl pyrrolidone in isopropanol, are available. These are not used unless absolutely necessary because of expense and the environmental problems caused by handling large volumes of flammable vapour.

The wetting stage is usually carried out in the same apparatus in which the dry powders were blended. Sufficient adhesive is added to form a damp, coherent mass, though overwetting should be avoided.

Granulation

The damp mass is now passed through a coarse sieve, usually of mesh size 1–2 mm, yielding roughly spherical particles or granules. This product is usually achieved mechanically, often by means of an oscillating granulator, in which a rotor, oscillating about its horizontal axis, passes the damp material through the screen. Alternatively, a comminutor, containing a number of rapidly revolving blades, may be used. Chapter 37 describes some commonly used granulation equipment.

Drying

The granules are now dried, the apparatus used being either a tray drier or, more usually, a fluidized bed drier. The resultant product will be a coarse, free-flowing solid. The process of drying is discussed in detail in Chapter 38.

Sizing

The size of granules at this point will usually be considerably larger than the size required for tableting. Also for the latter process, a relatively uniform size is needed to ensure that a constant weight flows into the die of the tablet press. Hence a comminution stage, followed by sieving, will normally be needed, the usual granule size for tableting being 350–700 μm.

Second blending

A second blending stage is now required, since at this point other important additives are incorporated.

The role of lubricants   A lubricant is almost invariably needed in a tablet formulation. As the granules are compressed and thus deformed, they exert a radial stress on the die wall, the magnitude of which can be great enough to prevent ejection of the tablet from the die. A lubricant is a substance which deforms easily when sheared between two surfaces and hence, when interposed between the tablet and die wall, provides a readily deformable film. Details of commonly used lubricants are given in Chapter 18.

The most effective are substances based on stearic acid and especially magnesium stearate, the hydrocarbon chains of which provide the deformable property. A consequence of this is that the granule surface is covered with a hydrophobic material, and this may lead to retarded disintegration of the tablet after ingestion. However, this can usually be counteracted by adding a wetting agent, e.g. sodium lauryl sulphate, to the formulation. In addition, the formation of interparticulate bonds, on which the integrity of the tablet depends, can also be decreased by the presence of a film of lubricant, and thus the tablet is weakened. For both these reasons therefore the minimum amount of lubricant is used.

Inadequate lubrication can be the cause of a number of tablet faults. Frictional forces at the die wall resist ejection of the tablet from the die. This can often be recognized by vertical scratches on the tablet edges. It can lead to tablet fragmentation on ejection and in extreme cases to damage to the press. Alternatively the tablet may tend to stick to the punch faces. This causes a build-up of powder on the faces which in turn will lead to a matt, dimpled appearance of the tablet face. This phenomenon, known as picking, may also occur with moist or sticky granules, a humid environment and is especially prone to happen if the tablet punches are engraved or embossed.

The role of glidants   One of the main reasons for granulation is to improve flow properties. However, the requirements for adequate flow are high, since the granules are required to fall uniformly into a confined space in a very short time. The purpose of the glidant is to promote flow. The most commonly used glidant is silica. It is believed to act by lodging in the surface irregularities of the granule, effectively smoothing its surface. Hence a finely divided grade of silica must be used. Details of this and other glidants are given in Chapter 18. Inadequate glidant action is detected by an unacceptable variation in tablet weight.

The role of disintegrants   In the course of compression, a particulate system with a high surface area is transformed into a solid mass of low porosity. Yet if the tablet is to liberate its active principle in the gastrointestinal tract, it is essential that the lumenal fluids gain access to the drug. If the bulk of the tablet is fairly soluble in water this is not difficult, but if not, it is possible that the tablet may pass through the gastrointestinal tract without yielding up the drug. The function of the disintegrant is to prevent this. It acts by causing the tablet to break up into small fragments, thereby increasing the surface area to which the dissolving fluid has access. The most commonly used disintegrants are described in Chapter 18.

The mechanism by which disintegrants act has in the past been the subject of some controversy. The various types of starch, which are still the most commonly used disintegrants, were believed to act by swelling when they came into contact with water. This disrupted the interparticulate bonds holding the tablet together and hence disintegration occurred. Whilst this may account for the disintegrant action of starch, it cannot explain the fact that certain other effective disintegrants do not swell in contact with water. These are believed to act by providing hydrophilic pathways within the tablet structure. When the tablet is immersed in water, the liquid is drawn up through these pathways by what is termed a 'wicking' mechanism, with the consequent rupture of interparticulate bonds. It is probable that the action of starch can also be attributed to this latter mechanism, the swelling of the starch grains being of secondary importance. A detailed discussion of disintegrant action is given by Lowenthal (1973).

Flavours   Taste masking in tablets is often achieved by using a sweet-tasting substance as diluent or by coating the tablet. However, it may be necessary to incorporate a flavouring agent, and as these are often thermolabile, they cannot be added prior to an operation involving heat. They are often added as spray-dried beads or, if oily, sprayed on to the granules as an alcoholic solution.

Colorants   Many tablets are coloured to aid identification and patient compliance. Whilst this is often achieved by coating the tablets, dyes can be added at the final mixing stage, usually as a water-insoluble precipitate with aluminium hydroxide, i.e. as the lake of the dye. Alternatively the water-soluble dye can be added to the granulating fluid, but this can lead to colour variation in the tablet (mottling) caused by migration of the dye during the drying stage.

Tablet production via fluidized bed granulation

Though a high proportion of all tablets are made by the wet massing process, there are a number of drawbacks to it. First, there are many stages involved, and hence the product must be moved from one piece of apparatus to another on several occasions. Thus production costs are increased. Second, the process involves the addition and subsequent removal of water. This too is an expensive procedure, but in addition the presence of water and heat can cause deterioration of substances susceptible to hydrolysis.

An attempt to reduce handling costs in the wet granulation process has been the introduction of fluidized bed granulation. In this, the drug and filler are loaded into a chamber through which a current of warm air is passed, which thoroughly blends the mixture. The binder solution is sprayed as a stream of droplets on to the fluidized powder, and thus granulation takes place as the particles are suspended in air. After granulation is complete, the spray is stopped but the fluidizing hot air is continued and the product dried as in a fluidized bed drier. Whilst this speeds up the process, it is still one which involves water and heat. Granules can be produced very effectively in this type of equipment and to some extent the granule size can be controlled.

Tablet production via spray drying

Granules can be produced directly from the spray-drying process. All the components of the formulation, diluent, binder, disintegrant and lubricant are suspended in a suitable vehicle to achieve a concentration of about 50–60% w/w. The slurry is then spray dried to produce nearly spherical granules of uniform diameter, 10–250 μm in size. The spray-dried product is usually free flowing. Spray-drying is normally only used on the very large scale and due to the very high capital cost, the advantages of this process are usually outweighed by the high investment involved in installing this specialized piece of equipment. As a consequence this process is little used except for the production of diluents.

Tablet production via precompression

This is an alternative to wet granulation and is employed where heat- or moisture-sensitive materials are involved. It is not widely used. The

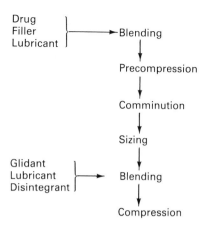

Fig. 39.2 Flow sheet of the precompression method of tablet production

process, sometimes known as slugging, is shown schematically in Fig. 39.2.

The constituents, after blending with some of the lubricant, are compressed into large tablets on a heavy duty press. These tablets (or slugs), which will lack the uniformity of weight and appearance normally required of tablets, are then broken down to granule-sized particles which are subsequently recompressed into the finished product. A variation on this technique is to squeeze the powder particles into a cake between rollers (roller compaction). Thus the process essentially replaces the wetting and drying stages of wet granulation with a preliminary compression stage.

Tablet production by direct compression

It has been repeatedly stressed that the great majority of solids need some preliminary treatment before they can be made into tablets. However, for those relatively few substances which need no prior manipulation, tableting is a simple matter. The steps are shown schematically in Fig. 39.3. The number of medicinal substances which can be tableted in this way is very small. Sodium and potassium chlorides and aspirin are the most common, but the promise of this method lies in the discovery of directly compressible fillers or diluents which produce good quality tablets without prior manipulation. The filler can be mixed with the drug without significantly reducing the compressional properties of the

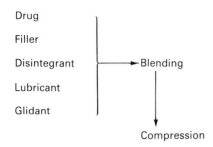

Fig. 39.3 Tablet production by direct compression

former. Since the amount of drug which can be added in this way is limited, the process is of greatest promise with potent substances where perhaps only a few milligrams are present in each tablet. In the last few years, a considerable number of direct compression diluents have been introduced. Details of some, together with their proprietary names, are given in Table 39.1.

Table 39.1 Direct compression diluents

Diluent	Proprietary name	Comments
Microcrystalline cellulose	Avicel PH	Very compressible; no lubricant needed
Microfine cellulose	Elcema	
Lactose; spray-dried	Zeparox	Highly compressible; good flow properties; high bulk density
Modified starch	Starch 1500	More useful as a disintegrant
Sucrose–dextrin coprecipitate	Dipac	Good flow properties; moisture-sensitive
Dextrose–maltose	Emdex	
Dicalcium phosphate	Emcompress	Insoluble in water; good flow properties

Advantages

The advantages of this process are obvious. Very few stages are involved, with a consequent reduction in appliance and handling costs. Furthermore as heat and water are not involved, stability is not affected. Also though additives such as lubricant and disintegrant are usually necessary, some direct compression diluents such as microcrystalline cellulose need neither, and hence costs are further reduced.

The requirements of a direct compression diluent

1 It should have good flow properties, so that uniform flow into the die is facilitated.
2 It should have a high bulk density. If the solid is light and fluffy, a relatively low weight of powder will fill the die, and after compression, the resultant tablet will be correspondingly thin.
3 The particle size should be such as to minimize segregation of the powder blend prior to compression. With wet granulated systems, the constituents of the mixture are stuck together during the blending stage, and hence cannot subsequently separate. In direct compression systems, separation may occur due, for example, to vibration. This is particularly prone to happen if the components of the mixture differ widely in particle size, and hence where possible the sizes of drug and diluent particles should be approximately equal. This matter is explored more fully in Chapters 32 and 37.
4 The substance should have a high capacity in that it is capable of considerable dilution with drug substances. There is no universally recognized method of measuring capacity, and consequently published data must be viewed with caution.
5 It should have a good compression pressure–tablet strength profile so that strong tablets are obtained at relatively low pressures.
6 The diluent should be physiologically inert, should not interfere with bioavailability, and should be compatible with the drug substance.
7 In the event of a defective batch of tablets being produced, the tablets should be capable of being broken down and recompressed. The structure of some direct compression diluents, e.g. spray-dried lactose, is lost on compression, and hence reworking may not be feasible.
8 The diluent should not be so expensive as to nullify the economic advantages of the direct compression process.

Disadvantages

Although the method is simple there are, however, limitations to the use of direct compression formulations. In particular, differences in particle size and bulk density between the diluent and the active ingredient may result and this can easily lead to stratification in handling and variation in drug content of the resultant tablets. From a quality control point of view, it is never certain how the powder mix will be handled before compression takes place, and if the mix is subjected to any form of vibration, e.g. on the back of a lorry, powder segregation could occur which would produce drug content variability. Static charges may develop on the drug during mixing which may prevent uniform distribution and inadequate mixing may result. Good earthing of mixers and blenders is thus essential.

TABLET COMPRESSION

Tablets are prepared by compressing a particulate solid in a die by the application of forces via two punches. The punches are termed the lower punch, the tip of which moves up and down within the die, but never actually leaves it, and the upper punch, which descends to penetrate the die and apply the compressive force, and then withdraws to permit ejection of the tablet. The die and punches are almost invariably made of hardened steel.

Compression sequence

Irrespective of the type of tablet press, the process of compaction can be divided into three distinct stages (Fig. 39.4).

1 The lower punch falls within the die, leaving a cavity into which particulate material can flow under the influence of gravity.
2 The upper punch descends, and the punch tip enters the die, confining the particles. Further punch movement applies the compressive force to the particles, which aggregate to form a coherent tablet.
3 The upper punch withdraws from the die and simultaneously the lower punch rises until its tip becomes level with the top of the die. The tablet is thus ejected from the die and removed from the tablet press.

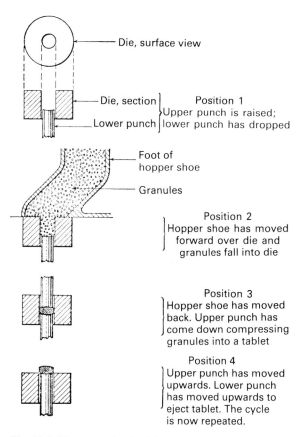

Fig. 39.4 Movements involved in tablet compression

This process demands that the particulate solid possesses good flow properties, is coherent, and yet will not adhere to the die wall and the punches of the press. As stated earlier, few substances possess all these properties, and so prior manipulation is almost always necessary.

Tablet compression machinery

There are two types of tablet press in common use.

The single stroke or eccentric press

This type possesses one die and one pair of punches. The particulate solid, contained in a hopper, is fed into the die by means of a shoe which moves to and fro over the die. The output of this type of press is 150–200 tablets per minute

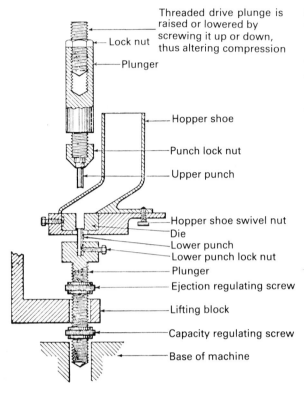

Threaded drive plunge is raised or lowered by screwing it up or down, thus altering compression

Lock nut

Plunger

Hopper shoe

Punch lock nut

Upper punch

Hopper shoe swivel nut

Die

Lower punch

Lower punch lock nut

Plunger

Ejection regulating screw

Lifting block

Capacity regulating screw

Base of machine

Fig. 39.5 Diagram of an eccentric tablet press

at a maximum, and so its use is limited to relatively small scale production or development work. A diagram of this type of press is given in Fig. 39.5.

The rotary tablet press

In this type, there are a number of dies and sets of punches. The former are set in a rotating disc or 'table', and the punches are set in tracks mounted above and below the table. The table and tracks rotate together, so that one die is always associated with one pair of punches. The vertical position of the lower punch in the die is governed by passage above cams, and the force is applied by the punches passing over and under pressure rolls. This is illustrated in Fig. 39.6.

Outputs of over 10 000 tablets per minute can be achieved by this type of press, the output being governed by the speed of rotation of the table and the number of sets of punches.

The cross-section of the die is usually circular, but is not necessarily so, and non-circular tablets are becoming more common, primarily as an aid to product identification.

Whilst punch faces may be flat, thereby giving cylindrical tablets, this is unusual. Bevelled and convex tablets, made with concave punches, are more frequently encountered, and the latter are essential if the tablets are to be coated. In addition, punches may be embossed, so that an identification mark, product name or manufacturer's logo appears on the tablet.

FUNDAMENTALS OF POWDER COMPRESSION

Measurement of force in a tablet press

Though Brockedon's patent for the compression of medicinal substances was issued in 1843, it was not for over 100 years that significant research into the production of tablets from powders took place. This was initially carried out by T. Higuchi and his group at the University of Wisconsin, and their series of publications entitled 'The physics of tablet compression' (Higuchi *et al.*, 1954) were the foundation of much of the research on compaction which has been carried out since then.

The reason for the delay in commencing fundamental research on tableting was probably an inability to measure accurately the compressing force. This parameter is a major influence on many tablet properties, e.g. strength and disintegration time, and so without knowledge of the applied force, meaningful studies on these tablet properties become difficult if not impossible.

Tableting research was transformed by the introduction of the so-called 'instrumented tablet machine' by Higuchi in 1954, in which strain gauges are attached to various parts of the press, enabling force to be measured accurately. In its simplest form, the strain gauge is a network of wires through which an electric current is passed. The wires are bonded very securely to, for example, the upper punch of a press. If a force is applied to the punch it deforms, the magnitude of deformation (i.e. strain) being governed by the applied force and the value of Young's modulus for the punch. The wire of the strain gauge is also deformed, and hence its electrical resistance changes. This results in a small voltage change,

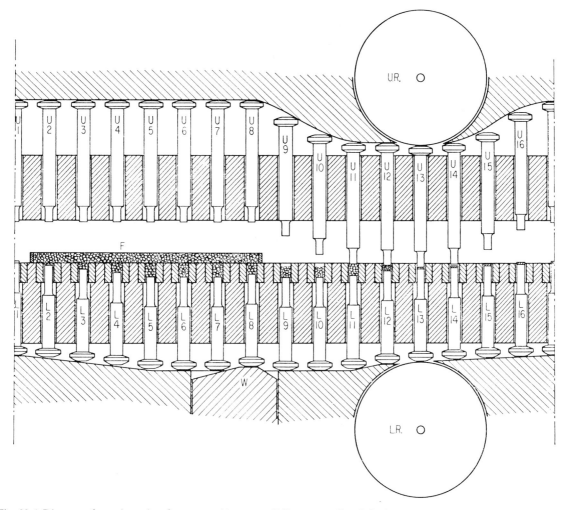

Fig. 39.6 Diagram of punch tracks of a rotary tablet press. U R, upper roller; L R, lower roller; W, capacity adjuster; F, feed frame with granules.
U1 to U8, upper punches in raised position; L1, lower punch at top position, tablet ejected; L2 to L7, lower punches dropping to lowest position and filling die with granules to an overfill at L7; L8, lower punch raised to expel excess granules giving correct capacity; U9 to U12, upper punches lowering to enter die at U12; L9 to L12, synchronized with U9 to U12 lower punches rising prior to compression; L13 and U13, upper and lower punches pass between rollers, and granules are compressed to a tablet; U14 to U16, lower punch rising to completely eject tablet at L16; U1 and L1, beginning of cycle

which can be amplified and recorded. The size of the signal from the strain gauge is proportional to the amount of deformation which in turn is a function of the applied force. Hence after appropriate calibration, the electrical signals can be expressed in terms of the applied force.

This concept is the foundation of much research on powder compaction. Rotary tablet presses have also been instrumented, and this, in addition to providing a research tool, permits automatic weight control in a production environment, since an incorrect fill of granules into the die gives an unacceptably high or low force. That particular tablet can thus be rejected. A further development has been the use of piezoelectric crystals as an alternative to strain gauges. The former emit an electric charge when compressed, the magnitude of which is proportional to the compressing force. Also the attachment of displacement transducers, which measure distance, enables punch position to be accurately determined. The signals from the various transducers may be fed into an oscillo-

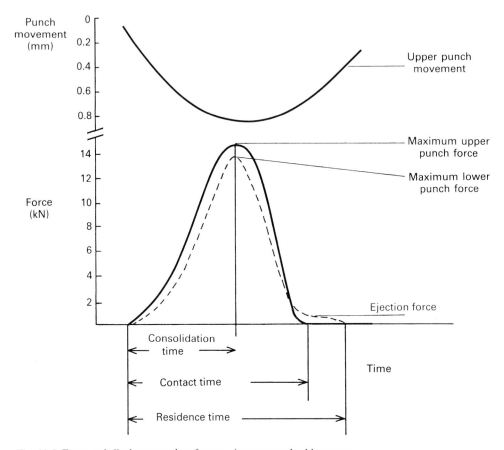

Fig. 39.7 Force and displacement data from an instrumented tablet press

scope, a chart recorder, or stored electronically and subsequently manipulated by computer.

A typical trace from an instrumented eccentric press is given in Fig. 39.7, which shows representations of upper and lower punch forces and the distance separating the punch faces. Considerable information can be derived from such a diagram, and it will be referred to several times in the remainder of this section.

The reader will already be aware that attractive forces exist between two particles. These forces may be non-specific, e.g. van der Waal's forces, or may be more specific in nature, e.g. brought about by molecules exhibiting intermolecular hydrogen bonding. However, irrespective of their nature, it is these forces which enable a coherent tablet to be formed, and an appreciation that their magnitude depends on the interparticulate distance is the key to understanding how tablets are formed,

and some of the problems which may arise during their manufacture.

Application of a force to particles in a die

Consider a number of particles present in a die and to which a force is applied. A series of events can then occur, perhaps sequentially, but there is a greater likelihood that some overlap will occur.

1 The particles will undergo rearrangement to form a less porous structure. This will take place at very low forces, the particles sliding past each other. This stage will usually be associated with some fragmentation, as the rough surfaces move relative to one another and rough points are abraded away.

2 The particles have now reached a state where further relative movement is impossible, though the porosity may still be considerable. A further

increase in applied force can then induce either particle fragmentation or deformation (or both). Which of these alternatives predominates will depend on the properties of the particulate material involved, but in either case, the net result will be a further decrease in porosity, and an increase in interparticulate contact.

As stated earlier, all structures exhibit mutual attraction, but between two particles of the mass of a powder particle, the force is so weak that it can be said to be significant only when the particles are touching or are very close to each other. Now if the particles are regarded as being spherical, it follows that they only touch at one point and thus the attraction is only significant at that point. Thus anything which increases the area of interparticulate contact must increase the strength of the aggregate or tablet.

Removal of the compressive force

If consolidation of the powder mass and an increase in the degree of interparticulate bonding has been brought about by fragmentation, then the removal of force should have no effect on the tablet, since there is no way in which the fragments can rearrange themselves to recombine into the original particles. However, purely fragmentary consolidation is unlikely to have occurred, and so the effect of force removal on deformed particles must be considered.

Deformation can be either elastic (reversible) or plastic (permanent) and the difference between the two, crucial in the consideration of tablet formation, is exemplified by the behaviour of a spring when subjected to an extensive, progressively increasing load (Fig. 39.8). Up to a certain point, the spring obeys Hooke's Law, in that the load and the degree of elongation are rectilinearly related, the reciprocal of the slope of the line in this diagram being termed Young's modulus. If such loads are removed, the spring returns to its former length, i.e. the deformation is totally reversible or elastic. However, consider the situation if a load in excess of E is applied. Extension will again take place, but the linear relationship is lost, and if the load is now removed, contraction will occur but at zero load the spring will still not have returned to its original length, i.e. it has been permanently deformed. Point E is termed the elastic limit.

The parallel between the Hookean behaviour of an extending spring with the compression of powder particles is not completely valid since with any particulate system, a point will be reached at zero porosity, when further application of force can bring about neither elastic nor plastic deformation. Neither, unlike the spring, is a particulate system anisotropic. None the less, it remains a useful analogy.

If the particles have deformed plastically, then removal of the compressing force will have no

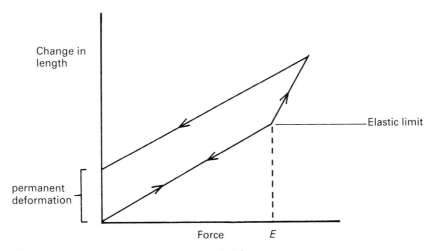

Fig. 39.8 Deformation of a spring by an applied force

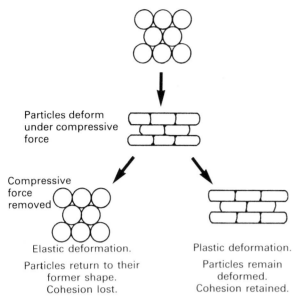

Fig. 39.9 Plasticity and elasticity in a particulate mass. (Reproduced from Armstrong, 1982 with permission of the copyright holder)

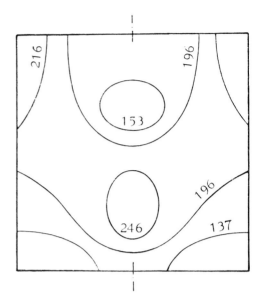

Fig. 39.10 Pressure distribution in a particulate mass. Contours are in N mm^{-2} (Reproduced from Train, 1957 with permission of the copyright holder)

effect, since interparticulate bonds which are formed as a result of increased particle contact will not be disrupted. However, if particles tend to revert to their former shape, coherence will be lost as a consequence of the reduction in the area of interparticulate contact (Fig. 39.9). Most particulate systems show some elastic and some plastic properties but it is obviously desirable that plastic deformation should predominate. How the degree of elasticity or plasticity present in a system can be measured and altered will be discussed later in this chapter.

Force transmission through a powder bed

Consider a group of particles in the die of an eccentric tablet press. Force is applied by means of a descending upper punch on the press, whilst the lower punch is passive and will have the force transmitted to it through the powder bed. The distribution of force within the powder bed was investigated by Train (1957), who found that the diminution of force did not proceed uniformly on descending through the bed, but formed a much more complex pattern, caused by the force being transmitted to, and reflected from, the die wall. Significant features are zones of high force at the periphery near the moving punch and much lower in the powder mass on its vertical axis. On the other hand, lower force zones occur on the same axis but much nearer the moving punch (Fig. 39.10).

The consequences of this on tablet strength can be profound. Particle deformation, whether elastic or plastic, will be proportional to the force applied, and as has been discussed, this deformation is an essential preliminary to the formation of interparticulate bonds on which tablet integrity depends. Thus the porosity of the tablet, and hence its strength, will vary within the tablet, and the weakest points in the tablet structure will be those that receive the lowest force, i.e. on the face of the tablet adjacent to the stationary punch and on the central axis near to the moving punch. The full consequences of this will be discussed later.

It should be noted that the above discussion assumes that only one punch is actively applying force to the powder mass whilst the other is stationary and passive. This is true in the case of an eccentric press, but with a rotary tablet press, both punches move and exert a force on the powder bed. The force distribution so obtained is thus different from that shown in Fig. 39.10, and results in two low density zones near the faces of the tablet, and a high density zone in approximately the centre of the powder mass.

The foregoing can be summarized by stating that because of its non-uniform density, some areas of a tablet are stronger than others. Furthermore after the compressing force is removed, elastic recovery will occur to a greater or lesser extent, which will result in a reduction in the strength of interparticulate bonds and an overall weakening of the tablet. It therefore follows that if the tablet is to be disrupted by elastic recovery, this is most likely to occur at its weakest point. This is just below the top surface, and is a phenomenon often encountered in tablet manufacture known as capping or lamination. With this explanation in mind, some observed effects associated with capping, and some pragmatic causes and solutions to the problem, can now be explained.

Capping was for many years considered to be due to the entrapment of air in the tablet, and even the production *in vacuo* of tablets exhibiting capping did little to dispel this theory. Neither did this theory explain why air should cause tablet fracture at one particular zone. However, by considering the non-uniform density distribution in the tablet, it can be seen that the weakness is not caused by the presence of air *per se*, but rather the relative absence of solid material in those parts of the tablet which have high porosity. If this air is compressed, it follows that the pores are now filled with air at elevated pressure, which will obviously assist in disruption of the tablet. Thus anything which obstructs the expression of air during compression will exacerbate capping though it is not the fundamental cause. Such factors include the clearance between punch and die, the speed at which the force is applied, and the presence of small particles in the granulation making passage of air through the tablet more tortuous.

Similarly, any stress which exceeds the breaking strength of the tablet will cause the tablet to break at its weakest point. A number of stresses occur when the tablet is removed from the die after compression. First, wear may occur at the point in the die where the tablet is compressed, i.e., the die is fractionally wider at this point than elsewhere. Thus when the tablet is ejected, it is forced

through an aperture of diameter slightly less than the tablet itself. This will obviously stress the tablet, and the interparticulate bonds may be overcome at their weakest point. As the tablet is extruded from the die, elastic expansion will occur not just in an axial direction but also radially. The latter occurs progressively, i.e., one segment of tablet is free to expand whilst the one below it is still constrained by the die. Disruption of some interparticulate bonds is an inevitable consequence.

Assessment of lubricant action

The reduction in applied force with descent through the powder bed is primarily due to force losses at the die wall and by interparticulate friction. Both of these factors are reduced by the presence of a lubricant, and so comparison of the force applied by the upper punch with that received by the lower punch affords a measure of lubricant efficiency. This method, first suggested by Higuchi and co-workers (1954), defines the force ratio (R) as the ratio between lower punch maximum force and upper punch maximum force, and can be derived from the data represented in Fig. 39.7. The maximum value of R is unity, and lubricants based on stearates usually exhibit R values greater than 0.95.

An alternative method of measuring lubricant action is to measure the force required to eject the tablet from the die after the compressing force is removed. This too can be obtained from Fig. 39.7.

Mathematical treatment of compression data

The data on which Fig. 39.7 is based have been used in a variety of ways to provide a mathematical representation of the compression process. For example, a number of equations have been derived linking the applied force to the density of the resultant tablet. The best known of these is the Heckel relationship:

$$\ln 1/(1 - D) = kP + A$$

where D is the apparent density of the tablet, P is the applied pressure and k and A are constants. The apparent density is derived from a knowledge of the tablet dimensions, and the latter can be obtained in turn from the displacement data in Fig. 39.7.

If the Heckel relationship is valid, then a graph of ln $1/(1 - D)$ vs P should be a straight line of slope k and intercept A on the ordinate. The equation has been used to distinguish substances which consolidate by fragmentation rather than deformation, and also as a means of assessing plasticity.

A totally different treatment is using the data from Fig. 39.7 to construct the so-called 'force-displacement curve'. In this, the force is plotted as ordinate and the corresponding punch position as the abscissa (Fig. 39.11). Calculation of the area enclosed by the curve has the units of force × distance which dimensionally is equivalent to 'work'. Therefore the force-displacement curve has been used to calculate the work expended in the compression of a solid. Further refinement of this technique enables a measurement of elasticity and plasticity to be made.

This has shown that the presence of a granulating agent causes a marked increase in the plasticity of the particulate mass, with a consequent increase in cohesion and tablet strength. The film of granulating agent between the particles can be regarded as a highly viscous liquid with a large yield value. Application of a force in excess of the yield value causes granules to deform. Reduction of the force to below the yield value leads to permanent deformation. A somewhat similar mechanism is believed to account for the properties of some direct-compression diluents, e.g. spray-dried lactose, which consists of small crystalline masses embedded in an amorphous and more easily deformed matrix.

STANDARDS OF QUALITY FOR COMPRESSED TABLETS

Pharmacopoeial tests

Like all other dosage forms, the tablet is subjected to those pharmacopoeial standards which deal with 'added substances' with respect to their toxicity, interference with analytical methods, etc. However, there are a number of procedures which apply specifically to tablets, and which are designed, in the main, to ensure that the patient receives a product containing the required amount of drug substance in a form which enables the latter to exert its full pharmacological action.

Such standards in the *British Pharmacopoeia* are: uniformity of diameter, uniformity of weight, content of active ingredient, uniformity of content, disintegration, and dissolution. In addition there are a number of quality control procedures, which, though widely applied, are not defined by the Pharmacopoeia. These will be discussed later.

Uniformity of diameter

If tablets containing the same amount of drug substance but made by different manufacturers differ greatly in size, the consumer may well doubt whether tablets of such dissimilar appearance are of the same potency. The purpose of this standard is to help to remove this doubt. For details of the test, the stipulated diameters for specific tablets and permitted deviations, the reader is referred to the current edition of the *British Pharmacopoeia*. Though only the diameter is specified and not the tablet weight, it is reasonable to expect that tablets of the same diameter will not differ markedly in weight. This test was

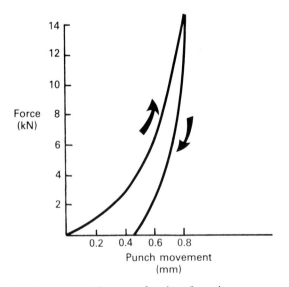

Fig. 39.11 Applied force as a function of punch movement in an eccentric press; a force-displacement curve

introduced into the *British Pharmacopoeia* of 1958, replacing a guide of recommended tablet diameters which had been issued for some years by the Association of British Pharmaceutical Industry. It does not apply to tablets which are enteric, film or sugar coated. The usefulness of this standard is currently the subject of debate: the USP has never had such a standard.

Uniformity of weight

This test is carried out by removing a sample of 20 tablets from a batch, weighing them individually and calculating the mean weight, which in turn governs the permitted deviations from the mean. These are given in Table 39.2.

Not more than two tablets are permitted to differ from the mean by greater than the stated percentage and no tablet by more than double that percentage. Other national pharmacopoeias have similar standards, perhaps differing in minor detail. This standard applies to uncoated and compression-coated tablets.

Failure to comply with this standard, with consequent rejection of the batch, may be due to

uneven feeding of granules into the die, or irregular movement of the lower punch, producing a die space of varying capacity.

Where the drug substance forms the greater part of the tablet mass, dosage is obviously linked to tablet weight, and compliance with this standard helps to ensure that uniformity of dosage is achieved. However, in the case of highly potent substances, where the bulk of the tablet is diluent, this is not the case. This point is exemplified by the work of Airth *et al.* (1967), some of whose findings are illustrated in Fig. 39.12. When the tablet contained some 90% of active ingredient, then a perfectly linear relationship was found between tablet weight and drug content. Where the active ingredient comprised only 23% of the weight of the tablet, the relationship was much less significant.

Content of active ingredient

To carry out this test, 20 tablets are chosen at random from a batch, powdered together, and an assay carried out on an aliquot of the resultant mixture, according to the method given in the relevant pharmacopoeial monograph. The latter also states the range for the content of active ingredient which is permissible, and this range can be modified if fewer than 20 tablets are available.

There are two points to note about this standard. The first is that though the test is called 'content of active ingredient', there is no test for activity *per se*, the assay measuring, by chemical

Table 39.2 Uniformity of tablet weight

Average weight of tablet	*Percentage deviation*
80 mg or less	10
More than 80 mg and less than 250 mg	7.5
250 mg or more	5

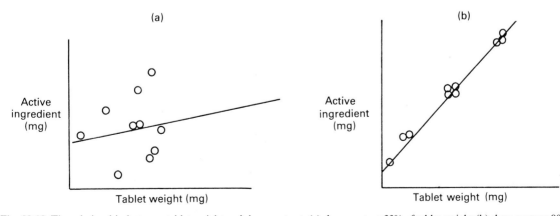

Fig. 39.12 The relationship between tablet weight and drug content: (a) drug content 23% of tablet weight (b) drug content 90% of tablet weight. (Reproduced from Airth, 1967 with permission of the copyright holder)

or physicochemical means, the amount of drug substance present. Possible therapeutic consequences of this are discussed elsewhere in this text (see particularly Chapters 8 and 9).

The second point is that the assay is carried out on a mixture obtained from 20 tablets, and thus the calculated content is the average content of those 20 tablets. Consider a hypothetical example, in which tablets were supposed to contain 100 mg of drug substance. Therefore 20 tablets would yield powder containing 2000 mg of drug. However, the same powder could be obtained from a sample of 10 tablets containing 150 mg plus 10 containing 50 mg or, in the extreme case, 10 tablets containing 200 mg plus 10 containing no drug whatsoever. Such high-dose tablets would almost certainly fail the uniformity of weight test described earlier. However, if the above calculation is now repeated, using a dose per tablet of 100 μg rather than 100 mg, then the potential therapeutic hazard of such a test will be apparent. Such tablets will comprise mainly diluent, and it is unlikely than a 100% variation in the weight of drug substance per tablet will necessarily be reflected in tablet weight. Consideration of some of the points in Fig. 39.12 will illustrate this. It is for this reason that a standard for uniformity of content was introduced.

Uniformity of content

This standard is designed to guard against the variability in drug content within a sample of tablets. At present, specific standards of uniformity of content are applied only to certain monographs, though the British Pharmacopoeia has a general statement that 'any tablets which when examined individually show gross deviation from the prescribed or stated content are not official'. 'Gross deviation' is not defined.

The general structure of the test is to assay 10 tablets individually. The drug content of nine tablets should fall within specified limits, whilst that of the tenth falls within specified wider limits. For example, in the case of Hyoscine Tablets BP, the content of nine must lie between 85 and 115% of the average content whilst the tenth lies within 80 and 120% of the average. The average content is determined by the assay procedure on a bulked

sample of 20 tablets, and in the case of Hyoscine Tablets BP should lie between 90 and 110% of the stated value. It thus follows that an acceptable sample can contain one tablet with an actual content as low as 72% or as high as 132% of its stated content.

The 1980 British Pharmacopoeia contains 14 monographs for tablets in which uniformity of content is specified, without exception those containing potent substances of dose a few milligrams or less. Non-compliance with this standard and that of 'content of active ingredient' will be due to incorrect weighing of ingredients, failure to achieve satisfactory mixing at the blending stage, or subsequent segregation of the components of the tablet formulation.

The USP has a general rule that if the stated dose of a drug in a tablet is less than in 50 mg, then a content uniformity test shall be applied. The structure of the test is similar to that in the BP, except that if one tablet lies outside the narrower limits, a further 20 tablets are assayed, all of which must lie within that limit.

Tablet disintegration and dissolution

Establishing the accuracy of the dose of a drug in a tablet is meaningless unless the drug can carry out its therapeutic function. In the majority of cases, this can only occur when the drug substance has dissolved in the fluids of the gastrointestinal tract. Dissolution rate depends on the surface area of the drug exposed to the dissolving fluid. The intact tablet has a low surface area, and hence breakup of the tablet into smaller particles is a necessary preliminary. Thus the overall rate of entry of the drug substance into the blood stream may be governed by the speed of absorption from the gut, the rate of dissolution of the drug substance or the speed of disintegration of the tablet.

Disintegration A test for tablet disintegration was first introduced into the seventh (1945) addendum of the BP 1932, and was modified several times until a test closely resembling the current procedure was introduced in 1955. The test provides a uniform means of agitating the tablet in an aqueous medium at body temperature, and a reasonably non-subjective end-point.

The disintegration chamber consists of a glass tube closed at the lower end by 2.00 mm aperture steel mesh. The tube is raised and lowered in a water bath at a constant frequency, so that at its highest point, the mesh remains below the surface of the water. For full details, the reader is referred to the current edition of the Pharmacopoeia. Commercial versions of this apparatus normally have six tubes.

The test is carried out by choosing a random sample of six tablets, placing one in each tube, adding a cylindrical plastic disc and agitating the tube in a water bath for 15 minutes. Disintegration is defined as 'that state in which no residue of the tablet, except fragments of undissolved coating, remains on the screen of the test apparaatus or, if any other residue remains, it consists of a soft mass having no palpably firm, unmoistened, core', and to comply with the standard, all tablets must normally disintegrate within 15 minutes.

There are, however, a number of exceptions. Coated tablets are expected to disintegrate within 60 minutes, either in water or 0.1 M hydrochloric acid, soluble tablets and dispersible tablets within 3 minutes in water at 19–21 °C, whilst effervescent tablets should disintegrate within 3 minutes when placed in a beaker of water at room temperature.

The disintegration properties of enteric coated tablets are studied by agitating the tablet for 2 hours in 0.1 M hydrochloric acid, during which time the tablets should show no sign of disintegration or cracking of the coat. This treatment is followed by agitation in pH 6.8 buffer, in which disintegration should be complete within one hour.

In addition 14 monographs for tablets have a standard for dissolution, and are thereby exempt from the standard for disintegration. There are a number of others to which the disintegration standard does not apply, for example, Aluminium Hydroxide Tablets BP, which are intended to be chewed before swallowing.

It must be stressed that the pharmacopoeial test for disintegration does not seek to mimic conditions in the human gastrointestinal tract with respect to fluid composition or intensity of agitation. Thus compliance with the standard is no guarantee of clinical efficacy. However, the converse is probably true in that a preparation which fails the pharmacopoeial test is unlikely to be fully efficacious. The disintegration time of a tablet is controlled by a number of experimental variables which are often interdependent. These include the type of granulating agent, the use of water-repellent lubricants, the type and amount of disintegrating agent and the force used to compress the tablet.

Dissolution   Whilst the test for tablet disintegration gives some control over those drugs whose bioavailability from tablets is governed by the rate at which the tablet disintegrates, it gives no information regarding those cases where the tablet disintegrates satisfactorily, but the rate-limiting step is the rate at which the active drug substance dissolves in the fluids of the gastrointestinal tract.

The realization that drug dissolution could affect bioavailability occurred in the 1960s when several instances were reported in which tablets, whilst meeting all pharmacopoeial requirements, failed to produce the expected therapeutic response. The British Pharmacopoeia Commission selected from all the tablet monographs in the BP 1973 those substances which might pose dissolution problems, perhaps because of low solubility, or which had been the subject of allegations of inequivalence, or where if inequivalence arose, serious therapeutic consequences might ensue. The first monograph stipulating a dissolution standard appeared in the 1977 addendum to the 1973 BP (Digoxin Tablets) and in the 1980 Pharmacopoeia, 14 tablets (and four capsules) are subject to such a standard.

The Pharmacopoeia stresses that in the majority of cases no attempt has been made to correlate dissolution results with *in vivo* data. The test is a measure of the proportion of drug dissolving in a stated time under standardized conditions *in vitro*. In a few cases, e.g. Digoxin Tablets BP, data have been obtained to establish that the *in vitro* dissolution standard correlates with *in vivo* performance.

The apparatus used in this test consists of a cylindrical steel basket into which the tablet (or tablets) is placed, and the basket is then rotated in a bath of dissolution fluid, the constitution of which is specified in the appropriate monograph. For details of the apparatus the reader is referred to the current edition of the BP. A sample is withdrawn from the dissolution fluid after a specified time (usually 45 minutes) and analysed by the method described in the monograph. Unless otherwise specified, not less than 70% of the stated content of the tablet should have dissolved. Five replicates are carried out, and if one of these fails to reach the standard, then five more tablets are tested, and now none should fail. Tablets which are subject to a dissolution standard need not be subjected to the test for disintegration.

The dissolution fluid is chosen bearing in mind the nature of the drug substance, and also the sensitivity of the assay procedure. Thus for example, 0.1 M hydrochloric acid is specified for bases such as chloroquine phosphate and quinine sulphate, a less acidic medium (pH 6.8 phosphate buffer) is specified for acidic substances such as phenoxymethylpenicillin, whilst water is suitable for neutral molecules such as digoxin. The latter also provides an example where the test is influenced by assay sensitivity, since 600 ml of water is used as a dissolution medium for six tablets. In this case, the dissolution data so obtained are obviously an average of the six tablets.

Whilst it is the intention of the *British Pharmacopoeia* to introduce a dissolution test only where dissolution problems are anticipated, the USP has adopted a totally different approach. Stating that the dissolution behaviour of oral solid dosage forms has been shown to be a useful criterion for controlling formulation and process variables, it proposes that except where such a standard would be inappropriate, all solid dosage forms shall be subject to a dissolution standard. The tablet disintegration test would thus ultimately be totally replaced.

Two methods are specified for carrying out the USP dissolution test. The first is a rotating basket method very similar to that of the BP. In the second, a paddle rotates in a bath of dissolution fluid. The composition of the latter, together with the method to be used, is specified in each monograph. Each monograph also specifies the amount (Q) which should dissolve in a stated time. Q is a percentage of the stated content of the

Table 39.3 Dissolution standards of the USP

Stage	Number of tablets to be tested	Criterion of acceptance
S_1	6	Each unit not less than Q
S_2	6	Mean of S_1 and S_2 not less than Q. None less than $Q - 15\%$
S_3	12	Mean of S_1, S_2 and S_3 not less than Q. Not more than 2 less than $Q - 15\%$.

Q is the amount which should dissolve in the specified time.

tablet, and the USP permits three stages of sampling, using up to 24 tablets. Details of this scheme are given in Table 39.3. If the tablets meet the specified standard at stage 1, then it is not necessary to proceed to stages 2 and 3.

The general dissolution requirement of the USP is 75% dissolved in 45 minutes, which is very close to the normal BP standard. In an attempt to reduce interlaboratory variation in dissolution testing, the USP suggests the use of standard discs of salicylic acid and prednisone as calibration devices for dissolution apparatus.

Non-pharmacopoeial tests

The previous section dealt with those standards which are mandatory if a tablet formulation is to be the subject of an official monograph. However, it must be clearly understood that the manufacturer may well apply tests to his product which are not stipulated by the Pharmacopoeia or may apply the pharmacopoeial tests but with higher standards. Thus, for example, a manufacturer may have his own 'in-house' standard for content uniformity or dissolution, even though there may be no such specification in the pharmacopoeia. It would be unlikely, in fact, for a product licence to be granted for a tableted drug unless such data were presented. There are also a number of tests, frequently applied to tablets, for which there is no pharmacopoeial requirement, but which will often form part of a manufacturer's own product specification. The two most important tests in this category involve the measurement of the tablet's ability to retain its physical integrity.

Crushing strength

This is often referred to as tablet 'hardness', but the latter term is a misnomer in relation to the manner in which this test is carried out. 'Hardness' implies that the tablet possesses a surface which is resistant to penetration, and whilst penetration tests have been carried out on tablets, this test normally consists of breaking or crushing the tablet by application of a compressive load. A number of devices have been designed to measure crushing strength. The simplest are hand-operated, the tablet being held between a fixed and a movable jaw. Typical examples of this type are the Monsanto tablet hardness tester, in which the force is applied via a screw-driven spring, and the Pfizer tester, in which a gripping action transfers force to the tablet. In experienced hands, these can give fairly reproducible results, but it has been found that the crushing strength so obtained is in part governed by the rate at which the force is applied. Therefore in more sophisticated testers, the load is applied at a more uniform rate by mechanical or electromechanical means, and so greater reproducibility is obtained. Examples in this category include the Schleuniger, Erweka, CT40 and Casburt testers. Even if the load is applied at a uniform rate, the variation in strength within a batch of tablets can be considerable. Also since crushing strength is dependent on tablet dimensions, comparing the strengths of tablets of different sizes is difficult. In an attempt to overcome these problems, the parameter 'tensile strength' is frequently used. This is given by the formula:

$$S_t = 2p/\pi \cdot d \cdot t \cdot (1 - e)$$

where S_t is the tensile strength, p is the crushing force, d is the tablet diameter, t is the tablet thickness, and e is the tablet porosity. This definition also compensates for the fact that porous tablets, having proportionally less interparticulate contact, will be expected to be weaker. A further development is to determine tablet 'toughness' in which the flexing of the tablet as a load is applied is also measured, analogous to force-displacement data obtained during tablet compression.

Resistance to abrasion

It is unlikely that in the normal life of a tablet it will be subjected to a compressive load large enough to fracture it. However, the tablet may well be subjected to a tumbling motion, e.g. during coating, packaging or transport, which whilst not severe enough to break the tablet, may abrade small particles from its surface. To examine this, tests to measure resistance to abrasion or 'tablet friability' have been devised. In all of these, the tablets are subjected to a uniform tumbling action for a specified time, and the weight loss from the tablets is measured. The Roche Friabilator is probably the most frequently encountered abrasion tester.

REFERENCES

Airth, J. M., Bray, D. F. and Radecka, C. (1967) Variability of uniformity of weight test as an indicator of the amount of active ingredient in tablets. *J. pharm. Sci.*, **56**, 233–235.

Armstrong, N. A. (1982) Causes of tablet compression problems. *Mfg Chem.* October, 64–65.

Higuchi, T., Nelson, E. and Busse, L. W. (1954) The physics of tablet compression. III, The design and construction of an instrumented tablet press. *J. Am. Pharm. Ass. (sci. Edn)*, **43**, 344–348.

Lowenthal, W., (1973) Mechanism of action of tablet disintegrants. *Pharm. Acta Helv.*, **48**, 589–609.

Schwartz, J. B. (1979) Optimisation techniques in pharmaceutics. In *Modern Pharmaceutics* (eds G. S. Banker and C. T. Rhodes), pp. 711–734, Marcel Dekker, New York.

Train, D. (1957) Transmission of forces through a powder mass during the process of pelleting. *Trans. Inst. Chem. Engrs.*, **35**, 258–266.

BIBLIOGRAPHY

Armstrong, N. A. and Morton, F. S. S. (1979) An evaluation of the compression characteristics of some magnesium carbonate granulations. *Pharm. Weekblad*, **114**, 1450–1459.

Augsberger, L. L. and Shangraw, R. F. (1966) Effect of glidants in tableting. *J. pharm. Sci.*, **55**, 418–423.

Banker, G. S., Peck, G. E. and Baley, B. (1980) Tablet formulation and design. In *Pharmaceutical Dosage Forms: Tablets, Volume 1* (eds H. A. Lieberman and L. Lachman), pp. 61–107, Marcel Dekker, New York.

de Blaey, C. J. and Polderman, J. (1970) The quantitative

interpretation of force-displacement curves. *Pharm. Weekblad*, **105**, 241–250.

Chowhan, Z. T. and Chow, Y. P. (1980) Compression behaviour of pharmaceutical powders. *Int. J. Pharm.*, 5, 139–148.

Cooper, A. R. and Eaton, L. E. (1962) Compaction behaviour of several ceramic powders, *J. Am. Ceram. Soc.*, **45**, 97–101.

David, S. T. and Augsberger, L. L. (1977) Plastic flow during compression of directly compressible fillers and its effect on tablet strength. *J. pharm. Sci.*, **66**, 155–159.

Goodhart, F. W., Draper, J. R., Dancz, D., and Ninger, F. C. (1973) Evaluation of tablet breaking strength testers. *J. pharm. Sci.*, **62**, 297–304.

Hess, H. J. E. (1978) Tablets under the microscope. *Pharm. Tech.*, **2**, 36–57.

Hiestand, E. N., Wells, J. E., Peot, C. B. and Ochs, J. F. (1977) The physical processes of tabletting. *J. pharm. Sci.*, **66**, 510–519.

Higuchi, T. and others, The physics of tablet compression, a series of 18 articles which appeared in *J. pharm. Sci.* from 1953 onwards.

Jarosz, P. J. and Parrott, E. L. (1982) Factors influencing axial and radial tensile strength of tablets. *J. pharm. Sci.*, **71**, 607–614.

Jones, T. M. (1978) Performulation studies to predict the compaction properties of materials used in tablets and capsules. *Acta Pharm. Tech.*, **6**, 141–159.

Lachman, L. and Sylwestrowicz, H. D. (1964) Experiences with unit-to-unit variations in tablets. *J. pharm. Sci.*, **53**, 1234–1242.

Matsuda, Y., Minamida, Y. and Hayashi, S. (1976) Comparative evaluation of tablet lubricants. *J. pharm. Sci.*, **65**, 1155–1160.

Pietsch, W. B. (1969) The strength of agglomerates bound by salt bridges. *Can. J. Chem. Engng*, **47**, 403–409.

Rippie, E. G. and Danielson, D. W. (1981) Viscoelastic stress-strain behaviour of pharmaceutical tablets. *J. pharm. Sci.*, **70**, 476–482.

Rudnic, E. M., Rhodes, C. T., Welch, S. and Bernardo, P. (1982) Evaluation of the mechanism of disintegrant action. *Drug Dev. Ind. Pharm.*, **8**, 87–109.

Scott, M. W., Lieberman, H. A., Rankell, A. S. and Battista, J. V. (1964) Continuous production of tablet granulations on a fluidised bed. *J. pharm. Sci.*, **53**, 314–320 and 320–324.

Sheth, B. B., Bandelin, F. J. and Shangraw, R. F. (1980) Compressed tablets. In *Pharmaceutical Dosage Forms: Tablets, Volume 1* (eds H. A. Lieberman and L. Lachman), pp. 109–185, Marcel Dekker, New York.

Shotton, E. and Obiorah, B. A. (1975) Effect of physical properties on compression characteristics. *J. pharm. Sci.*, **64**, 1213–1216.

Stenlake, J. B. (1981) The British Pharmacopoeia, 1980, scientific innovations. *Pharm. J.*, May 1981, 497–499.

Train, D. and Lewis, C. J. (1962) Agglomeration of solids by compaction. *Trans. Inst. Chem. Engrs*, **40**, 235–240.

Tablet coating

Tablet coating as a pharmaceutical unit process has origins which can be traced back to the time of the ancient Egyptians. Recognizably modern sugar coating processes arose in the middle of the nineteenth century as refined sugar became more widely available. The methods used for the sugar coating of pharmaceutical dosage forms have developed from the related technology of panning methods used to produce coated confectionery products.

Film coating of tablets in contrast is a relatively new technology dating back to the 1950s.

Types of tablet coating

There are three types in common use:

1 sugar coating
2 film coating
3 press coating (compression coating).

Of these the most important are sugar coating and film coating.

For historical reasons, sugar coating has been the most extensively employed method but is at present being superseded by film coating techniques. Most newly developed coated products are film coated.

Reasons for coating tablets

The reasons why tablets are coated are varied. The major reasons for tablet coating can be summarized as follows:

1 Protection of ingredients from the environment, particularly light and moisture.
2 Many drugs have a bitter or otherwise

unpleasant taste. Coating provides an efficient method of taste masking tablets. Tablets that are coated are also somewhat easier to swallow than uncoated tablets.

Both these factors aid patient compliance with dosage schemes.

3 Coloured coatings also mask any batchwise differences in the appearance of raw materials and hence allay patient concern over tablets of differing appearance.
4 Coloured coatings aid in the rapid identification of product by the manufacturer, dispensing pharmacist and patient.
5 Coating tablets facilitates their handling on high speed automatic filling and packaging equipment. Very often coating confers an added mechanical strength to the tablet core. Cross-contamination is also reduced in the manufacturing plant as 'dusting' from tablets is eliminated by coating.
6 Functional film coatings are used to impart enteric or controlled release properties to the coated tablet (see later in this chapter).

SUGAR COATING

Sugar coating may be visualized as the traditional method of coating tablets. It involves the successive application of sucrose-based solutions to tablet cores in suitable coating equipment. Conventional panning equipment with manual application of syrup has been extensively used although more specialized equipment and automated methods are now making an impact on the process.

Sugar coating was regarded in the past almost as much as an art form as an industrial process. However, much has been achieved in recent times in formalizing the process to make it compatible with modern documentary control required by good manufacturing practice (GMP).

Stages involved in the production of sugar coated tablets

Sugar coating is a multistage process and can be divided into the following steps:

1 sealing of the tablet cores
2 subcoating
3 smoothing (or grossing)
4 colouring
5 polishing
6 printing.

Sealing

Sugar coating is an aqueous process during which the tablet cores are thoroughly wetted by syrup applications. A tablet sealant is therefore applied to protect the tablet cores during this initial susceptible period from the action of water.

Tablet sealants are generally water-insoluble polymers or film formers applied from an organic solvent solution. Examples of tablet sealants are:

1 shellac — very commonly used and is best in combination with PVP which prevents hardening of the polymer on ageing,
2 cellulose acetate phthalate,
3 polyvinyl acetate phthalate,
(These two polymers are used at application levels insufficient to give an enteric effect.)
4 acrylate polymers.

The sealing stage must be conducted with some caution as over-application of tablet sealants can lead to disintegration problems.

Subcoating

Sugar coated tablets have a completely smooth profile with no visible edges remaining from the original tablet core (Fig. 40.1). To attain this shape the sealed tablet core must be built up to gain the desired profile. Tablet cores for sugar coating should have a small edge so as not to make the 'rounding' process more difficult than it need be (Fig. 40.2).

Fig. 40.1

Fig. 40.2

Subcoating can be accomplished by two methods, either

1 the application of a gum/sucrose solution followed by dusting with powder and then drying. This routine is repeated many times until the desired shape is achieved; or
2 the application of a suspension of dry powder in the gum/sucrose solution followed by drying. As above the procedure is repeatedly performed until the correct shape is evident.

The solution used is sucrose based and contains a gum such as gelatin, acacia or a starch derivative which aid in the adhesion of the powder fillers such as calcium carbonate or talc. If a coating suspension is used then the solids content is made as high as possible in order to reduce the drying time between each application.

Smoothing or grossing

After the correct profile has been attained then the subcoated tablets will almost certainly have a rather rough surface. They are made perfectly smooth by successive applications of dilute syrup. The tablets are subjected to drying air after each application.

Colour coating

Nearly all sugar coated tablets are coloured. The colours used are those colours permitted in the national legislation of the countries where the product will be sold. There are two groups of colouring substances generally used in coloured tablet coatings:

1 water-soluble dyes
2 water-insoluble pigments.

The use of water-soluble dyes is part of the traditional method of sugar coating tablets. However, their use demands a great deal of skill and patience and the process is prone to coating faults such as poor and uneven coverage and variation in colour from batch to batch.

Most modern sugar coating procedures utilize pigments such as the aluminium lakes or iron oxides. They are easier to use and permit comparatively fast colour coating times compared with soluble dye coating.

Polishing

After colour coating the tablets will require a separate polishing step for them to achieve an attractive appearance. This step is carried out in a clean pan but sometimes a wax or canvas lined pan is used. The tablets receive one or two applications of a wax dissolved in an organic solvent. Usually beeswax or carnauba wax is used.

In order to achieve a good finish recognition must be given to optimum temperature and humidity conditions.

Printing

The use of indented monograms on sugar coated tablet cores is not feasible because the considerable thickness of coating obliterates any core markings. Instead, if identification is required then this can be accomplished by printing. The printing process used is an offset rotogravure and this is used in conjunction with special edible printing inks (Lykens, 1979).

Process details

Typically tablets are sugar coated by a panning technique. The most simple form would be a traditional sugar coating pan (Fig. 40.3) with a supply of drying air (preferably of variable temperature and thermostatically controlled) and a fan-assisted extract to remove dust and moisture-laden air.

Methods of coating syrup application include:

1 manually using a ladle,
2 automatic control.

In modern equipment some form of automatic control is available for the application of coating syrups. These control devices allow programmed variation in dose volume, rolling time and drying time (see Fraade, 1983).

Traditional ladle application in conventional panning equipment is capable of achieving impressive results in skilled hands but this tech-

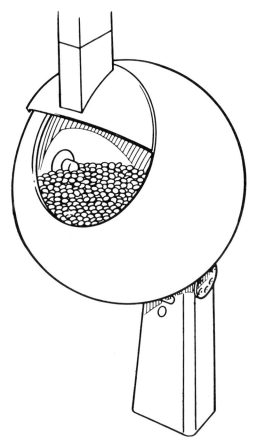

Fig. 40.3 Coating pan

nique is not easy to control in terms of modern GMP requirements.

Other more sophisticated equipment is available which overcomes the inherent disadvantages of the conventional pan, for example, poor drying capability. The various equipment listed below have efficient drying ability and are capable of some degree of automation:

1 Accela Cota — Manesty Machines, Liverpool, England,
2 Hi-Coater — Freund Company, Japan,
3 Driacoater — Driam Metallprodukt GmbH, Germany.

The following may be considered intermediate (with respect to efficient use of the drying air) between a conventional pan and the list above.

1 Pellegrini — Zanasi Nigris, Italy,
2 IDA — Dumoulin, France.

In these units the surface of the bed has been increased by efficient drum design but the drying air, as in the conventional pan, is still only acting on the surface of the bed.

Ideal characteristics of sugar coated tablets

First of all the tablets must comply with finished product specifications and any appropriate compendial requirements. Sugar coated tablets should ideally be of a perfectly smooth rounded contour with even colour coverage. Most manufacturers take advantage of the aesthetic appeal of a sugar coated tablet and polish to a high gloss. Any printing should be distinct with no smudging or broken print.

Fig. 40.4

Coating faults

These are usually associated with process defects. For example inappropriate drying conditions with dye-coloured tablets can lead to blotchiness on the final product.

FILM COATING

This is generally the more modern of the two major coating processes. Most newly launched coated products are film coated rather than sugar coated for the reasons highlighted in Table 40.1.

Process description

Film coating involves the deposition, usually by a spray method, of a thin film of polymer surrounding the tablet core. It is possible to utilize conventional panning equipment but more usually specialized equipment is employed to take advantage of the fast coating times and high degree of automation possible.

The coating liquid ('solution') contains a polymer in a suitable liquid medium together with other ingredients such as pigments and plasti-

Table 40.1 Major differences between sugar coating and film coating

Features	Sugar coating	Film coating
Tablets		
Appearance	Rounded (Fig. 40.1), with high degree of polish	Retain contour of original core, (Fig. 40.4). Usually not as shiny as sugar coat types
Weight increase due to coating materials	30–50%	2–3%
Logo or 'break' lines	Not possible	Possible
Process		
Operator training required	Considerable	Process lends itself to automation and easy training of operators
Adaptability to GMP requirements	Difficulties can arise	High
Process stages	Multistage process	Usually single stage
Functional coatings	Not usually possible apart from enteric coating	Easily adaptable for controlled release

cizers. This solution is sprayed on to a rotated, mixed tablet bed. The drying conditions permit the removal of the solvent so as to leave a thin deposition of coating material around each tablet core.

Coating solution formulation

Typically this comprises:

polymer
solvent
plasticizer
colorants.

Polymers

The fundamental ingredient in the formulation. Most commonly used are the derivates of cellulose such as hydroxypropylmethylcellulose (Fig. 40.5), methylcellulose and ethylcellulose. These have the advantages of forming clear, non-tacky, mechanically strong films from a wide variety of suitable solvents. They are widely available in a pure form

with adequate compendial control. Many of these polymers have had a long history of safe use in the food industry and therefore have a wide regulatory acceptance.

Acrylate-based polymers are also used in plain film coatings. However, other types are available in modifications designed to give gastric-insoluble films or controlled release properties.

Other more elderly film coating systems are occasionally encountered such as shellac or cellulose acetate phthalate in combination with PEG.

A recent development has been the introduction of fine particle suspensions of polymer, e.g. ethylcellulose, as a simple coating media. The film is formed by the combined action of plasticizer and drying heat on the individual polymer particles thus causing them to coalesce into a film.

Solvents

After the early development of film coating in the 1950s the polymers used for film coating were invariably dissolved in an organic solvent. Modern techniques have now tended to rely on water as

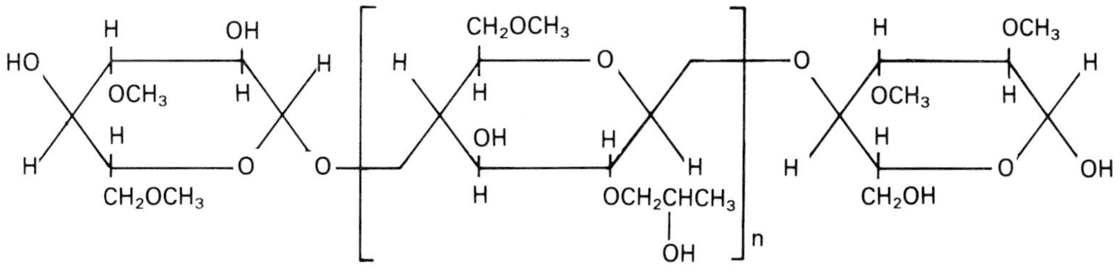

Fig. 40.5 Hydroxypropyl methylcellulose, structure

a solvent because of the significant drawbacks that readily became apparent due to the use of organic solvents. The disadvantages of organic solvents for the process can be listed below.

1 Environmental: the venting of untreated organic solvent vapour into the atmosphere is ecologically unacceptable whilst efficient solvent vapour removal from gaseous effluent is expensive.
2 Safety: organic solvents provide explosion, fire and toxic hazards to plant operators.
3 Financial: the use of organic solvents necessitates the building of flame- and explosion-proof facilities. Ingredient cost is also comparatively high and the associated costs of storage and quality control must also be taken into consideration (Hogan, 1983).

Plasticizers

Plasticizers are generally added to film coating formulae to modify the physical properties of the polymer to make it more usable in film coating. One important property is their ability to decrease film brittleness.

Commonly used plasticizers include PEG, propylene glycol, glycerol and its esters and phthalate esters. In general only water-miscible plasticizers can be used for aqueous based spray systems (Aulton *et al.*, 1981).

Colorants

As with sugar coated tablets, the colorants of choice are the water-insoluble pigments. Pigments overcome any colour variation problems encountered with dyes and their opaque properties lend themselves to the efficient colouring of the thin coatings used in film coating techniques. The use of pigments overcomes the specific incompatibilities that exist between some dyes and cellulosic systems.

Process details

The vast majority of film coated tablets are produced by a spray process. Generally the basic equipment listed under the sugar coating process details is suitable for film coating once suitably modified for the process change. Figure 40.6 shows the most widely used equipment for film coating, the Accela Cota. Modifications include provision of spray equipment and proper attention

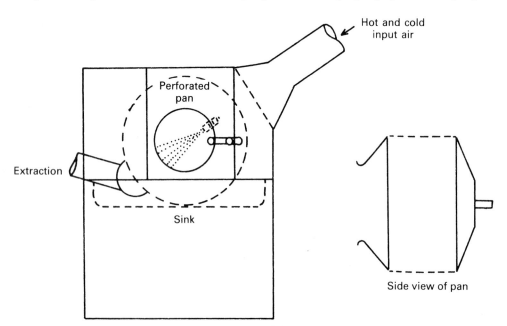

Fig. 40.6 Accela Cota, schematic

to drying air and mixing of the tablet bed. Indeed many of the units mentioned were designed with modern film coating techniques in mind. In addition, for film coating, fluidized bed equipment has made a considerable impact. Examples of such units are manufactured by:

1 Glatt AG, Switzerland and Germany,
2 Aeromatic AG, Switzerland.

Basic process requirements for film coating

These fundamental requirements are more or less independent of the actual type of equipment being used and include:

1 adequate means of atomizing the spray liquid for application to the tablet cores,
2 adequate mixing and agitation of the tablet bed. Spray coating relies upon each core passing through the area of spraying. This is distinct from sugar coating where each application is spread from tablet to tablet prior to drying,
3 sufficient heat input in the form of drying air to provide the latent heat of evaporation of the solvent. This is particularly important with aqueous-based spraying,
4 good exhaust facilities to remove dust and solvent laden air.

Ideal characteristics of film coated tablets

Film coated tablets should display an even coverage of film and colour. There should be no abrasion of tablet edges or crowns. Logos and break lines should be distinct and not filled in. The tablets must also be compliant with finished product specifications and any relevant compendial requirements.

Coating faults

These arise from two distinct causes:

1 Processing: for example, inadequate drying conditions will permit coating previously deposited on the tablet surface to stick against neighbouring tablets. When parted, this will reveal the original core surface underneath.
2 Formulation faults: film cracking or 'bridging'

of break lines are examples of this type. After taking due account of the mechanical properties of the film then reformulation will almost certainly be successful in overcoming the problem (Rowe, 1981).

PRESS COATING

The technology of press coating differs radically from the previously described sugar coating and film coating techniques. Press coating involves the compaction of granular material around an already preformed core (Fig. 40.7) using compressing equipment similar to that used for the core itself, e.g. Manesty Drycota.

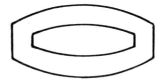

Fig. 40.7

From the greater sophistication of tablet compressing machinery of the 1950s arose the process of press coating. Originally the process had an obvious application for very water-sensitive tablet cores where a dry coating would be of enormous advantage. The granular coating material usually contains a high proportion of sugar to mimic the more conventional sugar coating techniques.

With the advent of film coating very soon after these developments, the process of press coating never did realize its full potential and has since been of decreasing importance. Today it is used mainly to separate chemically incompatible materials, one or more being placed in the core and the other(s) in the coating layer. However, there is still an interface of contact left between the two layers. In cases where even this is important then the process of press coating can be taken one stage further. It is possible to apply two press coatings to a tablet core using suitable equipment, e.g. Manesty Bicota. This equipment produces press coated tablets with perfect separation between active core and coating as these two can be separated by an inner inert coating.

ιulation and processing of the coating layer requires some care. Large or irregular sized agglomerates of granule will cause the core to tilt in the second die used for compression of the coating. Thus there is the possibility of an incomplete coating with the core visible at the tablet surface.

The disadvantages of the process arise from the relative complexities of the mechanism used in the compressing equipment.

FUNCTIONAL COATINGS

All the coatings described previously have been designed as a taste mask, as an identification aid or indeed for any of the reasons previously discussed for coating tablets. There are, however, tablet coatings produced which perform a pharmaceutical function such as conferring enteric or controlled release.

Enteric coating

This technique is used to protect the tablet core from disintegration in the acid environment of the stomach for one or more of the following reasons:

1 prevention of acid attack on active constituents unstable at low pH,
2 to protect the stomach from the irritant effect of certain drugs,
3 to facilitate absorption a drug preferentially absorbed distally to the stomach.

The following polymers are among those commonly used for the purposes of enteric coating:

1 cellulose acetate phthalate
2 polyvinyl acetate phthalate
3 acrylates.

Due to the possession of free carboxylic acid groups on the polymer backbone, they exhibit a differential pH solubility profile. These are almost insoluble in aqueous media at low pH but as the pH rises they experience a sharp, well defined increase in solubility at a specific pH, e.g. pH 5.2 for cellulose acetate phthalate.

Enteric coating is possible using both sugar and film coating techniques.

Enteric sugar coating

The sealing coat is modified to comprise one of the enteric polymers in sufficient quantity to pass the enteric test for disintegration. The subcoating and subsequent coating steps are then as for conventional sugar coating.

Enteric film coating

The enteric polymers listed are capable of forming a direct film in a film coating process. Sufficient weight of enteric polymer has to be used to ensure an efficient enteric effect. This is normally two or three times that required for a simple film coating.

Controlled release coatings

Film coating techniques are of great assistance in the production of tablets required to have a functional coating for the purposes of conferring a controlled release. The polymers used include:

1 modified acrylates,
2 water-insoluble celluloses, e.g. ethyl cellulose.

STANDARDS FOR COATED TABLETS

There are some differences between the requirements for coated and uncoated tablets in the general tablet monograph in the BP. For coated tablets, the requirement for uniformity of weight and diameter has been deleted. Also the disintegration test for coated tablets specifies a maximum disintegration time of 60 minutes in water but permits the test to be repeated in 0.1 M HCl should the tablets fail. As with uncoated tablets, if the individual tablet monograph requires a dissolution test, then the disintegration test may be justifiably omitted.

It is, however, common practice for a manufacturer to test the uncoated cores prior to coating, including in the test schedule parameters appropriate for an uncoated tablet.

The BP treats press coated tablets as for

uncoated tablets for the purposes of compendial control.

The BP disintegration test for enteric coated tablets directs that six tablets should withstand 2 hours in 0.1 M HCl without disintegrating but on replacing the fluid with pH 6.8 phosphate buffer all six should disintegrate within 1 hour.

COATING OF OTHER SOLID DOSAGE FORMS

In order to put coating in perspective it should be mentioned that solid dosage forms other than tablets are subjected to coating procedures for a variety of reasons. For example:

1 Gelatin capsules — both hard and soft elastic types — are occasionally enteric coated.
2 Granules and sugar seeds ('non-pareils') are frequently filled into hard gelatin capsules to produce a controlled release system. Here the drug is coated on to the outside of the particle and these are finally coated with a polymer which permits the slow diffusion of aqueous drug solution to the exterior.

REFERENCES

Aulton, M. E., Abdul-Razzak, M. H., and Hogan, J. E. (1981) The mechanical properties of hydroxypropyl methylcellulose films derived from aqueous systems. Part 1: The influence of plasticisers. *Drug Dev. Ind. Pharm.*, **7**, 649.

Fraade, D. J. (1983) *Automation of Pharmaceutical Operations*, Chapter 10, Pharmaceutical Technology Publications, London.

Hogan, J. E. (1983) Additive effects on aqueous film coatings, *Mfg Chem.*, **54**, 43.

Lykens, D. N. (1979) Edible printing inks. *Pharm. Tech.*, **3**(2), 56.

Rowe, R. C. (1981) The cracking of film coatings on film coated tablets — a theoretical approach with practical implications. *J. Pharm. Pharmac.*, **33**, 423.

BIBLIOGRAPHY

Banker, G. S. (1966) Theory and practice of film coating. *J. pharm. Sci.*, **55**, 81.

Delporte, J. P. (1981) Influence de quelques additifs sur les propriétés de resistance méchanique de films isolés d'hydroxypropylméthylcellulose de basse viscosité. *J. Pharm. Belg.*, **36**, 27.

Hogan, J. E. (1983) Additive effects on aqueous film coatings. *Mfg Chem.*, **54**, 43.

Porter, S. C. (1981) Tablet coating. *Drug and Cosmetic Ind.*, May 46, June 44, Aug. 40, Sept. 50.

Porter, S. C. (1979) Aqueous film coating: an overview, *Pharm. Tech.*, **3**(9), 55.

Rieckmann, P. (1963) Automation of dragee production, *Drugs Made in Germany*, **6**, 162.

Rowe, R. C. (1983) Coating defects — causes and cures. *Mfg Chem.*, **54**, 49.

Encapsulation

HARD GELATIN CAPSULES

Manufacture of hard gelatin capsule shells

The method used for the industrial manufacture of hard gelatin capsules (HGC) is basically the same as that described in the original patent. However, since then the process has been developed and is now undertaken on fully automatic machines housed in complex air conditioned buildings. As a result they are manufactured by only a small number of specialist companies who supply empty capsule shells to the pharmaceutical industry to fill with their own products. The two major producers in the world are the American companies, Eli Lilly and Parke Davis, who have both been making capsules since the turn of the century.

The first part of the process is the preparation of the raw materials. A concentrated gelatin solution is prepared in hot demineralized water in a jacketed pressure vessel. When the gelatin has completely dissolved a vacuum is applied to the solution to remove any entrapped air. Aliquots of this solution are dispensed into suitable containers and to them are added the required quantities of dye solutions and process aids such as preservatives. The viscosity of each mix is measured and adjusted to a target value. This parameter is used to control the thickness of capsule shell walls in production. The mixes are then transferred to heated storage hoppers on the manufacturing machines.

The manufacturing machines are approximately 10 m long and 2 m wide. They consist of two halves which are mirror images; on one half the caps are made and on the other bodies. The machines are divided also into two levels, an upper and a lower one. The moulds, called 'pins', are made of stainless steel and are mounted in sets on metal strips, called 'bars'. There are approximately 44 000 mould pins per machine. The machines are housed in large rooms, the humidity and temperature of which can be closely controlled.

The sequence of events in the manufacture of HGC shells is shown in Fig. 41.1. At the front end of the machine is a hopper, called a 'dip pan' or 'pot'. This holds a fixed quantity of the prepared gelatin solution at a constant temperature, between 45 and 55 °C. The level of solution is maintained by an automatic feed from the storage hopper. Capsules are formed by dipping sets of 'moulds', at room temperature, into this solution. A film is formed on the surface of each mould by gelling. The moulds are slowly withdrawn and then rotated during their transfer to the upper level of the machine in order to form a film of uniform thickness. Groups of 'pin bars' are then passed through a series of drying kilns in which large volumes of controlled humidity air are blown over them. At the rear of the machine the bars are transferred to the lower level and

travel through further drying kilns back to the front of the machine. Here in the automatic section, the dried films are removed from the moulds, cut to the correct lengths, the two halves joined together and complete capsules delivered from the machine. The mould pins are cleaned and lubricated for the start of the next cycle.

The machines are normally operated on a 24-hour basis 7 days per week only stopping for periods of maintenance. The output per machine is between 750 000 and 1 million capsules per day depending upon size.

The finished capsules now pass through a series of sorting and checking processes which can either be manual, mechanical or electronic to remove as many defective ones as possible. The quality levels are checked continuously using standard statistical sampling plans. If required the capsules are printed at this stage. This is performed on machines which use an offset gravure roll process with an edible ink. The information printed is usually either the product name or drug strength, the company name or some other identifying mark. The capsules are finally counted and packed for shipment preferably in heat-sealed aluminium

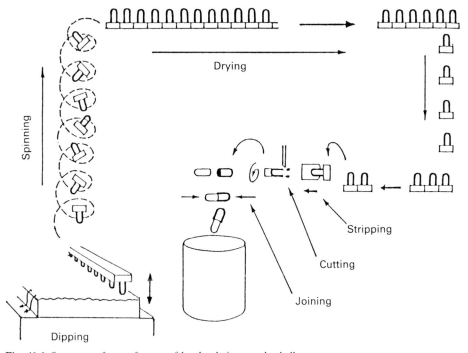

Fig. 41.1 Sequence of manufacture of hard gelatin capsule shells

foil sacs in cardboard cartons. In these containers capsules can be stored almost indefinitely provided that they are not subjected to localized heating or sudden temperature changes which will affect their moisture content.

The finished capsules have a moisture content of between 13.0 and 16.0%. This value can vary and it depends upon the conditions to which the empty capsules are exposed: at low humidities they will lose moisture and become brittle and at high humidities they will gain moisture and become soft. In suitable sealed containers the moisture content will be maintained at the optimum level.

The filling of hard gelatin capsules

The filling of hard gelatin capsules requires the same set of basic operations whether it is undertaken on the bench scale for extemporaneous dispensing or on industrial scale using high speed automatic machines. The capsule needs first to be taken apart, the body filled with the required quantity of material and the cap replaced on the body. The major difference between all of the many methods which are available is the way in which the dose of material is measured into the capsule body.

Bench-scale filling

There is a requirement for filling small quantities of capsules, from 50 to 10 000, in the community pharmacy, the hospital pharmacy or in industry either for special prescriptions or for clinical trials. There are several simple pieces of equipment available for doing this, e.g. the 'Feton' or the 'Labocaps'. They consist of sets of plastic plates which have predrilled holes to take from 30 to 100 capsules. Empty shells are fed into the holes either manually or with a simple loading device. The bodies are locked in their plate by a screw and the caps in their holder are removed. Powder can be filled into the capsules by placing it on the surface of the body plate and spreading and levelling it by means of a plastic spatula. The cap plate is then repositioned over the body one and the capsules rejoined together using manual pressure.

The uniformity of fill weight is very dependent upon good powder flow properties. It is difficult to achieve high fill weights. More sophisticated forms of this equipment are available which increases the powder packing within the body by using either mechanical agitation, e.g. Tevopharm CAP III or vibration, e.g. Zuma.

Industrial-scale filling

The machines for the large scale filling of hard gelatin capsules come in a large variety of shapes and sizes: varying from semi- to fully automatic, from continuous to intermittent motion and in output from 5000 per hour to 150 000 per hour. However, despite this apparent diversity they all use the same basic method of capsule handling and differ only in their powder dosing systems.

Capsule handling   Empty hard gelatin capsules are supplied in bulk containers. Thus it is first necessary for the machine to orientate them so that they are all pointing in the same direction, i.e. body first. To do this the capsules are loaded into a hopper and from there pass through tubes to a 'rectification' or 'aligning' section. Here the capsules are held in tight-fitting slots. A metal finger strikes them in the middle causing them to rotate and because the body is freer, it always having a smaller diameter than the cap, they do so with the body facing the direction of motion. The capsule is now fed into sets of holders or bushes, the diameters of which are designed so that the body can pass through the upper one but not the cap. This transfer is usually assisted by a vacuum. The cap and the body are thus separated. The caps are then moved to one side. The bodies pass under the dosing mechanism and are filled with material. The caps are then repositioned over the bodies and metal fingers are used to rejoin the two together to the correct closed joined length.

Dosing systems for powders   There are three basic methods which have been used for measuring the quantity of material to be filled into a capsule.

1 the auger or screw
2 the dosator
3 the tamping finger and dosing disc.

The auger This system is principally used on semi-automatic machines. Empty capsules are fed into a pair of ring holders. The caps are retained in one half and the bodies in the other. The bodies in their holder are passed under a powder hopper inside of which is a revolving auger or screw. Material is transferred into the bodies by the movement of the auger. The quantity of powder is dependant upon the speed of revolution and design of the auger, the quantity of powder in the hopper and the time the body is under the hopper. To obtain the best uniformity of fill weight it is necessary to fill the body as completely as possible.

The machine is semi-automatic because it requires a person to transfer the capsules from one operation to another: capsule feeding, filling and closing. Examples of machines which use this system are the Model No. 8 machine supplied by Elanco and Parke Davis. Their output is between 15 000 and 25 000 capsules per hour.

The dosator This system is used on fully automatic machines which can be either continuous or intermittent in motion. It is currently probably the most widely used system and is the one which has been referred to most in the literature. It consists of a dosing tube inside of which there is a spring loaded piston. The tube is plunged, open end first, into a powder bed. Material rises up in the tube to the piston to form a plug of powder. This can be consolidated further by applying a compression force to the piston. The assembly is then raised and positioned over the capsule body. The piston is lowered ejecting the powder plug into the capsule. The fill weight can be varied by adjusting the position of the piston inside the dosing tube or altering the depth of the powder bed.

Examples of machines which use this system are:

1 intermittent motion: Zanasi, Pendini, Macophar, Bonapace. Their outputs range from 5000 to 60 000 capsules per hour.
2 continuous motion: MG2, Zanasi, Farmatic. Their outputs range from 30 000 to 150 000 per hour.

The tamping finger and dosing disc This system is used on fully automatic machines which all have an intermittent motion. The dosing disc forms the base of a revolving powder hopper. The disc has a series of accurately drilled holes in it. Powder plugs are formed in these holes by sets of metal rods, tamping fingers which are lowered into them through the powder bed. The plug is formed in five positions. At each one the fingers push material into the holes before they index onto the next position. At a sixth position the powder plugs are pushed out and into the capsule body. The fill weight can be varied by the depth of the powder bed and the relative movement of the tamping fingers and the thickness of the dosing disc.

The machines which use this system are the Höfliger Karg manufactured by Robert Bosch and the Harro Höfliger. Their outputs range from 6000 to 180 000 capsules per hour.

Other systems Other systems for dose measurement have been used but with only limited success. The 'Accofil' system used for filling powder vials was incorporated into a capsule filling machine by the American company Perry Industries Inc. The dose of material is measured in a device similar to a dosator with the material being sucked into it to form a plug and then being blown out into the body. The Japanese company Osaka have developed a system in which the body passes under a powder hopper. Inside the hopper there is a vibrating plate which 'fluidizes' the powder causing it to flow into the bodies. In practice it would appear that both machines work with free-flowing powders but have a drawback in being unable to achieve the fill weights required with low density materials.

SOFT GELATIN CAPSULES

Production of soft gelatin capsules

Soft gelatin capsules are produced using an encapsulation machine and a rotary die process. An overall view of the apparatus is shown in Fig. 41.2. Normally, two tanks of liquid feed material to the encapsulation machine; one contains a mass of molten gelatin, at 60 °C, and the other contains the medicinal liquid fill material at 20 °C. For bicoloured capsules two gelatin containers are used to produce the two parts of the shell.

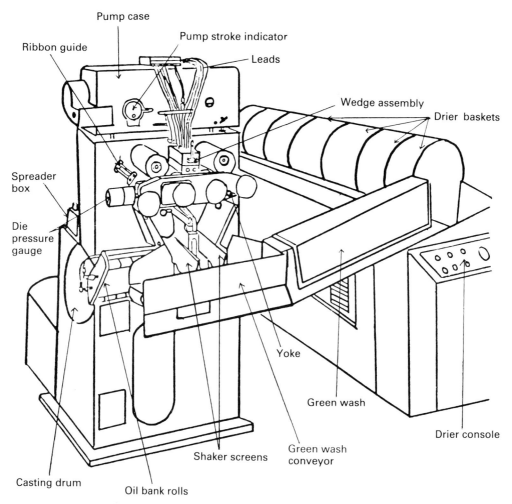

Fig. 41.2 Diagram of a soft gelatin encapsulation machine

The gelatin formulation consists of gelatin (35–50%), a plasticizer (e.g. glycerol 15–30%, sorbitol or propylene glycol) and water. Other materials such as preservative (potassium sorbitate, methyl, ethyl and propyl parabens), dyes, opacifiers and flavours may also be present. See Chapter 19 for further formulation details.

The liquid fill material consists of a liquid drug or solid drugs dissolved or dispersed (with suspending agents e.g. beeswax or hydrogenated vegetable oil) in vehicles or combinations of vehicles such as mineral oil, vegetable oils, triglycerides, glycol, polyols and surfactants. Again the reader is referred to Chapter 19 for extra information.

The molten gelatin flows down two heated pipes through two heated spreader boxes onto two large cool casting drums maintained at 16–20 °C where flat solid ribbons of gel are formed. The two ribbons are fed between mineral oil lubricated rollers and then into the encapsulation mechanism, see Fig. 41.3.

Medicinal liquid fill material (usually at room temperature) in the other tank flows under gravity through a tube leading to a multiplunger positive displacement filling pump. Accurately metered volumes of the liquid fill material are injected through the wedge (heated to 37–40 °C) between the gelatin ribbons as they pass between the die rolls. The injection of liquid forces the gelatin to expand into the pockets of the dies which govern the size and shape of the capsules. The

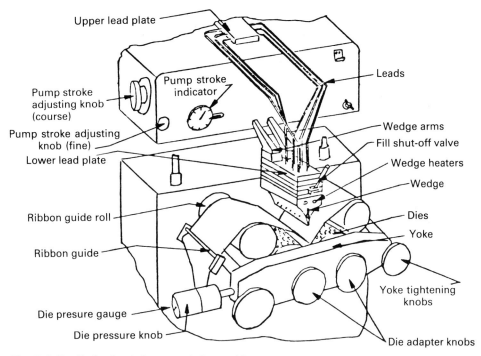

Fig. 41.3 Detail of soft gelatin encapsulation machine

ribbon continues to flow past the heated wedge and is pressed between the die rolls where the capsule halves are sealed together by the application of heat (37–40 °C) and pressure. The capsules are cut out automatically from the gelatin ribbon by the dies, and are transported through a naphtha wash to remove surface lubricating oil.

The capsules are passed through a rotating basket, infra-red dryer and are then spread onto trays to complete the drying process in a tunnel-corridor using air at a relative humidity of approximately 20%. The capsules are inspected for quality, washed again in naphtha if necessary, graded according to size specification and are packaged for distribution.

Storage of soft gelatin capsules

Capsules containing oils as liquid fills are potentially stable in temperate climates in packs which are not good barriers against moisture ingress. Products containing hygroscopic liquids, however, should be protected against moisture and be packed in containers such as glass bottles with screw caps and waxed wad seals.

Temperature as well as humidity can play an important role in the stability of soft gelatin capsules. Exporting soft gelatin capsules to hot climate areas can probably cause deformation, leaking or melting if the temperature climbs over 40 °C for long periods. This applies even in packs which provide good protection against moisture ingress. For good stability the temperature should be maintained below 30 °C.

CAPSULE STANDARDS

Products filled into gelatin capsules have to comply with the requirements of the official compendia. There are over 30 pharmacopoeias in the world and of these 27 have either monographs or set limits for capsule products. The monographs take the general form of a description followed by a series of tests. These are designed to set official minimum acceptable performance standards, i.e., that the product has a known, uniform, stable quantity of active ingredients in a form which is biologically available to the patient. There are many different tests described, however, and there are only two which are common to them all; the uniformity of fill weight and the disintegration test.

Hard gelatin capsules

Uniformity of fill weight test

This test is used as a simple means of estimating the content of active ingredient per capsule. It is based upon the assumption that the active ingredient is homogeneously dispersed through the contents of a batch of capsules. The test involves weighing a specific number of capsules, emptying out their contents, reweighing the shells and calculating the weight of the fill. A test criterion is applied to the results which can be of two types; a single or a double limit. In the former, all weight must be within a pair of limits and in the latter a proportion can be outside an inner limit but all must be within an outer one. The limits are sometimes varied depending upon the weight of the contents. For example, the *European Pharmacopoeia* uses a sample of 20 capsules. For those products which have a mean weight of less than 300 mg, at least 18 of the results must be within ±10% of the mean weight and the remainder must be within ±20%. If the product has a mean weight of 300 mg or more, then the limits are 7.5% and 15% respectively.

In carrying out the determination of fill weight, care must be taken to remove all of the contents from the shells before they are reweighed. Little difficulty is experienced in completely removing powders, granules and pellets. However, more care must be taken with liquid or pasty products and the pharmacopoeias usually recommend the washing of the shells with a solvent to remove the last traces. Soft gelatin capsules need to be cut open to remove their contents and care must be taken to retain all parts of the shell for reweighing. During industrial manufacture, the gross weights of a product in a hard gelatin capsule are used for in-process control. This can be done because the shell weight normally makes only a small contribution to the total variation; due to the fact that the ratio of shell weights to content weight is in the order of 1 : 4 or 1 : 5 and the total variation is derived from the sum of the squares of the individual variations. Some pharmacopoeias use both the gross and net weights of capsules. The Indian Pharmacopoeia has a sequential type of test. Initially the gross weights of a small sample (10) are determined and a tight test criterion is applied. If the sample does not meet this requirement, the test is repeated on the net weights of a further larger sample (20) and a lesser test criterion applied. Thus a capsule product which has weight uniformity will be accepted with the minimum of effort whereas products which are less uniform will have a more searching test applied.

Most pharmacopoeias do not have separate limits for the uniformity of content of capsules but include them in either the general tests or the individual monographs for the active ingredients. The USP XX introduced in 1982 a new type of test which combines a weight uniformity with a content uniformity test. It also breaks new ground in using a statistical measure of uniformity, the relative standard deviation, thus giving a better indication of how good a batch is in relationship to the standard.

Disintegration test

This test is used to indicate whether a capsule will release its contents *in vivo*. The experimental conditions used attempt to simulate gastric conditions. They are carried out in a liquid, usually water, at 37 °C which corresponds to body temperature. The sample is agitated in some way to simulate stomach movements. The tests can be divided up into two types depending upon the method of sample agitation.

The simplest method uses a conical flask. The test medium and the sample are placed in the flask which is held in a water bath and the contents swirled. The end point is usually described as the start of release of the contents. The other method uses a transparent tube with a metal mesh base. Sets of these tubes are oscillated up and down in the test medium. The end point is taken as the time at which all the contents have passed through the mesh. This test was originally designed for tablets, and capsules do not perform in it very well because of their different physical nature. The capsule, as it disintegrates, first splits and then the contents empty out, usually leaving a mass of gelatin. This adheres to the mesh and often makes determination of a finite end point difficult. Extra care needs to be taken in performing this test to ensure that the temperature limit is closely adhered to. Temperature fluctuations do not significantly affect tablet disintegration but they do affect capsules. Gelatin is not soluble at temperatures below about 30 °C and as the temperature falls towards this value there is a marked decrease in solubility.

Dissolution tests

The disintegration test was the first attempt to devise a simple *in vitro* bioavailability assessment. It has now been superseded in some pharmacopoeias by the dissolution test which measures the rate at which the active drug passes into solution. The USP was the first pharmacopoeia to introduce such a test. In the USP XXI there are two methods; the rotating basket and the paddle method. Dissolution test procedures were originated for tablets and like the disintegration tests problems can occur. For example, in the rotating basket method, the gelatin can adhere to the mesh so occluding some of the holes; in the paddle method the capsules tend to float so that they need to be weighed down by a piece of stainless steel wire.

Soft gelatin capsules

Uniformity of fill weight test

This is as for hard shell capsules.

Disintegration test

The compendial disintegration apparatus is used where tubes oscillate up and down for 30 minutes in the test medium, i.e. as for hard gelatin capsules. The capsules pass the test if no residue remains on the screen of the apparatus or, if a residue remains, it consists of fragments of shell or is a soft mass with no palpable core.

Dissolution tests

These are as for hard shell capsules if the liquid fill is hydrophilic. In the case of oil fills, the compendial rotating basket or rotating paddle dissolution apparatus is not suitable since the oil floats on the surface and gives a non-relevant profile. Attempts have been made (not successfully) to introduce a flowthrough test to satisfy compendial requirements.

BIBLIOGRAPHY

Cole, G. C. (1982) Capsule Filling. *Chem. Eng.* **383**, 473–477.
Jones, B. E. (1982) The manufacture of hard gelatin capsules. *Chem. Eng.* **380**, 174–177.
Jones, B. E. and Törnblom, J.-F. (1975) Capsules in the pharmacopoeias. *Pharm. Acta Helv.* **50**, 33–41.
Lachman, L., Leiberman, H. A. and Kanig, J. L. (1976) *The Theory and Practice of Industrial Pharmacy*, 2nd edn. Lea & Febiger, Philadelphia.

Design and operation of clean rooms

The ultimate objective in pharmaceutical manufacturing is the assurance that a product will be of a quality appropriate to its intended use. The quality of the product will always be influenced by the facilities available for its manufacture. A primary aim must be the prevention of sources and routes of contamination of the product. This involves not only the careful planning and design of the manufacturing facility, but also the implementation of effective physical and biological monitoring, both at the time of commissioning and at regular intervals during subsequent use. The operation of the facility requires trained personnel following clearly defined protocols. Adequate documentation at all stages of manufacture, storage and distribution are essential. These ideals are embodied in the *Guide to Good Pharmaceutical Manufacturing Practice* (Department of Health and Social Security 1983).

The requirements for sterile product manufacture are even more stringent, with the need for special care and precautions to eliminate particulate and microbial contamination. In parenteral products particles could, if inert, cause occlusion of blood vessels or, if reactive, could induce inflammatory, thrombositic, antigenic, pyrogenic or even neoplastic responses. Elimination of micro-organisms is essential to reduce the loading on any sterilization processes and thereby increase the probability of sterilization being achieved. Control of microbial contamination is also necessary to eliminate pyrogens and toxic bacterial debris from the product since these will not be removed by the sterilization process.

Definitions

For manufacturing purposes it is necessary to distinguish between two types of sterile product. One type is prepared in a clean fashion, transferred to its final container, sealed, and sterilized by an appropriate method. These are referred to as 'Terminally Sterilized' and require preparation in a clean area. Products that are not terminally sterilized are aseptically processed from sterile materials, or sterilized by filtration, before final packing in sterile containers. These are referred to as 'Aseptically Prepared' and require preparation in an aseptic area. In this context a clean area is a room or suite of rooms with defined environmental control of particulate and microbial contamination, constructed and used in such a way as to reduce the introduction, generation and retention of contaminants within the area. An aseptic area is a room or suite of rooms or special area within a clean area designed, constructed, serviced and used with the intention of preventing microbial contamination of the product.

Sources of contamination

Micro-organisms and inert particles are derived from similar sources and the design of clean and aseptic areas necessitates an understanding of the possible sources of contamination. These have been discussed fully in Chapter 27 but those aspects relevant to clean rooms are repeated briefly here.

Atmosphere

The atmosphere is unable to support microbial growth and has no inherent flora. However, it is invariably heavily contaminated with particles and micro-organisms are associated with many of these. Since a high proportion of dust particles in outside air originate from soil they may carry soil organisms. These include spore bearing bacteria, *Bacillus* and *Clostridium*, yeasts and moulds. Indoor air may also contain organisms of human origin such as *Staphylococcus* and β-haemolytic *Streptococci* on particles of skin or clothing. These will also occur in droplets expelled into the atmosphere from the respiratory tract by talking, coughing and sneezing. The rate at which dust particles settle from the air depends, among other factors, on the particle size, the amount of air movement and the humidity. Most particles in still outdoor air are between 0.1 and 1 μm and are therefore small enough to be retained for a very long time by Brownian movement. Air currents produced by ventilation, draughts or activity will disturb dust and reduce sedimentation of particles. Contamination is lower in damp atmosphere than in dry atmosphere due to sedimentation of particles and organisms in droplets. Organisms free from particles, especially yeasts and mould spores, are commonly found in indoor and outdoor air. These sediment slowly in still air and are kept suspended by air movement.

Operator

The skin, hair and clothing of the operator are potent sources of particulate and microbial contamination. Organisms found on the skin and transmitted on skin particles include *Staphylococcus*, diphtheroids, lipophilic yeasts and dermatophytic fungi. Since these organisms often reside in the deep layers of the skin they may not be removed by normal washing. Poor personal hygiene can result in the presence on the skin of coliforms and other intestinal bacteria. Open wounds are a source of saprophytic and pathogenic organisms. Emission of particles and micro-organisms from the skin is greatly influenced by skin flexing and abrasion and thus by the activity of the individual. Such movement also serves to liberate particles that are dispersed on clothing and hair.

Raw materials

Raw materials may account for a high proportion of the microbial and inert particulate contamination introduced into pharmaceutical products. Drugs which are obtained from natural sources are frequently contaminated with a variety of micro-organisms. These may be saprophytic bacteria, yeasts and moulds if the material is of plant origin, or if the material is from animal sources the contaminating organisms may be pathogenic bacteria or bacterial spores. Processing of the material may significantly modify the level and type of contamination. Synthetic drugs are generally free from contamination when prepared and if properly stored should remain so. Water is a material that is often taken for granted but it can be a prime source of particulate contamination, and if incorrectly processed, stored or distributed may be a source of Gram-negative bacteria such as *Pseudomonas*. Packaging materials and closures are a particularly troublesome source of particulate contamination especially in the preparation of parenteral solutions.

Equipment

Sources of particulate and microbial contamination may be inherent in the design of processing equipment. Dust may also be generated by the equipment during use. Work surfaces and external surfaces of equipment are also potential sources of contamination due to sedimentation of particles and droplets from the atmosphere.

ENVIRONMENTAL CONTROL

Environmental cleanliness standards

Environmental cleanliness is defined in terms of the maximum number of airborne particles greater than a defined particle size that are permitted in a given volume of air. Two systems exist for the classification of environmental cleanliness. These are the British Standard 5295:1976 and the United States Federal Standard 209b: 1973. The two systems are compared in Table 42.1. As the US Federal Standard is in Imperial Units and the British Standard is in metric units both equivalents are given, the converted figures being in parentheses.

It can be seen that the British Standard Class 2 for environmental cleanliness closely approximates to US Federal Standard Class 10 000 and is the standard applicable to clean areas. The more stringent British Standard Class 1 approximates to US Federal Standard Class 100 and is the standard applicable to aseptic areas.

Air flow

There are two main methods of controlling atmospheric contamination, both involving filtration processes to remove dust particles and micro-organisms.

Conventional flow

Filtered air is pumped into the room to produce a positive pressure (plenum) compared to the exterior and in a turbulent fashion to scavenge particles already present, flush them out, and so

Table 42.1 Environmental cleanliness standards

Particle size	Maximum number of particles greater than stated size per specified volume					
	British Standard 5295:1976			US Federal Standard 209b		
	Class	No. per m³	No. per ft³	Class	No. per m³	No. per ft³
0.5 5	1	3000 0	(86) (0)	100	(3500) (0)	100 0
0.5 5 10	2	300 000 2000 30	(8495) (57) (0.08)	10 000	(350 000) (2300) (N/A)	10 000 65 N/A

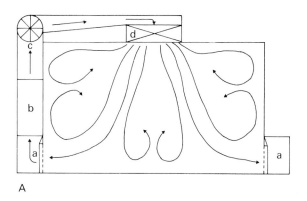 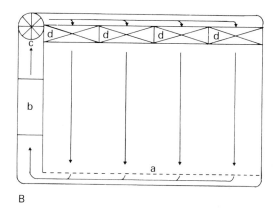

A   B

Fig. 42.1 Schematic diagrams of air flow types: (A) conventional flow (B) unidirectional vertical flow. (a) Outlet, (b) air conditioning unit, (c) fan, (d) HEPA filter

maintain clean conditions. Air enters the room through filters in the ceiling or high up in a wall and leaves through carefully sited outlets fitted low down on the opposite wall or in the floor at a distance from the inlets (Fig. 42.1A). Conventional air flow is defined in terms of the number of air changes per hour (Table 42.2).

Unidirectional flow (laminar flow)

Here the room is continually swept by a cushion of filtered air. The total air within the room moves, ideally with uniform velocity, along parallel flow lines which may be either vertical or horizontal. Air enters the room through a bank of filters which comprises one complete wall or ceiling, and exits through a bank of outlets comprising the opposite wall or floor (Fig. 42.1B). Laminar air flow is defined in terms of air velocity (Table 42.2). The complete laminar flow room has little practical application in pharmaceutical product manufacture as its benefits in the case of

the horizontal room are limited to the area immediately in front of the filters, and the vertical room is too expensive.

With both conventional and unidirectional flow types the air supply must be so balanced as to provide a minimum positive differential pressure between the clean area and adjoining uncontrolled area of 1.5 mm water gauge (w.g.) (0.06 inch w.g.) in the British Standard specification and 0.05 inch w.g. (1.3 mm w.g.) in the US Standard.

A typical system for supplying clean air involves the following.

1. *Intake of fresh air.* This should be through an intake situated well above ground level and away from chimneys to exclude most of the pathogen-containing dust particles found at street level.
2. *Prefiltration.* This consists of a coarse filtration to remove large particles and protect the main filters.
3. *Temperature adjustment.* The air is passed over

Table 42.2 Air flow standards

Air flow type	British Standard 5295:1976				US Federal Standard 209b	
Conventional	≮ 20 air changes per hour				≮ 20 air changes per hour	
	ft min⁻¹		m sec⁻¹		ft min⁻¹	m sec⁻¹
Unidirectional (laminar)	Horizontal	Vertical	Horizontal	Vertical		
	(84 ± 20)	(56 ± 10)	0.45 ± 0.1	0.30 ± 0.05	90 ± 20	(0.48 ± 0.10)

coils through which steam or refrigerant is circulated to permit thermostatic control of the air temperature.

4. *Humidification*. The air is passed through a fine atomized spray of demineralized water to increase the humidity to an acceptable level. Drying of the air, if required, is achieved by passing it over beds of desiccant or condensing the vapour in a cooling unit.

5. *Final filtration*. Final filtration is achieved through a High Efficiency Particulate Air (HEPA) filter, positioned at or as close as possible to the inlet to the room.

The complete ventilation system must be designed so that all filters, and other components are accessible for maintenance and replacement from outside the clean area.

Laminar flow units For aseptic processing, rooms with conventional filtered air flows and with contained laminar flow units at working points are usually more convenient than laminar flow rooms. Laminar air flow units providing Class 1 (Class 100) (see Table 42.1) conditions are of two types, horizontal and vertical, depending upon the direction of air flow. In the vertical unit a fan passes air down through the HEPA filter into the work area and the air exits, often with the aid of a second fan, through a perforated work surface (Fig. 42.2A). In the horizontal unit the HEPA filter is at the rear of the work area and air from the fan passes from back to front through the filter, exiting at the front of the unit (Fig. 42.2B). Where product protection is the primary concern, as in aseptic processing, the horizontal unit is satisfactory. If in addition to product protection there is a requirement to protect the personnel from the product the horizontal unit is clearly unsuitable and the vertical unit must be used. Guidance on the choice, commissioning, maintenance and use of laminar flow units is given in Health Equipment Information No. 67.

Air filtration

Types of air filter

Fibrous filters These are composed of slag wool, long-staple cotton wool, glass wool, or oil-wetted glass fibre. When loosely packed they may be used for prefiltration, removing 99% of particles down to 5 μm at an average air velocity of 22.5 ft min^{-1} (0.12 m sec^{-1}). When compressed into felts and presented as pleated sheets they are able to remove 99.9% of particles down to 1 μm at similar average air velocities.

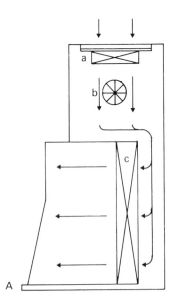
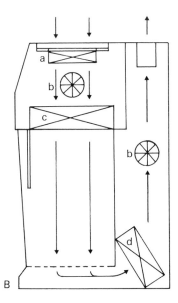

Fig. 42.2 Schematic diagrams of laminar flow units: (A) vertical (B) horizontal. (a) Pre-filter, (b) fan, (c) HEPA filter, (d) exhaust filter

HEPA filters   These are composed of various fibres bonded with resin or acrylic binders. The original HEPA filters were constructed of cellulose and asbestos but the health risks associated with asbestos have led to the demise of this material and its replacement with glass fibre and ceramic materials. The filter consists of a continuous sheet of filtration material, pleated, with a corrugated separator placed between each pleat, and sealed into a rigid metal frame. Efficient gaskets are used to ensure that air cannot leak past the filter material or past the filter unit when it is mounted in its trunking. HEPA filters are capable of removing 99.99% of particles down to 1 μm at an average air velocity of 100 ft min^{-1} (0.54 m sec^{-1}). filters are capable of removing 99.99% of particles down to 1 μm at an average air velocity of 100 ft min^{-1} (0.54 m sec^{-1}).

Filter efficiency

The British Standard requires filter efficiency of not less than 99.995% for a Class 1 environment and not less than 99.95% for a Class 2 environment when tested in accordance with BS 3928:1969. For Class 1 laminar flow units a filter efficiency of 99.997% is required. In this test an aerosol is produced from a solution of sodium chloride, to generate a known concentration of sodium chloride particles of a controlled size upstream of the filter. Retention efficiency is evaluated by sodium flame photometry downstream of the filter.

The US Standard requires a HEPA filter to have an efficiency of not less than 99.97% to mono-size 0.3 μm particles of dioctyl phthalate (DOP) smoke. In this test DOP is thermally vaporized upstream of the filter to produce an aerosol of particles which are detected downstream of the filter using a suitable photometer.

Temperature and humidity

These are obviously parameters which are governed by the process requirements. BS 5295 suggest a suitable temperature for working conditions as 20 ± 2 °C (68 ± 3.5 °F) while the US Federal Standard 209b recommends a temperature of 72 ± 5 °F (22.2 ± 2.8 °C). The British Standard suggests that the humidity should be controlled and maintained at a relative humidity of 35–50% while the US Standard recommends a relative humidity of not more than 50%.

BUILDING DESIGN, CONSTRUCTION AND USE

Siting

Clean rooms are best sited within a larger structure since this prevents wind movement being translated to the walls. Outside walls should not form part of the clean room because of possible damp transmission and movement due to wind force. Precautions must be taken against differential settlement leading to cracking of the floor and building. This may be achieved by providing very stiff ground beams, exaggerated floor loadings or by designing independent floor panels with allowance for movement between them. With the latter the joints between the panels should be located in non-critical areas such as under walls or in corridors outside the room. The clean room should be remote from main corridors, stairways or lifts which provide airways for particulate and bacterial transmission. It is important to design the clean room to be the smallest practical size bearing in mind the operations to be undertaken and the number of people likely to be employed in the area. Present day fire regulations limit the volume of a room to around 4000 m³, buildings exceeding this needing to be subdivided by permanent fire walls. Ceiling height is thus an important factor. If false ceilings are used adequate sealing is required to prevent contamination from the space above them.

Floors

These must be flat, smooth, impervious, easily cleaned and disinfected, and be constructed to minimize microbial and particulate contamination. The finish of the floor is dependent upon the type of operation being carried out, the risk of spillage, and the chemical nature of the material likely to be spilled. There are two basic types of floor material — flexing and non-flexing.

Flexing floor materials are made of synthetic elastomers of which the most commonly used are non-slip grades of polyvinylchloride (PVC). This is usually applied in sheets with the seams welded to eliminate pockets of contamination. Natural rubber has been used in the past but is light-sensitive and has a limited life. A flexing floor material has a theoretical advantage over the rigid floor in that it gives to the foot and the large area of contact reduces abrasion. PVC flooring is easily cleaned, easily repaired, relatively cheap and simple to install, and is quiet and comfortable to walk on. It will absorb vibrations and can be made electrostatically resistant or conductive. However, it is easily scored, hard particles can be ground in, and it will deform and flow under concentrated load such as equipment legs.

Non-flexing floors are generally made of hard inorganic filler substances in a matrix material. The classic floor of this type was quarry tiles set in cement, with expansion joints of ebonite to prevent cracking. Some problems were experienced with cleaning but these have been largely overcome with the development of corrosion-resistant cements. Concrete with a hard finish of terrazzo (cement and crushed marble) or other ground and polished surfaces is also suitable particularly in areas where frequent washing in necessary. When concrete is used it must be adequately sealed with a material resistant to chemicals, solvents and cleaning fluids. Modern sealing materials include epoxy resins, poly-urethane, acrylates and isocyanates. Flooring types based on asphalt and bitumen are generally not used because they tend to flow under pressure and are easily damaged by solvents. Non-flexing flooring has the disadvantages of being cold, noisy, tiring to walk on, slippery when wet, and expensive.

Walls and ceilings

Dividing walls must be made of non-inflammable or fire-resistant materials and covered with a smooth impervious and washable finish. The first generation of clean rooms used materials such as stainless steel, glass and enamelled steel selected regardless of cost. Modern practice is to use the most cost effective material. If the building struc-

ture is rigid and there are no vibrations a hard gloss-finish paint will provide an adequate surface finish, although it must be non-flaking and must retain some flexibility to absorb movement of the underlying material, which may be wood, plaster or steel sheet. Care is required with plaster walls which are easily damaged by impact. To reduce fungal growth, up to 1% of a fungistat such as 8-hydroxyquinoline, pentachlorophenol or salicyl-anilide may be added to the paint. Epoxy resin paints and polyurethane paints are also used although cracking and peeling can be a problem with these materials. If high humidity is likely to occur in the clean area glazed bricks or tiles, adequately sealed, are the materials of choice. Laminated plastic cladding and PVC sheeting are also suitable materials. PVC has the advantage that it can be sealed at joints either by feathered tape or by heat welding. It is also possible to build up a surface sheet by repeated application of a sprayed solution of PVC in a volatile solvent. This is ideal since there are no seams and the material can be carried over joins in partitioning, wall fittings etc. to give a perfect seal.

The theoretical ideal internal shape for a clean room in order to minimize regions where dust could collect would be a sphere. This is clearly an impractical shape for a room, but a good practical approximation can be achieved by ensuring the absence of all sharp corners. All wall to wall joints, wall to ceiling joints, and wall to floor joints should therefore be coved. Care should be taken to ensure that the coving itself does not create additional dust-collecting ridges. Wherever possible part glazing of walls with flush-fitting, well-sealed glass panels is recommended since this provides good visibility and permits adequate surveillance of the area. Heat losses and noise can be reduced by double glazing, the inner sheet being fixed and the outer being openable for cleaning. Clean and aseptic areas are best finished in pastel shades since a totally white area, although conveying the impression of cleanliness, can cause glare and be uncomfortable to work in for long periods.

Doors and windows

Doors and windows should fit flush with the walls. Decorative architraves and frames, ledges and pelmets should be excluded. All wood surfaces should be painted with a hard gloss finish. Windows, if required at all, are solely to provide illumination and are not for ventilation. They should therefore be non-openable. Except where a positive pressure airflow is being maintained, doors should be well fitting. Doors should be self-closing, hinges should be concealed and protruding door handles should be omitted. Sliding doors cause less air disturbance but are difficult to hang without creating dust traps and are therefore not recommended. Passage of materials and personnel into the clean area should be via an air lock designed with an interlock so that only one side may be opened at any time.

Services

Pipes, ducts and cables that need to be brought into a clean area should be installed either in deep cavity walls or preferably above a false ceiling where they can be accessible for maintenance. Exposed pipes, ducts, cables etc. should not be present in the clean room. All pipes passing through the walls of the room should be effectively sealed and either flush-fitting and easily cleaned or boxed in with low particle shedding materials. Gas cylinders should be excluded and all gases should be piped from outside the area. Only essential switches and sockets should be installed in the clean area and those should fit flush to the wall and be capable of being cleaned and disinfected. Modern touch-sensitive switches are preferable to the traditional toggle type. Non-essential switches such as room lighting switches and isolators should be installed outside the clean area. Lights are best fitted above close fitting and adequately sealed transparent panels in a false ceiling, with external access for maintenance.

Wherever possible sinks and drains should be avoided in clean areas. In aseptic areas sinks and drains should be excluded except where absolutely essential, e.g. in the preparation of radiopharmaceuticals. Drains should be vented to outside air, fitted with rodent screens, and incorporate efficient, deep-seal type traps that can be easily cleaned. They should preferably be fitted with an efficient means of *in situ* disinfection and be sited downstream of the air flow. Floor channels should

be avoided, but where these are essential they should be open, shallow, easily cleaned and connected to drains outside the clean area. Where fitted, sinks should be of stainless steel construction with no overflow or trap. The water supply to the sink should be of at least potable quality.

Furniture and equipment

The furniture in a clean area should be kept to an absolute minimum, working benches should be fitted with a hard top, free from imperfections, impervious to liquids and capable of vigorous cleaning and disinfection. Stainless steel, glass and some laminated plastics are suitable materials for work bench construction. Stools and trolleys should be of simple design and construction to minimize trapping of dust and organisms. They should be made of smooth, low particle-shedding impervious materials and should be able to withstand cleaning and disinfection. Storage cupboards, drawer units, and shelves should be excluded unless demonstrated to be absolutely essential. Fixtures and fittings should be kept to the minimum, and projections and recesses should be eliminated or minimized. Communication with the clean area should be via speak panels rather than telephones.

Only essential equipment should be installed in or taken into a clean area. All equipment should be designed, constructed and installed so that it may be easily dismantled, cleaned, disinfected or sterilized as necessary. Equipment and furniture should be arranged within the area to provide the lowest possible impedance to the air flow and the best possible air flow characteristics.

Personnel

The quality of any pharmaceutical product prepared in clean or aseptic conditions is very much dependent upon the personnel involved in its manufacture. The operators must therefore be responsible individuals, carefully selected and specially trained for sterile product manufacture. The operator is a major source of microbial and particulate contamination; the majority of contamination found in a clean room results from personnel entering and using the room. Operator-borne contamination can be controlled by limiting the number of operators in the clean area, restricting their movement, and isolating them from the product and the environment with suitable protective clothing.

All personnel should be trained in the principles of good manufacturing practice. This must include training in hygiene, emphasizing the need for high standards of personal hygiene and cleanliness. An understanding of sources and types of contamination and their control, especially operator-borne contamination, is also necessary. Persons likely to constitute a greater than normal contamination risk, e.g. carriers or sufferers of communicable diseases, must not be employed in clean or aseptic areas. Operators should be instructed and encouraged to report any condition such as skin lesions, wounds, respiratory infections, or gastrointestinal disorders that could result in the dissemination of abnormal numbers or types of organisms. Regular medical inspection of staff is therefore highly desirable. Access to clean and aseptic areas should be restricted to authorized persons, all non-essential personnel and visitors being excluded.

Protective clothing

Protective clothing is designed to prevent contamination from the body and everyday clothing from being transmitted to the clean or aseptic area and must therefore completely isolate the operator from the environment. It must be constructed of material which is of tight weave, non-linting, non-particle shedding, easily cleaned and non-inflammable. Operator discomfort is reduced if the material has antistatic properties and is porous to water vapour. Ceramic-based terylene, nylon, and modified polyethylene fabrics are usually used for clean room clothing. Cotton and linen are unsuitable. All protective clothing must be capable of being laundered without showing any detrimental changes. Clothing required in aseptic areas must also be able to withstand sterilization.

Normal laboratory overalls are of little value since they only cover a limited area and are too loosely fitting to provide adequate enclosure. The main garment should fit correctly to permit free movement, and be designed to be put on and taken off easily without becoming contaminated. The one-piece coverall, tight fitting at the neck, wrists and ankles, is the most convenient garment. This should be comfortable and loose fitting to reduce abrasion. It should be constructed with double seams and without external pockets. Fastening should be by means of zips which should be protected by inner or outer flaps. 'Velcro' fastenings may be preferred to zips but these may degenerate and release particles with repeated use. Two-piece garments may be preferred since they fit more closely. The lower part of the jacket or smock must be tucked into the trousers, and the trouser bottoms tucked into the foot covers.

The head must be covered with a one-piece head cover designed to totally enclose the hair and beard. The cover must be elasticated to ensure a close fit above the eyebrows and along the sides of the face to the point of the chin, and must extend onto the shoulders to allow it to form a good seal with the neck of the suit. In aseptic areas the head cover is worn in conjunction with a facemask of non-linting material or synthetic fibre designed to prevent the shedding of droplets by the operator.

Foot covers, designed to fit over shoes and totally enclose them, should be worn. The base of the covers should be hardwearing and resistant to abrasion.

Disposable gloves should be worn. These should be sufficiently strong to prevent puncturing but thin enough to allow sensitivity to touch. They should be sufficiently comfortable and elastic to permit free movement and the cuff should be close fitting and long enough to provide a good seal for the sleeves of the jacket. Gloves require to be packaged and lubricated to facilitate application, but must be particle free.

Protective clothing for use in clean and aseptic areas should be restricted to use in these areas only. Clothing should be changed regularly and particularly on every occasion that the operator enters the area. Protective clothing should be laundered to the highest possible standard and by a method which does not produce particulate contamination. Soaps and detergents must be selected to be compatible with the clothing material and care must be taken to prevent cross-contamination from linting and particle producing materials such as cotton. Clothing should be carefully checked for damage after processing and then each item should be conveniently packaged, preferably in double bags. For aseptic areas protective clothing must be sterilized and the outer package should include a means of indicating that it has been subjected to a sterilization process. The usual sterilization processes for clothing are autoclaving in a porous loads sterilizer or ethylene oxide sterilization. Protective clothing must be routinely monitored for particulate contamination.

Cleaning and disinfection

Clearly defined and rigorously enforced cleaning and disinfection procedures are an essential element in the operation of clean and aseptic areas. The objective of these procedures is the removal of microbial and particulate contamination that arises in the area during normal use. Daily cleaning should take place immediately after the work shift ends and involves cleaning of all work surfaces and floors. More thorough cleaning of the room should be arranged on a weekly basis. In the case of an aseptic room an additional procedure is required to disinfect the areas of the room that are not easily cleaned and disinfected by swabbing. This involves fumigation of the room with formaldehyde vapour at high relative humidity for a 12-hour period, and is undertaken on a weekly or monthly basis depending on the extent to which the room is used. Cleaning materials should be selected to be compatible with the surfaces being cleaned and should not cause corrosion or leave a residue. Suitable cleaning agents are the alkaline detergents and non-ionic and ionic surfactants. All cleaning materials, i.e. swabs, mops etc., should be designated to a particular clean area and heat sterilized before and after use. Cleaning materials should always be stored dry to prevent microbial growth and all cleaning solutions should be maintained at 65 °C during use.

Sodium hypochloride and organochlorine compounds at concentrations of 50–100 parts per million free chlorine, quarternary ammonium compounds at 0.1–0.2%, 70% ethanol or isopropanol, and 1% w/v formaldehye solution are all suitable disinfectants for use on work surfaces in clean areas. Cetrimide or chlorhexidine in 70% alcohol are suitable for use as skin disinfectants.

TESTING OF CLEAN AND ASEPTIC ROOMS

The tests applied to clean and aseptic areas can be divided into two categories: commissioning tests, usually carried out in the unmanned state, designed to confirm that the room meets the required design specification, and monitoring tests carried out with the room in operation and manned to assess the performance of the room during normal use.

Commissioning tests

British Standard 5295 lists the tests and procedures which should be used to commission a clean or aseptic room. The data from commissioning tests are recorded and used as the reference for subsequent monitoring.

Final filter installation test This is done to demonstrate that the filter is not damaged and that the filter mounting frame does not leak at the gasket flange or the connection to the ducting.

Induction leak test This test demonstrates that particles cannot enter the room from leaks in construction joints or by back-streaming from openings.

Filter efficiency test The British Standard recommends membrane sampling and subsequent microscopic examination for validating filter efficiency. However, there are practical problems with this technique since it cannot be used for the precise location of leaks, and does not give instantaneous or continuous readings. In practice, aerosol photometers and the generation and detection of DOP smoke or sodium chloride crystals are usually used for these tests.

Particulate contamination control test This is used to demonstrate that the number and size distribution of particles in the clean room air do not exceed the levels specified for the particular class of room. Microscopic techniques and direct reading light scattering photometers (Royco

Instruments Inc., California, USA) are used in this type of test.

Air pressure test   This test determines the differential pressure between the clean area and adjacent areas. This is usually measured using a sensitive manometer.

Temperature and humidity tests   These tests demonstrate that the specified limits can be achieved and maintained. Particular attention is paid to positional variations within the room and to time-dependent variations during operation. Measurements are usually made with a sling psychrometer, repeat readings being taken after 30 seconds' whirling of the instrument until stable wet and dry bulb temperatures are obtained.

Air flow tests   These are performed to demonstrate either in a laminar flow room or unit that the air velocity and uniformity of flow comply with the required standard or in a conventional flow room that the number of air changes is as specified. Air flow within ducts can be measured with a pitot tube and manometer. Using a suitable pattern of test holes within the supply ducting, the air flow rate can be obtained by measuring the velocity head. This technique is mostly used in 'conventional flow' rather than 'laminar flow' areas. Air change rates can be demonstrated by tracer gas decay rate or smoke decay rate methods. At terminal HEPA filter housings and in laminar flow areas an electronic anemometer is the most useful method of measurement. This device, operated by a capacitance transducer, integrates the speed of vane movement with time and presents a direct reading of air velocity in ft min^{-1} or m sec^{-1}. Air flow patterns throughout all parts of the room are observed using smoke tubes, with particular attention being paid to examining areas around openings.

Noise level tests   Noise level measurements are taken within the area both of the general background sound without any laminar flow units operating and also with any such ancillary equipment switched on. The measurements are taken 1 metre from air inlets and at work benches. The US Standard simply states that the maximum noise level acceptable shall be stated, while the British Standard stipulates a maximum level of 65 dB(A) except by agreement between the clean room manufacturer and the user.

Lighting test   The quality of the general illumination within the area and also at the work bench is measured using a portable photoelectric photometer. Recommended lighting levels at the work surface are <300 lux (28 ft candles) for the British Standard and 100–150 ft candles (1076–1614 lux) for the US Standard.

The US Federal Standard 209b lists similar commissioning tests for filter integrity and retention characteristics, and for air quality, but does not include tests for integrity of construction joints or uniformity of air flow.

Microbiological tests   These determine the microbial contamination resulting from the introduction of personnel into the area. It has not been possible to date to establish official standards for microbial contamination on the same basis as those for particulate contamination. This is because of the difficulties in recovering and culturing micro-organisms from the air, the variety of counting techniques that are available, and the statistical problems associated with sampling procedures. The *Guide to Good Pharmaceutical Manufacturing Practice* (DHSS, 1983) suggests levels for the maximum number of viable organisms per cubic metre of less than 1 for laminar flow units, 5 for aseptic (Class 1) rooms, and 100 for clean (Class 2) rooms. It is recommended that these conditions should be achieved throughout the room when unmanned, and be maintained in the immediate surroundings of the product whenever the product is exposed. Microbiological tests should include the following.

Settle plates   A nutrient agar plate is exposed to the atmosphere in the sampling area for a predetermined period and then incubated and the colonies counted. Although simple and inexpensive, the settle plate cannot be recommended for quantitative evaluation of airborne bacteria since it collects chiefly those particles large enough to be pulled by gravity or impacted by air turbulence on to the collecting surface. Airborne particles that are too small to settle out quickly may not be collected, and if the turbulence varies the yields will also vary. These disadvantages of the settle plate can be overcome by causing a stream of air at high velocity to impinge upon the surface of the plate resulting in the particles leaving the air stream and remaining on the surface. Alternatively the particles may be collected on a membrane filter. These methods have the added advantage of permitting defined volumes of air to be tested.

Agar contact plates and swabs These are used to measure the microbial contamination on surfaces. With agar contact plates the nutrient agar is present against the surface to be examined, removed, and incubated. The method is particularly useful for determining types and numbers of organisms on operators' gloved hands and on work surfaces. Alternatively, wetted sterile swabs can be wiped over the surface, placed in nutrient broth or buffer solutions, and plate counts carried out.

Process simulation tests The product is substituted with a nutrient broth or a material of similar consistency and appearance to the product which will initate and maintain the growth of low numbers of common micro-organisms. The test should simulate the most difficult and demanding aspects of the process, and is often carried out at the end of the production run when the contamination levels in the environment would be expected to be highest. The WHO has indicated an acceptable contamination level for process simulation testing to be 0.3% although the Parenteral Drug Association suggests that manufacturers should strive for less than 0.1%.

Sterility tests These are required to be carried out on all products that are prepared aseptically and must be performed on each batch of the product.

Monitoring tests

The tests used in commissioning a clean or aseptic area should be repeated regularly to ensure that the design conditions are maintained. The British Standard recommends minimum intervals for repeat testing. Air pressure, temperature, and humidity measurements should be recorded continuously. Particulate contamination should be determined daily for aseptic (Class 1) rooms and weekly for clean (Class 2) rooms. Tests for air flow velocity and uniformity should be carried out at 3-monthly intervals. Tests for filter efficiency should be conducted yearly. Tests should also be repeated after repairs or maintenance. Settle plates, agar contact plates and swabs, and sterility tests should be carried out during each work shift.

It is recommended that process simulation tests should be conducted at 3-monthly intervals.

THE OPERATION OF CLEAN AND ASEPTIC ROOMS

This involves the recognition of three main areas as follows.

'Black' or 'dirty' areas

These are areas where particle and microbial control is almost impossible and comprise external corridors, storage areas for operators' outdoor clothing, stores of raw materials and containers, offices etc. These are situated on the periphery of the production unit and are well insulated from the preparation areas.

'Grey' or 'semi-clean' areas

These are areas where high standards of hygiene and cleanliness operate and where some attempt is made to minimize particulate and microbial contamination. They comprise washing facilities for apparatus and containers, sterilization areas, some sections of the changing rooms for operators etc.

'White' or 'clean' areas

These comprise the final preparation areas where full environmental control is operational and special protective clothing is worn by the operator. The area may be a Class 1 (aseptic) room, or a Class 2 (clean) room possibly with laminar flow units installed at terminal operation points such as filling lines.

The routine flow of all materials and personnel must be from black to grey to white and subsequently to grey and to black. Only when the product is in its final sealed container is it permitted to leave by the latter route. A physical barrier such as a low wall on an air-lock must be provided to delineate the boundary where one area ends and another begins to prevent thoughtless movement between areas. The facility is designed

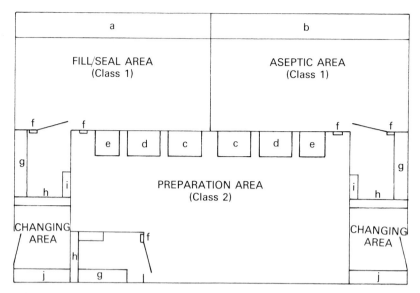

Fig. 42.3 Diagrammatic representation of a unit for the manufacture of terminally sterilized and aseptically prepared pharmaceutical products. (Materials storage, container washing, final packaging, quality control and bond storage areas are not shown.) (a) Vertical laminar flow units / bench, (b) horizontal laminar flow units / bench, (c) double-ended autoclave, (d) double-ended hot air oven, (e) transfer hatch, (f) viewing / speech panel, (g) gown racks, (h) step-over barrier, (i) wash basins / dryers, (j) clothing storage

so that all movement of personnel and materials from black to grey to white areas is against the air flow. A typical manufacturing facility is illustrated in Fig. 42.3.

Entry of personnel into a clean or aseptic area must be through a changing room fitted with interlocked doors. The number of operators using the changing room at any one time should be strictly controlled and movement should be slow and methodical and be kept to a minimum. The changing room for a clean room is in two sections, divided by a step-over wall. The personnel entering the changing room will have already changed out of their outdoor clothing and will be wearing standard laboratory or factory protective clothing. This clothing is removed in the first section of the changing room. The second section is equipped with a handwashing sink with foot-operated tap controls and preferably a foot or elbow operated hot air drier. After thorough scrub-up the operator puts on the clean room clothing starting with the footwear, then the head covering, the overall and finally the gloves, and proceeds directly to the clean room. For an aseptic area the changing room may be in three sections, each separated by step-over barriers. Standard

protective clothing is removed in the first section. In the second section the operator puts on slippers, scrubs-up, and puts on the sterile head cover and face mask. After rewashing and drying the hands and arms the operator enters the third section, puts on the sterile coverall or suit, over-boots and disposable gloves, and then enters the aseptic area. Clothing for the aseptic area is double wrapped and sterilized in a porous loads autoclave which in a large manufacturing unit may be double ended and interlocked, with one end opening directly into the changing room.

All materials entering the aseptic area must be sterile. Entry into the aseptic room is preferably through a double ended interlocked autoclave or hot air sterilizer. Alternatively the sterilized double wrapped materials can be passed into the aseptic room through a double ended interlocked exchange hatch. The outer wrapping is removed in the hatch by the person placing the pack in it, and the inner wrapping is then removed in the aseptic area by the operator. Solutions can be transferred from the clean manufacturing area via sterilized tubing through a $0.22 \ \mu m$ membrane filter, into a sterile vessel in the aseptic room. An exit route is provided for finished products and equipment from the aseptic room to an adjacent clean area. The aseptic process itself should be fully documented and conducted by carefully selected and highly trained operators in a controlled and methodical manner so as to prevent particulate and microbial contamination.

REFERENCES AND BIBLIOGRAPHY

British Standard 2831: 1971. Methods of test for air filters used in air conditioning and general ventilation.

British Standard 3928: 1969. Method for sodium flame test for air filters (other than air supply to I.C. engines and compressors).

British Standard 5295: 1976. Environmental cleanliness in enclosed spaces. Part 1: Specification for controlled environment clean rooms, work stations and clean air devices. Part 2: Guide to the construction and installation of clean rooms, work stations and clean air devices. Part 3: Guide to operational procedures and disciplines applicable to clean rooms, work stations and clean air devices.

British Standard 5726: 1979. Specification for microbiological safety cabinets.

Department of Health and Social Security (1983). *Guide to Good Manufacturing Practice*. HMSO, London.

Federal Standard 209b (1973). *Clean Room Work Station Requirements, Controlled Environment*. GSA Business Service Centre, Boston, USA.

Groves, M. J. (1973) *Parenteral Products*. William Heinemann Medical Books, London.

Health Equipment Information No. 67, Feb. 1977.

Kay, J. B. (1980) Manufacture of pharmaceutical preparations. In: *Textbook of Hospital Pharmacy* (Eds M. C. Allwood and J. T. Fell), pp. 71–143. Blackwell Scientific Publications, Oxford.

Sterilization practice

Quality assurance in sterilization processes

In the manufacture of sterile products it is not sufficient simply to subject the product to a sterilization process. It is important to remember that sterility cannot be instilled into the product at the end of the manufacturing process but must be planned into each stage of the process. Some of the essential elements involved in the quality assurance of a sterile product are:

1 selection of raw materials that contain low levels of microbial contamination. A limit on the level of contamination should be set and monitoring of materials carried out to ensure compliance with the limits.
2 manufacture of the product by trained and responsible personnel under carefully controlled and monitored conditions designed to eliminate microbial contamination (see Chapter 27).
3 selection of a suitable sterilization protocol based on a knowledge of the type, resistance and probable number of contaminants, and on the maximum acceptable risk of failing to achieve sterility. The method must be selected on the basis of the maximum permissible damage to the product and its container. The suitability and efficiency of the protocol must be established before it is adopted, and such validation should be repeated at regular intervals and whenever modifications are made to equipment or procedures.

4 adequate in-process control of the sterilization process together with tests on the final product. Permanent records of all controls and tests should be kept as part of the batch record. Records of routine testing and maintenance of sterilizing equipment are essential.

5 correct storage and use of the product to prevent recontamination.

Guidance on sterile product manufacture is provided in the *Guide to Good Manufacturing Practice* (DHSS, 1983) and the *Guide to Good Manufacturing Practice for Sterile Single-use Medical Devices and Surgical Products* (DHSS, 1981), Guidance on the testing and maintenance of sterilizers is given in Health Technical Memorandum (HTM) No. 10.

METHODS OF STERILIZATION

Methods of sterilization in current use may be categorized as:

1 Processes utilizing increased energy. These include moist and dry heat, the combination of heat and bactericidal chemicals, and radiations.

2 chemical processes using bacterial gases.

3 physical removal of organisms by filtration.

Moist heat sterilization — autoclaving

Moist heat in the form of saturated steam under pressure is the most reliable method of killing micro-organisms.

Steam is described as saturated when it is at a temperature corresponding to the liquid boiling point appropriate to its pressure (see Chapter 30). Several characteristics of dry saturated steam contribute to its high efficiency as a sterilizing agent. A large proportion of its heat energy, around 80%, is in the form of latent heat. When saturated steam condenses it liberates all its latent heat immediately. This occurs in a sterilizer whenever the steam touches the cool surface of an article inside. The latent heat that is given to the article makes a major contribution in raising it to the sterilization temperature. Since all the sensible heat is retained by the condensate there is no fall in temperature of the surroundings. The condensed

water also hydrates any micro-organisms present rendering them more sensitive (see Chapter 25).

When saturated steam condenses it contracts to an extremely small volume. In consequence a region of low pressure is created and more steam is drawn into the area to re-establish the pressure. This property ensures rapid penetration and is of particular importance in the sterilization of bulky porous loads such as dressings.

Wet or saturated steam is steam containing droplets (water fog) produced by secondary cooling. Although wet steam has the same lethal properties as dry saturated steam, condensation is reduced and less latent heat is available resulting in reduced heating-up times. Water fog can also saturate the load with free water and may interfere with steam penetration.

Superheated steam is steam not in equilibrium with its source. This can occur if steam is heated out of contact with water at constant pressure or if the pressure is reduced at constant temperature. Superheating may be produced unintentionally by running autoclave jackets at higher temperatures than the chamber, by lagging reducing values thereby lowering the pressure but maintaining high temperature, or by producing localized superheat from the heat of hydration of dry cotton fabrics. Superheated steam is no more efficient at transferring heat, penetrating the load, or destroying organisms than hot air at the same temperature.

In turbulent conditions air steam mixtures can form so that at a given total pressure only the partial pressure of the steam controls the temperature. For example if 90% of steam at 121 °C is mixed with 10% air to a final pressure of 15 p.s.i. the final temperature will be 118 °C ($\equiv$ 13.5 p.s.i. dry saturated steam).

Autoclaves

The design of any autoclave must therefore ensure that the load is permeated with dry saturated steam, that the formation of supersaturated steam is efficiently minimized and that air is eliminated both from the chamber and the load (if porous). Design of autoclaves is the subject of British Standard 3970:1966.

Downward displacement autoclaves These are usually horizontal although smaller units may be vertical. Steam is generated externally at high pressure and reduced via reducing valves to the autoclaving pressure. Separators are used to remove water droplets and minimized super-heating of the steam. Steam is admitted to the top of the chamber via a baffle. Since the steam has a lower density than air at the same temperature the air will be displaced downwards via a drain. Condensation will also be removed via the drain. The drain is fitted with a 'near to steam' trap capable of discharging air and condensate while retaining saturated steam in the chamber. Precautions are taken to prevent back syphoning from the drain into the autoclave chamber. Provided that the chamber is sufficiently lagged a steam jacket is not necessary with this type of autoclave, but if one is used care must be taken to avoid superheating. Temperature measurement is taken at the drain, as near to the chamber as possible. Air and condensate removal will be completed when this temperature is equivalent to that of dry saturated steam at the operating pressure. Temperature control during the steri-lizing period is by regulation of the steam pressure. At the end of the sterilization period the autoclave contents are allowed to cool to zero gauge pressure and air is admitted to the chamber via a bacteria-proof filter. Safety controls are fitted to ensure that the autoclave cannot be opened during the sterilization cycle or until the contents have cooled to below 80 °C.

Air ballasted autoclaves In recent years glass containers have been replaced with plastic containers particularly for infusion fluids. Heat sterilization can cause softening of the plastic, and distortion of the containers can occur during the pressure drop at the end of the sterilization cycle. Some modern designs of autoclave compensate for the pressure drop by introducing warmed compressed sterile air to the chamber at the end of the cycle. This is termed gas ballasting.

Spray cooled autoclaves A large load of bottled fluids can take a considerable time to cool to 80 °C because of its large heat capacity and the poor rate of heat transfer through and from the glass walls. A significant reduction in the cooling time can be achieved if the bottles are sprayed with a fine mist of distilled water droplets. Breakage of bottles is minimized if the droplet size is sufficiently small. Some autoclaves are now fitted with spray cooling devices with or without gas ballast. Spray cooling is not without its prob-lems and contamination of bottled fluids, usually resulting from inadequate closures, has been reported.

High vacuum autoclaves There are consider-able problems in using downward displacement autoclaves for sterilization of porous loads due to the time required for air removal, and the conden-sation which results in the need for drying of the load at the end of the cycle. These problems have been overcome by the development of the high vacuum or porous loads autoclaves. In these air is removed by reducing the vacuum pressure by means of an oil-sealed or water ring pump, often backed by a thermocompressor and cold water condenser. In the initial prevacuum stage of the cycle air is removed from the load and chamber either by evacuation of the heated chamber to about 15 mmHg absolute pressure followed by continuous application of the vacuum, or by alter-nate steam injection and evacuation (pulsing) until negligible residual air levels are reached. Steam is immediately and rapidly admitted to the operating conditions, usually 134 °C, 32 p.s.i with a holding time of 3–3.5 minutes. During the post-vacuum stage, steam is quickly removed by rapid evacu-ation to 50 mmHg. The vacuum is maintained for a variable period, usually 3–5 minutes, depending on the condensate retention of the load, in order to produce a dry load. Sterile air is then admitted to the chamber until the pressure reaches atmos-pheric. The total cycle time should not exceed 30 minutes. These autoclaves must be fitted with devices to determine faulty air removal and leakage of air into the chamber.

Continuous autoclaves Autoclaves are normally operated in a discontinuous mode and industrial production of sterile bottled fluids is often limited by the autoclave capacity and speed of throughput. These problems may not be wholly solved by simply increasing the number and size of the auto-claves. Similar problems in the canning and dairy products industry have led to the development of continuous sterilizers of which the 'Stock-Amsterdam Hydromatic' is a typical example.

This consists of a large (up to 50 ft high) vertical closed tower containing three interconnecting sections:

1 a water-filled column for preheating containers leading to

2 a central steam-filled sterilizing column leading to

3 a final water-filled cooling column, sometimes with additional sequential spray cooling and container drying sections.

The pressure of the steam in the central column is counterbalanced by the hydrostatic pressure in the other columns, which also seals the central section. The sterilizing temperature is therefore infinitely variable. Containers are laid horizontally on carriers and move through the columns on an ascending and descending chain belt, the holding time at any stage being governed by the conveyor chain speed.

Protocols for autoclaving

The time at temperature cycles recommended in the *British Pharmacopoeia* are given in Table 43.1. It must be remembered that since these cycles have evolved by trial and error rather than being based on a quantitative mathematical approach they are not equivalent in their lethal efficiencies. For example, the *D* values for *B. stearothermophilus* NCTC 8919 spores in aqueous suspension at 121 °C and 115 °C are 2 minutes and 10 minutes respectively. A cycle of 15 minutes at 121 °C will have an IF of $10^{7.5}$ against these spores whereas a cycle of 30 minutes at 115 °C will only have an IF of 10^3. In general, the highest temperature, compatible with the material to be processed, should be used. Other combinations of time and temperature may also be used if they can be demonstrated to be as effective. Since these are time at temperature cycles sufficient time must be

allowed for every part of the load to reach the required temperature before timing is commenced. This heating up time must be determined for each type of load and added to the required holding time

Heating with a bactericide

This method can be used for aqueous solutions and suspensions of medicaments that are unstable at autoclaving temperatures. The bactericide at the required concentration is included in the preparation which is then distributed into the final sealed containers and heated for sufficient time to ensure that the whole of the contents of each container is maintained at 98–100 °C for 30 minutes. Recommended bactericides for injections are 0.2% w/v chlorocresol or 0.002% w/v phenyl mercuric nitrate or acetate. In ophthalmic solutions chlorocresol cannot be used but 0.01% w/v benzalkonium chloride, chlorhexidine, or thiomersal may be used as alternatives to phenyl mercuric salts. The bactericide is selected on the basis of its freedom from toxicity and its compatibility with the product, the container, and the closure. The toxicity of the bactericide precludes the use of this technique for many types of injections and for intravenous injections where the single dose exceeds 15 ml.

Low temperature steam with formaldehyde (LTSF)

The use of saturated steam at sub-atmospheric pressure (low temperature steam) in combination with formaldehyde has been suggested for the sterilization of heat-sensitive porous loads and equipment. The aim of the process is to expose the load within the sterilizer chamber to a homogeneous mixture of monomeric formaldehyde gas and dry saturated steam at the chosen temperature. The apparatus used is similar in design to the high vacuum autoclave. Careful control of the autoclave jacket temperature is necessary to minimize condensation and polymerization of formaldehyde in the chamber. In a typical LTSF cycle air is first removed from the chamber and the load by evacuation and steam pulsing. This also humidifies the load. In the 'formalizing' stage

Table 43.1 Time at temperature cycles recommended in the *British Pharmacopoeia* 1980 for moist heat sterilization

Temperature (°C)	Pressure (p.s.i.)	Minimum holding time (min)
115–118	10–12.5	30
121–124	15–18	15
126–129	20–24	10
134–138	30–40	3

formaldehyde gas generated from vaporized formalin or by heating paraformaldehyde in di-iso-octylphthalate is admitted to the evacuated chamber. Evacuation and admission of formaldehyde gas is repeated to ensure impregnation of the gas into the load. The chamber is then evacuated and the sterilizing dose of formaldehyde is admitted along with dry saturated steam to the required temperature/pressure level, and these conditions maintained for the sterilizing period. Layering of formaldehyde gas in the chamber may be minimized by pulsing the formaldehyde gas/steam mixture. At the end of the sterilizing period evacuation and steam pulsing is carried out to ensure efficient removal of the formaldehyde and sterile air is finally admitted to the chamber.

Protocols for LTSF sterilization

The factors that determine the optimum conditions for LTSF sterilization are still under investigation and consequently there is a wide range of protocols in existence. Concentrations of formaldehyde between 3.3 mg l^{-1} and 100 mg l^{-1} have been used at temperatures ranging from 65 to 80 °C. The accepted protocol for LTSF sterilization in the UK is exposure for 2 hours to a formaldehyde concentration of 25 mg l^{-1} in combination with dry saturated steam at 73 $\pm$ 2 °C (0.35 $\pm$ 0.03 bar).

Dry heat sterilization

Dry heat sterilization is usually carried out in a hot air oven. The design and performance characteristics of the oven are specified in British Standard 3421:1961. It should be electrically heated, thermostatically controlled and provided with a fan or turbo blower to provide a continuous forced circulation of air. The oven should have automatic process control and the door should be interlocked so that the operating cycle cannot start before it is secured and it cannot then be opened until the cycle has been completed. Safety controls against electricity supply failure and overheat are also included.

Heat is transferred from the source to the articles in a hot air oven by conduction, convection and radiation. Conduction along

shelves is of minor importance because of the small area of contact between the product and the shelf. Heaters are arranged all around the chamber to maximize the amount of heat radiated from the walls, but articles near the walls will screen others in the oven. It is important, therefore, to make maximum use of direct transfer of heat from the air by providing the forced circulation, restricting the size of the articles to be sterilized, and loading the articles to permit the optimum air circulation. Before loading the oven is preheated to the required temperature to minimize the heating up time of the load. Heating up times are variable and often very long. For each type of load trials must therefore be conducted with thermocouples inserted in various parts of the load to determine the heating up time, which is then added to the holding time. Articles for hot air sterilization require careful packaging since no attempt is made to sterilize the air entering the oven at the end of the cycle.

Continuous hot air sterilizers

Prolonged heating up times, holding times and cooling times combine to make hot air sterilization a very time consuming and energy intensive process. Continuous hot air sterilizing processes have been developed using forced convection ovens and infra-red ovens. These processes operate at high temperatures (>180 °C) and have the advantage of short heating up times. The articles to be sterilized are passed through the oven on a conveyor belt to give high output.

Protocols for dry heat sterilization

Dry heat is less efficient as a sterilizing agent than moist heat (see Chapter 25) and as a consequence higher temperatures and longer exposure times are required. There is considerable variation in the time at temperature cycles that are recommended. Examples of these cycles are given in Table 43.2. The *British Pharmacopoeia* recommends 150 °C for 1 hour for non-aqueous liquid preparations but this is generally considered to be barely adequate. Many pharmaceutical preparations cannot be subjected to the temperatures given in Table 43.2 and require alternative time at temperature cycles

Table 43.2 Time at temperature cycles for dry heat sterilization

Source	Temperature (°C)	Minimum holding time (min)
Medical Research Council Memorandum No 41 (1962)	160	60
	170	40
	180	20
British Pharmacopoeia (1980)	160	60
	180	11

to be established. Other combinations of time and temperature can be used for hot air sterilization provided they are shown to be as effective.

Radiation sterilization

Radiation sterilization is a low temperature process and may therefore be a useful alternative to other low temperature processes such as ethylene oxide for the sterilization of thermobile materials. Types of ionizing radiation, their mechanisms of action and the factors affecting their bactericidal activity have been discussed in Chapter 25. Only two types of radiation are used in sterilization, electromagnetic (ultraviolet and gamma) and particulate (high energy electrons). Ultraviolet radiation at wavelengths between 240 and 280 nm is bactericidal but has poor penetrating ability. It has been used to sterilize air and water in thin layers but is not an acceptable source of sterilizing radiations for medical devices or drug materials.

Gamma irradiation

The primary source of gamma rays used for sterilization is the radioactive isotope of cobalt ^{60}Co. This is produced by exposing natural cobalt to neutrons in a reactor, and has a half-life of 5.3 years. The radiation from ^{60}Co consists of two protons (1.33 and 1.17 MeV) and one electron (0.31 MeV) giving a total emission per disintegration of 2.81 MeV. Modern sterilization facilities contain between 10^6 and 2×10^6 Ci of radioactive source material. It is possible that ^{60}Co will eventually be replaced by caesium-137 which is a product of the disintegration of uranium. ^{137}Cs

has a lower energy output (0.66 meV) than ^{60}Co. Elaborate and expensive precautions must be taken to protect the environment and the operator from the effects of radiation. The radiation chamber is surrounded by concrete. The isotope in the form of pellets is enclosed in a number of double, stainless steel tubes, and when not in use are submerged in water. Articles are packed in boxes of standard size which are suspended from a monorail and conveyed in and out of the irradiation chamber in such a manner as to ensure that all parts receive the same dose. Different doses can be given by varying the exposure times. Gamma emission is continuous, and this together with the high capital and replacement costs renders the method only suitable for large scale use.

High energy electrons

These are particles accelerated to high energy (5–10 MeV) in electron accelerators. At these energy levels the electron penetration is satisfactory and problems of induced radiation in the product are minimal. The dose rate in the electron accelerator is higher than that in the gamma source and sterilizing doses can be achieved very rapidly. Protection of environment and operators against electron radiation is required as for gamma radiation.

Protocol for radiation sterilization

The accepted sterilizing dose is 2.5 Mrad (25 kGy). Since, unlike heat, the effects of radiation are cumulative, the sterilizing dose can be given in divided doses.

Other methods utilizing increased energy

Irradiation with laser light has been suggested as a possible method of sterilization and promising bactericidal activity has been demonstrated with a 50 W unfocused CO_2 laser. Since the exposure times are extremely short, of the order of 0.01 s, there is very little temperature rise, and the method could be applicable to thermolabile substances. The use of radio frequency generated plasma of argon, helium, oxygen and nitrogen as sterilizing agents has also been considered. The penetrating capacity of both the laser beam and the plasma is limited and restricts their potential use to the sterilization of surfaces and thin films.

Gaseous sterilization

Although many chemicals exhibit antimicrobial activity the requirements for adequate penetration and efficient removal of the agent mean that only chemical vapours are of use in sterilization. Of these, ethylene oxide is the most widely used.

Ethylene oxide sterilization

The properties of ethylene oxide and the factors affecting its antimicrobial activity are detailed in Chapter 25. Concentration, temperature, relative humidity and exposure time are critical and require careful control during the sterilization process. Care must also be taken to avoid occlusion of micro-organisms in the load and to ensure adequate gas penetration.

Commercial sterilizers consist of a heated chamber which is gas tight and able to withstand high pressure and vacuum. This is connected to a high efficiency vacuum pump for extracting the air before, and the gas mixture after, sterilization. An expansion chamber and heat exchanger are used to vaporize and warm the gas which is admitted to the chamber via a baffled inlet. A means of maintaining a relative humidity of at least 33% in the chamber is also provided. The toxicity and flammability of ethylene oxide is taken into account in the design of the sterilizer and automatic process control is provided. The load is either preconditioned for 24 hours at a humidity in excess of 60% or a prehumidification stage is included at the beginning of the cycle. The chamber is heated to the required temperature and an initial vacuum is drawn to remove air from the load without drying it. Ethylene oxide and water vapour are admitted via the expansion chamber and heat exchanger to the required concentration, relative humidity, and pressure. The sterilizing conditions are maintained for the required holding time often with pulsing. High vacuum is then drawn and held for sufficient time to ensure removal of the gas from the chamber

and the load, and sterile air is admitted. A post-sterilization quarantine period of at least 24 hours is required for removal of trace amounts of ethylene oxide from the load.

Protocols for ethylene oxide sterilization

These must be determined individually for each product by means of standard product loads containing reliable biological test pieces. Concentrations of ethylene oxide between 450 and 1500 mg l^{-1} have been used. Temperatures range from 25 to 60 °C depending on the product with chamber pressures between 2 and 10 p.s.i. Ethylene oxide sterilization is a slow process and requires exposure times up to 36 hours at lower temperatures. Holding times of the order of 3 hours have been used at higher temperatures.

Filtration sterilization

Thermolabile solutions may be sterilized by filtration through suitable bacteria-proof filters. Sterilization by filtration differs from other sterilization processes in that micro-organisms are physically removed and not destroyed. Bacteria-proof filters are available in a variety of types including porous porcelain ceramic filters, asbestos/cellulose pads, sintered glass filters and membrane filters. A description of filtration mechanisms and the construction and characteristics of filters is given in Chapter 31. Filters such as asbestos or cellulose pads that may release fibres or particles are unsuitable for pharmaceutical use except as prefilters. Membrane filters are most frequently used for filtration sterilization. High filtration rates, together with low fluid retention and minimal solute absorption, resulting from the high and uniform porosity, are features of membrane filters. Furthermore, since these function primarily as screen filters rather than as depth filters there is less risk of organisms being trapped in the filter matrix and 'growing through'. Membrane filters are available in a range of pore sizes from 0.025 μm to 14 μm. A pore size of 0.2–0.22 μm is recommended for sterilization by filtration. The range of constituent materials that are available permits the selection of a membrane filter that is compatible with a particular product.

Filtration can be carried out under negative or positive pressure. Negative pressure is limited to a maximum of one atmosphere differential pressure and is likely to cause foaming of the filtrate. Positive pressure filtration is carried out using air or nitrogen gas pressure in the upstream side of the filter. Differential pressure is limited only by the design and construction of the equipment. When using membrane filters for heavily contaminated solutions the use of a depth filter upstream as a prefilter will minimize clogging of the membrane and will enable the filtration process to attain an absolute retention efficiency to the specified size and yet have high particle holding capacity. Filters are produced in a variety of sizes: 13 and 25 mm diameters will cope with syringe volumes while 45 mm, 90 mm and 142 mm diameters will handle volumes of 300 ml, 5 litres and 20 litres respectively. For large volume filtration, multiple plate systems and pleated cartridge filters are available. Filters for filtration sterilization together with any downstream distribution apparatus must be sterilized and this is usually by autoclaving at 121 °C or by ethylene oxide.

Filtration sterilization involves filtration of the solution through a sterilized filter unit followed by aseptic distribution of the filtered solution into previously sterilized containers and subsequent aseptic closure of the containers. It is an aseptic process and must therefore be carried out by skilled operators under aseptic conditions. Filtration does not lend itself to in-process validation by reliable physical or chemical methods and therefore sterility tests must be carried out on all products sterilized by filtration.

Selection of sterilization method

With sterilization methods employing increased energy and chemicals there is always the possibility that the process will have a damaging effect on the material being sterilized. The selection of a sterilization method is therefore a compromise between the maximum acceptable risk of failure to achieve sterility and the maximum permissible damage to the product and its package. Where practicable heat sterilization is the method of choice.

Moist heat sterilization is applicable to a wide variety of aqueous preparations for parenteral and non-parenteral administration. It can also be applied to natural rubbers and many plastics including PVC and nylon. Glassware and equipment can be autoclaved provided that there is adequate steam penetration and exposure to moisture is not deleterious. Autoclaving is the most effective method for sterilizing surgical dressings and the high vacuum autoclave in particular satisfies the essential requirements for total air removal and prevention of excessive condensation. When materials are damaged by the presence of moisture, e.g. oils, ointment bases, waxes and powders, sterilization by dry heat is often possible. This is usually the method of choice for glassware, syringes and surgical instruments and equipment.

Overheating, and thus the risk of product degradation during heat sterilization, may be minimized by considering an integrated lethality approach to the calculation of sterilization protocols. Also, since the Arrhenius parameters for drug degradation and lethality are usually markedly different it may be possible to reduce the amount of drug degradation, without significantly affecting lethality, by using high temperature, short time protocols in place of low temperature, long time protocols. High temperature, short time (HTST) treatment of 15–45 seconds at 130 °C and ultra-high temperature (UHT) treatment of 2–3 seconds at 140–150 °C are used for most heat sterilization of thermosensitive food products and could be applicable to some pharmaceuticals.

Many materials are unable to withstand the temperatures used in heat sterilization and require the use of 'cold sterilization' techniques. Ethylene oxide has been used for the sterilization of thermolabile powders, some plastics and rubbers, surgical instruments, e.g. bronchoscopes and cytoscopes, surgical dressings and woollen blankets. The gas must of course be capable of penetrating to all parts of the material to be sterilized. LTSF sterilization (described above) is also applicable to the sterilization of woollen blankets and some surgical instruments. Since ethylene oxide and formaldehyde are highly reactive chemicals it is necessary to establish that no toxic reaction products are formed during sterilization. The reliability of gaseous sterilization methods is questionable due to the critical conditions required and the difficulties in monitoring these conditions, and the methods are only recommended where more reliable methods are not practicable.

The alternative 'cold sterilization' method, radiation, is extremely reliable, but it too suffers from the disadvantage of including degradation in a wide variety of materials. Aqueous solutions of pharmaceuticals cannot be radiation sterilized due to the extensive degradation brought about by the radiolysis products of water. The method is used for large scale sterilization of plastic disposable Petri dishes and surgical equipment, surgical instruments, dressings (particularly adhesive dressings), and sutures.

When terminal sterilization by any of the above methods cannot be used, sterilization by filtration and aseptic processing is the only applicable method.

STERILIZATION CONTROLS

In a sterilization process the probability of a viable organism remaining is greatly reduced and designing the process to have a high inactivation factor ensures that there is high probability of achieving sterility. Quality assurance of the process depends upon integrating and controlling the process variables. In a process such as autoclaving where the parameters for sterilization are clearly defined and can be accurately measured by instruments the process is best controlled by physical monitoring. In ethylene oxide and LTSF processes the kinetics of inactivation are less understood and additional parameters such as gas penetration and absorption are involved. In these processes all the parameters cannot be integrated by physical methods and biological sterilization indicators are essential. Where reliable physical and chemical validation of the process is not possible, as in filtration sterilization, product testing assumes an important role in sterilization control.

Sterilization controls are of two types, in-process controls and product controls. In-process controls are discussed here whilst the philosophy of product testing (sterility tests) is discussed in

Chapter 26 and methodology is discussed in Chapter 28.

In-process controls

Physical measurements

In moist and dry heat sterilization, measurement and recording of temperature is essential. Mercury or volatile liquid distance reading thermometers have been frequently used for temperature measurement in sterilizers. However, their sensitivity is not great and they require recalibrating at regular intervals. The use of thermocouples is preferred. Chromel/alumel (Type K) thermocouples with potentiometric measurement are normally used, since they allow permanent printed records to be prepared using suitable recorders, and are able to control automatic switching systems. Resistance thermometers and thermistors are very sensitive to temperature changes but are not generally sufficiently robust or corrosion resistant for use in autoclaves. Temperature should be recorded at the coolest part of the load or loaded chamber (usually the drain) for autoclaves and gaseous sterilizers and at the part of the load with the longest heat-up time for hot air ovens.

Pressure measurement is normally by means of bourdon type pressure gauges although pressure transducers are being increasingly used in modern sterilizers.

At the pressure and temperature used for sterilization there is no satisfactory method of measuring the relative humidity or of determining the degree of saturation of steam either in the chamber or in the load. Dew point hygrometers are either affected by the presence of free water droplets, inoperable under pressure, or incapable of withstanding high temperature. Direct calorimetry of samples from the chamber is too slow and unreliable to be of value.

A physical method for indirectly assessing the efficiency of filters is available. This calculates the maximum pore size from the pressure necessary to force the first bubble of air through the filter when it is wetted with a liquid of known surface tension. The British Standard 1752:1963 describes a bubble pressure test of this type.

Physical measurements of sterilization processes are only meaningful if the instruments are carefully calibrated initially, well maintained and regularly checked during use, and used intelligently.

Chemical indicators

These rely on the ability of the sterilization process to change the chemical and/or physical nature of a particular chemical. A good indicator is designed to measure directly whether the sterilization conditions have been achieved, although some only show that a particular article or batch has been through the process and do not indicate whether or not the process was successful.

Browne's tubes The most commonly used chemical indicators for heat processes are Browne's tubes (A. Browne, Leicester, Ltd). These are small sealed tubes containing a reaction mixture and an indicator. Exposure to high temperature completes the reaction producing a change in the colour of the indicator. Different types are available for different heat sterilization processes:

Type 1 (black spot) for moist heat sterilizers operating at up to 126 °C.
Type 2 (yellow spot) for high vacuum moist heat sterilizers operating at 130 °C or more.
Type 3 (green spot) for dry heat hot air sterilizers operating at 160 °C.
Type 4 (blue spot) for dry heat infra-red conveyor ovens operating at 180 °C.

All four types change from red through yellow brown to green, the latter colour only being achieved after a specified time at the given temperature. Browne's tubes have the advantage of being cheap and convenient and a number can be distributed easily within a load. However, the colour change is brought about equally by moist and dry heat and therefore in the case of moist heat sterilization processes they will not indicate problem conditions such as superheating. Furthermore, as the chemical reaction involved can also occur, albeit slowly, at low temperature as well as at high temperature, defined storage conditions and indicator shelf life are essential.

Crystal indicators Indicators developed using crystals of substances that melt at sterilization temperatures (i.e. witness tubes) serve no useful purpose since they give no indication of time of exposure and are equally affected by moist and dry heat. A development of the witness tube utilizes 2,4-dinitrophenylhydrazone impregnated on to filter paper/aluminium foil laminated strips. When melted the liquid travels along the paper strip, the distance travelled indicating the time that the strip was maintained at or above temperature. A variety of test papers and tapes are available which use temperature-sensitive or thermochromic inks, and change colour on reaching the sterilization temperature. The time of heating that is required is not critical and therefore the colour change can only be used to distinguish between treated and untreated items and cannot indicate the success of the treatment.

Heat-sensitive tape Heat-sensitive tape is used quantitatively in the Bowie-Dick test. This is a test to determine that all air has been removed from dressings and that subsequent steam penetration has been even and rapid. A standard dressings pack containing a pattern of autoclave tape in its centre is exposed to a normal sterilization cycle. The tape is examined for uniformity of colour change, the presence of air resulting in a pale region in the centre of the pattern. It must be emphasized that this is not a time at temperature indicator.

Royce sachet The Royce sachet is a chemical indicator for ethylene oxide sterilization. This consists of a polythene sachet containing magnesium chloride, HCl, and bromophenol blue indicator. A given concentration–time exposure to ethylene oxide results in the formation of ethylene chlorohydrin and a colour change from yellow to purple. Indicators consisting of papers impregnated with chemothermochromic inks have also been developed to use with ethylene oxide and LTSF but their reliability is unproven.

Chemical dosimeters Chemical dosimeters give an accurate measure of the radiation dose absorbed and are considered to be the best technique currently available for controlling radiation sterilization. These are manufactured from red polymethyl methacrylate or nylon polyvinyl chloride produced in the form of a slide which can be inserted directly into a visible light spectrophotometer to determine the optical density change induced by the radiation. These are placed in areas where the dose is expected to be at a minimum. Their useful range is 0.1–5.0 Mrad. Qualitative indicators made of radiosensitive chemicals impregnated in plastic are also available. The indicator changes from yellow to red during irradiation, but since the colour change occurs at relatively low doses these can only be used to differentiate between irradiated and non-irradiated items. They are insufficiently accurate and are not quantitative, and must not be confused with the chemical dosimeters described above.

Biological indicators

Biological indicators consist of a suitable organism deposited on a carrier and distributed throughout the sterilizer load. At the end of the sterilization process the units are recovered and cultured to determine the presence or absence of survivors. It is argued by proponents of biological indicators that, unlike physical and chemical monitors, the biological indicator measures sterilization processes directly and is able to integrate all sterilization parameters. The selected organism should possess high and reproducible resistance to the sterilizing agent, ideally produce log-linear survivor curves, and be genetically stable, readily characterizable and non-pathogenic. Conditions for growth and harvesting of the organisms, the preparation and storage of the indicator, and recovery of survivors must be carefully standardized and rigidly controlled. It has been argued that the indicator should ideally be in a form similar to the item being sterilized, e.g. in aqueous suspension for moist heat sterilization of aqueous solutions, in sand for dry heat sterilization of powders. Alternatively the product itself could be used as the suspending medium but the effects of the product

on the resistance and recovery of the organism would need to be established.

The organisms used as biological indicators are usually resistant bacterial spores. The following are the most widely used.

B. stearothermophilus and *B. coagulans* dried on filter paper or PVC strips or in aqueous suspensions (for moist heat);

B. subtilis var. *niger* and *Cl. sporogenes* dried on aluminium foil, glass, stainless steel strips or sterile washed sand (for dry heat);

B. pumilus and *B. sphaericus* dried on filter paper on aluminium foil (for radiation);

B. subtilis var. *niger* dried on aluminium foil or PVC strips (for ethylene oxide).

An ideal organism and carrier for LTSF have not yet been established although those used for autoclaving have been with variable success.

The number of spores that should be present in the indicator is debatable, most commercially available units containing between 10^5 and 10^7 or more. A minimum of ten indicators distributed throughout the load is recommended where biological monitoring is essential, i.e. in ethylene oxide and LTSF sterilization, and then they should only be used in conjunction with physical measurements. The variables that effect spore resistance (see Chapter 25) indicate the need for strict quality control and regular checking of biological indicators.

In cases where a bubble test cannot be applied or is not practical the efficiency of filters for sterilization can be measured directly by filtering a known volume of solution containing a known number of organisms and measuring the bacterial retention capacity of the filter. The *Pharmaceutical Codex* describes a test of this type which uses *Serratia marcescens* as the test organism. *Pseudomonas diminuta* and spores of *B. subtilis* var. *niger* are used as alternative test organisms.

REFERENCES AND BIBLIOGRAPHY

British Pharmacopoeia (1980) Pharmaceutical Press, London.
British Standard 1752:1963. Specification for laboratory sintered or fritted filters.
British Standard 3421:1961. Performance of electrically heated sterilising ovens.
British Standard 3970:1966. Specification for steam

sterilisers. Part 1: Sterilisers for porous loads. Part 2: Sterilisers for bottled fluids.
Department of Health and Social Security (1980) *Pressure Steam Sterilisers*. Hospital Technical Memorandum 10. HMSO, London.
Department of Health and Social Security (1981) *Guide to*

Good Manufacturing Practice for Sterile Single-use Medical Devices and Surgical Products. HMSO, London.

Department of Health and Social Security (1983) *Guide to Good Manufacturing Practice*. HMSO, London.

MRC Memorandum No. 41 (1962). Medical Research Council, London.

Perkins, J. J. (1969) *Principles and Methods of Sterilization in Health Services*, 2nd edn. Charles Thomas Publishers, Springfield, Illinois, USA.

Pharmaceutical Codex (1979). Pharmaceutical Press, London.

Russell, A. D., Hugo, W. B. and Ayliffe, G. A.J. (1982) *Principles and Practice of Disinfection, Preservation and Sterilisation*. Blackwell Scientific Publications, Oxford.

Packaging technology

PACKAGING MATERIALS

Packaging types, styles and systems can be broadly defined by the material of construction, e.g. glass, plastic, metal, rubber, paper, etc., and the process used for fabrication, e.g. blow moulding, injection moulding, etc.

Glass and glass containers

Glass has had a successful history for pharmaceutical products in that it offers transparency, sparkle, easy cleaning, effective closuring and reclosuring where applicable, high speed handling, good rigidity and stackability and is, by the selection of the correct type of glass, generally inert. The two main disadvantages, fragility and heavy weight, have partially been reduced by surface coatings to increase the surface lubricity and careful design. The latter includes the avoidance of sharp angles and the use of adequate radii. Plastic coated or plastic sleeved containers are likely to allow even thinner glass containers to be produced. The specific gravity of glass normally lies between 2.25 and 2.5 whereas most plastics are well below 1.5 (PVC is 1.4–1.45).

Glass is basically of three types, neutral glass, (type I), surface treated soda glass (type II) and soda or alkali glass (type III). These materials may be converted into components by pressing, blowing in a mould or by the shaping of glass cane (tubular containers). Typical composition of type I (neutral) and type III (soda or alkali) glass are as follows.

	Type I	Type III
Silica	66–74%	66–75%
Lime	1–5%	6–12%
Soda	7–10%	12.5–19%
Alumina	4–10%	1–7%
Boric oxide	9–11%	—

In type I glass, the alkaline element is largely eliminated by the use of boric oxide to neutralize the oxides of potassium and sodium. Neutral glass has a higher melt temperature, around 1750 °C, has a narrower working temperature range which together with the higher cost of boric oxide and greater likelihood of imperfections usually means a cost of two to three times that of soda glass for containers made by the blow moulding process.

Surface treated glass (type II) is made by treating the hot surface of type III (soda) glass with sulphur dioxide, ammonium sulphate or in some countries ammonium chloride. This neutralizes some of the surface alkali radicals producing a more neutral surface. The process, which may also be referred to as sulphuring or sulphating, invariably leaves a hazy surface bloom (normally sodium sulphate) hence washing is essential prior to use. Soda glass (type III) is the most widely used material where extraction of alkali metal ions is not critical to the product. All glass types are available in clear (white flint) and amber with other colours, including green, being produced as special makings. Although the majority of all glass containers are made by a blow moulding process, vials, ampoules and cartridge tubes, produced by 'shaping' glass softened by heat after a length is cut from glass cane, find wide application for pharmaceutical and cosmetic products.

Metal and metal containers

Metal, mainly as tin plate or aluminium, was at one time widely used for rigid containers for tablets, capsules, pastilles, powders and even liquid products. A significant part of this usage has been lost to other materials over the last 10 years. Light flexible gauges of metal (aluminium, tin and tin-coated lead) were widely used for collapsible tubes. Thin gauges of aluminium are widely used as foil in combination with other support or heat sealing polymer films. Although all the above uses for metals still exist, there has been a gradual reduction in use of metal other than for foil and for aerosols. In addition to containers, tin plate, aluminium and aluminium alloy have been widely employed for ancillary components including closures. Although the use of tin plate and certain types of aluminium screw closures have reduced, the special aluminium alloy developed for rolled on and rolled on pilfer proof closures has remained in use mainly due to recent events related to security and tamper evidence.

The production of collapsible tubes made by a process known as impact extrusion has been fairly static recently, first due to the growth in plastic tubes, and more recently due to the introduction of a multi-ply lamination, once known as 'Glaminates'. Metal collapsible tubes in the UK are largely made in aluminium (plain or lacquered) with a few in pure tin. As aluminium work hardens during impact extrusion (i.e. it becomes less flexible and more springy) aluminium tubes have to undergo an annealing process to ensure that the metal becomes flexible and capable of being shaped and folded. If any interaction between the product and metal is likely an internal protective lacquer usually based on vinyl or epoxy resins can be added. As metal tubes have a shoulder bearing an orifice (which takes a closure) and an open end (through which the contents are filled and after which the metal is folded and crimped), they have in effect two closures and two areas of seal. Whilst the dispensing end can be sealed with a blind nozzle and/or a screw cap to make a good seal, the folded metal is less reliable in terms of searching or mobile products. The fold can therefore be improved by the addition of a latex or heat seal band. Although the number of folds in the filling end can also be varied (e.g. saddle back (triple) fold, double fold, etc.) the longer tube length required for the former (say + 9 mm) will add to the cost.

Tubes with elongated nozzles and a controlled orifice size are used for eye ointments. Nearly all caps on metal tubes are wadless, being plastic and moulded in polyethylene and polypropylene.

Plastics and plastic containers

Types and uses

The past 30 years has seen a significant expansion in the use of plastic from a few thermoset caps and the odd container (for menthol cones and shaving sticks) to a point where plastics have become a major packaging material. Plastics used now are mainly related to the thermoplastic resins. The most economic four are polyethylene (low, medium and high densities), polyvinyl chloride (unplasticized and plasticized), polypropylene (homopolymer and copolymer) and polystyrene (general purpose and impact modified). Other selected materials find specialized usages for containers, devices, components, plies or coatings. These include nylon (PA), arcylonitrile butadiene styrene (ABS), styrene acrylonitrile (SAN), poly-carbonate (PC), polysulphone, polyvinylidene chloride (PVdC), polymonochlorotrifluoroethylene (PCTFE), polyester (PET) and polytetrafluoro-ethylene (PTFE). Plastic resins or polymers offer many attributes, in choice of material and grade, processes of fabrication and decoration, a wide selection in design, and physical and chemical properties, all on an economical basis.

Disadvantages

Plastics in theory appear to have certain disadvantages, i.e. possible extraction, interaction, adsorption, absorption, lightness and hence poor physical stability, all are permeable to some degree to moisture, oxygen, carbon dioxide, etc., most exhibit electrostatic attraction, allow penetration of light rays unless pigmented black, etc. It is necessary to be aware of other possible negative features. These include:

1 *stress cracking*: a phenomenon related to low density polythene and certain stress cracking agents such as wetting agents, detergents and some volatile oils;
2 *panelling or cavitation*: whereby a container shows inward distortion or partial collapse due to absorption of gases from the headspace, absorption causing swelling of the plastic, or dimpling following a steam autoclaving operation;
3 *crazing*: a surface reticulation which can occur particularly with polystyrene and certain

chemical substances (isopropyl myristate first causes crazing which ultimately reaches a state of total embrittlement and disintegration);
4 *poor key of print*: certain plastics such as the polyolefins need pretreating before ink will key. Additives which migrate to the surface of the plastic may also cause printing problems;
5 *poor impact resistance*: both polystyrene and PVC have poor impact resistance. This can be improved by the inclusion of impact modifiers such as rubber in the case of polystyrene and methyl methacrylate butadiene styrene for PVC. However, both increase the permeability of each.

The majority of these effects can be either overcome or minimized by one means or another. An industrial example will illustrate the point.

It was required to pack a nasal spray formultaion in a plastic squeeze bottle which was available world-wide. This immediately called for a low density polyethylene pack. The product, however, contained a volatile preservative system which both dissolved in LDPE and was lost from it by volatilization, thereby immediately suggesting that a conventional squeeze pack was unsuitable. The LDPE bottle was, however, enclosed in a PVC blister impermeable to the volatile preservative and fitted with a peelable foil lid (also impermeable). As a result of this combination the loss of preservative was restricted to less than 5% of the total, i.e. preservative soluble in the LDPE, and preservative in the air space of the PVC blister reached a point where equilibrium was achieved between product, LDPE and the surrounding air space.

Additives

Since plastics still tend to be seen as relatively new materials, those used for ophthalmic solutions and injectables have a specific extractives procedure to pass. However, knowledge of the constituents which may be found in a plastic material are equally important. The constituents fall into four categories, the polymer, residues associated with the polymerization process, additives (those constituents added to modify the plastic in a specific way) and any processing aids (which are used to assist any part of the process). The list of residues, additives and processing aids varies according to plastic involved. Natural polyethylenes usually are low in residues and are only likely to contain a small quantity of an antioxidant. Polyvinylchloride on the other hand invariably contains a stabilizer to restrict any degradation which may occur during the heat processing.

The residues, additives and processing aids which may be used, and therefore possibly extracted from, a plastic include the following:

Monomer residues	Modifiers
Catalysts	Emulsifiers
Accelerators	Antioxidants
Solvents	Mould release agents
Extenders	Lubricants
Fillers	Stabilizers
Slip additives	Colourants — pigments and
Antislip additives	dyes
Antistatic agents	Whiteners and opacifiers
Antiblocking	UV absorbers
agents	Flame retardants
Plasticizers	Light excluders (e.g. carbon
Release agents	black)

Let it be said that most plastics will only include a few of the constituents listed above. However, depending on the additive used other properties of the plastic can be changed, e.g. fillers such as chalk or talc are likely to increase moisture permeation.

Fabrication of plastics

Unlike glass plastic containers and components can be fabricated by a far greater number of processes. These include injection moulding, injection and extrusion blow moulding, injection stretch and extrusion stretch blow moulding, thermoforming, scrapless forming process (SFP), reaction injection moulding (RIM), solid phase pressure forming (SPPF), all of which mainly relate to thermoplastic resins. Designs, rate of moulding and cost all vary according to the process chosen and the number of moulds involved, i.e. single or multiple cavity. Irrespective of the process, all moulding operations operate to a 'cycle' whereby the basic resin is heated, softened, shaped in a mould or moulds, and cooled to a temperature at which the article can be handled without distortion. Virtually all plastics shrink in the moulding/cooling operation and allowance has to be made for this. Subsequent to moulding, plastics can be decorated or printed by another wide range of processes, i.e. silkscreen, dry offset letterpress, hot die stamping, cliche or tampon printing, therimage, letraset, or labelled by heat-sensitive, self-adhesive labels or plain paper labels using a special adhesive. Knowledge of both the fabrication and decoration of plastics is essential when a plastic material is to be used in contact with a pharmaceutical product.

Paper and board

The use of paper-based materials (cellulose fibre) remains a significant part of pharmaceutical packaging in spite of the fact that paper is rarely used on its own for a primary pack. However, the list of paper usages covers labels, cartons, bags, outers, trays for shrink wraps, layer boards on pallets, etc. and combinations of paper, plastic and foil which are discussed separately. Cartons are used for a high percentage of pharmaceutical products for a number of reasons, increasing display area, providing better stacking for display of stock items, and the collating of leaflets which would otherwise be difficult to attach to many containers. Cartons also provide physical protection, especially to items like metal collapsible tubes. Cartons therefore tend to be a traditional part of pharmaceutical packaging. Fibreboard outers either as solid or corrugated board also find substantial application for bulk shipments.

Regenerated cellulose film, trade names Cellophane and Rayophane, are still used as an overwrapping material for either individual cartons or to collate a number of cartons. However, it is being substantially replaced by orientated polypropylene film. Although paper, even when waxed, has relatively poor protective properties against moisture, both paper and board (ointment, pill and tablet boxes) were widely used for primary packs up to 20–25 years ago, particularly for dispensing operations.

Films, foils and laminates

The development of plastic films (early 1950s onwards) as distinct from regenerated cellulose film based on viscose, and the process of laminating two or more plies selected from films, cellulose coatings, foil and paper, has seen an ever increasing use of the various combinations. These materials fall into different roles such as supportive, barrier, heat seal and decorative. Paper for example is usually a supportive ply which can readily be printed to give decorative appeal. Aluminium foil even in the thinnest gauges (particularly when laminated or coated with a plastic ply) offers the best barrier properties which are not approached even by the most impermeable plastics. Metallization, a relatively new process whereby particles of metal are laid down on to a surface under vacuum, can significantly improve the barrier properties of a material but these do not approach the properties of pure foil. The reflective properties of both metallization and foil can add to the decorative appeal of a pack. Plastics, either as films or coatings, can be used for decoration, flexibility, to provide various barrier properties, heat sealability, see-through properties (i.e. transparency) and to protect the other plies within the lamination.

In terms of cost, paper/plastic (paper/LDPE or paper/PVdC) or single plies of coated regenerated cellulose film or coated polypropylene represent the more economical materials which can be used for strip packs, sachets, overwraps, etc. Although in general, costs increase as the number of plies increase, newer techniques such as coextrusion, where a number of plastic plies are extruded in combination, can produce complete laminations cheaper than those produced by individual bonding. However, lamination bonding is still essential for plies containing paper and foil as these materials cannot be extruded.

Usages for films, foils laminations are numerous, e.g. sachets, diaphragm seals for bottles, strip packs, blister packs, liners for large containers, overwraps, flow wraps, liners for boxes either attached (e.g. Cekatainer and Hermetet cartons) or loose bag-in-box systems and bags. Each of the above is likely to use different materials or combinations of materials for a number of reasons. For example, a blister pack consists of a thermoformed tray with a lid make from board, paper, foil, film with coatings which will either tenaciously adhere to the tray, and act as a push-through material or be peelable so that the lid can be peeled back to gain access to the contents. The thermoformable portion, i.e. the tray, can again be made from a single material, e.g. polystyrene, polyvinyl chloride, polyester, etc., or be a combination, e.g. PVC coated with PVdC, PVC/PVdC/PE/PVdC/PVC, PVC/PCTFE (i.e. Aclar).

The thermoforming operation whereby a heated and softened plastic ply or sheet is drawn into a cooled mould can be done by vacuum, positive air pressure, mechanically by a die, or a combination of these. If thicker foil is incorporated into the basic web to give a combination of nylon or polypropylene/40–50 μm foil/PVC or polyethylene, then cold forming whereby a web is stretched without perforating can be carried out. Foil blisters, as these are known, when sealed with a foil lid can provide an hermetic pack, i.e. a pack which excludes virtually any exchange of gases between the product and the surrounding atmosphere. Similar protection can be achieved by using a foil bearing laminate for a strip pack. In this case the foil laminate is either stretched by the insertion of an item in the 'pocket area' when it is held against a recess in a heat sealing roller or the pocket area is prestretched prior to reaching the intermeshing heat sealing roller position. In all cases the blister or pocket has to be especially designed for the item to be filled if the maximum economy of material and machine is to be achieved. The volume and area of a blister pack is very product/machine dependent and whilst it may be practical to put an item in a larger size of blister or pocket (at additional cost in material and possible slower production speed), it is usually impossible to make packs smaller, without technical risks being taken, e.g. product sticking to foil lid in a blister pack; product causing pocket to perforate in a strip pack, etc.

Both blister and strip packs appear to offer a reasonable degree of child resistance particularly if the materials are opaque (opinion based on actual recorded poisonings or accidents).

Rubber-based components

Rubber components may be made from either natural or synthetic sources. As the majority of rubber usage is related to the closuring of sterile products (aqueous or oil-based and freeze-dried or powdered solids). Although natural rubber is being replaced by synthetics it offers advantages in terms of reseal (multidose injections), fragmentation and coring (descriptions for the means by which particles are created when a needle is passed through a rubber) but is poorer in respect to ageing, multiple autoclaving, extractives, moisture and gas permeation and absorption of preservative systems. Synthetic rubbers tend to reverse all of the above properties and some formulations actually contain natural rubber in order to improve resealability, fragmentation and coring. However, most rubber formulations are relatively complex and may contain one or more of the following: vulcanizing agents (many of which are sulphur based), accelerators, fillers, activators, pigments, antioxidants, lubricants, softeners or waxes.

The main types of rubber used for pharmaceutical products include natural rubber, neoprene, nitrile, butyl, chlorobutyl, bromobutyl and silicone. Of these silicone is the most expensive and although the most inert is readily permeable to moisture, gases and absorbent to certain preservatives.

As indicated above rubber components are likely to contain more additives than plastics. They are therefore tested by basically similar extractives and product contact procedures before they are utilized for injectable or i.v.-type products.

Rubber gaskets are also found in aerosols and metered dose pump systems.

CLOSURES

Functions of a closure

Closures may be required to perform any of the following functions:

1 to provide a totally hermetic seal. This is a closure which permits no exchange between the contents and the outside of the pack, e.g. a fused glass ampoule.
2 to provide an effective microbiological seal, e.g. rubber bung and metal overseal. Since rubber is permeable to moisture and gases to some

degree, a bacteriological seal may not be strictly hermetic.
3 to provide an effective seal which is acceptable to the product, i.e. a closure which is not hermetic or a total guarantee against bacterial ingress but adequate for the product.

The USP XXI classifies certain degrees of permeation by reference to *tight* or *well closed* containers. The test which uses a dried desiccant and storage at 20 °C and 75% RH tests the whole container and expresses the moisture gain against the content volume of the container per day, i.e. *tight* containers — not more than 1 in 10 containers exceeds 100 mg per day per litre and none exceeds 200 mg per day in moisture permeability; *well closed* containers — not more than 1 in 10 containers exceeds 2000 mg per day per litre and none exceeds 3000 mg per day per litre in moisture permeability.

The USP also provides a similar classification system for unit dose containers for capsules and tablets, and high density polyethylene bottles, as detailed below.

(a) Single unit dose packs:
Class A — if not more than 1 in 10 exceeds 0.5 mg per day and none exceeds 1 mg per day.
Class B — if not more than 1 in 10 exceeds 5 mg per day and none exceeds 10 mg per day.
Class C — if not more than 1 in 10 exceeds 20 mg per day and none exceeds 40 mg per day.
Class D — those outside the above the limits.
(b) High density polyethylene (HDPE), containers for tablets and capsules. Pass if not more than 1 in 10 exceeds 10 mg per day per litre and none exceeds 25 mg per day per litre.

Providing a 'seal' frequently depends on the marriage of a hard material with a softer more resilient material so that the former makes a physical impression on the latter. Closures generally require consideration of the following factors

1 to be resistant and compatible with the product and the product/air space. Note — product contact will vary according to how pack is

stood; upright, upside down, on side, intermittent contact during transportation, movement, etc.;

2 if of a reclosable variety, to be readily openable and effectively resealed;

3 to be capable of high speed application where necessary for automatic production without loss of seal efficiency;

4 to be decorative and of a shape which blends in with the main container;

5 to offer such additional functions as may be deemed necessary — to aid pouring, metering, administration, child resistance, tamper evidence, etc.;

6 to prevent or limit exchange with the outside atmosphere, to a permissible level. Note — as well as moisture exchange, this may have to cover gases, vapours and actual liquid seepage or leakage.

Although a closure can be affected by various basic means, i.e. adhesion, heat sealing, welding, crimping, mechanical impression, interlocking, stapling, sewing, etc., the majority of systems are related to physical compression or heat sealing.

The *physical compression systems* include:

1 screw caps — in metal or plastic; prethreaded or rolled on with or without a wadding system (i.e. wadless);

2 plug in — a friction push in fit;

3 push over — where a flanged or raised ring portion is pressed over a bead or lip.

Some closuring systems endeavour to combine one or more of these systems and thereby achieve a multiple seal, for example, a seal may press externally on a sealing surface and also on an internal bore. Wadless thermoplastic caps using a 'crab's claw' seal or a skirted bore seal are becoming increasingly popular.

Wadded screw caps either contain a wad plus a facing, a disc of resilient platic or have a flowed-in plastic compound. The wad may be of compocork, feltboard, pulpboard or expanded polyethylene, faced with such materials as aluminium foil, tin foil (expensive), polyethylene, a vinyl material or PVdC (Saran). The latter which has good barrier properties and is reasonably inert, is now the most widely used. Foil or waxed foil is slightly preferable if a higher barrier material is required. The wadding materials mentioned above are occasionally used, usually waxed, on their own. Plasticized PVC, polyethylene or foamed polyethylene have also found selective usage. Flowed-in linings although slightly inferior in barrier properties and inertness, offer production line advantages in that there is no wad to fall out whereby a pack is left without an effective closure. Wadless caps also have this same advantage. The knowledge required in order to understand closuring systems is frequently under-rated.

Rolled on (RO) and rolled on pilfer proof (ROPP) aluminium alloy metal caps have always been popular for the security of export products. The RO and ROPP closure consists of a plain metal shell containing a wadding or flowed-in system, which is placed over the container neck and top pressure applied to give a good impression on the wad. Whilst the pressure is still held, the threads are formed by a mechanical inwards pressure. In the case of the pilfer proof closure an additional perforated collar is rolled under a lower bead. This type of closure system is capable of maintaining an excellent seal and does not suffer from the occasional tearing of the wad facing found when a conventional screw cap is applied to a substandard bottle finish. In the case of a rubber wad it also avoids any watchspring affect. However, a RO or ROPP cap does require a slightly higher standard for the quality of the bottle neck.

Determination of closure efficiency

Closure efficiency, i.e. the ability to prevent undesirable exchanges between the product and the outside atmosphere, can be determined by numerous methods:

1 placing a desiccant in a pack stored under high RH and detecting any moisture gain.

2 putting liquid inside the pack, storing at high temperature and low RH and then detecting any moisture loss as a reduction in weight.

3 holding empty pack under water, applying a vacuum and observing for leakage or liquid ingress. Adding a dye and a wetting agent to the water may assist detection of leaks.

4 putting liquid in the pack, inverting and applying vacuum. A poor seal is detected by liquid seeping or leaking out.

5 checking that cap-removal torque (assumes quality of bottle and cap) is satisfactory. Torque can be time-temperature related particularly on plastic bottles — hence measurement should be made against a standard condition and test period.

6 checking on compression 'ring' seal in cap liner when system contains a liner or lining compound. If indentation by bottle surface on liner is not uniform or continuous a faulty seal can occur. This can be assisted by 'painting' (magic marker) the bottle surface before applying the cap to the specified torque.

The above tests cover those carried out to establish that a closure is satisfactory in a development programme and those which can be used in production monitoring as part of on-line quality control. Some closuring systems using ratchet tamper evidence closures or rolled pilfer proof seals have two release torques — that to release the cap from the bottle sealing surface and the torque required to 'break' the tamper evident feature.

Heat seals

As indicated earlier another widely used method of sealing is heat (direct and indirect). To achieve an effective and permanent heat seal the two sealants must be compatible (partly compatible sealants can be used to give a peelable seal). Four factors have to be controlled: temperature, pressure, dwell (the length of time that temperature and pressure is applied) and the cooling period. Contamination of any area of seal (for example, with product) should be avoided although certain plastics will seal better than others in the presence of a contaminant. The main heat sealants include polyethylene (low density), wax coatings, PVdC, Surlyn ionomer, selected vinyl-based products and certain types of modified polypropylene. Conditions of sealing vary according to the heat sealant with the majority sealing between 75 °C and 150 °C. The total effectiveness of the seal is also dependent on other variables such as seal width, seal pattern, pack shape, the presence of creases or stress lines (particularly if product area is overfilled or undersize) etc. The seal is usually checked by vacuum (carried out under water probably containing a dye plus a wetting agent) to see if ingress occurs and by the force required to pull apart the seal.

Other sealing methods

Sealing of plastics can also be achieved by other techniques, such as ultrasonics, high frequency welding, hot air welding and sealing by other heat sources (flame, infrared, induction, etc.).

Suffice it to say that closuring is a most essential part of both primary and secondary packs.

FILLING

Packaging lines

Products packed on production lines cover such items as unit and multidose packs, closable and non-reclosable packs, sterile products produced aseptically or by terminal sterilization or non-sterile products with or without a degree of microbiological control, preformed containers which have to be filled and sealed, etc., or those packed by a form fill seal process, etc. Packaging lines may be fairly conventional and involve unscrambling, cleaning, filling, closuring, labelling, cartoning (probably with leaflet insertion), outerization and finally palletization or be selective to a specialist operation, e.g. blister and strip packaging. Additional operations which may be carried out on a production include printing, batch coding and expiry dating, the incorporation of administration aids, etc. Glass bottles other than those used for the more critical types of product (injection, eye drops or similar sterile products) are normally manufactured and packed clean and then subjected to pressurized air and vacuum as a final cleaning process (for fibres) prior to filling.

The total efficiency and hence profitability of a packed product depends not only on the type of pack and the material selected but also on the production line operation and the packaging equipment chosen. For example the filling speed for a tablet will depend on the characteristics of the tablet; the size, shape, fragility, resistance to powdering if uncoated, surface lubricity, etc. and the type of pack chosen. For a non-fragile easy flowing tablet, filling speeds for a wide mouthed container (100s, could be 20 000 tablets per minute, with 5000 for a blister pack and 2000 for a strip pack. Choosing a narrow mouthed container irrespective of the material used could reduce the filling speed to below 10 000 tablets per minute.

Organization of packaging lines

The organization of a production line involves several factors which ultimately may affect output. These include labour, planned maintenance, staff training, on-line quality control (QC), facilities for batch coding and expiry dating where relevant, constant delivery of an adequate supply of materials to the agreed specification on to the line, and removal of finished product from the line. Also required are clearly defined procedures for cleaning, start up and close down of the line plus full documentation on both procedures and materials to be handled (including reclamation, verification, reconciliation), environmental control, which all form part of good manufacturing practice (GMP), and of course the actions to take should one piece or part of a machine break down. On a line performing a number of separate functions (i.e. unscrambling, feeding, filling, closing, labelling and cartoning) each following operation should be capable of higher output speeds than the former. Intermediate holding areas, like a revolving table top may also be placed between certain functions should, say, the capper unit temporarily need attention. In this way the first part of the filling operation can still continue provided the alteration or adjustment to the capper can be carried out relatively quickly. The rest of the line with the higher output capability can then cope with the backlog of containers.

Packaging of certain products

The method of packaging obviously depends on the type of material to be packed. *Solid items* such as tablets and capsules are counted by, for example, resolving disc, slat counter, breaking a beam of light, etc. *Powder or granular products* may be filled by volume using an auger (powder held in a rotating screw), a filling cup, or by weight using a bulk feed plus trickle top-up. In the case of very small quantities a dosator which dips into a constant level of powder held in a reservoir can be employed. Whatever the process of fill, observations have to be made as to whether the filling process changes the characteristics of the powdered product, e.g. separation due to vibration, impaction due to compression, etc. *Cream and ointment type products* are either filled volumetrically by a piston-type filler or auger. *Liquid products* are also widely filled by a piston filler, a volume cup method using a pressure or gravity feed or where a rigid non-collapsible container is involved, by vacuum. In this process two tubes are lowered into the bottle and a seal made by a gasket on the container neck. When a vacuum is drawn on the vacuum tube, liquid flows through the filling tube until the liquid reaches the level of the vacuum tube. The flow then cuts off. This process provides a clean fill, detects containers which are faulty (contain holes or have a dipped or uneven sealing surface) and of course it operates a no container, no fill feature. However, it is not ideally suited to frothing or more viscous liquids. A container which would collapse under a relatively low vacuum can be filled by vacuum, provided it is placed in an outer container, and then sealed so that a vacuum can be drawn internally and externally to the pack.

Aerosols

Aerosols fall into a category of their own. They use a variety of materials (metal, glass, coated glass or plastic as containers and combinations of metal, plastic and rubber for the valve) and offer a form of packaging where the product and pack cannot be separated. In fact an aerosol only comes into existence once it has been filled with a product and pressurized with a propellant. The latter may be either an inert gas or a halogenated hydrocarbon. Pharmaceutical aerosols by and large can be divided into metered dose aerosols where the total volume usually does not exceed 50 ml, and topical applications with a volume of 100 ml plus.

Metered dose aerosols, many of which are used

to treat asthmatic or bronchial conditions, are required to produce a product with a fine particle size, i.e. significant part of the cloud below 7 μm. This can be achieved by using powder or liquid aerosols where breakup is assisted by the propellant formulation and the valve. Attempts to produce a fine particle cloud using inert gases with a breakup system have so far fallen short of the standard required. The recent criticisms on the use of fluorocarbon propellants and their possible attack on the ozone layer has led to considerable innovation with trends towards separating the product from the pressurized part of the system. As a result a number of bag-in-can, or piston systems have been developed. Although such systems will dispense a solid or liquid product they will now provide sufficient breakup to give a true aerosol type of dispensing.

Parenterals

Parenterals can normally be divided into small volume parenterals (SVP), e.g. injections, and large volume parenterals (LVP), e.g. i.v. injections and dialysis solutions. Although the size of containers varies between SVP and LVP the range of materials used, i.e. glass, plastic, rubber, is common to each. The background required for the development of a parenteral shares the same phases as other products. However, greater emphasis has to be placed on the packaging material and the sterilization process, hence the points made below.

Glass Glass can be sterilized by dry heat, steam, ethylene oxide, but is discoloured by gamma irradiation.

Rubber Rubber can be sterilized by steam, ethylene oxide subject to adequate aeration to remove residues, but has to be very carefully checked if irradiation is used as both unacceptable physical and chemical changes may occur. Rubber generally will not withstand dry heat.

Plastics Only a few plastics will withstand dry heat.

Sterilization Sterilization is possibly by steam, ethylene oxide, gamma irradiation and a process not mentioned previously — accelerated electrons — which is in essence a milder form of gamma irradiation. This rather sweeping statement has to

be supported by adequate testing as each case has to be considered in the end on its own merits. In the case of ethylene oxide treatment, degassing may be a critical stage since residues of ethylene oxide, ethylene glycol (hydrolysed ethylene oxide) and epichlorhydrin (if chloride ions are present) are all of a toxic nature. Gamma radiation can cause physical (due to molecular cross-linking) and chemical changes to a plastic.

Labelling

If the pack is not already printed, labelling normally follows closuring. Although the preferred labelling system is reel-fed self-adhesive labels in Europe and the UK with limited use of plain labels and adhesive and heat seal labels, this is not necessarily the case in other countries. The USA, for example, is more orientated towards heat seal (reel-fed and cut singles) than any self-adhesive system.

Both self-adhesive and heat seal labels may contain constituents which may prove to be migratory when adhered to certain plastics. Inactivation of benzalkonium chloride when self-adhesive labels have been applied to LDPE has been recorded.

QUALITY CONTROL OF PACKAGING

In the UK, pharmaceutical products are broadly controlled by guidelines related to good manufacturing practice (GMP and the 'Orange' Guide) and good laboratory practice (GLP). These cover all stages in the discovery, development, production and sale of a pharmaceutical entity and the means of providing records and documentation literally from inception to ultimate withdrawal from the market preferably when it has been superseded by a more effective drug and had a successful use in history. Many of the aspects are related to quality assurance and quality control. However, any approval of a new drug discovery must involve thorough attention to detail with the effective recording of information through all initial evaluation stages of drug preformulation, formulation, clinical and safety evaluation, packaging development, formal stability, leading into a production/marketing operation. In terms of packaging this should mean that any 'container' used for excipients or drug entities is identified, recorded and cleared for use at all stages. This should also include the storage of intermediates, and all tests irrespective of whether they are of investigational or formal nature coupled to the procedures which control the pack, e.g. a product is to be stored in a glass bottle with a plastic cap with a liner/facing.

1 Glass bottle should be described in type, amber/white flint, type of glass (type I, II, III, etc.), closure type (e.g. screw neck) and cleared as meeting a provisional specification in terms of dimensions, quality, etc.
2 The closure should be defined terms of material (black phenol formaldehyde and wadding, i.e. pulpboard faced with a 20 g m^{-2} Saran) and identified and cleared in terms of material, dimensions, quality, etc.

If these materials are then used for a test at least the on and off torques should be recorded within say one hour of application. Identifying the climatic conditions (temperature and RH) may in certain circumstances need recording, e.g. in the packing of a moisture-sensitive product. This information and the associated documentation — probably a laboratory note book — is all part of GLP. The recording, examining and passing the bottles prior to acceptance for any type of test combines GLP with GMP with quality control. To put testing into perspective no test should be performed without good knowledge of the pack, the product and how these two items were assembled. For example, moisture gain by a sensitive product coupled with the finding of loose caps immediately poses the questions 'Were the caps adequately tightened?', 'Are the bottles and caps satisfactory?'. These questions cannot be answered unless a disciplined approach is used and adequate detail recorded. This attitude should apply to all developmental work as well as more important items such a clinical trial supplies, human volunteer studies, etc. Tests between products and packs which are carried out to define a suitable pack/product are usually termed either feasibility or investigational studies. Once this stage has been completed, coupled with development of analytical

methods and analytical data usually from accelerated storage tests, there should be a high confidence that the pack/product combination chosen has an acceptable shelf life or stability profile. The final proof that this opinion is correct lies with the formal stability programme where the packed product is produced in the pack to be sold (or a near replica of it), by the final product method and placed on test for a period of up to 5 years. The storage conditions in such a programme may range from 4 to 50 °C with challenges associated with low and high RH, light, etc. with analytical periods of 0 (initial), 3, 6, 9, 12, 18, 24, 30, 36, 48 and 60 months. Certain regulatory bodies, e.g. the FDA may dictate the number of batches to be put on test; i.e. this is a minimum of three in the USA, using three distinct batches of the basic drug substance.

'Analysis' normally involves purity, identification of degradation products, loss or gain of moisture, if relevant, microbial levels, effectiveness of preservative system, any exchange, interaction, adsorption, absorption between product and pack, and last and not least assessment of appearance, flavour, smell, etc. as these aspects are sometimes more readily quantified by an observer than a pure chemical analytical method. Specific analytical methods are essential for the main drug entity. Since certain drugs degrade according to an Arrhenius plot a range of test temperatures are chosen, i.e. 4 °C, 15 °C, 25 °C, 35 °C (or 37 °C), 45 °C. The temperatures most often chosen are 25 °C and 37 or 38 °C, to equate with temperate and tropical parts of the world. However, it should be emphasized that most medicines finish up in the bathroom or kitchen (preferably high up out of the reach of children) hence even home conditions can be particularly severe whilst the product is used or simply stored. Although disposal of drugs is recommended for dispensed medicines after the course of treatment has been completed both these and OTC products are inevitably stored for longer periods.

The procedures and controls for drug development are both intense and rigorous, and the same type of control is maintained throughout production, marketing, etc. finishing up by the monitoring of any complaints and/or adverse reactions. Products once launched are also sampled say one batch in 50 and put on a further stability test — known as ongoing or existing product stability to ensure that the shelf life profile is maintained. Any change following launch to processes, pack or product is not only similarly monitored but needs further input from packaging expertise.

Packaging development whether carried out by a formulator or a special packaging section has to have a thorough knowledge of all packaging materials, packaging processes, basic test procedures as applied to paper, plastic, glass, metal, laminations, etc. and devise programmes which provide the level of confidence that is essential between product and pack. In many cases this will involve packs which act as devices or separate devices and user/patient type tests designed to establish functional efficiency and/or what will go wrong under conditions of misuse.

The ultimate of all pack clearance procedures is a pack specification which becomes the lead document for purchase and clearance of future deliveries of packaging materials.

Whereas quality assurance is the establishing of procedures which maintain quality, quality control is the actual testing activity. For instance incoming packaging materials are first examined as a bulk delivery, then sampled on a statistical sampling basis and finally examined in terms of variables and attributes for critical, major and minor faults to agreed acceptable quality levels (AQLs). Since examination covers dimensional, aesthetic and functional aspects plus identification (particularly relevant with plastics) it ensures that the material specified has been received. With production lines becoming faster, stoppages due to repairs, malfunction, etc. have become more critical as ineffective and inefficient production can significantly affect costs. As an alternative to the statistical sampling of deliveries arriving in house two other options are:

1 a random sampling taken at the point of manufacture which is isolated and identified so that it can be checked by the user;
2 purchasing on warrantee certification which confirms that the quality specified is met as per agreed statistical testing scheme operated by the manufacturer.

With many items where a high quality of cleanliness is essential sampling of the bulk delivery may lead to an additional risk of particulate or microbial contamination. In such circumstances the alternative schemes indicated above may be used in order to maintain the integrity of the incoming stock. Inspection and quality control plays a further role with ongoing stock inspection, control on production lines, i.e. of the packaged product and the monitoring of finished (saleable) warehoused stock. As mentioned earlier the final success of any product and its pack can only in the long run be equated to sales and complaints.

A catalogue of test procedure, is given in part (c) of the bibliography of this chapter.

BIBLIOGRAPHY

(a) General reading on packaging

The reader is referred to the general reading list given in Chapter 12.

(b) More specific reading on pharmaceutical packaging

Cooper, J. (1974) *Plastic Containers for Pharmaceuticals. Testing and Control.* World Health Organisation (WHO), Geneva.
Dean, D. A. (1978) The use of aluminium foil in pharmaceutical packaging. *Mang Chem. Aerosol News*, Feb, pp. 51–61.
Dean, D. A. (1983) *Packaging of Pharmaceuticals Packages and Closures.* IOP, Melton Mowbray.
Dean, D. (1984) Pharmaceutical Packaging — present and future trends. *Mang Chem. Aerosol News*, March 10th, pp. 282–284.
FDA (1983) *Code of Federal Regulations* (CFR). Food and Drugs Administration (FDA), Washington, DC.
Griffin, N. I. and Sacharow, S. (1975) *Drug and Cosmetic Packaging,* published by Noyes Data Corporation, New York.
HMSO (1978) *WHO Expert Committee on Specificators for Parmaceutical Preparations,* 26th Report. HMSO, London.
Remington's Pharmaceutical Science, 16th edition, 1980, Chapters 80 and 81.
Ross, C. F. (1975) *Packaging of Pharmaceuticals Products, Sterilisation and Safety.* Institute of Packaging (IOP), Stanmore, Middlesex.
Swinbank, Colin (1983) *Packaging of Chemicals and other Industrial Liquids and Solids.* IOP, Melton Mowbray.

(c) Bibliography of test procedures and standards for packaging materials and containers which may be used for pharmaceutical products

BP 1980, Plastic containers, Appendix XIX, pages A200–202.

BP 1980, Containers for injections, Appendix XVIIIB, page A197.

BS795: 1983. Ampoules (BSI).

BS 1679 (being updated) Containers for pharmaceutical dispensing (in 7 parts). British Standards Institute (BSI).

BS 2006: 1984. Collapsible tubes, published by the British Standards Institute (BSI).

BS 5321: 1985. Reclosable pharmaceutical containers resistant to opening by children (BSI).

Desk Diary Institute of Packaging (annually), for list of BSI standards on packaging and packaging materials.

DIN 58363: 1980. Transfusion, infusion; infusion containers and accessories; infusion bags and bottles made from plastic. Published by DIN, West Germany.

EP (1983) 2nd edn, section VI. Container materials used for the manufacture of containers — plastic, silicone and glass.

USP XXI 1985, Containers, pages 1233–1241.

USP XXI 1985, Packaging — child safety, pages 1330–1333.

Index